Contents

Calorie, Fat & Carbohydra[...]

Diet Guides & Counters

Weight Control Tips

✔ Eat Sensibly

- Avoid fad diets. Eat 3 sensible meals daily with adequate fruit and vegetables.
- Limit fats and high-fat foods, sugar, soda and alcohol.

(Sample Diet Plan ~ Page 11)

✔ Exercise Daily

- Get active and exercise every day!
- Include muscle-strengthening exercises. You'll lose more fat and keep it off. You'll also feel and look better, and you can eat a little more food. *(Exercise Guide, Page 13)*

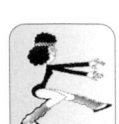

✔ Reshape Eating Behaviors

- Be aware of eating habits and behaviors that lead to overeating.
- Also focus on social and emotional situations that lead you to snack compulsively. *(Extra notes - Page 14)*

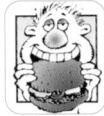

✔ Keep a Food & Exercise Diary

- A diary helps you see exactly what you eat and drink, and how much you exercise.
- An excellent motivator and proven weight loss aid. Keeps you honest!

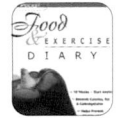

✔ Arrange Moral Support

Gain the support of family and friends. Get extra professional help if required, from your doctor, dietitian, psychologist, exercise trainer, or slimming group. Beware of family saboteurs who discourage you from adopting a healthier lifestyle!

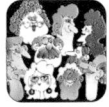

DOCTOR CHECK-UP
Ask your doctor to check you for high blood pressure, diabetes, and high blood cholesterol.

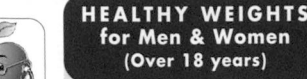

HEALTHY WEIGHTS
for Men & Women
(Over 18 years)

Based on weights with least risk of disease or death from heart disease, diabetes, stroke and cancer.

Based on Body Mass Index - range 20-25.

BMI calculated as: $\dfrac{\text{Weight (kg)}}{\text{Height (m)}^2}$

Height (No Shoes)		Healthy Weight Range
Ft Ins		Pounds
4'7"	~	86-108
4'8"	~	88-110
4'9"	~	92-114
4'10"	~	97-121
4'11"	~	99-123
5'0"	~	101-127
5'1"	~	105-132
5'2"	~	110-136
5'3"	~	112-140
5'4"	~	114-145
5'5"	~	119-149
5'6"	~	123-156
5'7"	~	127-158
5'8"	~	129-162
5'9"	~	134-167
5'10"	~	138-173
5'11"	~	143-178
6'0"	~	145-182
6'1"	~	149-187
6"2"	~	156-193
6'3"	~	158-198
6'4"	~	162-202
6'5'	~	170-211
6'6"	~	172-215
6'7"	~	175-220

Body Fat Distribution & Health

Moderate amounts of body fat do not compromise health. Excess fat above the hips carries a far greater health risk than fat on or below the hips - better to be a 'pear-shape' than an 'apple-shape'.

Abdominal obesity greatly increases the risk of developing diabetes, heart disease, high blood fats, hypertension, stroke, sleep apnea, arthritis and some cancers. So-called **'cellulite'** carries no extra health risk.

Waist Circumference directly reflects the increased health risk of abdominal obesity. Waist size associated with a high health risk:
Men ~ Over 40 inches **Women** ~ Over 35 inches

Body Mass Index (BMI)

BMI is a general (but not specific) indicator of body fatness. Although BMI alone is not diagnostic, the higher the BMI, the greater the health risk of developing diabetes, high blood pressure and heart disease. BMI does not apply to heavily muscled persons. BMI is used in a different way for children.

Check Your BMI: Find your height (no shoes) – look across the row to the weight nearest your own. Then track down to BMI.

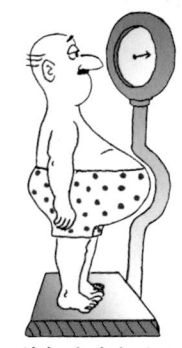

Abdominal obesity
greatly increases
the risk of ill-health
and earlier death.

Ht	WEIGHT (LBS) ~ ADULTS													
5'1"	100	106	111	116	122	127	132	137	143	148	153	158	185	211
5'2"	104	109	115	120	126	131	136	142	147	153	158	164	191	218
5'3"	107	113	118	124	130	135	141	146	152	158	163	169	197	225
5'4"	110	116	122	128	134	140	145	151	157	163	169	174	204	232
5'5"	114	120	126	132	138	144	150	156	162	168	174	180	210	240
5'6"	118	124	130	136	142	148	155	161	167	173	179	186	216	247
5'7"	121	127	134	140	146	153	159	166	172	178	185	191	223	255
5'8"	125	131	138	144	151	158	164	171	177	184	190	197	230	262
5'9"	128	135	142	149	155	162	169	176	182	189	196	206	236	270
5'10"	132	139	146	153	160	167	174	181	188	195	202	207	243	278
5'11"	136	143	150	157	165	172	179	186	193	200	208	215	250	286
6'0"	140	147	154	162	169	177	184	191	199	206	213	221	258	294
6'1"	144	151	159	166	174	182	189	197	204	212	219	227	265	302
6'2"	148	155	163	171	179	186	194	202	210	218	225	233	272	311
6'3"	152	160	168	176	184	192	200	208	216	224	232	240	279	319
6'4"	156	164	172	180	189	197	205	213	221	230	238	246	287	328
BMI	19	20	21	22	23	24	25	26	27	28	29	30	35	40

BMI Classification:

BMI Below 19
Underweight

BMI 19-24.9
Healthy Weight
(Low Health Risk)

BMI 25-29.9
Overweight
(Moderate Health Risk)

BMI 30-40
Obese (High Health Risk)

BMI Over 40
Morbid Obesity
(Very High Risk)

Interactive BMI Calculator
www.calorieking.com

Calories & Weight Loss

Calories in Food

Calories in food are derived from protein, fat and carbohydrate. Alcohol also provides calories. Vitamins, minerals and water provide no calories.

Calorie Values Per Gram

Fat/Oil	~ 9 Calories
Carbohydrate	~ 4 Calories
Protein	~ 4 Calories
Alcohol	~ 7 Calories

Note that fats have over double the calories of protein and carbohydrate. The higher the fat content of food, the higher the calories.

Sample Calculation

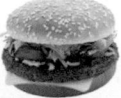

QUARTER POUNDER® WITH CHEESE has 530 calories derived from:

30g Fat (x 9 cals/gram)	= 270
38g Carbohyd.(x 4 cals/gram)	= 152
27g Protein (x 4 cals/gram)	= 108
Total Calories	**= 530**

Calorie Levels for Weight Loss

Commence with a calorie-controlled diet that allows a moderate weight loss of $1/2$ - 1 pound per week. Weight loss is usually much larger in the first few weeks due to extra fluid losses.

Note: It is better to increase exercise rather than lessen food calories too drastically.

Suggested Calories for Weight Loss

Women:	Non-active	1000 - 1200
	Active	1200 - 1500
Men:	Non-active	1200 - 1500
	Active	1500 - 1800
Teenagers:		1200 - 1800

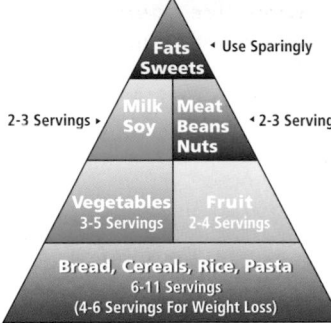

The Food Guide Pyramid emphasizes eating a wide variety of foods from the 5 major food groups. For weight loss, make lowfat choices and eat the lower number of servings.

Examples of Serving Size

Bread & Cereal Group:
- 1 slice bread
- $1/2$ bun, small bagel or English muffin
- 4 small crackers or 1 tortilla
- 1 oz ready-to-eat cereal
- $1/2$ cup cooked cereal, rice or pasta

Fruit Group:
- 1 medium apple, orange, banana
- $1/2$ cup canned fruit
- $1/4$ cup dried fruit
- $3/4$ cup fruit juice
- $1/4$ medium avocado

Vegetable Group:
- 1 cup raw leafy vegetables
- $1 1/2$ oz raw chopped vegetables
- $1/2$ cup cooked vegetables
- $1/2$ - $3/4$ cup vegetable juice

Meat & Alternatives Group:
- 2-3oz (cooked) lean meat/poultry/fish
- 2 eggs or 7oz tofu or $1/4$ cup nuts
- 1 cup (cooked) dried beans or chickpeas
- 4 Tbsp peanut butter

Milk & Alternatives Group:
- 1 cup (8 fl.oz) milk, soy drink, yogurt
- $1 1/2$ oz cheese or $1/2$ cup cottage cheese

Portion Size Counts!

Food portion size is critical to controling calorie intake for weight control.

Super-sized food servings have become more common when eating out and in the home. This can mean a day's worth of calories being consumed in one meal; or a snack being equivalent to a full meal.

It is easy to underestimate portion size of foods and drinks, and unwittingly consume excess calories – even if the fat content is low or even zero!

To more accurately estimate portion size of different foods, weigh and measure your food with food scales, measuring spoons and cups. Better control of calories will result.

For a visual idea of portion sizes, visit www.CalorieKing.com. See examples (fries and cola) on this page.

Allow for Extra Calories in Packaged Food

The actual weight of packaged foods is usually 5-10% more than the label net weight (the minimum legal weight) - and in some cases up to 50% more. However, manufacturers calculate the calories based on the net weight. For actual calories, weigh the product and calculate the extra calories. **For extra details see www.CalorieKing.com**

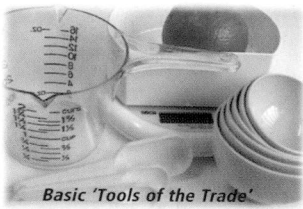

Basic 'Tools of the Trade'

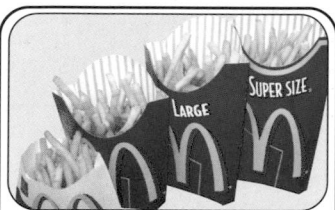

Fries

Fries	Cal	Fat	Carb
Small	210	10	26
Medium	450	22	57
Large	540	26	68
Super Size	610	29	77

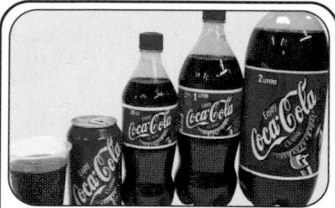

Cola

Cola	Cal	Fat	Carb
8 fl.oz Cup	100	0	25
12 fl.oz Can	150	0	37
20 fl.oz Bottle	250	0	63
1 Liter Bottle	400	0	100
2 Liter Bottle	800	0	200

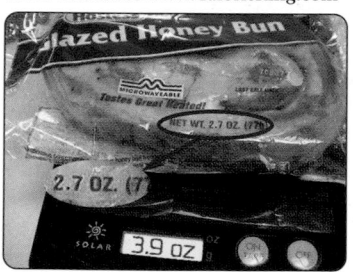

Fat Percent Explained

Percent Fat Calories
(Percent of Calories from Fat)

While health authorities recommend that not more than 30% of our total food calories should come from fat, it is not implied nor even recommended that you eat only those foods with less than 30% calories from fat.

Our normal diet is made up of foods that are either well above or below 30%. Only on average should the total diet be less than 30% calories from fat.

Some higher fat foods such as avocados, nuts and seeds, are highly nutritious and favor lower blood cholesterol levels. **Moderation is the aim . . . not elimination.**

Nevertheless, knowing the percent of calories from fat can be useful in spotting high-fat foods and drinks.

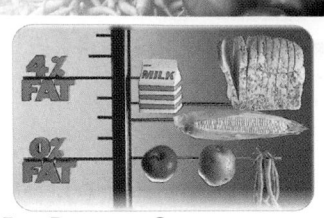

Fat Percent Content
(Percent of Fat in Food)

Don't be fooled by promotion of foods claiming to have a low percent of fat. It's **serving size and total grams of fat that count.**

For example, whole milk with 3.5% fat sounds low (3.5g fat/100ml) but an 8fl.oz cup contains 8g fat (and 2 cups contain 16g fat).

Icecream with 10% fat seems high, yet a large scoop (3fl.oz) has only 5g fat. (Low-fat icecream has less than 2g fat/serve.)

❖   ❖   ❖

Also note that the percent of fat in a food is not the same as the percent of calories derived from fat.

Foods with a low percent of fat can still have a high percent of calories derived from fat - as shown below.

For example, around 50% of total calories in whole milk comes from fat - yet whole milk has less than 4% fat. Low fat/light milk with less than 1% fat has only 18% of total calories from fat - a much better choice.

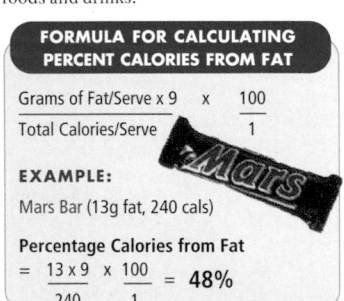

FORMULA FOR CALCULATING PERCENT CALORIES FROM FAT

$$\frac{\text{Grams of Fat/Serve} \times 9}{\text{Total Calories/Serve}} \times \frac{100}{1}$$

EXAMPLE:

Mars Bar (13g fat, 240 cals)

Percentage Calories from Fat

$$= \frac{13 \times 9}{240} \times \frac{100}{1} = \mathbf{48\%}$$

FAT CONTENT & FAT PERCENT OF MILK

	Whole Milk	Reduced Fat	Low-Fat (light)	Non-Fat Skim
Percentage Fat	▶ 3.5%	2%	1%	0%
Fat (Grams) in 8 fl.oz Cup	▶ 8g	5g	2g	0g
Calories	▶ 150	120	100	95
Percent Calories From Fat	▶ 48%	38%	18%	0%

Recommended Fat Intake

Americans consume too much fat with many having over 40% of total calories from fat - either as fat or oil, or as fat in foods and drinks. A range of 20-30% is healthier.

Fat Intake – Healthy Ranges

Children	30-60g
Teenagers (Active)	40-80g
Women	30-60g
Men: Active	40-80g
Heavy Activity/Athlete	80-120g

The chart below recommends maximum fat intake for different calorie levels.

MAXIMUM DESIRABLE FAT INTAKE (Daily)

Calories	Fat	% Fat Cals
1200 cals	30g fat	23%
1500 cals	40g fat	24%
1800 cals	50g fat	25%
2000 cals	60g fat	27%
2200 cals	70g fat	28%
2500 cals	80g fat	29%
2800 cals	90g fat	29%
3000 cals	100g fat	30%
3500 cals	117g fat	30%
4000 cals	135g fat	30%

Infants Fat Intake

Infants and toddlers under 3 years should not be restricted in their fat intake because much larger volumes of food would be required to guarantee adequate calorie intake and growth. Whole milk should be used rather than light milk (1%) or nonfat milk. Similarly, a high fiber diet is also not suitable for infants.

Calories Versus Fats

For successful weight control it is important to be aware of both fats and calories in foods. It widens your choices at the supermarket and when eating out.

While choosing more lowfat foods is wise, it does not guarantee that total calories will be reduced, particularly if portion size is not limited.

It is a mistake to think that eating lowfat or fat-free foods allows you to eat double the quantity.

Be aware that lowfat and fat-free cakes, cookies and ice cream are **not calorie-free.** Nor are soda drinks, fruit juices, beer, alcoholic spirits, sugar and sugar candy which are also fat-free. Bread, rice and pasta also have negligible fat.

Carbohydrate Calories Count

It is also a fallacy that carbohydrate calories don't count. Carbohydrates in excess of body needs can still be converted to and stored as body fat - particularly in women in their child-bearing years.

Total Calories Count!

Ultimately, **it is food portion size and total calories that count** whether from fat, carbohydrate or protein. Remember, cows get fat on grass!

FOOD LABEL MEANINGS

FDA Nutrition Claim Definitions
(All are on a Per Serving Basis.)

Low Calorie: 40 calories or less

Light or Lite: One third fewer calories or, 50% or less fat than regular product

Fat-Free: Less than half a gram of fat

Low-Fat: 3 grams or less of fat

Reduced-Fat: 25% less fat than regular product

Fewer or Less Calories: At least 25% fewer calories than regular product

Hints to Reduce Fat

Meats & Poultry

- **Choose lean cuts** of meat with little marbling. Choose the white meat of chicken and turkey, and extra lean ground beef.
- **Trim all visible fat** from meat and remove the skin from poultry. Removal of fat after cooking is okay (to prevent dryness).
- **Eat modest portions** (3-4 oz cooked weight) of meat, poultry or fish. **Add extra** beans, lentils, tofu, tempeh, vegetables, potatoes, rice, pasta, bread, or tortillas.
- **Avoid high-fat meat products** such as salami, bacon, sausage and franks. Choose lowfat and fat-free brands. Choose lean luncheon meats (90% or more fat-free).
- **Broil or bake.** Avoid frying. Allow casseroles to cool and skim off surface fat.

Fish & Seafood

- **Choose fresh or frozen fillets**, and canned fish (in water pack).
- **Avoid fried fish**, frozen fish in batter, canned fish in oil.

Fats & Oils

- **Use minimal amounts** of all types of fat and oil. All are high in calories.
- **Choose** 'light' and 'reduced fat' spreads but still use sparingly. Check the Fats and Spreads section of this book for lower fat brands.
- **Use minimal amounts** of oil when stir-frying. Use no-stick sprays like *Pam*.

Salad Dressings & Sauces

- **Avoid regular mayonnaise and oil dressings.** Choose 'light', 'reduced fat' or 'fat-free' brands (Check salad dressings section of this book).
- **Choose** lowfat or fat-free sauces. Most tomato-based pasta sauces are lowfat but avoid 'pesto', 'alfredo', cheese and 'creamy' sauces.

Milk, Dairy, Soy Drinks

- **Choose** lowfat or skim milks and yogurts. Avoid full-cream milk, cream, *Half & Half* coffee creamers.
- **Soy Drinks:** Choose lowfat brands.
- **Cheese:** Choose fat-free, lowfat and fat-reduced (e.g. cottage, part-skim ricotta). Cheese substitutes can still be high in fat.
- **Icecream:** Choose lowfat and fat-free brands, frozen yogurt, sorbet, sherbet and ices. Limit regular icecream to a small serving. Avoid rich high-fat icecreams.

Frozen Meals & Entrees

- **Choose lowfat varieties** such as *Lean Cuisine*, *Healthy Choice* and *Weight Watchers*. Add extra vegetables.

Soups

- **Choose lowfat brands.** Avoid high-fat ramen noodle blocks/soup.

FRYING ADDS FAT!

The greater the surface area of potato exposed to fat or oil, the higher the fat content.

Whole Potato (3 oz)
Nil Fat, 65 Cals

Roast Potato (3 oz)
5g Fat, 155 Cals
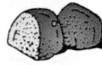

Fries (Large, 3 oz)
12g Fat, 220 Cals
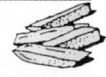

Fries (Small, 3 oz)
15g Fat, 265 Cals
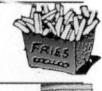

Potato Chips (3 oz)
30g Fat, 450 Cals

Bread, Bagels, Crackers

- **All breads are suitable** as well as pita, bagels, English muffins and rice cakes. Avoid croissants, sweet rolls, danish pastry and doughnuts. **Avoid** fat-soaked toast and garlic bread.
- **Choose lowfat crackers** such as graham, saltines, matzo, bread sticks, crispbreads. **Avoid** regular cheese or butter crackers.

Cereals, Pasta, Noodles, Rice

- **Most cold and hot cereals** are low in fat and nil in cholesterol. Avoid granola made with hydrogenated oils.
- **Choose** plain pasta or rice. Avoid dishes made with cream, butter or cheese sauces. **Avoid** high-fat ramen noodle blocks/soups.

Fruits & Vegetables

- **Choose all types.** (Note: Avocados contain no cholesterol. Their fat and fiber can help lower blood cholesterol). Use mashed avocado on bread in place of fat.
- **Choose** dried beans, lentils, chick peas, baked beans.
- **Avoid** french-fried potatoes and regular potato salad. Avoid vegetables made in butter, cream or sauce.
- **Avoid** deli-style salads made with high fat dressings. Choose lowfat brands. Use lowfat and fat-free salad dressings.

Snacks, Cookies, Candy

- **Avoid** high-fat snacks such as potato chips, corn/tortilla chips, cheesy balls, buttered popcorn, chocolate and carob bars.
- **Choose** fat-free potato chips and tortilla chips made with *olestra* (such as *Wow!* brand) but still limit quantity.
- **Choose** plain popcorn, lowfat cookies and muffins, hard candy, jelly beans, fruit rolls and frozen fruit bars and popsicles.
- **Choose** fresh and dried fruits, vegetables. Limit nuts and seeds if overweight.

Desserts/Sweets

- **Avoid high-fat desserts,** such as fruit pies, pastries, cheesecake, cheese board.
- **Choose** fresh fruits, fresh fruit salad, lowfat custard and lowfat yogurt. Use yogurt in place of cream or ice cream.
- **Avoid** regular icecream. *Choose* lowfat brands but still limit quantity.
- **Choose** sugar-free gelatin desserts such as *Jell-O* (sugar-free package).

Fast-Foods & Take-Out

Check the Fast-Foods Section of this book for actual fat counts and wise selections.

- **Delis:** Choose sandwiches/bread rolls, pitas with lowfat fillings and plain salad. Limit meat/cheese to small portions. Request half quantities.
- **Avoid high-fat deli salads.** Choose plain salads and add your own lowfat dressing. Eat more fruit.
- **Chicken & Fish:** Avoid deep-fried chicken or fish, BBQ chicken with fat or skin, chicken nuggets. Choose broiled or baked chicken breast without fat or skin.
- **Hamburgers:** Choose medium size, lower fat burgers. Avoid bacon. Have a side salad (without dressing).
- **Pizzas:** Avoid sausage/pepperoni. Choose vegetarian topping and modest quantity of cheese. Eat a moderate serving. Eat extra salad and fruit.
- **Desserts:** Avoid apple pie, danish, choc chip cookies. Choose lowfat muffins (e.g. *McDonald's*), fresh fruit or fruit salad.
- **Avoid regular shakes and sundaes.** Choose lowfat milk, lower fat shakes (such as *McDonald's*), and orange juice, but choose smaller sizes.

Hints to Reduce Sugar

- While reducing the amount of fat is an important dietary focus for weight control, sugar intake also needs to be watched.
- Many overweight, inactive persons consume over 500 calories of refined sugars per day (equivalent to over 30 level teaspoons) -
- significant amount in weight control terms. Halving this amount would be reasonable and worthwhile.

Note: Naturally occurring sugars in fruits, vegetables and milk are fine when consumed in normal recommended amounts.

- Most sugar in our diet is 'hidden' in processed foods such as soft drinks, fruit drinks, candy, cookies, cake, jam, sauces, icecream, desserts, canned foods, and breakfast cereals.

Certainly enjoy moderate quantities of these foods, but for serious weight control, look for 'low calorie', 'diet' or sugar-free alternatives. Be careful not to substitute sugar-rich foods with high-fat foods which might boost calories even more!

- Sugar-free sweeteners such as *Equal, DiabetiSweet, NutraSweet, Splenda, Sweet'n Low* and *Stevia* make it easy to reduce sugar in drinks and recipes. (Most recipes can be adapted to contain less sugar with little effect on taste or quality.)

- The body can obtain sufficient sugar for its needs from carbohydrate rich foods such as bread, rice, spaghetti and other pasta, potatoes, corn, fruit, vegetables, beans, nuts, seeds and lactose in milk.

These foods are also rich in other nutrients. Refined sugar is referred to as 'empty calorie' because it supplies calories but negligible nutrients and no fiber.

DIFFERENT FORMS OF SUGAR

Be aware that sugar comes in different forms. Check the label.

- Sugar
- Brown Sugar
- Dextrose
- Fructose
- Corn Syrup
- Honey
- Maple Syrup
- Sucrose
- Confectioners' Sugar
- Glucose
- Malt, Maltose
- High-Fructose Corn Syrup
- Molasses
- Turbinado Sugar

SUGAR CONTENT OF SOME COMMON FOODS

	Teaspoons of Sugar
Coca Cola or *Pepsi*, 12 fl.oz	10
20 fl.oz size	17
Iced tea, sweetened, 12 fl.oz	8
Choc malted Milk, 12 fl.oz	4.5
Honey Smacks Cereal, 1 oz	4
Popcorn, caramel, 1 cup	3.5
Chocolate Bar, 1.5 oz	6
M&M's, 1.7 oz pkg	7
Cake, sponge, jam-filled	8
Choc Chip Cookie, 1 oz	2
Donut, iced	6
Apple Pie, 1 piece	7
Jell-O, 1/2 cup	4.5
Jam, 1 Tbsp, 20g	2.5
Syrup, maple, 1 Tbsp	3

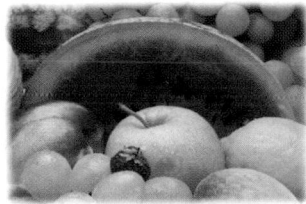

Reach for fresh fruit when you want to snack instead of candy or snack products rich in sugar and fat.

Sample Diet Plan - 1200 Calories

For Overweight Persons. Please Check With Your Doctor.
(Menu contains approximately 30-35 Grams Fat)

 Breakfast (approx. 250 cal)

1 Small Fruit or ½ oz Dried Fruit

Plus Cereal: 1½ oz Dry (high fiber)

or 1 cup cooked Oatmeal

Plus Milk (from daily allowance)

Milk Allowance (160 calories)

2 cups Skim Milk or 1½ cups Lowfat (1%) Milk
or equivalent Soy Drink, Yogurt, Cheese, Tofu

Fat Allowance (140 calories; 15g Fat)

4 tsp Fat or 6-8 tsp Diet Margarine or 3 tsp Oil
or 1½ Tbsp Mayonnaise or ½ medium Avocado
or 1½ Tbsp Peanut Butter or 30g Nuts/Seeds

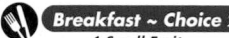 **Breakfast ~ Choice 2**

1 Small Fruit

Plus 1 Egg (no added fat)

or ¾ oz Cheese

or 2 oz Cottage Cheese

or 1 oz Lean Bacon

Plus 1 Toast or ½ Muffin (English)

 Lunch (approx. 440 calories)

2 slices Bread (2 oz) or 1 medium Roll or Bagel
or 4 Crispbreads/Crackers or 6" Pita

Plus 2 oz lean Meat, Chicken or Turkey

or 3½ oz Tuna (in water) or 2½ oz Salmon

or 1 oz Cheese or ½ cup (4 oz) Cottage Cheese

or ½ cup (4 oz) Ricotta Cheese (lowfat)

or ½ cup (4 oz) Fruit Yogurt (lowfat)

or ½ cup (4 oz) Bean Salad

Plus Large Salad (Oil-free dressing)
Plus 1 small Fruit or ½ oz Dried Fruit

 Dinner (approx. 360 Calories)

Soup (fat-free)

Plus 3 oz lean Meat (cooked weight)

or 4 oz Chicken Breast (no skin)

or 3 oz Chicken Thigh/Leg (no skin)

or 5 oz Fish (grilled, no fat)

or ¾ cup (6 oz) Beans (Soy, Baked, Haricot etc)/Lentils

or Lowfat Entree (e.g. Lean Cuisine) or Recipe Dish

Plus 1 small Potato or ½ cup Rice/Pasta or 1 slice Bread
Plus 2-3 servings Vegetables/Salad
Plus 1 small Fruit + Diet Gelatin Dessert

 Between Meals Water, Coffee, Tea, Diet drinks,

Fruit from main meals; Raw vegetable pieces, Milk from Allowance
Note: Take a multivitamin/mineral supplement daily while dieting.

Exercise & Weight Control

- Persons who exercise regularly **lose more weight** and keep it off longer than non-exercisers.

- Exercise also improves general health and well-being. **Mood, confidence and self-esteem** are enhanced by a sense of control and accomplishment.

- **Exercise increases the metabolic rate** of the body even for hours after exercise - a good way to 'wake up' a sluggish metabolism and burn extra fat.

  Exercise compensates for any decrease in metabolic rate with increasing age and also in some heavy smokers when they stop smoking.

- **Strength training** further builds muscle and aids body reshaping. You can also eat more food!

Note: It is muscle which burns fat. Each extra pound of muscle burns an extra 100 calories daily ~ even while you sleep! Weight from exercised muscles is okay. It is surplus fat that is potentially harmful.

- **Avoid injury** by beginning with walking, low impact aerobics, or weight-supported exercise (e.g. swimming, cycling). Avoid competitive sports.

- **How Much?** Start with 10 - 20 minutes/day and progress to 30-45minutes/day - even if broken into 5-10 minute lots. It all adds up! **Aim to achieve 250-500 calories of exercise daily.**

  Also walk up stairs instead of using lifts. Take a brisk walk at lunch. Use an exercise bike, treadmill or stair machine while watching TV.

- **How Often?** While aerobic fitness requires only 3 - 4 sessions weekly, **weight control is a daily event which requires daily exercise.**

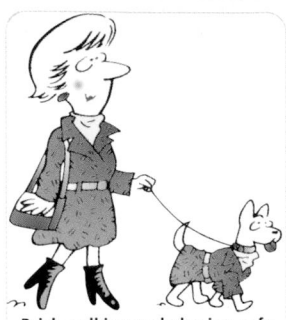

Brisk walking each day is a safe and effective way to keep trim and fit. Try it - you'll like it!"

Strength-training with light weights helps to retain or rebuild muscle tissue and enhances weight control.

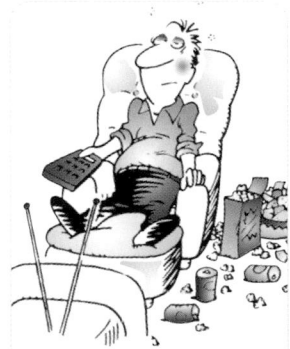

Middle-age spread has little to do with getting older. Too little exercise is the main culprit.

Daily exercise and sensible eating can minimize middle-age spread.

TV CAN BE FATTENING!

Many adults and children watch over 20 hours of television per week and indulge in high-fat snacks at the same time - potent contributors to obesity.

Are you a TV couch potato? Limit your TV hours and plan healthy physical activities. At least use an exercise bike or treadmill while watching TV!

Calories Used in Exercise

LIGHT	MODERATE	HEAVY
4 Calories/Minute	**7 Calories/Minute**	**10 Calories/Minute**
Walking, slow	Walking, brisk	Walking (power), Jogging
Cycling, light	Cycling, moderate	Cycling (vigorous), Spinning
Gardening light	Swimming, crawl	Swimming, strenuous
Golf, social	Weight-training, light	Weight-training, heavy
Tennis, doubles	Tennis, singles	Wrestling/Judo, advanced
Housework, cleaning	Racquetball, beginners	Racquetball, advanced
Calisthenics, Yoga	Aerobics, light	Tae Bo, Kick Boxing
Ten Pin Bowls	Football, Grid Iron	Football, training
Ping-pong, social	Basketball, Baseball	Basketball (Pro)
Ice Skating	Walking Downstairs	Climbing Stairs, Skipping
Aquarobics	Snow Skiing (downhill)	Skiing (cross country)
Skate Boarding	Shoveling snow	Aquarobics, advanced
Line/Square Dancing	Dancing (vigorous)	Dancing (strenuous), Zumba

Note: Only those sports or activities that are sustained over a period of time (e.g running) qualify for heavy exercise. Stop-start sports such as tennis are considered 'moderate'.

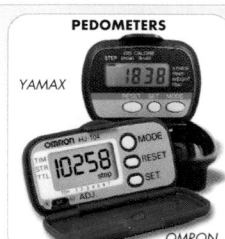

PEDOMETERS

YAMAX

OMRON

10,000 STEPS PER DAY

A pedometer can motivate you to be more active every day.

Different models count steps, miles and even calories used. It clips to your belt or waist band and registers each step.

Aim for 8,000 - 10,000 steps per day, instead of an average of only 3,000 - 4,000 steps.

Extra information: www.CalorieKing.com
Ordering Details ~ Page 303

WALKING PROGRAM

Weeks	Distance To Walk	Time Taken	Calories Used (140lb Person)
Weeks 1-2 ▶	1 mile	20 mins	140 calories
Weeks 3-5 ▶	1.5 miles	28 mins	200 calories
Weeks 6-8 ▶	2 miles	35 mins	250 calories
Weeks 9-10 ▶	2.5 miles	45 mins	310 calories
Weeks 11+ ▶	3.5 miles	60 mins	420 calories

Reshaping Eating Behaviors

- Eating is a behavior that is largely controlled by people with whom we live or socialize, places in which we carry out our lives, and our emotions. Become aware of those situations that commonly lead to extra food being eaten.

- We may also be unaware of 'bad' eating habits that can lead to excess calorie intake; e.g. eating quickly, large mouthsful, eating when tense or bored, finishing a large serving of food when not hungry.

Hints to help uncover and correct those 'bad' eating habits include:

- **Don't eat while engaged in other activities**; for example, watching TV, reading. Eat only at the table, not at the fridge or while standing.

- **Don't eat quickly.** Chewing slowly allows time to register a feeling of fullness. Don't use fingers, only utensils. Cut food into smaller pieces. Don't load your fork until the previous mouthful is finished.

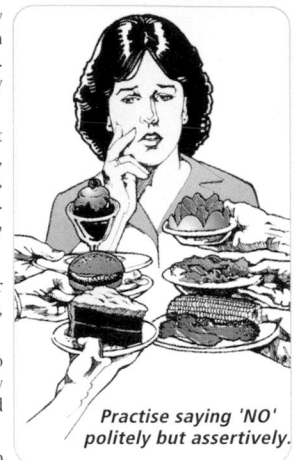

Practise saying 'NO' politely but assertively.

- **Don't purchase problem high calorie foods.** Shop from a set list to prevent impulse buying. Avoid shopping with children.

- **Buy snack foods** in the smallest package. The larger the serving size or package, the more you are likely to eat or drink.

- **Plan meals in advance. Stick to a set menu.**

- **Plan a strategy to avoid uncontrolled eating** and drinking at social events, or when your emotions urge you to binge.

  Rehearse repeatedly in your mind exactly what you will do in such situations. Remind yourself several times each day that you are in charge of your actions and that you can be strong-willed. Seek counseling or coaching on various strategies.

- **Promise yourself** that when you feel the urge to snack, you will engage in some activity that will distract you away from food (e.g. go for a walk, brush your teeth, phone a friend.)

  If you eat out of boredom, find some new hobby or interest that gets you out of the house. Even enrol in an adult education class.

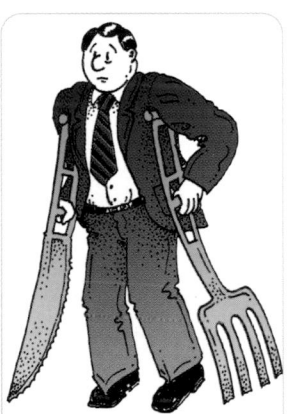

Do you use food as an emotional crutch? If so, professional counseling may be helpful.

The Value of a Food Diary

The food diary is the most powerful proven aid for dieters. Persons who keep a food and exercise diary not only lose more weight they also keep it off. Here are some of the reasons:

- Recording your eating and exercise habits jolts you into realizing just what you do eat and drink each day; and also whether you exercise sufficiently.

- **Helps you identify problem foods** and drinks with excessive calories and fat.

- **Helps identify moods,** situations and events that lead to excessive eating of unwanted calories. You can then plan to overcome or avoid them.

- **Prevents 'calorie amnesia'**, the forgetfulness that leads to rebound weight gain after successful weight loss. Recording puts you back on the right track.

- **Helps you develop greater self- discipline.** You will think twice about over indulging if you have to record it - especially if someone checks your diary regularly. It certainly keeps you honest!

- **Motivates you** to carefully plan your meals and to exercise each day.

- **Serves as a check system** for your doctor, dietitian or counselor to assess your progress and make recommendations.

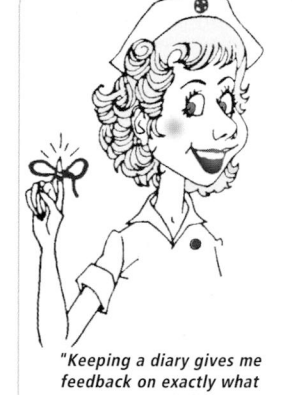

"Keeping a diary gives me feedback on exactly what I eat each day. It helps prevent 'calorie amnesia' and reminds me to exercise each day. It's a must for successful weight control!"

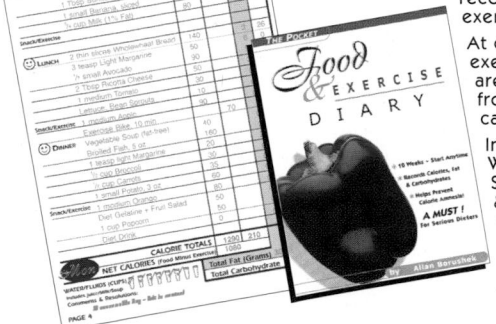

Sample Page from The Pocket Food & Exercise Diary, a 10-week diary to record food and exercise.

At day's end, exercise calories are deducted from food calories.

Includes Weekly Summary Page & Progress Checklist.

EXTRA DETAILS ~ SEE PAGE 304

Diabetes Guide

What is Diabetes?

Diabetes is a disorder in which the body cannot make proper use of carbohydrates (sugar and starches).

- After digestion, sugar and starches are changed into **glucose** - the simplest form of sugar that is vital to body cells for energy and growth.

- **Insulin** is the hormone which acts like a key that opens the door to body cells and allows glucose to enter.

- **Without sufficient insulin**, unused glucose builds up in the blood and passes into the urine. This produces symptoms of frequent urination, continual thirst and tiredness.

- **Untreated diabetes** increases the risk of damage to nerves and blood vessels. This, in turn, increases the risk of heart disease, stroke, blindness, kidney damage, foot ulcers and gangrene, impotence and other complications.

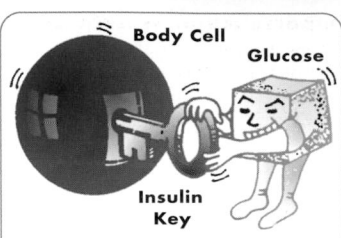

*Insulin acts like a key.
It opens the door to body cells
and allows glucose to enter.*

*Some persons with diabetes (Type 1) have
too few or no keys and require
insulin injections.*

*Others (Type 2) have ample keys but
'mis-shapen' key holes (insulin resistant)
- particularly if obese and inactive.*

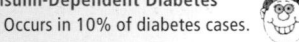

TYPE-1 DIABETES

Insulin-Dependent Diabetes

- Occurs in 10% of diabetes cases.
- Usually children and young adults.
- Pancreas gland produces little or no insulin. Daily insulin injections are necessary, plus:
- Regular meals with even carbohydrate distribution to match insulin dosage. Regular exercise and weight control are also important.

WARNING SIGNALS

- Frequent urination
- Continual thirst
- Rapid weight loss
- Unusual hunger
- Extreme weakness/fatigue
- Nausea, vomiting, irritability

TYPE-2 DIABETES

Non-Insulin Dependent

- Occurs in 90% of diabetes cases.
- Occurs mainly in adults - particularly in overweight and inactive persons.
- Insulin is produced but body cells resist its action and glucose cannot enter cells.
- Usually treated with diet and exercise. Sometimes requires medication (pills or insulin injections).

WARNING SIGNALS

- Any Type-1 symptom
- Blurred vision
- Excessive itching
- Skin infections with slow healing
- Tingling/numbness in feet

Diabetes Guide

Importance of Weight Control

- **Type-2 diabetes** occurs 2-3 times more often in overweight persons - particularly if inactive.

- Such persons do not usually lack insulin. Rather, their insulin is less effective. As obesity develops, muscle and other body cells may resist insulin in varying degrees. The resultant build-up of blood glucose may lead to diabetic symptoms.

- **Weight loss alone** often corrects this condition in Type-2 diabetes. If overweight, try a moderate diet of 1200-1500 calories **plus daily exercise.**

  Within several weeks, body cells can lose their resistance and become sensitive once again to the effects of insulin. Insulin and blood glucose levels may normalize, and symptoms may disappear.

  Further, the need for oral antidiabetic drugs might be prevented or much lessened in dosage. **So, give diet and exercise a fair go** - and maintain them to keep symptoms under control.

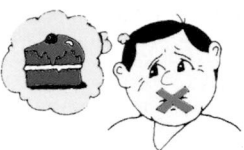

Modest weight loss and daily exercise can greatly improve control of Type-2 diabetes.

Managing Diabetes

Don't battle diabetes alone. Establish a partnership with your doctor, dietitian, certified diabetes educator and pharmacist. For extra support, contact the *American Diabetes Association* 1-800-342-2383.

Hints to keep blood glucose within safe limits:

- **Control your diet.** Know what and when you will eat. Seek referral to a dietitian for expert advice.

- **Exercise regularly.** It assists weight control and can improve sensitivity of body cells to insulin. Plan exercise into your daily routine.

- **Monitor your blood glucose** at home and work - ideally with a portable blood glucose meter. It will help you become familiar with your blood glucose patterns, and the effects of diet, exercise and medication. **Insulin pumps** can also help control blood glucose levels around the clock.

- **Don't skip prescribed insulin or oral medication.** If on insulin, know what action to take if hypoglycemia (low blood glucose) occurs. Also educate family and friends.

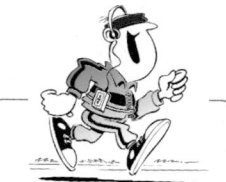

Get Moving! Everyday, do at least 30 minutes of moderate intensity exercise. It's the key to improving insulin sensitivity.

Add strength-training 3-4 times a week to double the benefits.

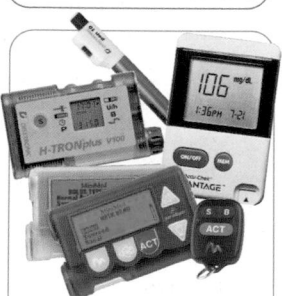

Blood glucose meters, insulin pumps and pens can greatly improve control of diabetes and lifestyle choices.

Diabetes ~ Diet Hints

Guidelines for choosing a healthy diet apply equally to persons with or without diabetes. Eating a wide variety of foods with the emphasis on low-fat, high fiber and low in refined sugars, is recommended.

However, actual food quantities, as well as when you eat, will also influence control of blood glucose. Your dietitian will individualize a diet plan to suit your food preferences, lifestyle and medical status. Here are a few hints:

- **Maintain a healthy weight.** If overweight, even a modest weight loss plus daily exercise can help to normalise blood glucose in Type-2 diabetes.

- **Don't skip meals.** If you take insulin or an oral hypoglycemic agent, regular meals are important.

- **If on insulin**, eat meals at the same time each day. Eat a similar amount of food at each meal. Even distribution of carbohydrate over the day will make best use of the available insulin and prevent wide variations in blood glucose levels.

- Note: Take your rapid-acting insulin no more than 15 minutes before eating. Regular and combination insulins are best taken with about 30 minutes between insulin injection and breakfast.

- **Choose wholegrain breads, cereals and pasta.** Eat fresh fruits, vegetables and legumes. These foods contain more fiber and slow the release of glucose into your blood after a meal.

- **Limit foods high in saturated fat and cholesterol.** Enjoy fish, soy foods, and other foods rich in omega-3 fats. *(See Fats & Cholesterol Guide, Pages 265-269)*

- Avoid sugars and foods high in added sugar particularly if overweight. Small amounts of sugar as part of a meal may occasionally be okay. Check with your dietitian. Use *Equal*, *Splenda* and *NutraSweet*-sweetened foods and drinks.

- **Foods (and supplements) rich in antioxidant vitamins C, E and beta-carotene**, as well as omega-3 fats, magnesium, zinc and chromium may help prevent long-term complications of diabetes (such as damage to small blood vessels and nerves). Be sure to check with your doctor.

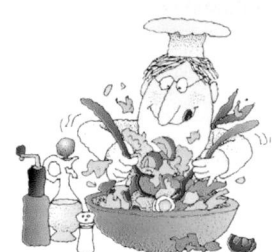

Eat a well-balanced diet, high in fiber-containing foods and low in fat.

NEW BLOOD SUGAR LEVEL FOR DIAGNOSING DIABETES
(Adopted by American Diabetes Assoc.)

Blood Sugar Levels
Previously: 140 mg/dL
New: 126 mg/dL

Everyone 45 and older should have a blood test every 3 years.

Excess Alcohol
contributes to obesity, diabetes, and high blood pressure.

The risk of hypoglycemia (low blood sugar) and drug interactions with alcohol is also increased.

Carbohydrates & Diabetes

- **Carbohydrate foods** in their more natural forms are an important part of a healthy diet. They provide energy, fiber, vitamins, minerals, protein and water. Carbohydrates are found mainly in cereal grains, fruit, vegetables and milk. Animal flesh foods contain negligible amounts. A healthy diet of at least 2000 calories is based around carbohydrate foods and should provide over 50% of total calories - whether or not we have diabetes. Lower calorie diets for weight control will have as little as 40% carbohydrate calories.

- **Carbohydrates include** sugars, starches and fibers. Sugars and starch provide energy to body cells. Even though fiber is not digested, it benefits the body - more so in diabetes. *(See Fiber Guide ~ Page 276)*

  The **various forms of carbohydrate** affect blood glucose levels in different ways; and it is difficult to predict the effect of particular foods, sugars or meals, simply by their actual carbohydrate content. Thus, the **same amount** of carbohydrate from different foods may affect blood sugar differently. It depends on many factors.

  For example, fiber can slow digestion and absorption of sugars by acting as a physical barrier or by forming a gel. Both fiber and fat also slow the emptying rate of the stomach into the intestines where further digestion and absorption takes place. The physical form of food (solid, puree, liquid) also matters - the more natural the better.

  Generally, raw foods rather than cooked foods, and whole-foods rather than ground-up foods, are more slowly absorbed.

- **Sugar: Small amounts** eaten as part of a meal, may not adversely affect blood glucose in persons with good blood glucose control. Nevertheless, minimal amounts of sugar are encouraged for nutritional and weight control reasons.

Glycemic Index

- Glycemic index (GI) indicates how fast a carbohydrate-containing food is digested and how much it causes blood glucose to rise (glycemic response).

Slower Acting Carbohydrates

These foods are more slowly digested and absorbed. They help maintain more even blood glucose levels. Use these foods regularly but still limit quantities for weight control. Examples:

- Dried beans, peas, lentils
- Nuts and seeds
- Wholegrain breads, pita
- Bran cereals, oats
- Barley, buckwheat, bulgur
- Spaghetti, pasta, Basmati Rice
- Fresh fruit: apples, avocados, bananas (firm), cherries, grapefruit, grapes, olives, oranges, peaches, pears, plums
- Vegetables: sweet corn, yam
- Milk, yogurt, soy drinks

Quicker Acting Carbohydrates

These foods more rapidly raise blood glucose levels. Eat in moderation.

- White bread, rice cakes, bagels, croissants, doughnuts
- Low fiber cereals: Cornflakes, *Rice Krispies, Froot Loops*
- White potato, white rice
- Watermelon, ripe bananas, cantaloupe, pineapple
- Glucose drinks and candy

Diabetes & Carbohydrate Distribution

- **For people with diabetes**, regular meals with even distribution of carbohydrate over the day are important for good control of blood sugar levels.

- **Smaller amounts of food** eaten more frequently result in steadier, more even blood glucose levels. (Be sure to control your weight.)

Recommended daily eating patterns for good blood glucose control:

1. **Three Meals & Three Snacks ~**
   Best for persons on insulin (Type-1 diabetes) with normal blood glucose variations.

2. **Three Meals ~**
   Best for Type-2 diabetes (especially if overweight).

Note: If blood sugar levels show excessive variations see doctor and dietitian.

- **Your doctor or dietitian** will select the level of calories and carbohydrate most appropriate to your weight, medication and activity. (Regular blood glucose checks will provide feedback on the level of control.)

- **Amounts of carbohydrate** in the guide below provide an average of 50% of total calories. **A rough rule of thumb is: 13 grams of carbohydrate per 100 calories.**

At calorie levels above 2000, carbohydrates approach 50-60% of total calories.

At lower calorie levels used for weight loss (1200-1500 calories), carbohydrates account for as little as 40% of total calories. This is because protein has nutritional priority.

These carbohydrate quantities (and percentages) apply equally to persons with or without diabetes.

IDEAL CARBOHYDRATE DISTRIBUTION
For Type-1 Diabetes (Insulin Dependent)

3 MEALS & 3 SNACKS
Balanced Blood Sugar Levels

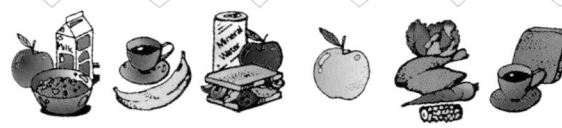

GUIDE TO CARBOHYDRATE DISTRIBUTION

Daily Total Calories		Daily Total Carbohyd.	Percent Carbohyd. Cals	Each Main Meal (3)	Between Meals (3)
1200 Cals	~	120g	40%	30g	10g
1500 Cals	~	170g	45%	40g	15g
2000 Cals	~	250g	50%	60g	25g
2500 Cals	~	345g	55%	70g	45g
3000 Cals	~	450g	60%	90g	60g

Unexplained Weight Gains

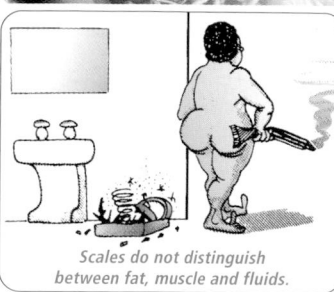

Scales do not distinguish between fat, muscle and fluids.

Body Fluid Changes

Body weight fluctuates from day to day. This is mainly due to changes in body fluids which make up around 70% of total body weight. It can be affected by changes in hormone levels, dietary factors such as salt and carbohydrate, and even exercise.

Weight change over several weeks is more likely to reflect changes in levels of fat and muscle rather than fluid. Unfortunately, the scales do not distinguish between weight changes due to water, fat or muscle. This is why **we shouldn't allow every fluctuation in weight to rule our lives.**

To limit fluid retention, avoid salty foods and go easy on the salt shaker. Eating sufficient fruit and vegetables supplies extra potassium which counteracts sodium and encourages fluid loss. However, **do not limit water intake.** Be sure to drink at least 6-8 glasses of water and other fluids per day.

When dining out, be aware that the extra pound or two that might show on the scales the next morning is not the result of a small dietary indiscretion. It is more likely due to fluid retention resulting from more highly seasoned and salty food.

Monthly hormonal changes in women can also account for a build-up of fluids of several pounds prior to menstruation.

Menopausal Weight Gains

Most women gain an average of 4-5 pounds in the years leading up to the menopause - usually in their middle to late 40's. This can occur even when exercise and eating habits have not changed significantly.

With hormonal changes occurring at that time, body fat also tends to be redistributed from thighs, buttocks and hips to the breast and stomach areas (a greater health risk).

Be sure to eat wisely and continue daily physical activity including strength-training to maintain or build muscles - and to boost metabolism and self-esteem.

Underactive Thyroid

Thyroid hormone is secreted into the blood-stream by the thyroid gland in the neck. When insufficient thyroid hormone is made, metabolism and body processes slow down and weight gain can occur.

Symptoms of hypothyroidism can be subtle and easily overlooked as signs of normal aging. **Early symptoms** may include fatigue, muscle weakness, sluggishness, a swollen tongue that you keep biting, and a puffy face.

As metabolism continues to slow, **further signs can include** chronically cold hands and feet, slow reflexes, constipation, dry skin and coarse hair, brittle nails, heavy menstrual periods, slower pulse, and a husky voice.

Depression-like symptoms may also develop such as forgetfulness, loss of interest, mood swings and irritability.

Weight gains of as much as 10-20 pounds (mainly fluid) can occur, as well as a **raised blood cholesterol level.**

The condition is more common in women, especially following pregnancy, around menopause, or after age 60.

A simple blood test through your doctor can detect hypothyroidism. It is easily treated in most cases with thyroid hormone pills.

Adults 35 and older should have a TSH (thyroid stimulating hormone) test every 5 years. Testing when pregnant is also wise.

Tips For Overweight Kids & Teens

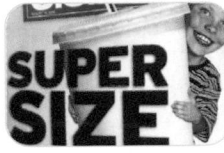

The XL Generation

Some 15% of American kids and adolescents are overweight; and childhood obesity has doubled over the last 20 years. Diabetes, high blood pressure and high cholesterol are major problem areas for overweight children and adolescents, as are depression, low self-esteem, sleep apnea and bone joint problems.

To address this problem, cooperation is required between kids, parents, schools and regulators. Weight control is a family and community affair.

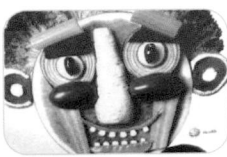

Some simple tips to get started:
≫ Watch Soda Intake!

Limit soda and sugary drinks to one serving on the weekends soda should not be an everyday beverage. Try water instead. When at fast-food restaurants or using a soda fountain, choose small servings with ice or choose diet soda instead. Schools should provide water and restrict access to soda. Parents need to supervise kids at the soda fountain!

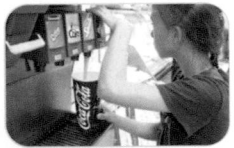

≫ Say "No" to Super-Sizing!

Portion sizes are on the increase, and for just a few cents, meals can be up-sized - with loads more calories. Choose sensible portion sizes when dining out and at home. Use smaller plates and choose smaller packages.

≫ Limit Between-Meal Snacking

Watch out for high-fat and high-calorie snacks. Choose fresh fruit and vegetables instead. Keep your eye on portion sizes and limit foods like chips and candy to parties and special occasions.

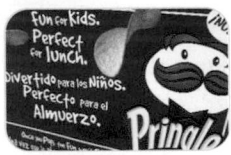

≫ Cut back on Fast-foods and Eating Out

Many more calories are consumed when you eat out. Healthy meals prepared at home are best for the whole family.

≫ Get Moving!

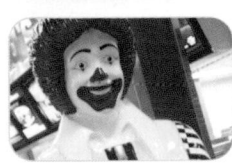

Kids need at least 60 minutes of physical activity every day. Limit time spent in sedentary activities, such as playing computer games or watching TV - as well as the accompanying snacks! Include exercise in family activities. Note: When kids watch TV in a motionless trance, they burn even less calories than if simply sitting, reading or talking.

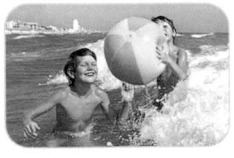

For extra information and tips see
www.CalorieKing.com

- Calorie and fat values have been rounded off.
  Calories - to the nearest 5 or 10 calories.
  Fat - to the nearest half gram.
  Note: Trace amounts of fat (less than 0.3 grams per serving) have been treated as zero.

- Because manufacturer's figures on labels are rounded off, figures in this book may differ slightly from the label. Serving sizes may also vary.

- Food product formulations change from time to time, and hence the need to regularly update this type of publication. Many products also come and go. Check the food label for any changes.

- **Seek Professional Advice:** This book is intended for educational purposes only. It is not a substitute for professional advice.

- **Feedback Welcome:** Please contact the author directly with your queries, and suggestions for foods to be included in future editions.

  Write to: Allan Borushek (Dietitian)
  PO Box 1616, Costa Mesa CA 92628
  Email: allan@calorieking.com

- **Free Information Service:** Check the author's website for new food product updates.

www.calorieking.com

C ~ **Calories**
F ~ **Fat (grams)**
Cb ~ **Carbohydrate (grams)**

Abbreviations

tsp	=	teaspoon
Tbsp	=	Tablespoon
oz	=	ounce(s)
c	=	cup
fl.oz	=	fluid ounce(s)
g	=	gram(s)
<1	=	less than 1

Volume Measures

3 tsp	=	1 Tbsp
2 Tbsp	=	1 fl.oz
1/2 cup	=	4 fl.oz
1 cup	=	8 fl.oz or 16 Tbsp
2 cups	=	1 Pint
2 Pints	=	1 Quart

(All measures are level)

Note: 8 oz weight is not the same as 8 fl.oz volume (space occupied). Dense foods weigh more per set volume. Examples:
  1 cup popcorn weighs 1/2 oz
  1 cup milk weighs 8 1/2 oz
  1 cup pudding weighs 10 oz

Metric Conversion

1/2 oz	=	14 grams
1 oz	=	28.4 grams
2 oz	=	57 grams
3 1/2 oz	=	100 grams
1 fl.oz	=	30 mls
1 cup (8 fl.oz)	=	240 mls
33 fl.oz	=	1 liter (volume)

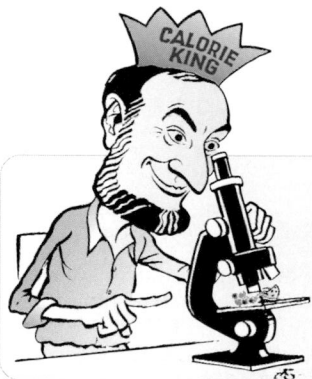

SOURCES OF INFORMATION

- U.S. Dept. of Agriculture
- Food Manufacturers
- Food Industry Boards & Councils
- Independent laboratory analysis
- Scientific publications
- Overseas food composition tables
- Author extrapolations

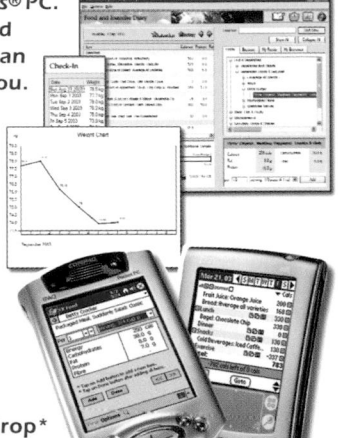
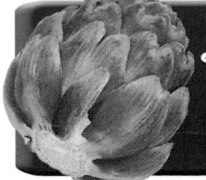

Quick Guide C F Cb

Cow Milk ~ Average All Brands

Whole (3.5% fat):

	C	F	Cb
2 Tbsp, 1 fl.oz	20	1	1.5
1 Glass, 6 fl.oz	110	6	8.5
1 Cup, 8 fl.oz	150	8	12
1 Pint, 16 fl.oz	300	16	23
1 Quart, 946 ml	600	32	46

Reduced-fat (2% fat):

	C	F	Cb
2 Tbsp, 1 fl.oz	15	0.5	1.5
1 Glass, 6 fl.oz	90	4	8.5
1 Cup, 8 fl.oz	130	5	13
1 Pint, 16 fl.oz	260	10	26
1 Quart, 946 ml	520	20	52

Light/Lowfat (1% fat):

	C	F	Cb
2 Tbsp, 1 fl.oz	12	0.3	1.5
1 Glass, 6 fl.oz	75	2	8.5
1 Cup, 8 fl.oz	120	2.5	14
1 Pint, 16 fl.oz	240	5	28
1 Quart, 946 ml	480	10	56

Light/Lowfat (1/2% fat):

	C	F	Cb
2 Tbsp, 1 fl.oz	12	0.1	1.6

Fat Free/Skim:

	C	F	Cb
2 Tbsp, 1 fl.oz	10	0	1.5
1 Cup, 8 fl.oz	90	0.5	13
1 Pint, 16 fl.oz	180	1	26
w. Replace (Oatrim Fiber): 1 cup	85	0	12

Protein-Fortified:

	C	F	Cb
2% fat, 1 cup	140	5	14
1% fat, 1 cup	120	3	14
Skim, 1 cup	100	0.5	14

Acidophilus: Average All Brands

	C	F	Cb
Reduced Fat (2%), 1 cup	130	5	13
Lowfat (1%), 1 cup	100	2	13

Buttermilk: Average All Brands

	C	F	Cb
Reduced Fat (2%), 1 cup	120	5	10
Low Fat (1%), 1 cup	100	2.5	12
Oak Farms (1%), 1 cup	100	2.5	12

Lactose-Reduced:

	C	F	Cb
Reduced Fat: Lactaid, 1 cup	130	5	12
Dairy Ease 100, 1 cup	130	5	12
Lowfat, Lactaid, 1 cup	110	2.5	13
Fat Free Lactaid/Lucerne, 1 cup	80	0	13
Lactaid with Soy Protein	110	0	13

Soy/Non-Dairy Drinks

~ See Page 27 ~

Goat/Sheep Milk, Kefir

Goat's Milk (Meyenberg):

	C	F	Cb
Whole, 1 cup, 8 fl.oz	140	7	11
Light/Lowfat (1%), 8 fl.oz	90	2.5	9
Evaporated, reconst., 8 fl.oz	145	8	11
Kefir: Alta Dena, 1 cup, 8 fl.oz	240	4.5	41
Nancy's, fruit flavors, avg, 1 cup	200	8	25
Steve's Kefir Peach, 1 cup	220	9	25
Sheep's Milk: Whole, 1 cup	265	17	13

Canned & Dried Milk

	C	F	Cb
Condensed: Reg. 2 Tbsp, 1 fl.oz	130	3	22
Lowfat (Eagle), 2 Tbsp	120	1.5	23
Fat Free (Eagle), 2 Tbsp	110	0	24
Evaporated: Whole, 2 Tbsp	40	3	3
Whole, 1/2 cup	170	10	13
Lowfat (Carnation), 2 Tbsp, 1 oz	25	0.5	3
1/2 cup	110	3	12
Fat Free, 2 Tbsp, 1 oz	25	0	4
Dried: Whole, 1/4 cup, 1 oz	150	8	11
Skim/Nonfat, 1/3 cup	80	0	12
Made-up, 1 cup, 8 fl.oz	80	0	12
Buttermilk, sweetcream, 1 oz	110	2	3
Nonfat, 1 Tbsp	25	0	3

Whey Drink

	C	F	Cb
Acid: Dry, 1 Tbsp, 3g	10	0	2
Fluid, 1 cup, 8 fl.oz	60	0	13
Sweet: Dry, 1 Tbsp, 8g	25	0	6
Fluid, 1 cup, 8 fl.oz	65	1	13
Nutri Mil: Orig./Low Fat 8 fl.oz	80	3	11
Chocolate, 8 fl.oz	110	3	19
Fat Free (Calcium Enriched)	60	0	11

Flavored Milk Drinks

Chocolate Milk
Average All Brands: Per Cup, 8 fl.oz

	C	F	Cb
Whole Milk (3.3%): 1 cup	225	9	26
1 Pint	450	18	52
Reduced Fat (2%), 1 cup	190	5	26
Lowfat (1%), 1 cup	160	3	26

Brands ~ Flavored Milk
Ready-To-Drink: Per 8 fl.oz Unless Indicated

	C	F	Cb
Albertson's, lowfat	170	2.5	30
Bodywise, nonfat	180	0	35
Borden Dutch Choc., 1 cup	220	8	28
Bosco	230	8	33
Brown Cow Farm, 1 cup	250	8	39
Deans'Chug': Regular	220	9	26
Lowfat, 1 cup	160	2.5	27
Dominick's Lowfat, 1 cup	170	2.5	28
Golden Guernsey, 1 cup	130	2.5	15
Grocers Pride Choc D'Lite, 1 cup	120	3	22
Hershey's: Fat Free Chocolate	165	0	31
Reduced Fat Chocolate/Strawb.	200	5	31
White Chocolate	130	5	12
MilkShake, avg, 8 fl.oz	285	8	44
Hood, Lowfat (1%)	150	2	27
Horizon Organic	160	2.5	27
Knudsen	200	3	32
Kroger (3.25% milk)	220	9	28
Lactaid (1%)	160	3	26
Land O'Lakes, lowfat (0.5%)	150	1.5	35
Meadow Gold (3.5%)	230	8	31
Nesquik: 16 fl.oz bottle	460	16	62
Choc., Fat Free, 16 fl.oz bottle	320	0	62
Double Choc., 16 fl.oz bottle	460	18	60
Reduced Fat Banana, 8 fl.oz	200	5	30
Very Vanilla, 8 fl.oz	220	8	29
Oak Farms, 1 cup	210	8	26
Parmalat (2%)	180	5	28
Ralph's	240	3	34
Sobe Love Bus Chocolate, 8 fl.oz	140	1	28
Viva, Lowfat	130	2.5	26
Yoo Hoo Choc Drink, 9 fl.oz	150	1	33

Bottled Coffee
See Coffee Section: Page 166

Shakes & Smoothies

Smoothies
Made Up Ready-To-Drink
(8 fl. oz Milk/Soy + Fruit): Per 12 fl.oz

	C	F	Cb
Average all types: w. Whole Milk	300	8	50
+ Icecream, 1 scoop	400	13	62
with Nonfat Milk	240	0	50

Freshens; Jamba Juice; TCBY:
See Fast-Foods Section

Shakes
Regular:

	C	F	Cb
Chocolate, 10 fl.oz	360	11	58
Vanilla/Strawberry, 10 fl.oz	320	9	53

Burger King; McDonald's: See Fast-Foods

Cocoa-Chocolate Mixes
Add extra cals/fat/carbohydrate for milk

	C	F	Cb
Alba '66 Milk Choc, 1 pkg	60	0	14
Carnation Cocoa Mixes:			
Chocolate Rich, 3 Tbsp/1 pkg	110	1	24
Milk Chocolate, 3 Tbsp	110	1	24
w. Mini Marshmallows, 1 oz pkg	110	1	24
Malted Milk Original, 3 Tbsp	90	2	15
70 Calorie Cocoa Mix, 3 tsp	70	0.5	15
Fat-Free, 2 Tbsp/1 pkg	25	0	4
No Sugar, 1 pkg	50	0.5	8
Land O' Lakes: Per 1¼ oz Pkg			
Choc.Mint/Raspb./Supreme	160	5	25
Nestle Hot Cocoa Mix, 1 oz	110	1	23
w. Marshmallows, 1 oz	120	1	23
French Vanilla	120	3	22
Nesquik Powder (Nestle): Per 2 Tbsp			
Choc.; Dble Choc; Strawberry	90	0.5	19
Chocolate, No Added Sugar	40	1	7
Ghirardelli: Per 2 Heaping Teaspoons			
Choc. Mocha/Hazelnut/Dble Choc	80	1.5	21
Pralines & Creme, 2 Tbsp	90	0	23
Ovaltine Cocoa Mixes, 4 tsp	80	0	20
Swiss Miss Cocoa Mixes:			
Milk Chocolate, 1 oz pkt	110	1.5	22
w. Marshmallows, 1.2 oz pkg	140	3	22
Choc. Sensation, 1.25 oz pkg	150	4	27
Lite, 1 pkg	70	0	18
Diet Cocoa Mix, 1 pkg	25	0	4
Hot Cocoa Mix, 1 pkg (0.6 oz)			
with calcium, no added sugar	60	1	10
Sugar Free	60	0	10
Fat Free, 0.53 oz	50	0	9
Vending Machine, 1.34 oz pkg	145	2	24
Weight Watchers: Hot Cocoa Mix	70	0	10

Soy & Non-Dairy Drinks

Soy ~ Ready-To-Drink

Per 1 Cup Serving (8 fl.oz)	C	F	Cb
Cereal Match, 1 cup	100	3	17
Eden Blend: 1 cup	120	3	18
Edensoy: Original, 1 cup	130	5	13
Extra, Vanilla	150	3	23
Carob	170	4	27
Light: Original, 1 cup	95	2	14
Vanilla	120	2	21
8th Continent: Chocolate (lowfat)	140	3	23
Original, Lowfat	80	3	8
Vanilla, Lowfat	90	3	11
Hain Soy Supreme: Original	80	3	9
Vanilla, 1 cup	100	3	12
Harmony Farms: Regular, 1 cup	80	3	10
Enriched; Vanilla, 1 cup	100	3	14
Health Source: All flavors	150	1.5	23
Health Source Plus	160	1	17
Soy Protein Shake	100	1	4
Health Valley: Soy Moo	110	0	21
It's Soy Delicious: Vanilla	110	1	22
Awesome; Chocolate	120	2	22
Lifeway: Soy Treat, Apple; Caramel	160	4	23
Naked Juice: Choc Soy Shake	210	2	38
Vanilla Soy Shake	170	1	33
Odwalla Future Shake: Chocolate	160	3	27
Vanilla al'monde	190	6	24
Pacific: Ultra, Plain/Vanilla	150	5	20
Original unsweetened	100	5	5
Enriched (Soy Isoflavin): Plain	90	2.5	14
Vanilla, 1 cup	110	2.5	16
Fat Free: Plain	70	0	14
Vanilla	90	0	17
Select (Soy Isoflavin), Plain	100	2.5	13
PowerDream: Mango Passion	320	5	65
Java Jolt, Chai, Vanilla Blast	250	5	42
X-treme Chocolate	260	5	48
Silk (White Wave): Plain, regular	100	4	8
Plain, unsweetened	90	4	5
Chai, Mocha	140	3	20
Chocolate	140	3.5	23
Coffee Soylatte, 1 cup	170	3.5	29
11 oz Bottle	220	5	38
Spice Soylatte, 11 oz bottle	200	6	27
Vanilla	100	3.5	10
Silk Creamer, 1 Tbsp	15	1	1
SoyDream: Orig./Enriched 8 fl.oz	130	4	17
Carob/Chocolate Enriched	210	4	37
Vanilla; Vanilla Enriched	150	4	22
Soy Fusion: Berry, 1 cup	120	1.5	24

Soy Nice: Per 1 Cup (8 fl.oz)	C	F	Cb
Natural, 8 fl.oz	70	3.5	2
Original	80	3	6
Chocolate, 1 cup	110	3	17
Vanilla	100	3	11
SunSoy: Chocolate, 1 cup	155	3.5	26
Creamy Original, 1 cup	95	4	8
Vanilla, 1 cup	105	3.5	12
Ultra Slim-Fast: Juice-based			
With Soy, all flavors, 11 oz can	220	1	46
Vitasoy: Refrigerated: Crmy Orig.	100	4	9
Rich Chocolate	160	4	23
Smooth Vanilla	110	4	11
Long Life: Creamy Original	110	4	11
Classic Original	120	4.5	11
Green Tea Soy Drink	120	4	13
Rich Chocolate	160	4	24
Unsweetened Original	80	4	5
Vanilla Delight	120	4	11
Light: Original	60	2	7
Chocolate	110	2.5	18
Vanilla Soy Drink	90	2	14
WestSoy: Plus, Plain, 8 fl.oz	130	3	17
Plus, Vanilla	130	3	19
100% Organic: Original (2% fat)	130	3.5	18
Unsweetened, Plain	90	4.5	5
Unsweetened, Vanilla	100	4.5	5
Nonfat: Plain	70	0	11
Vanilla	80	0	14
Lite: Plain, 1 cup, 8 fl.oz	90	1.5	15
Chocolate	130	1.5	25
Vanilla	110	1.5	19
Lowfat: Plain	90	1.5	14
Chocolate	140	3	24
Strawberry	160	3	25
Vanilla	120	1.5	21
Chai: Original, 8 fl.oz	130	3	25
Smoothies, all flavors, 8 fl.oz	140	1.5	28
Soy Shakes: Choc; Vanilla	170	3.5	30
Vigor Aid: Vanilla	230	5	37
Chocolate	260	5	42
Juice Bar: average all flavors	120	1.5	24
Vitamite 100: 1 cup, 8 fl.oz	110	5	14
Wild Oats: Original, 1 cup, 8 fl.oz	100	3.5	12

Rice & Cereal Drinks • Yogurt

Soy Powder Mix   C   F   Cb

(1 oz (1/4 cup) mix makes 1 cup, 8 fl.oz)

	C	F	Cb
Better Than Milk: Original, 1 oz	100	2.5	16
Light, 1 oz	80	0.5	13
Joy Soy: Extra (Carob/Van.), 2 T.	80	3	11
Revival Soy Shakes (Per Packet):			
Plain; Chocolate Daydream	110	1.5	2
Flavors, average: with Fructose	225	2	33
Unsweetened or Splenda	130	2	4
Soyagen: Reg./No Sugar, 1 oz dry	130	6	12
Carob, 1 oz dry	130	6	13
Soy Protein Isolate, 1 oz dry	95	1	0
Soy Quik (Ener-g), 1 oz dry	100	4.5	8

Rice & Cereal Drinks

	C	F	Cb
Almond Breeze: Original, 8 fl.oz	60	3	8
Vanilla, 8 fl.oz	90	3	16
Amazake: Almond Light, 8 fl.oz	110	2	20
Horchata: *Don José,* 8 fl.oz	140	4	25
Kerns, Aguas Frescas, 8 fl.oz	140	3	26
Eden Blend: Rice & Soy, 1 cup	120	3	18
Eden Rice: 1 cup, 8 fl.oz	110	3	21
Hain Rice Supreme: Lowfat Orig.	100	3	16
Lowfat Cinnamon, 8 fl.oz	130	3	22
Pacific Foods: Multigrain, 8 fl.oz	150	2	31
Naturally Oat: Original, 1 cup	110	1.5	21
Vanilla, 1 cup, 8 fl.oz	130	1.5	24
Naturally Almond: Original, 1 cup	70	2.5	10
Vanilla, 1 cup, 8 fl.oz	90	2.5	15
Pacific Rice: Lowfat, Plain, 1 cup	90	2	18
Fat Free: Plain, 8 fl.oz	80	0	18
Cocoa, 8 fl.oz	100	0	21
Vanilla, 8 fl.oz	110	0	24
Rice Dream: Carob, 1 cup	150	2.5	32
Chocolate; Enriched, 1 cup	170	3	36
Vanilla/Vanilla Enriched, 1 cup	130	2	28
Original/Original Enriched, 1 cup	120	2	25
Westbrae: Rice: Plain/Van., 8 fl.oz	110	2.5	20
Wild Oats: Vanilla, 1 cup, 8 fl.oz	120	2	26
Original, 1 cup, 8 fl.oz	100	2	20

Rice/Nut Drink Mixes

	C	F	Cb
Better Than Milk: Light, 19g	70	0.5	14
Original, 23g	100	2.5	16
Nut Quik, 2 Tbsp powder, 18g	110	9	3
Rice Moo, 2 Tbsp powder, 19g	72	0	17
Solait, 3 Tbsp powder, 22g	80	1.5	13
Sun's Up, 2 scoops, 40g powder	160	2	36

Quick Guide

Yogurt   C   F   Cb

Average All Brands: Per 8 oz Cup

	C	F	Cb
Plain Yogurt: Whole, 8 oz	180	7	11
Lowfat	140	4	16
Nonfat	110	0	18
Fruit Flavored: Whole, 8 oz	250	6	38
Lowfat	230	3	32
Nonfat, regular	150	0	32
Nonfat, no sugar added	120	0	32
Goat's Milk Yogurt-Same as Regular Yogurt			

Yogurt ~ Brands

	C	F	Cb
Alex Rod: Fat Free, all flav., 8 oz	70	0	12
Albertson's (Lowfat):			
Swiss, avg. all flavors, 8 oz	280	2.5	54
Fruit on the Bottom (lowfat):			
average all flavors, 8 oz	260	2.5	49
Alta Dena (Lowfat): Plain, 8 oz	170	4.5	20
Fruit flavors, average	280	2.5	53
Fruit on the Bottom: Cherry Van.	270	2.5	55
Other flavors, average	220	2.5	40
Nonfat: Plain, 8 oz	110	0	17
Flavors, average	190	0	39
America's Choice: Swiss Style	210	2.5	41
Nonfat, all flavors, 8 oz	100	0	15
Berkeley Farms: Per 8 oz Cup			
Lowfat: Boysenberry/Cherry	230	2.5	46
Raspberry	220	2.5	43
Strawberry, Lemon, Vanilla	270	2.5	52
Nonfat: Average all flavors	100	0	16
Breyers: Light n' Lively, 4.4 oz	135	1	27
Lowfat: 1% fat, all flavors, 8 oz	220	2	41
1.5% fat, plain, 8 oz	125	0.5	22
Smooth & Creamy, 8 oz	230	2	45
Brown Cow: Per 8 oz			
Cream Top: Plain	170	10	12
Chocolate	250	8	39
Creamy Coffee, Vanilla	210	9	25
Fruit Flavors, average	230	8	35
Lowfat: Plain	130	3	18
Flavors, average	220	3	41
Non Fat: Plain	115	0	17
Fruit Flavors, average	190	0	39
Cabot: Plain, 8 oz	140	4	16
Flavors, 8 oz	220	3	42
Cascade Fresh: Lowfat, 6 oz	140	2	23
Fat Free, all flavors, 6 oz ctn	110	0	20
Whole Milk, 8 oz	170	8	12

Yogurt ~ Brands (Cont)

	C	F	Cb
Colombo			
Light, all flavors, 8 oz	110	0	20
Classic, avg. all types, 8 oz	220	3	41
Fat Free, Plain, 8 oz	110	0	16
Continental: Nonfat, 8 oz ctn			
Fruit on the Bottom, 8 oz	190	0	38
Vanilla	190	0	38
Crowley: Lowfat Blueberry, 8 oz	240	2.5	48
Dannon: Plain (Natural), 8 oz	170	8	14
Danimals: Super Creamy, 4 oz	120	1	18
Squeezable, 2 oz	140	5	20
Drinkable, 3.3 fl.oz	120	0	22
Fruit Blends: Blueberry, 6 oz	170	1.5	33
Strawberry Blueberry, 4 oz	110	1	21
Fruit on the Bottom,			
average all flavors, 6 oz ctn	160	1.5	29
Frusion Smoothie: 10 fl.oz bottle	280	3.5	53
la Creme: Avg. all flavors, 4 oz	150	5	21
Mousse, all flavors 2.6 oz	120	5	15
Light 'n Fit (0% Fat):			
average all flavors, 6 oz	90	0	17
Creamy, avg. all flavors, 6 oz	120	0	16
Smoothie, 7 fl.oz bottle	80	0	15
Natural: avg. all flavors, 6 oz	160	2.5	22
Sprinkl'ins: All flavors, 4.1 oz ctn	120	1.5	22
Whipped: avg. all flavors, 4.6 oz	160	3	28
Dominick's: Lowfat, 8 oz	230	2	40
Fruit on the Bottom, avg, 8 oz	230	2	40
Fat Free 80 Calories, 8 oz	80	0	13
Plain: Lowfat, 8 oz	130	2.5	15
Nonfat, 8 oz	120	0	17
Friendship: Regular type, 6 oz	190	5	31
Grocer's Pride: Lowfat, 4.4 oz	140	1.5	28
Hood: Fat Free, Plain, 8 oz	130	0	18
Flavors, average, 8 oz	190	0	40
Horizon Organic			
Whole Milk: Vanilla, 8 oz	220	6	32
Lowfat, fruits, avg, 6 oz cup	160	2	30
Fat Free: Plain and Simple, 6 oz	80	0	13
Vanilla, 6 oz	130	0	24
Fruit On The Bottom, avg, 6 oz	140	0	27
Fruit, Blended, 6 oz	160	2	30
32 oz Ctn: Plain, 1 cup, 8 oz	110	0	15
Vanilla, 1 cup, 8 oz	170	0	32

Jerseymaid (Vons)	C	F	Cb
Fruit on the Bottom, 8 oz	240	2.5	46
Prestirred (lowfat), average	240	2.5	46
Plain, lowfat, 8 oz	140	3.5	18
Jell-O: Spaceship, 4 oz	110	1	22
Helios: Kefir Organic, 1 cup	120	5	13
Jewel: Lowfat, average, 8 oz	250	2.5	48
Kemps: 100 Calories Nonfat, 5 oz	100	0	22
Classic Lowfat, 6 oz	160	1.5	30
Free Nonfat, 6 oz	90	0	22
Knudsen: 70 Calories, 6 oz	70	0	11
Free, average, 6 oz	170	0	33
Kroger: Per 8 oz Ctn			
Lite (Nonfat) avg. all flavors	100	0	16
Lowfat: Plain, 8 oz	150	4	17
Flavors, avg, 8 oz	250	2.5	47
Fruit on the Bottom,			
avg. all flavors, 8 oz	220	3	40
Lactaid: Lowfat Vanilla, 8 oz	240	2.5	45
La Yogurt			
Fruit Flavors, average, 6 oz	170	2	32
Light, average all flavors, 6 oz	70	0	12
Light n' Lively			
Free 50 Calories, 4 oz	50	0	8
Free 70 Calories, 6 oz	70	0	11
Free (Regular) 6 oz: Vanilla	160	0	32
Strawb. Fruit/Peach/Lem./Berry	170	0	34
Strawberry/Raspberry	180	0	36
Kidpack/Multipack, avg 4.4 oz	140	1	28
Lucerne			
Low Fat: Plain, 8 oz	150	3.5	18
Fruit flavors, avg, 8 oz	240	2.5	47
Vanilla	230	2.5	43
Fat Free: Plain, 8 oz	130	0	19
Light Fat Free, fruit, 8 oz	120	0	22
YoCups, avg all flavors, 4 oz	130	1	27
Yo On The Go, 2.25 oz tube	80	2	13
Meadow Gold: Plain, 8 oz	160	5	16
Flavors, average, 8 oz	250	4	42
Mountain High			
Original: Plain, 8 oz	190	8	18
Fat Free Plain, 8 oz	120	0	20
Fat Free: Plain, 8 oz	110	0	19
Flavors, average, 6 oz ctn	110	0	29
Low Fat: Plain/Vanilla, 8 oz	150	2	22

Yogurt (Cont)

Brands (Cont)   **C**   **F**   **Cb**

Mystic Lake Dairy (Goat Milk Yogurt)

Item	C	F	Cb
Plain, 1 cup, 8 oz	120	6	9

Nancy's: *Per 8 oz Serving*

Item	C	F	Cb
Whole Milk: Honey, plain, 8 fl.oz	180	8	17
w. Fruit Cup, avg, 9.5 oz	230	8	29
Low Fat: Plain/Lemon/Vanilla, avg	140	3	16
Other flavors, average	180	3	28
Nonfat: Plain, 8 oz	120	0	17
Maple, Vanilla (8 oz ctn)	160	0	27
w. Fruit Cup, avg, 9.5 oz	165	0	29
Vanilla (32 oz ctn), swtn'd, 8 oz	220	0	40
Soy Cultured: (6 oz ctn): Plain	145	3	25
Berry flavors, avg.	150	3.5	24
Vanilla	120	3	19
Kiwi-Lime; Mango, avg.	170	3	33
Old Home: 100 Cal., Nonfat, 6 oz	100	0	20
Velvet Delight, avg., 6 oz	240	7	39

Pavel's: Original Russian, 8 oz 140 8 10

Item	C	F	Cb
Lowfat Vanilla, 8 oz	120	4	12
Nonfat Russian, 8 oz	110	0	15
Mountain Dairy, 6 oz	150	1.5	27

Publix: Light, average, 8 oz 130 0 21

Item	C	F	Cb
Fruit on the Bottom, avg, 8 oz	250	2.5	43
Fat Free: Plain, 8 oz	140	0	23
Swiss Style (lowfat), 8 oz	240	2.5	41

Redwood Hill Farm (Goat Milk Yogurt)

Item	C	F	Cb
Fruit flavors, average, 8 oz	180	5	28
Vanilla, 8 oz	190	6	28
Plain, 8 oz	120	6	9

Silk (Soy): Plain, 1 cup, 8 oz 120 2.5 22

Item	C	F	Cb
Vanilla, 6 oz ctn	120	2	23
Other flavors, average, 6 oz	170	2	31

Sky Hill Napa Valley: Plain, 8 oz 130 8 8
Snackwell's: Nonfat, 6 oz 160 0 36

Stater Bros:

Item	C	F	Cb
Nonfat, average all flavors, 8 oz	130	0	14
Yo2Go, 2.25 oz tube	80	2	13

Stonyfield Farm (Organic)

Item	C	F	Cb
Whole Milk: Plain, 1 cup, 8 oz	180	9	16
French Vanilla, 6 oz	185	6	27
6 oz Cups: Vanilla, Mocha	190	6	27
Other flavors, avg	170	6	24
Lowfat: Plain, 6 oz	90	1.5	13
Flavors, average, 6 oz	140	1.5	25
4 oz cup pkg	100	1	19
Nonfat: Plain, 8 oz cup	100	0	15
Other flavors, avg. 8 oz	160	0	32
O'Soy: 4 oz Multipack, avg	110	1.5	19
Fruit On Bottom, 6 oz, Vanilla	150	2	26
Other flavors, 6 oz, avg	170	2	33
YoBaby, 4 oz ctn	110	4	15
YoSqueeze, 2 oz tube	60	1	11

Stop & Shop: **C**   **F**   **Cb**

Item	C	F	Cb
Blended Lite, 8 oz	120	0	20

"TCBY" Fat Free (Fantasies):

Item	C	F	Cb
Banana Creme Pie, 6 oz	110	0	18
White Chocolate, 6 oz	90	0	12

Trader Joe's

Item	C	F	Cb
Nonfat: Regular 8 oz	190	0	40
French Village, Vanilla, 8 oz	170	0	32
Organic Vanilla, 8 oz	160	0	27
Lowfat, average, 8 oz	230	2.5	44
Organic Low Fat, average, 6 oz	150	2.5	24
Cultured Soy, all varieties, 6 oz	140	2.5	28

Wallaby (Organic):

Item	C	F	Cb
Lowfat, avg. all flavors, 6 oz	150	2.5	24
WholeSoy: Plain, 6 oz ctn	140	2.5	24
Other flavors, avg, 6 oz ctn	150	2.5	24
YoFarm: All flavors, avg, 8 oz	220	6	37

YoCrunch: Lowfat w. Toppings, 6.5 oz cup

Item	C	F	Cb
Oreo Cookies	190	4	35
Peach/Strawb./Rasp. w. Granola	220	2	46
Strawberry w. Nestlé Crunch	240	6	41
Vanilla w. Choc Crunch/Reese's	240	7	39

Yoplait: *Per 6 oz*

Item	C	F	Cb
Fruit Flavors, 6 oz	170	1.5	33
Coconut Cream Pie, 6 oz	190	3	34
Lemon Burst, 6 oz	180	1.5	36
Pina Colada, 6 oz	170	3	33
Light (Fat Free): Fruit, 6 oz	100	0	19
Ban./Lemon Crm Pie; Very Van.	110	0	20
Custard Style, all flavors, 6 oz	190	3.5	32
Go-Gurt, 2.25 oz tube	80	2	13
Grande: 99% fatfree; Plain, 8 oz	130	0	19
Avg. all flavors, 8 oz	250	2.5	48
Trix, avg., all flavors, 4 oz	120	1.5	23
Whips!, 4 oz ctn	140	2.5	25
Yumsters, 4 oz	120	2	21

Yogurt Drinks & Probiotics

Item	C	F	Cb
Actimel (Dannon) Probiotic, 3.3 fl.oz	90	2	16
Alta Dena, Drinkables, 1 cup	220	0	46
Carbolite, 8 fl.oz	85	2	8
Dannon, Danimals, 3.4 fl.oz bottle	90	1.5	16
Glen Oaks, all flavors, avg, 1 cup	250	4	46
Nouriche, all flavors, 11 fl.oz	290	0	60
Old Home, Yog. Smoothies, 10 fl.oz	290	3.5	57
Stonyfield Farm, 10 fl.oz	250	3	48
WholeSoy, 12 fl.oz bottle	210	3	35
Wow Cow, 8 fl.oz	80	0	16
Yo Soy, 8 fl.oz	80	4	4
Yonique, 6 fl.oz: Pina Colada	190	4	30
Peach; Banana; Guava	170	2	30

Icecream & Frozen Yogurt

Quick Guide

Icecream

C **F** **Cb**

Vanilla: *Average All Brands*
Other flavors ~ See Brand Listings.

Regular Icecream (10% fat):
(Examples: *Borden/Hood*)

	C	F	Cb
3 fl.oz scoop	100	5	12
1/2 cup, 4 fl.oz	130	7	16
1 Pint, 16 fl.oz	520	28	62
1/2 Gallon (4 Pints)	2100	112	248

Rich (16% fat):

	C	F	Cb
3 fl.oz scoop	130	8	13
1/2 cup, 4 fl.oz	170	10	17
1 Pint	690	40	68

Super-Rich (20% fat): (*Haagen-Dazs/Ben & Jerry's*)

	C	F	Cb
3 fl.oz scoop	200	14	16
1/2 cup, 4 fl.oz	270	18	21
1 Pint	1100	72	84

Reduced Fat/Light (6% fat):
(*Breyer's Light/Hood Light*)

	C	F	Cb
3 fl.oz scoop	100	3	14
1/2 cup, 4 fl.oz	140	4	18
1 Pint	560	16	72

Low Fat (less than 4% fat):
(*Healthy Choice/Weight Watchers/Snackwell's*)

	C	F	Cb
3 fl.oz scoop	90	2	17
1/2 cup, 4 fl.oz	120	2.5	22
1 Pint	480	10	88

Fat Free: (*Baskin-Robbins FF/Borden FF/ Breyers FF/Dreyers FF/Hood FF)*)

	C	F	Cb
3 fl.oz scoop	75	0	17
1/2 cup, 4 fl.oz	100	0	22
1 Pint	400	0	88

Soft Serve: Regular, 1/2 cup

	C	F	Cb
	140	5	20
1 cup	280	10	40
Nonfat, 1/2 cup	90	0	23
1 cup	180	0	46

Quick Guide

Frozen Yogurt

C **F** **Cb**

Average All Brands

	C	F	Cb
Hard: Lowfat, 1/2 cup	140	3	26
Nonfat, 1/2 cup	110	0	29
Soft: Lowfat, 1/2 cup	120	2.5	28
Nonfat, 1/2 cup	100	0	30

Brands: *See Icecream & Ices Section*

Quick Guide

Gelato/Ices

C **F** **Cb**

	C	F	Cb
Gelato: Per 1/2 Cup			
Milk base: Vanilla	200	15	18
Choc. Hazelnut	370	29	26
Water base: 1/2 cup	100	0	25
Ice (Milk base): Average all flavors			
Hard (4% fat), 1/2 cup	100	3	15
Soft Serve (3% fat), 1/2 cup	110	2	19
Shaved Ice: Average, 12 fl. oz	160	0	40
Sherbet: Average, 1/2 cup	120	2	28
Sorbet: Fruit (no fat), 1/2 cup	120	0	30
Fruit Ice Pops	80	0	20

Tofu Frozen Desserts: See Page 35

Sundaes

C **F** **Cb**

	C	F	Cb
Denny's Sundaes:			
Single Scoop, no topping	195	14	14
Double Scoop, no topping	385	27	29
Banana Split	930	43	121
Toppings: Blueberry, 2 oz	70	0	17
Chocolate, 2 oz	340	25	27
Fudge, 2 oz	215	10	31
Strawberry, 2 oz	80	1	17
McDonald's Sundaes:			
Hot Fudge Sundae, 6.3 oz	340	12	52
Oreo® Cookie McFlurry™	570	20	82
Toppings: Nut/Sundae, 1/4 oz	40	3.5	2

Icecream Bars & Pops

See Pages 36-38

Icecream Cones & Cups

C **F** **Cb**

Average All Brands

	C	F	Cb
Wafer Cone/Cup, average	20	0	4
Sugar Cone, average	40	0	9
Waffle Cone:			
Small	60	0	11
Large	100	1	22
Brands:			
Oreo Chocolate Cone	50	0	10
Comet Sugar Cone	50	0	11
Keebler Sugar Cone	45	0	11

Icecream & Frozen Yogurt (Cont)

Baskin-Robbins: See Page 190 (Fast-Foods)

Brands	C	F	Cb
Alta Dena: *Per 1/2 Cup*			
Golden Honey Vanilla	160	10	17
Honey Chocolate	160	9	19
Atkins: *Per 1/2 Cup*			
Endulge, average all flavors	130	11	6
Baskin-Robbins: *See Page 190 (Fast-Foods)*			
Ben & Jerry's: *Per 1/2 Cup*			
Butter Pecan	290	21	20
Cherry Garcia; Vanilla	250	15	26
Chocolate For A Change	270	17	36
Chocolate Fudge Brownie	280	14	33
Choc. Chip Cookie Dough	280	16	33
Chubby Hubby	330	21	32
Chunky Monkey; Coffee Heath	310	19	30
Coffee For A Change	240	15	21
Concession Obsession	310	19	32
Everything But The . . .	320	19	30
Fudge Central; Van. Heath Bar, avg.	300	18	31
Half Baked	280	14	34
Honey, I'm Home!	260	15	29
Karamel Sutra	290	15	33
Makin' Whoopie Pie	270	14	33
Mint Chocolate Cookie	270	16	26
New York Super Fudge Chunk	310	20	30
Nutty Waffle Cone	310	19	31
Oatmeal; One Sweet Whirled	280	16	32
One Sweet Whirled	280	15	33
Peanut Butter Cup	380	26	29
Peanut Butter Me Up	330	21	28
Phish Food	280	13	38
Pistachio Pistachio	280	19	21
S'mores	260	12	34
The Full Vermonty	260	16	27
Triple Caramel Chunk	290	17	32
Uncanny Cashew	290	19	27
Vanilla For A Change	240	16	21
Vanilla Caramel Fudge	280	16	32
World's Best Chocolate	280	17	27
World's Best Vanilla	250	16	21
Frozen Yogurt: *Per 1/2 Cup*			
Cherry Garcia Yogurt	170	3	32
Choc. Fudge Brownie Yogurt	190	3	36
Half Baked Yogurt	210	3.5	39
Phish Food Yogurt	230	5	42
Sorbet: Average all flavors	120	0	30
Bars/Pops: *See Page 36*			

Blue Bunny	C	F	Cb
Fat Free, No Added Sugar: *Per 2.5 oz*			
Brownie Sundae; Burgundy Cherry	105	0	23
Caramel Toffee Crunch	110	0	24
Average other flavors	90	0	20
Reduced Fat, No Added Sugar: *Per Serving*			
Banana Split; Butter Pecan	135	6	16
Cherry Vanilla; Double Strawb.	125	4	18
Exquisite Mint; Tin Roof	145	6	20
Neopolitan; Vanilla	120	5	16
Rocky Road; Turtle Sundae	155	7	20
Frozen Yogurt, 6 fl.oz	75	0	13
Bars/Pops: *See Page 37, 38*			
Bon Bon's			
Vanilla w. choc. coating, 20 pces	200	14	17
8 pieces	330	23	27
Bresler's: *Per 1/2 Cup*			
All Flavors Icecream: average	230	12	23
Royal Cremes, average	260	16	24
Royal Lites, average	220	0	49
Breyers: *Per 1/2 Cup*			
Fat Free: Average	90	0	2
Lactose-Free: Vanilla	130	7	14
Light: Average	130	4.5	0
All Natural: Banana Fudge Chunk	170	9	21
Butter Pecan	170	11	14
Cherry Van.; Choc.; Coffee, avg.	150	8	16
Choc. Chip; Mint Choc. Chip	165	10	17
Cookies 'n Cream	165	9	18
Dulce de Leche	155	7	21
Extra Creamy Chocolate/Vanilla	160	8	19
French Vanilla	160	10	15
Mocha Almond Fudge	180	10	20
Peach; Strawberry	130	6	18
Peanut Butter & Fudge	180	10	17
Vanilla; Van./Choc./Strawberry	150	8	16
Wild Berry Swirl	145	8	16
Other varieties, average	160	8	18
Light: Average all flav., 1/2 cup	120	4	18
Parlor Pints: Chips Ahoy	160	8	18
Creasicle	130	5	20
Heath English Toffee; Reese's	180	9	22
Hershey's; Almond Joy, avg.	170	8	21
Klondike Icecream Sandwich	160	7	21
Mint w. Oreo; Oreo, avg.	165	8	20
Sponge Bob Squarepants	160	7	21

Brands (Cont)   **C** **F** **Cb**

Breyers (Cont): *Per 1/2 Cup*

	C	F	Cb
Homemade: Double Choc Fudge	180	9	23
Neopolitan	150	8	17
Vienetta: All flavors, avg., 1 slice	190	11	19
Frozen Yogurt: Average, 1/2 cup	140	4.5	22
No Sugar Added	105	4.5	13

Carvel Icecream ~ See Page 195

Colombo: *Per 1/2 Cup*

	C	F	Cb
Frozen, Soft Serve: Nonfat var.	100	0	22
Slender Sensations varieties	60	0	11
Lowfat: Old Worlde; Cookies	120	2.5	20
Other varieties, avg.	95	0	21
Sorbet: Vanilla	140	0	29
Other flavors	95	0	24

CremaLita (Soft Serve)

Calories will vary with density (air in product) and serving size.
Best to weigh product and calculate on 25 cals per 1 oz weight.

	C	F	Cb
Vanilla: Small (4 fl.oz cup),			
If 2 1/2 oz weight	60	0	14
If 4 oz weight*	100	0.5	23
If 6 oz weight*	150	1	35
(*) Most common weights			
Medium (8 fl.oz cup), 11 oz wt	275	1.5	63
Chocolate: Small, 6 oz weight	160	1	36

Dairy Queen/Brazier ~ See Page 199

Dannon Frozen Yogurt: *Per 1/2 Cup (4 fl.oz)*

	C	F	Cb
Light Soft, all flavors, average	90	1	21
Light 'N Crunchy, all flavors, aver.	110	1	23
Pure Indulgence, all flavors, aver.	150	3	25

Dolewhip (Soft Serve): *Per 1/2 Cup (4 fl.oz)*

	C	F	Cb
Chocolate; Vanilla	100	3	18
Fruit flavors, average	80	0.5	16

Dreyers: *Per 1/2 Cup*

	C	F	Cb
Starburst Sherbet, avg. all flav.	150	2.5	30
Whole Fruit Sorbet: Coconut	140	3	28
Other varieties, average	145	0	35
Fat Free Icecream: Avg. all flav.	110	0	25
Grand Icecream: Cracker Jack	170	9	20
Dexter's Lab.; French Van. Pie	160	7	21
Scooby Doo!	160	8	16
Ultimate Caramel Cup	170	8	22
Grand Light Icecream: Vanilla	100	3	15
Mocha Almond Fudge	120	5	16
Average other flavors	115	4	17

Dreyers (Cont): *Per 1/2 Cup*

	C	F	Cb
Dreamery: Banana Boogie	290	17	27
Black Raspberry Avalanche	270	16	27
Caramel Toffee Bar Heaven	290	16	32
Cashew Praline	280	16	30
Cherry Chip ba da Bing	280	15	33
Chocolate Almond Bar	300	17	32
Choc Peanut Butter Chunk	310	18	29
Cool Mint	300	17	32
Deep Dish Apple Pie	280	15	34
Dulce de Leche, Caramel	270	14	32
Grandma's Cookie Dough	300	17	32
New York Strawb. Cheesecake	260	15	27
Nothing But Chocolate	280	14	34
Strawberry Fields	220	12	26
Tiramisu	260	13	31
Ultimate Mudslide	260	15	28
Homemade: Chocolate	150	7	19
Grovestand Peach	120	5	17
Mint Chocolate Chunk	160	8	18
Old Fashion Butter Pecan	150	9	15
Strawberries and Cream	130	6	17
Vanilla	140	7	15
Vanilla Custard	150	8	17
Candy Bar: Twix; Milky Way, 1/2 c.	170	8	21
Frozen Yogurt: Vanilla	100	2.5	19
Other flavors, avg., 1/2 cup	120	4	19
Fat Free, average all flavors	90	0	20

Edys: *Per 1/2 Cup*

	C	F	Cb
Banana Split; Choc. Fudge Mousse	160	8	19
Cherry Choc; Van./Choc.; Espresso	150	8	17
Choc. Fudge Sundae; Dble Fudge	170	9	19
Ice Cream Sandwich	150	7	19
Grand Light: Vanilla	100	3	15
Butter Pecan; Choc. Almond	120	5	16
Chiquita 'N Chocolate	110	5	13
Choc. Fudge Mousse	110	3	17
Cookie Dough; P'nut Butter Cups	130	5	18
Cookies 'n Cream; Rocky Road	120	4	18
French Silk	130	4.5	19
Fat Free: Average all flavors	115	0	25

Eskimo Pie: *Per 1/2 Cup*

	C	F	Cb
Reduced Fat: Butter Pecan	140	7	16
Choc. Marshmallow	130	4	23
Neopolitan; Vanilla	110	4	18
Fudge Ripple	120	4	19

Bars: See Page 37

Icecream & Frozen Yogurt (Cont)

Brands (Cont) **C** **F** **Cb**

Friendly's
	C	F	Cb
Icecream: Chocolate Almd Chip	170	10	18
Forbidden Chocolate	150	9	14
Fudge Nut Brownie	200	11	23
Vanilla Choc. Strawb.; Vanilla	150	8	16
Vienna Mocha Chunk	180	11	19
Frozen Yogurt: Per 1/2 Cup			
Regular flavors, average	150	4	24
Lowfat flavors, average	120	3	20
Sundaes: Per 3 Scoops			
Apple Pie	700	30	98
Candy Shop Satisfaction Snickers	810	35	100
Dble Deluxe Caramel Fudge Blast	700	30	98
Cyclones: Per 12 fl.oz			
Fudge Brownie	790	25	127
Reese's Peanut Cup	880	43	100

	C	F	Cb
Frostline (Soft Serve): Chocolate	90	2	20
Vanilla, 1/2 cup	90	3	18

Frusen Gladje: Per 1/2 Cup
	C	F	Cb
Butter Pecan	280	21	16
Chocolate	240	17	17
Chocolate Choc. Chip	270	18	21
Mocha Chip; Praline & Cream	280	18	22
Strawberry	230	15	20
Swiss Choc. Candy Almond	270	19	18
Vanilla	230	17	16
Vanilla Swiss Almond	270	19	18

Gelatida: Per 1/2 Cup
	C	F	Cb
Almond Biscotti	150	3	26
Amaretto Chocolate	150	4.5	23
Average other flavors	130	2	22

Godiva: Per 1/2 Cup
	C	F	Cb
Belgian Dark Chocolate	280	17	26
Choc Hazelnut Truffle	350	23	31
Choc Raspberry Truffle	290	16	32
Chocolate Cheesecake	310	17	36
Chocolate w. Chocolate Hearts	330	20	32
Classic Milk Chocolate	290	18	28
Pecan Caramel Truffle	320	19	32
Vanilla Caramel Pecan	290	16	33
Vanilla w. Choc. Caramel Hearts	310	18	32
White Choc. Raspberry	260	12	32

Good Humor: Per 1/2 Cup
	C	F	Cb
Light: Coffee	110	3	18
Choc. Chip, Toffee Bar Crunch	130	4	20
Cookies n' Crm; Praline Alm. Crnch	130	3	21
Vanilla, Vanilla Choc. Strawb.	110	3	19

Haagen-Dazs
C **F** **Cb**
Icecream, Sorbet, Frozen Yogurt: *See Pg 209*
Bars: *See Page 37*

Healthy Choice: Per 1/2 Cup
	C	F	Cb
Brownie Bliss	125	2	25
Cookies 'N Cream	130	2	24
Double Karma; Happy Together	140	2	29
Jumpin' Java	130	2	25
Peanut Butter Cup	110	2	19
Praline & Caramel; Rocky Road	130	2	25
Vanilla; Mint Choc Chip	100	2	18
Other flavors, average	120	2	18
Lowfat, No Sugar Added: Vanilla	90	2	18
Coffee Almond Fudge	110	2	20
Chocolate Fudge Brownie	115	2	20
Mint Chocolate Chip	100	2	18

Hood: Per 1/2 Cup
	C	F	Cb
Regular Icecream: Avg. all flavors	150	8	17
Light Icecream: Creamy Vanilla	110	3.5	18
Raspb. Swirl; Heavenly Hash, avg	130	3.5	22
Other flavors, average	140	5	22
No Sugar Added, Lowfat Icecream:			
Vanilla Dream; Classic Trio	100	2.5	14
Choc Frenzy; Mocha Madness, avg	120	2.5	19
Chocolate Chip	120	4	16
Fat Free Icecream: Avg. all flavors	100	0	23
Dble Brownie; Heavenly Mash	120	0	27
Frozen Yogurt: Reg., avg. all flav.	150	8	17
Nonfat: Strawb., Old Fashion. Van.	110	0	24
Other flavors, average	120	0	27
Icecream Bars: *See Page 37*			

I Can't Believe It's Yogurt: *See Page 211*

Jerseymaid (Vons): Per 1/2 Cup
	C	F	Cb
After Dinner Mint; Cookies & Crm	170	9	19
Choc Chip; Mint Choc Chip	160	9	17
Heavenly Hash; Nut Chunky Choc.	170	8	22
Mocha Almd Fudge; Rocky Road	160	7	20
Neopolitan; Vanilla	140	7	16
Strawberry	140	6	18

Brands (Cont)

	C	F	Cb
Kilwin's: Per 1/2 Cup			
Butter Pecan	190	13	16
Butter Pecan Yogurt	130	6	17
Chocolate	170	10	17
Average other flavors	190	10	20
Fat Free Icecream, avg. all flavors	100	0	23
Topping: Caramel	160	4.5	31
Fudge	110	6	28
Luigi's Real Italian Ice			
Cherry/Lemon Cup, avg., 6 fl.oz	110	0	27
Oberweis Dairy			
Icecream: Per 1/2 Cup			
Chocolate; Marshmallow	220	10	29
Peach; Strawberry	190	10	24
Udderly Truffles; Peanut Butter	295	20	26
Average other flavors	240	15	23
Low Fat Icecream, average	140	2.5	28
Sugar Free Icecream, 1/2 cup	205	15	15
Icecream Cakes: Per Slice			
Black Forest, 4.2 oz	325	17	40
Celebration, 4 oz	370	21	42
Strawberry Torte 6", 3.2 oz	285	15	35
Icecream Pies: Per Slice			
Brownie Ala Mode, 4.4 oz	415	20	55
Key Lime; Moolata Mocha	360	20	41
Peppermint, 3.9 oz	375	17	51
Summer Dream; Turtle	445	25	51
Rice Dream (Non Dairy): Per 1/2 Cup			
Vanilla Carob/Choc/Cappuccino	150	6	23
Other varieties	170	8	26
Sealtest: Per 1/2 Cup			
Butter Pecan	160	9	16
Choc. Chip Cookie Dough	160	8	20
Fudge Royal; Heavenly Hash	150	7	20
Vanilla/Choc. Strawberry	140	7	16
Snackwell's: Per 1/2 Cup			
Brownie; Rocky Road; Praline	140	2	28
Vanilla	100	2	18
Soy Delicious (Organic): Per 1/2 Cup			
Quarts: Twisted Vanilla Orange	120	2	24
Choc Peanut Butter	150	5	23
Mocha Fudge	150	3.5	27
Other flavors, avg	140	4	23
Pints: Per 1/2 Cup			
Almond Pecan	160	5	24
Choc Almond/P'Nut Butter	150	5	24
Other flavors, average	130	3	25

	C	F	Cb
Soy Dream (Non-Dairy): Per 1/2 Cup			
Butter Pecan	160	10	17
Chocolate Fudge Brownie	150	8	20
Mint Chocolate Chip	150	9	19
Average other flavors	140	6	20
Starbucks: Per 1/2 Cup			
Caramel Cappuccino	240	12	30
Classic Coffee; Italian Roast	230	12	26
Coffee Almond Fudge; Java Chip	250	13	29
Mud Pie	240	11	32
White Chocolate Latte	280	15	31
Lowfat: Mocha Mambo; Latte	170	3	30
Bars: See Page 38			
Stonyfield Farm (Organic): Per 1/2 Cup			
Icecream: Chocolate	265	18	22
Decaf Coffee; Vanilla, avg	260	18	21
Other flavors, average	260	16	26
Frozen Yogurt: Nonfat Choc.; Raspb.	100	0	21
Nonfat Vanilla; Decaf Coffee	90	0	19
Nonfat Vanilla Fudge Swirl	110	0	23
Lowfat: Creme Caramel	120	1.5	23
Choc Mint; Mocha Almond	130	3	22
Sweet Nothings (Non-Dairy/Fat Free)			
Average all flavors, 1/2 cup, 3 oz	120	0	28
TCBY: Per 1/2 Cup			
Frozen Yogurt: Nonfat, all flavors	110	0	23
96% Fat Free, all flavors	135	3	23
No Sugar Added, all flavors	95	0	20
Hand-Dipped Icecrm: Butter Pecan	260	20	17
Chewy Chocolate Fudge	270	16	27
Chocolate Chocolate; Pralines	215	13	21
Choc. Chunk Cookie Dough	210	14	18
Lemon Meringue Pie	235	12	29
Oatmeal Raisin	220	12	25
Vanilla Bean	195	13	17
Very Berry Strawberry	185	11	19
White Macadamia; Mint Choc.	250	16	23
Sorbet, 1/2 Cup	95	0	24
Tasti D-Lite (Soft Serve)			

Tasti D-Lite (Soft Serve)
Calories will vary with density (air in product) and serving size.
Best to weigh product and calculate on 25 cals per 1 oz weight.

	C	F	Cb
Vanilla: Small (4 fl.oz cup), 6 oz wt	180	4	35
Medium (8 fl.oz cup), 11 oz wt	330	7	64
Tofutti Non-Dairy Dessert: Per 1/2 Cup			
Low Fat Supreme: Average	110	2	25
Too Toos: Vanilla S'wich	215	10	28
Van. Choc. Swirl/Chip S'wich	230	11	30

Icecream Bars & Pops

Brands (Cont)	**C**	**F**	**Cb**
Premium: Vanilla	190	11	20
Better Pecan; Alm. Bark	220	13	22
Choc. Cookie Crunch	210	11	26
Chocolate Supreme	180	11	18
Van. Fudge; Wildberry	190	9	24
Cutie Pies: Average, 67g bar	250	19	18
Teddy Fudge: 52g bar	70	1	19
Turkey Hill: *Per 1/2 Cup*			
Black Cherry	140	7	18
Butter Pecan	170	11	16
Choco. Mint Chip, Cookies 'n Crm	160	10	17
Neapolitan, Vanilla & Choc.	150	8	18
Rocky Road	170	8	23
Vanilla, Vanilla Bean	140	8	16
Lite: Choco Mint Chip	140	5	19
Cookies 'n Cream	130	5	21
Vanilla & Choc., Van. Bean	110	3	18
Weight Watchers: *Per 1/2 Cup*			
Cookie Dough Craze	140	3.5	24
Oh! So Very Vanilla	120	2.5	20
Positively Praline Crunch	140	3	25
Reckless Rocky Road	140	3	23
Triple Chocolate Tornado	150	3.5	26
Bars: Smart Ones, See Page 38			
WholeSoy Glace: *Per 1/2 Cup (70g)*			
Mocha Fudge	130	4	21
Swiss Chocolate	180	9	21
Strawberry	150	6	20
Vanilla Bean	190	9	25

Bars & Pops			
Per Bar/Serving			
Baby Ruth (Nestlé)	180	12	15
Baskin Robbins: Tiny Toons	140	17	20
Cappuccino Blast, average	120	4	20
Sundae Bar, Pralines 'n Cream	280	17	28
Ben & Jerry's: One Sweet Whirled	260	16	27
Cherry Garcia: Icecream Bar	240	16	23
Yogurt Bar	250	11	35
Chocolate Fudge Brownie	230	11	28
Cookie Dough: 89ml Bar	330	19	36
110ml Bar	410	24	45
Phish Stick: 89ml Bar	260	16	29
110ml Bar	290	17	33
Vanilla Heath Crunch	320	21	32
Big Bear: See Klondike			
Big Ed's Super Saucer, 10 fl.oz	420	28	32
Borden: Sundae Cone	210	10	27
Twin Pops	60	0	14

Per Bar/Serving	**C**	**F**	**Cb**
Bon Bons (Nestlé): Milk Choc., (8)	330	23	27
Dark Chocolate, 8 pces	310	21	26
Bounty: all varieties	70	5	7
Butterfinger Bar, 2.5 oz	190	13	16
Breyers: Natural Strawb. Fruit Jce	120	0	30
Fruit Bars: All Natural, 1.75 fl. oz	45	0	11
No Sugar Added, 1.75 fl. oz	20	0	5
Soft Caramel Magnum Bar	375	23	38
Soft Frozen Lemonade Cup	295	0	74
Soft Frozen Strawberry Cup	265	0	66
Carnation: Orange Sherbet, 3 oz	90	1	19
Icecream Cup: Choc., 3 fl.oz	140	8	16
Strawb., Vanilla, 3 fl.oz	100	6	12
Choc./Vanilla Malt, 12 oz	270	6	48
Sundae Cup, all types, 5 fl.oz	210	9	30
Chipwich Jr: Choc. Chip S'wich	240	10	35
Chiquita: Swirls, all flavors	80	3	12
Cool Creations: Mini Sandwich	110	5	14
Cookies & Cream Sandwich	240	11	34
Pops, all types, 2 oz	60	0	14
Mickey Mouse: 2.5 oz Bar	120	8	10
Creamsicle: Sugar-free pops	25	0	15
Orange, 2.8 fl.oz	110	3	20
Crunch (Nestlé): King, 4 oz	270	19	21
Reduced Fat, 2.5 oz	130	7	14
Regular Icecream Bar, 3 oz	200	14	16
Crystal Light: Cool 'n Creamy	50	2	7
Dole Bars: Coconut, 4 oz	210	7	33
Fruit Juice, reg., 1.75 oz	45	0	11
No Added Sugar, 1.75 oz	25	0	6
Fruit 'n Juice: Small, 2.5 oz	70	0	16
Pine-Coconut, 4 oz	150	4	27
Other flavors, 4 oz	120	0	28
Dove Bar: Almond	340	22	30
Bite Size, 5 pces, average	350	22	36
Caramel Pecan	350	35	35
Mocha Cashew; Van. Milk Choc.	260	17	25
Peppermint	390	17	31
Vanilla Dark Choc; Cookie	340	21	35
Single Vanilla Dark	200	12	24
Dreyers: Icecream Bars, average	250	17	22
Fruit Bars, 3 fl.oz	90	9	23
Smoothie Bars, average	95	0	21
Sundae Bar, 4 fl.oz	240	11	31
Whole Fruit Bars, 1.75 fl.oz	60	0	16
Drumstick (Nestlé): Chocolate	320	17	36
Choc. Dipped	320	16	40
Original Vanilla	340	19	35
Vanilla Caramel/Fudge	360	20	39

Per Bar/Serving	C	F	Cb
Eskimo Pie: Arctic Madness, 2.5 oz	230	15	23
Bars: Milk/Dark Choc, 50g	160	11	15
Fudge Bar, 55g	60	1	11
Reduced Fat varieties	120	8	13
Crispy Bar, 47g	130	8	13
Pecan, 51g	190	15	12
Big Bar, 99g	300	20	26
Icecream Sandwich, 65 g	160	4	27
Cones, 74g	210	12	24
No Sugar Added: Bar, 49g	120	8	13
Pudding Bar, 59g	90	1.5	13
Flintstones: Push Up Sherbet	100	2	20
Push Up Pebbles, 2.75 oz	120	6	15
Cool Cream, 2.75 oz	90	2	18
Frosty Dreams (Nestlé)	100	2	19
Frosty Pops (Nestlé)	40	0	11
Froz-Fruit: Cherry	60	0	15
Strawberry	80	0	20
Fruit A Freeze: Coconut	130	5	20
Lime	65	0	16
Banana; Strawberry	90	1.5	19
Dark Choc-Dipped Strawberry	90	3.5	14
Fudge Bar (Nestlé)	110	1	23
Fudgesicle: Fudge Bar (1)	45	0.5	9
Fat Free (1)	60	0	13
Fudgetastics: Sticks Sundae	220	15	37
Godiva: Pecan Caramel Bar	380	23	39
Good Humor: Bubble Play	105	0	26
Candy Center Crunch	315	23	24
Chocolate Eclair	225	11	30
Great White	70	0	18
Hyper Stripe	80	0	19
Number 1	200	11	21
Premium Vanilla	260	17	23
Reese's Peanut Butter Cup	315	21	27
Strawb. Shortcake; Tstd Almd	230	10	35
Cones: Giant King	395	21	44
King	255	13	30
Premium Sundae	265	15	29
Strawberry Shortcake	235	10	34
Sundae Twist	165	2.5	29
Sandwiches: Premium Vanilla	190	7	29
Giant Mississippi Mud	300	14	37
Giant Neapolitan/Vanilla	260	10	37
Premium Cookie	295	13	41
Haagen-Dazs: Vanilla & Almonds	320	12	22
Caramel & Almond Crunch	310	21	27
Caramel Pecan Nut Cluster	420	16	31
Chocolate & Dark Chocolate	290	20	23
Chocolate Fudge & Almonds	210	23	25

Per Bar/Serving	C	F	Cb
Haagen-Dazs (Cont):			
Chocolate Sorbet Bar	80	0	20
Coffee & Almd; Cookies & Crm	310	12	23
Dulce De Leche (Caramel)	300	19	28
Raspb. Sorbet & Van. Yogurt	90	0	21
Tres Leches; Raspb. Cheesecake	310	22	24
Vanilla Caramel & Pecans	360	26	27
Vanilla & Dark Chocolate	280	20	22
Vanilla & Milk Chocolate	280	20	20
Health Smart (Blue Bunny), avg.	80	0	18
Healthy Choice: Fudge Bar	75	1	13
Caramel Swirl Sandwich	145	3	27
Fudge Swirl Sandwich	145	3	27
Strawberry & Cream	80	1.5	13
Vanilla Sandwich	130	3	24
Hood: Chocolate Eclair, 1 bar	150	10	14
Cooler Cup, 2.1 oz	80	1	18
Crispy Bar	180	13	15
Fabulous Fudgies, 1 bar	100	3	19
Fabulous Fudge P'nut Butter	110	4	17
Fudge Bar	100	1	21
Hendrie's Cherry Choc. Dips	120	9	11
Hoodsie Cup Van./Choc.	100	5	12
Orange Cream Bar	90	2	18
Rockets, each	120	5	18
Vanilla Bar	160	12	11
Icecream Sandwich (Nestle)	170	6	26
Jell-O: Pop Bars	31	0	7
Jigglers, all varieties, 6 oz	215	1.5	50
Pudding Bars	80	2	13
Klondike: Choco Taco, 4 fl.oz	300	16	35
Dark Chocolate Crunch, 2.5 fl.oz	140	8	15
Heath, 5 fl.oz	295	20	26
Krunch, 5 fl.oz	280	19	25
Mini's Vanilla Icecream, 3 fl.oz	170	11	15
Movie Bites, 4.5 fl.oz	320	22	26
No Sugar Added Red. Fat, 4 fl.oz	180	9	21
Oreo, 3 fl.oz	160	10	17
Original, 5 fl.oz	280	19	24
Planters Caramel & Peanut	310	20	28
Reese's Peanut Butter, 2.9 fl.oz	220	15	20
Slim-a-Bear, 5 fl.oz	270	15	31
Cones: Big Bear Sundae Cone	315	17	36
Big Bear Vanilla Sundae Cone	300	17	31
Oreo Cone	250	12	32
Cup, Sundae, 6 fl.oz	280	17	26
Sandwich: Big Bear	190	7	28
Giant Cookie w. Hershey's	470	20	66
w. Oreo Cookies	230	9	34

Icecream Bars & Pops (Cont)

Per Bar/Serving	C	F	Cb
Kool-Aid Pops	40	0	10
Krispy Frostick	150	10	13
Juice Flavored Sticks	50	0	13
M&Ms Cookie Icecream S'wich	220	11	29
Mars Almond Bar	210	14	20
Matterhorn Cone, 10 fl.oz	510	38	19
Milky Way: Choc, Reduced Fat	140	7	19
Caramel Swirl, 1 bar	180	10	21
Snack Bar, Vanilla/Chocolate	70	4	9
Minute Maid Fruit Juice Pops	60	0	15
Nestlé Icecreamers: Push Up Pop	90	1.5	19
Crunch: 1.7 oz bar	140	8	15
Multipack, 2.2 oz bar	230	16	18
Shock Tarts, 1 pop	45	0	11
Tiger Tails, 1 pop	60	0	15
Drumstick: S'Mores	290	16	33
Strawberry Cheesecake	260	12	34
Original	280	15	33
Oreo: Big Stuf, 1 sandwich	240	10	33
Cookies n' Cream, 1 bar, 59g	180	12	18
Pathmark: Vanilla w. choc. coat.	150	10	14
Polar Bar: Vanilla w. choc. coat.	240	18	15
Choc. Chip Cookie Dough	450	28	48
Pops (water/juice), average	60	0	14
Popsicles: Big Stick Ice Pops	70	0	17
Creamsicle Pop	70	2	13
Crispy Cones, 2.5 fl.oz	150	7	20
Fudgesicle Fudge Pop	90	1.5	16
Firecracker Super Hero; Fruit Shot	40	0	10
Minis Icecream Pop	190	13	18
Rainbow Floats, 1.75 fl.oz	60	1.5	11
Sponge Bob Squarepants Pop Up	90	1.5	17
Scribblers Icecream: 2 pces	130	7	15
Juice Pops, 2 pces	60	0	16
Ice Pops: 1 pce	45	0	11
Sugar-Free, 1 pce, 1.9 oz	15	0	3
Reese's: Peanut Butter Icecream	160	11	22
Rice Dream: Pies, all flavors	320	18	40
Bars: Strawberry	250	13	31
Chocolate, Vanilla	270	15	32
Choc/Vanilla Nutty	270	18	23
Safeway Select Coffee Almd Bar	270	17	26
Silhouette *(The Skinny Cow)*			
Cookies 'N Cream Bar	120	1.5	23
Fat Free Fudge Bar	90	0	19
Sandwich, Lowfat, avg. all flav.	140	2.5	23
Sundae Cups: Chocolate	130	1	29
Vanilla Strawberry	120	0	27
Van. w. Choc. Fudge Topping	130	0.5	29

	C	F	Cb
Slim-Fast: Fudge Bar	110	1.5	22
Icecream Sandwich: Vanilla	130	1	27
Chocolate	130	1.5	27
Smart Ones *(Weight Watchers):*			
Chocolate Mousse	40	1	9
Chocolate Treat	100	0.5	20
English Toffee Crunch	110	6	12
Giant Fudge Bar, 76g	80	0	20
Mocha Java	80	1.5	20
Orange Vanilla Treat	40	0.5	10
Vanilla Lowfat Sandwich	150	3	28
Snackwell: Icecream Sandwich	90	1.5	18
Yogurt Bars, 1 bar, 80g	120	2	22
Snickers: Icecream Bar	180	11	18
Pralines n' Creme	220	13	22
Icecream Bar (The Big One)	250	15	25
Snack, 4 bars	390	25	38
Soy Delicious: Big Buddy	240	8	42
s/w Li'l Buddy, Vanilla	265	14	32
Mocha/Mint Mania (choc coated)	265	14	32
Mint Choc Chips	260	10	41
Bars: Creamy Fudge	140	4	25
Creamy Vanilla	250	13	31
Vanilla & Almond	300	17	32
Soy Dream *(Non-Dairy):*			
Dreamwich Vanilla	130	6	15
Heavenly Pies: Mocha; Vanilla	290	14	40
Lil' Dreamers: Choc; Vanilla	60	3	7
Rocket Bars: Choc; Vanilla	220	12	29
Starbuck's Frappuccino Bars, avg.	130	2	25
Starburst: Juice Bars	20	0	5
Super Sundae Bar, 86g	310	20	26
Sweet Freedom *(Blue Bunny)*			
Fudge Lites, 1.75 fl. oz	45	0	9
Citrus/Fruit Ice Lites, 1.75 fl. oz	25	0	6
Icecream/Krunch Lites, 1.4 oz	105	6	11
Icecream Sandwiches, avg.	160	2	32
Sugar Free Bomb Pops, 2 fl. oz	30	0	8
Sugar Free Pops, 1.9 oz	15	0	4
Vanilla Sundae Cone, 3 oz	255	13	30
3 Musketeers: 2 fl.oz bars	170	10	21
Snack Bar, regular	60	4	16
Tandem *(Nestlé)* Sandwich	380	21	39
Twin Pop *(Nestlé)*	60	0	14
Twix Bar	180	10	19
Vitari Soft Serve, 4 fl.oz, average	80	0	20
Welch's: Fruit Juice Bars, 92g	80	0	19
Tropical Coolers, 92 bar	45	0	11
No Sugar Added, 1 bar	25	0	6
Fruit Smoothie, 1 ctn	240	0	59

Cream & Creamers

Quick Guide

Cream | C | F | Cb

Average All Brands

	C	F	Cb
Half & Half Cream: 1 Tbsp, 0.5 oz	20	2	0.5
2 Tbsp, 1 oz	40	4	1
Light, coffee/table (20% fat): 1 T.	30	3	0.5
2 Tbsp, 1 oz	60	6	1
Medium (25% fat), 2 Tbsp, 1 oz	40	4	0.5

Sour Cream:

	C	F	Cb
Regular, 1 Tbsp, 0.5 oz	30	3	0.5
1 cup, 8 oz	490	48	8
Lowfat/Light, 1 Tbsp, 0.5 oz	20	2	1.5
2 Tbsp, 1 oz	40	2.5	2
Half & Half, 1 Tbsp, 0.5 oz	20	2.5	0.5
Fat Free, 2 Tbsp, 1 oz	20	0	3
Fat Free: (HeluvaGood), 2 Tbsp	20	0	6
(Kroger), 2 Tbsp, 1 oz	25	0	5
(Naturally Yours; Oak Farm), 2 T.	20	0	3
(Knudsen), 2 Tbsp, 1 oz	35	0	6

Sour Cream Substitute:

	C	F	Cb
(Albertson's/ IMO), 2 T., 1 oz	60	5	2
(Tofutti) Sour Supreme, 1 oz	50	5	1

Whipping Cream:

Heavy (37% fat):

	C	F	Cb
1 Tbsp fluid/2 Tbsp whipped	50	5	1
1/4 cup whipped	100	11	2
1/2 cup fluid/1 cup whipped	400	44	8

Light (30% fat):

	C	F	Cb
1 Tbsp fluid/2 Tbsp whipped	45	4,5	0.5
1/2 cup fluid/1 cup whipped	350	37	4

Coconut Cream/Milk

Coconut Cream (Canned),

	C	F	Cb
Plain/unsweetened, 2 Tbsp, 1 oz	70	6	4
1/2 cup, 4 oz	280	24	16
Sweetened: Coco Lopez, 1 oz	120	5	20
1/2 cup, 4 oz	480	20	80

Coconut Milk (Canned):

	C	F	Cb
Natural Value: Reg., 1/4 c., 2 fl.oz	90	9	1
Lite, 1/4 cup, 2 fl.oz	55	5	1
Thai Kitchen: Reg., 1/4 c., 2 fl.oz	125	7	3
Lite, 1/4 cup, 2 fl.oz	50	3	2
Premium, 2 fl.oz	125	12	3
Coconut Water (center), 1 cup	45	0.5	9

Whipped Toppings

Average All Brands

	C	F	Cb
Cream (Pressurized): 2 Tbsp	20	2	1
1/4 cup	45	4	2
1/2 cup	90	8	4
Cream Toppings: Jewel, Lite, 2 T.	20	1	2
Cool Whip: Extra Creamy, 2 T.	25	1.5	2
Lite, 2 Tbsp, 9g	20	1	2
Free, 2 Tbsp, 9g	15	0	3
Non Dairy, 2 Tbsp	22	2	2
Kraft: Whipped, 2 Tbsp	20	2	1
Real Cream, 2 Tbsp	20	2	1
Reddi-Wip: Original, 2 T., 8g	20	2	0
Original Light, 2 Tbsp	15	1	1
Non-Dairy, 2 Tbsp, 8g	20	1.5	2
Extra Creamy, 2 Tbsp, 8g	30	3	0.5
Fat Free, 2 Tbsp, 8g	10	0	2

Non-Dairy Coffee Creamers

Powder *Coffee-Mate/Cremora/N-Rich:*

	C	F	Cb
Regular, 1 tsp	20	2	1
1 heaping tsp	25	2	2
Fat Free, 1 tsp	10	0	2
Lite, 1 tsp	10	0.5	2
Flavors: 1 1/3 Tbsp	60	3	9
Fat Free: Average, 1 1/3 Tbsp	50	0	11

Liquid/Refrigerated: *Per Tablespoon*

Coffee-Mate Non-Dairy Creamer:

	C	F	Cb
Plain: Regular/Plain, 1 Tbsp	20	1	2
Fat Free, 1 Tbsp	10	0	2
Lite, 1 Tbsp	10	0.5	1
Flavors: All flavors, 1 Tbsp	40	2	5
Fat Free, all flavors, 1 Tbsp	25	0	5
Crème de la Soy (Westsoy):			
Original, 1 Tbsp	20	1.5	2
Amaretto; French Vanilla, 1 T.	25	1	4
Hood (Non Dairy), 1 Tbsp	25	0	5
International Delight: 1 Tbsp	35	1.5	6
Fat Free flavors, 1 Tbsp	30	0	7
Mocha Mix: Original, 1 Tbsp	20	1.5	1
Fat Free, 1 Tbsp	10	0	1
Lite, 1 Tbsp	10	0.5	1
Morningstar, 1 Tbsp	40	1.5	7
Rich's Coffee Rich: Regular, 1 T.	25	1	2
Light	15	0.5	0.5
Rich's Farm Rich: Regular, 1 Tbsp	20	1	2
Light/Fat Free	10	0	0.5
Silk (White Wave) Creamer, 1Tbsp	15	1	1
French Vanilla, 1 Tbsp	20	1	3

Fats, Spreads & Oils

Butter & Margarine

Average All Brands

	C	F	Cb
Regular: 1 tsp (5g)	35	4	0
1 Pat (5g)	35	4	0
1 Tbsp, approx. $^1/_2$ oz	100	11	0
2 Tbsp, 1 oz	205	23	0
1 Stick, $^1/_2$ cup, 4 oz	810	92	0
1 Pound, 2 cups, 16 oz	3240	368	0
Light (Regular) 40% Fat:			
1 tsp, 5g	17	2	0
1 Tbsp, $^1/_2$ oz	50	6	0
2 Tbsp, 1 oz	100	11	0
Whipped Butter (Regular):			
1 tsp (4 g)	27	3	0
1 Tbsp (10g)	70	7.5	0
1 Stick, $^1/_2$ cup, $2^2/_3$ oz	570	60	0
Whipped Light Butter 40% Fat:			
1 tsp, 5g	10	1	0
1 Tbsp, 9g	35	3.5	0
2 Tbsp, 18g	70	7	0
Unsalted: Same as Regular			

Clarified Butter

	C	F	Cb
100% Fat: 1 Tbsp, $^1/_2$ oz	130	15	0
2 Tbsp, 1 oz	260	30	0

Flavored Butter/Spread

Average All Brands

	C	F	Cb
Honey Butter (60% Fat):			
1 Tbsp, $^1/_2$ oz	90	7	4
Downey's, 1 Tbsp, $^1/_2$ oz	60	1	11
Garlic Butter (80% Fat):			
1 Tbsp, $^1/_2$ oz	100	11	0
Macadamia Butter *(Atkins)*, 1 T.	125	12	2.5
Sweet Cream Butter:			
Regular, 1 Tbsp	100	11	0
Stick (70% Fat), 1 Tbsp	90	10	0
Tub (60% Fat), 1 Tbsp	80	9	0

Other Spreads & Fats

	C	F	Cb
Copha, Dripping, Lard, Suet, Shortening:			
1 Tbsp, $^1/_2$ oz	120	13	0
Chicken, Duck, Goose Fat:			
1 Tbsp, $^1/_2$ oz	115	13	0

Light & Reduced Fat Spreads

Per 1 Tbsp, $^1/_2$ oz (Unless Stated)

	C	F	Cb
Benecol: Spread, 1 Tbsp, 14g	80	9	0
Light, Spread, 1 Tbsp, 14g	45	5	0
Blue Bonnet Homestyle (48% Veg Oil)	60	7	0
Breakstone's Whipped Butter	60	7	0
Brummel & Brown: Spread	45	5	0
Chiffon: Whipped, 1 Tbsp	70	7	0
Country Crock (Shedd's): Regular	60	7	0
Light; Calcium & Vitamins	50	5	0
Country's Delight (70% Veg.)	90	10	0
Country Morning: Light	50	6	0
Downey's Honey Butter	60	1	0
Dutch Farms: 52% Veg. Spread	70	7	0
Fleischmann's: Soft Spread	80	9	0
Original	80	9	0
Fat Free Spread	5	0	0
'I Can't Believe It's Not Butter': Reg.	90	10	0
Light; Sweet Cream	50	6	0
Imperial: Diet, 1 Tbsp	50	6	0
Jewel: Soft Spread	60	7	0
Unbelievably Butter	90	9	0
Kraft: 'Touch of Butter' (bowl)	50	6	0
Land O'Lakes: Fresh Buttery Taste	80	8	0
Honey Butter	90	7	4
Light Butter Whipped	35	3.5	0
Light Butter	50	6	0
Mazola: Diet	50	6	0
Mother's; Mrs Filbert's, 1 Tbsp	70	8	0
Miracle: Soft	60	7	0
Stick	70	7	0
Nucoa: HeartBeat Margarine	25	3	0
Olivio: Vegetable Spread	80	8	0
Parkay: Squeeze, 1 Tbsp	80	9	0
Stick, $^1/_3$ Less Fat	70	7	0
Tub, 1 Tbsp	60	7	0
Tub, Light/Soft Diet	50	6	0
Whipped	70	7	0
Promise: Regular	90	10	0
Extra Light	50	6	0
Buttery Light	45	5	0
Ultra, w. Canola Oil	35	4	0
Smart Balance: Regular, 1 Tbsp	80	9	0
Light, 1 Tbsp	45	5	0
Smart Beat: Fat Free	10	0	3
Take Control: Regular Spread	80	8	0
Light Spread	45	5	0
Weight Watcher's: Light, all types	45	4	2

Fats, Spreads & Oils

Butter Substitutes

	C	F	Cb
Bake It Perfect (Fat Free Spread), 1 T.	5	0	0
Best O'Butter, 1/2 tsp	4	0	0
Butter Buds, 1 serving, 1/2 tsp	4	0	0
Butterlike Saute Butter, 1 Tbsp	35	2	0
Butter Sprinkles (Watkins), 1 tsp	5	0	0
Earth Balance, Non GMO, 1 tsp	35	3.5	0
Molly McButter, 1/2 tsp	5	0	0
Mrs Bateman's Baking Butter, 1 T.	35	1	0
Natural Touch Soy, 1 Tbsp.	85	5.5	5

Spreads Comparison

Mayonnaise: Regular, 1 Tbsp	100	11	0
Light, average, 1 Tbsp	50	5	1
Fat Free, 1 T.	10	0	3
Miracle Whip (Kraft):			
Regular, 1 Tbsp	70	7	2
Light, 1 Tbsp	40	3	3
Free, 1 Tbsp	15	0	3
SmartBeat Dressing: 1 Tbsp	10	0	3
Extra Listings for Mayonnaise & Dressings			
~ See Page 95 ~			
Avocado, mashed, 1 Tbsp	25	2.5	2
Peanut Butter, 1 Tbsp	100	8	3.5
Nutella, 1 Tbsp	100	5.5	12

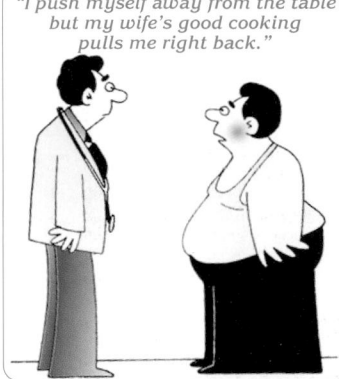

"I push myself away from the table but my wife's good cooking pulls me right back."

Animal Fats/Lards

Average All Types

Beef Tallow/Drippings, Lard (Pork), Chicken, Duck, Goose, Turkey.	C	F	Cb
1 Tbsp (13g)	115	13	0
2 1/4 Tbsp, 1 oz	255	28	0
1 cup, 7 1/4 oz	1850	205	0
1/2 pound, 8 oz	2040	227	0
Ghee/Butter Oil: 1 Tbsp, 13g	110	13	0
2 1/4 Tbsp, 1 oz	250	28	0

Vegetable Shortening

Average All Types (example, *Crisco*)

1 Tbsp, 0.44 oz	113	13	0
2 1/4 Tbsp, 1 oz	250	28	0
1 cup, 7 1/4 oz	1810	205	0

Vegetable Oils

Includes almond, avocado, canola, corn, coconut, flaxseed, grapeseed, linseed, mustard, olive, palm, peanut, rice-bran, safflower, sesame, sunflower, soybean, wheatgerm. Note: Oil is 100% fat.

1 tsp, 5g	45	5	0
1 Tbsp, 1/2 oz	120	14	0
2 Tbsp, 1 oz	250	28	0
1 cup, 7 3/4 oz	1930	205	0

Fish Oils

Average All Types (Includes cod liver, herring, salmon, sardine):

1 Tbsp, 1/2 oz	125	14	0

Cooking Sprays / Squeezes

Cooking Sprays (Pam, Mazola, I Can't Believe It's Not Butter, Weight Watchers, Wesson):			
Per serving	2	0	0
2-3 second spray	6	1	0
I Can't Believe It's Not Butter	0	0	0
Parkay Buttery Spray	0	0	0
Squeeze (Parkay), 1 Tbsp, 0.5 oz	70	8	0

Olestra (Olean)

Olestra (Olean)	0	0	0

Olean is *Proctor & Gamble's* brand name for olestra - a no-calorie cooking oil that gives snacks (like potato chips, tortilla chips and crackers) taste and texture without adding fat or calories.

Cheese

Quick Guide   **C** **F** **Cb**

Firm/Hard Cheeses
(American, Cheddar, Colby, Coon, Swiss)

	C	F	Cb
Regular Cheese:			
1 oz slice/piece	110	9	0.5
8 oz package	880	72	4
16 oz (1lb) package	1760	144	8
Cubes: 1" cube, 3/4 oz	55	5	0.5
1 1/4" cube, 1 oz slice	110	9	0.5
Diced: 1 cup, 4 1/2 oz	500	40	2
Grated: 1 Tbsp, 1/4 oz	27	2	0
Shredded:			
1/4 cup, 1 oz	110	9	0.5
1 cup, 4 oz	440	36	4
Sliced: 1 thin (3 1/2" sq.), 3/4 oz	85	7	0.5
Rectangular (7"x 4"x 1/8"), 1 1/2 oz	165	14	1
Round (3 1/4" diam. x 1/8"), 3/4 oz	85	7	0.5
Semi-circular, 1 1/4 oz			
(5 1/2" long, 3 1/2" radius, 1/8"thick)	140	11	0.5
Light: Average All Brands, 1 oz	80	5	0.5
Fat Free: Average All Brands, 1 oz	50	0	2
Lowfat: Average All Brands, 1 oz	50	1.5	1

Cheese   *Per 1 oz Unless Indicated*

	C	F	Cb
American:			
Regular, 1 slice, 1 oz	110	9	1
Kraft, 0.7 oz slice	60	4	1
Grated, 1 Tbsp, 1/4 oz	23	2	0
Light: *Borden,* 1 oz	70	4	0.5
Land O'Lakes, 1 oz	70	5	0.5
Smart Beat, 0.6 oz slice	35	2	0
Kraft, (2% Milk), 0.7 oz slice	45	3	1
Fat Free: *Kraft,* 0.75 oz slice	30	0	2
Alpine Lace, 1 oz	45	0	2
HealthyChoice, Singles, 0.7 oz	25	0	2
Weight Watchers, 3/4 oz	30	0	3
Babybel (Laughing Cow), 1 oz	90	7	0
Crumbled, 1/2 cup, 2 1/2 oz	250	20	1
Dorman's Castello, 1 oz	135	12	1
Bonbel (Laughing Cow), 1 oz	100	8	0
Mini, 3/4 oz	75	6	0
Brick, 1 oz	100	8	0
Brie, 1 oz	95	8	0
Cabot Vermont Ched., 50% light	70	4.5	1
Camembert, 1 oz	90	7	0
Caraway, 1 oz	105	8	1

	C	F	Cb
Cheddar: (Also see 'Quick Guide')			
Regular, 1 oz	110	9	0.5
Reduced Fat/Light, 1 oz	80	5	0.5
Weight Watchers, 1 oz	80	5	1
Fat Free: *Alpine Lace,* 1 oz	45	0	2
Weight Watchers, 1 sl., 3/4 oz	30	0	3
Cheese Balls (Kaukauna), 1 oz	100	7	0.5
Cheese Nut, Average, 1 oz	100	7	2
Cheese Logs, Average, 1 oz	100	7	0.5
Cheshire, 1 oz	110	9	1.5
Colby, Regular, 1 oz	110	9	0.5
Reduced Fat (Alpine Lace), 1 oz	80	5	1
Colby-Jack, 1 oz	110	9	0.5
Cottage Cheese: *Average All Brands*			
Creamed (4% milk fat): 2 Tbsp, 1 oz	30	1	1
1/2 cup, 4 oz	120	5	4
w. fruit, 1/2 cup, 4 oz	130	4	15
Reduced Fat (2%), 2 T., 1 oz	25	0.5	1
1/2 cup, 4 oz	100	2	4
Low Fat (1%), 2 Tbsp, 1 oz	20	.5	1
1/2 cup, 4 oz	80	1	3
Fat Free/Non Fat, 2 Tbsp, 1 oz	20	0	1
1/2 cup, 4 oz	80	0	3
Borden Dry Curd (0.5%), 1/2 c., 4 oz	80	0	0
Friendship: Low Fat P'apple, 4 oz	120	1	17
Non Fat Plus Peach, 1/2 c., 4 oz	110	0	15
Pot Style, 1/2 cup, 4 oz	90	3	3
w. Pineapple, 4 oz	140	4	16
Hood Fruit Stirs, avg, 110g ctn	200	2.5	24
Knudsen: 1.5% Fruit, 4 oz	110	2	12
Free: Non Fat, 1/2 cup, 4.3 oz	80	0	7
Lowfat, 4 oz	85	2	4
Cottage Doubles, avg, 5.5 oz ctn	150	2.5	18
4% Milk Fat, 1/2 cup, 4.3 oz	120	5	5
Light N' Lively: Garden Salad, 4 oz	90	2	5
Peach and Pineapple,			
1/2 cup, 4.3 oz	120	1	14
Cream Cheese: *See Page 45*			
Edam: Regular, 1 oz	100	8	0
Farmer (Friendship), 2 Tbsp, 1 oz	50	3	0
Feta: Regular, *Frigo,* 1 oz	100	8	1
Crumbled, 1/2 cup, 2 1/2 oz	190	15	2.5
Reduced Fat (Alpine Lace),	60	4	1
Fontina (Sargento/Classica), 1 oz	110	9	0.5
Gjetost (Goat's Milk, fresh), 1 oz	85	7	0.5
Sargento, 1 oz	130	8	12
Goat's Milk: Soft: *Chevre,* 1 oz	70	6	0.5
Chavril, 3 Tbsp, 1 oz	60	4.5	0.5

Goat's Milk Cheese (Cont)	C	F	Cb
Semi-Soft: 1 oz	100	8.5	1
Hard: Sargento, 1 oz	130	10	0.5
Gorgonzola, 1 oz	110	9	0.5
Galbani Dolcelatte, 1 oz	95	8	1
Gouda, 1 oz	100	8	0.5
Gruyere, 1 oz	115	9	0
Havarti, 1 oz	120	11	0
Italian (Classica Italiano), 1 oz	110	10	1
Jarlsberg, 1 oz	100	7	1
Jarlsberg Lite shredded, 1 oz	70	4	1
Kefir, 2 Tbsp, 1 oz	60	4	1
Limburger, 1 oz	90	8	0
Mascarpone, 1 oz	130	13	1
Mexican (Sargento Recipe Blend), Shredded, 1/4 cup, 1 oz	110	9	1
Monterey, 1 oz	105	8.5	0
Monterey Jack: regular, 1 oz	110	9	0
Light Naturals (Kraft), 1 oz	80	5	0
Alpine Lace , Monti-Jack Lo, 1 oz	80	5	0
Weight Watchers, 1 oz	90	6	1
Mozzarella:			
Regular: Kraft/Dorman's, 1 oz	90	7	0.5
Land O'Lakes/Polly-O, 1 oz	80	6	0.5
Shredded, 1/4 cup, 1 oz	80	6	0.5
Light: Polly-O Lite, 1 oz	60	2.5	0.5
Kraft Light Naturals, 1 oz	80	5	1
Sorrento Lite, 1 oz	60	3	0.5
Part Skim (Alpine Lace), 1 oz	70	5	0.5
Polly-O, 1 oz	90	6	0.5
Fat Free: Healthy Choice, 1/4 c., 1oz	45	0	1
Polly-O, 1 oz	35	0	1
Kraft, shredded, 1/4 cup, 1 oz	50	0	2
Muenster: Regular, 1 oz	110	9	0
Reduced Fat (Dorman's), 1 oz	80	5	0
Neufchatel: Dominick's, 1 oz	70	6	2
Philadelphia, 1 oz	70	6	0.5
Flavored: Fruit/Herbs	80	7	1
Chocolate (Hickory Farms), 1 oz	110	8	1
Parmesan: Fresh/Block, 1 oz	110	7	1
Shredded/Grated, 1 Tbsp	22	1.5	0
Grated (Packaged): 1 Tbsp	26	2	0
1 oz quantity	130	9	1
1/2 cup, 1-3/4 oz	230	16	2
w. Romano (Frigo), grated, 1 oz	130	9	1

Note: Packaged grated and shredded Parmesan have more calories (per unit weight) than block Parmesan due to a lower moisture content.

	C	F	Cb
Pizza, shredded:			
Frigo, 1/4 cup, 1 oz	90	7	1
Lowfat (Frigo), 1 oz	65	3	1
Port Du Salut, 1 oz	100	8	0.5
Port Wine (Hickory Farms), 1 oz	100	7	2.5
Pot (Sargento), 1 oz	25	0	1
Provolone: Regular, 1 oz	100	8	1
Reduced Fat, Alpine Lace, 1 oz	70	5	1
Pub (Hickory Farms), 1 oz	95	7	1
Quark: 40% fat, 1 oz	47	3	1
20% fat, 1 oz	32	1.5	1
Skim/Nonfat, 1 oz	22	0	1.5
Queso Anego/Asadero/Blanco	105	9	1
Queso Chichuahua/De Papa	110	9	2
Ricotta Cheese:			
Whole Milk, 2 Tbsp, 1 oz	50	3.5	1
1/2 cup, 4-1/2 oz	225	16	4.5
Part Skim, 2 Tbsp, 1 oz	40	2.5	1
1/2 cup, 4-1/2 oz	180	12	4.5
Light/Low Fat, 2 Tbsp, 1 oz	100	5	1
1/2 cup, 4-1/2 oz	100	2.5	5
Fat Free, 1/2 cup, 4-1/2 oz	100	0	4
Knudsen 'On The Go': Lowfat, 4oz	90	2	4
Free (Non-Fat), 4 oz container	80	0	6
Baked Ricotta, 2 oz portion	130	9	3
Romano: Block/Loaf, 1 oz	110	8	1
Grated (Pkg), 1 oz	120	9	1
1 Tbsp	26	2	0.5
Roquefort, 1 oz	105	9	0.5
Slim Jack (Dorman's), 1 oz	90	7	1
Sheep's Milk (Hollow Rd Farm)	45	3	1
Smoked: Sargents, Smokestick	100	7	1
Hickory Farm, Smoky Lyte, 1 oz	80	6	1
Stilton, 1 oz	118	10	1
String (Frigo/Kraft/Sargento), 1 oz	80	5	1
Light String-Ums, 1 stick	60	2.5	0.5
String Lite (Frigo), 1 oz	60	2	1
Mootown Light (Sargento), 1 stick	50	2.5	0.5
Swiss: Regular, 1 oz	110	9	1
Reduced Fat: Alpine Lace, 1 oz	90	6	1
Dorman's/Kraft Light Naturals, 1oz	90	5	1
Weight Watchers, 3/4 oz slice	30	0	2
Taco Cheese, shredded, 1/4 cup	110	9	1
Tilsit (Sargents), 1 oz	100	7	0.5
Tybo (Dorman's/Sargents), 1 oz	100	7	0.5
Vermont (Churny), 1 oz	100	9	1
Wensleydale, 1 oz	108	9	0
Whey Cheese, 1 oz	125	8	9

Cheese (Cont)

Cheese Products

	C	F	Cb
Cheese Food:			
Average all flavors: 3/4 oz slice	70	5	1.5
1 oz slice	90	6	2
Alouette: Fr. Onion/Garl.,2 T., 0.8oz	70	7	1
Light Garlic, 2 Tbsp, 0.8 oz	50	4	1
Cracker Barrel Cheddar, 1.1 oz	100	8	4
Delico: Alouette Cajun, 2 T, 0.8 oz	70	7	1
Garden Vegetable, 2 T, 0.8 oz	60	6	1
Handi-Snacks:			
Cheez 'n Breadsticks, 1 pkg	130	7	11
Cheez'n Pretzels, 1 oz pkg	110	7	11
Cheez'n Crackers, 1.1 oz pkg	130	8	10
Mozzarella Stringchse Stick, each	80	6	0.5
Healthy Choice Amer. Singles, 1 sl.	30	0	2
Heluva Good Cheese:			
American, 1 slice	45	5	2
Cheddar w. H/radish, 2 Tbsp, 1oz	90	7	3
Jalapeno: Avg., all brands, 1 oz	90	7	2
Kraft: American grated,1T., 0.2 oz	25	2	1
Singles, 1 slice, 3/4 oz	70	6	1
Free Singles, 1 slice, 0.7 oz	40	3	3
Pimento Spread, 2 Tbsp, 1.1 oz	80	6	3
Velveeta (Process Cheese Spread)			
Regular, 3/8" slice, 1 oz	100	6	3
Light, 3/8" slice, 1 oz	60	3	3
Rip-Ums, 1 strip, 0.75 oz	80	7	0.5
String-Ums (Lite), 1 stick	60	2.5	0.5
Lifeway: Farmers Cheese, 2 oz	75	5	2.5
Precious: String Chse Stuffsters, 1 oz	70	4.5	1
Roka Blue, 2 Tbsp, 1.1 oz	80	7	2
Rondele: Soft Spread., 2 T, 1 oz	100	9	1
Light, 2 Tbsp, 0.9 oz	60	4	2
SmartBalance: Crmy Cheddar, 1 sl.	40	2	2
Spreadery: Vermont, 2 Tbsp, 1 oz	80	5	3
Neufchatel, all flavors, 2 T, 1 oz	80	7	1
Velveeta: Cheese, 1 slice, 1 oz	100	6	3
Light, 1 oz	60	3	3
Shredded, 1/4 cup, 1.3 oz	130	9	3
WisPride: Hickory Smoked Cup;			
Port Wine Ball/Cup, 2 T., 1.1 oz	100	7	4
Light, 2 Tbsp., 1.1 oz	80	3	5

Cheese Whiz (Sauce)

	C	F	Cb
Regular, 2 Tbsp, 33g	90	7	2
Light, 2 Tbsp, 33g	80	3	6
Squeezable, 2 Tbsp, 33g	100	8	4

Cheese Substitutes

Per 1 oz Unless Indicated

	C	F	Cb
Almond Rella (Nu Soya):			
Cheddar; Garlic & Herb, 1 oz	70	3.5	3
Borden Taco-Mate, 1 oz	100	7	2
Delicia American Colby	80	6	1
Dorman's Lo Chol	100	7	1
Formagg: Cheddar, 1 slice, 0.7 oz	60	4	0.5
American Wh./Yellow, 1 sl. 0.7oz	60	4	0.5
Mozzarella (Old World), 1 oz	60	3	1
Parmesan Grated, 1 Tbsp, 1/4 oz	22	1.5	1.5
Provolone (Vintage), 1 oz	60	3	1
Swiss White, 1 slice, 0.7 oz	60	4	0.5
Frigo: Cheddar; Mozzarella, 1 oz	90	7	1
Georgio's: Imitation Cheddar;			
Mozzarella., shredded, 1/4 c., 1 oz	90	7	1
Golden Image: American 1 slice, 0.7 oz			
Mild Cheddar, 1 slice, 0.7 oz	70	5	1
Harvest Moon : Per 1/4 Cup, 1.3 oz			
Shredded: American; Cheddar	120	9	3
Mozzarella	110	9	3
Nu Tofu: Mozzarella, 1 oz	70	4	2
Fat Free: Mozz./Ched./Jack, 1 oz	40	0	2
Sargento Classic Supreme:			
Cheddar, shredded, 1 oz	90	6	2
Mozzarella, shrd 1/4 cup	80	6	0.5
Smart Beat, Fat Free, 0.6 oz sl.	35	0	3
Soya Kaas: Regular, 1 oz	70	5	1
Fat Free, all varieties, 1 oz	40	2	1
Soyco: Almond/Oat/Rice Slices,			
1 slice, 0.7 oz	40	2	1
Veggy Singles, 1 slice, 0.7 oz	40	2	1
Grated Parmesan, 2 tsp, 5g	15	0.5	0
Tofu Rella, avg. all varieties, 1 oz	80	5	1
Tofutti Better Than Cream Cheese	80	8	1
Weight Watchers: Fat Free Slices,			
All varieties, 3/4 oz slice	30	0	3
Grated Italian Topping, 1 Tbsp	20	0	2
White Wave, Soy A Melt:			
Cheddar/Mozz./Mont. Jack, 1 oz	80	5	1
Fat Free, 1 oz	40	0	3
Singles: Amer./Mozzarella, 3/4 oz	60	4	1
Yves Good Slice,3/4 oz slice, avg.	35	2	1

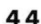

Cream Cheese

	C	F	Cb
Regular/Soft: 2 Tbsp, 1 oz	100	10	1
3 oz pkg	300	30	2
w. Chives/Herbs/Pimento, 1 oz	90	9	0.5
w. Fruit/Strawb./P'apple, 1 oz	90	8	5
Lox, 1 oz	90	9	0.5
Philadelphia® (Kraft): Per 2 Tbsp			
Original, 1 oz	100	10	1
1/3 Less Fat, 1 oz	70	6	1
Light: Plain, 1 oz	60	4.5	2
Strawberry, 0.7 oz	70	7	1
Fat Free, 1 oz	25	0	2
Flavored: Blueberry/Raspberry, 1 oz	95	8	5
Strawberry, 1 oz	90	8	4
Garden Vegetable, 3 oz	95	9	2
Snack Bars: avg, all types (1)	190	11	20
Whipped: Regular, 2 Tbsp, 0.7 oz	70	7	1
Mixed Berry, 2 Tbsp, 0.7 oz	70	6	3
Alpine Lace: Fat Free, 2 T., 1 oz	30	0	1
Weight Watchers, 2 Tbsp, 1 oz	40	2.5	1

Dips/Spreads ~ Per 2 Tbsp (1 oz)

	C	F	Cb
Avocado/Guacamole	50	4	4
Baba Ghannoush (Eggplant/Sesame)	70	6	2
Best Foods Dippin' Sauce: Per 2 Tbsp			
Honey Mustard Madness	60	2	10
Rockin' Ranch	90	6	8
Totally BBQ	110	12	1
Birdseye No Fat Veggie Dip, 1.1 oz	25	0	5
Breakstone's Sour Cream, all flav.	50	4	4
Chalco: Quéso Quesadilla; Cotija	120	10	0
Fresco, 2 Tbsp, 1 oz	70	8	0
Chi-Chi's: Con Quéso, 2 Tbsp	90	7	4
Hot/Medium/Mild/Acante, 2 T.	10	0	2
Cool Cuts: Carrot & Ranch	60	4	5
Celery & Peanut Butter	170	14	9
French Onion Dip, avg. all brands	60	6	3
Frito Lay: Chili Cheese; Jalapeno	50	3	3
French Onion	60	5	4
Bean/Jalapeno Bean	40	1	6
Guacamole, 2 Tbsp, 1 oz	50	4	4
Guiltless Gourmet: Nacho Dip	25	0	5
Other varieties	30	0	5
Heluva Good Cheese: Chse 'N Salsa	80	3	3
Clam/French Onion	50	5	2
Bacon/Homestyle/Ranch	60	5	2
Light Fr. Onion/Jalapeno Cheddar	40	2	3
Hummus: 2 Tbsp, 1 oz	50	1	5
1/2 cup, 4.5 oz	220	4.5	23
Hy-Top Pimiento, 1 oz	90	8	3

Dips/Spreads (Cont)

Per 2 Tbsp (1 oz)

	C	F	Cb
Kaukauna Nacho Cheese	90	7	4
Knudsen Nacho Cheese	60	4	3
Sour Cream Bacon & Onion	60	5	2
Sour Cream French Onion	50	4	2
Kroger The Big Dipper; all flavors	60	5	2
Kraft: Average all flavors, 2 Tbsp	60	5	4
Philly flavors:			
Bacon & Cheddar	60	5	3
Average other flavors	55	4.5	3
Fat Free: Strawberry	25	0	3
Garden Veges	30	0	2
Lay's Lowfat Sr. Cream, Onion	40	1	0
Louise's: (Fat Free) Honey Mustard	40	0	0
Sour Cream & Onion/White Chse	25	0	0
Luisa's Fiesta Dip, 2 Tbsp	35	2	3
Marie's: Reg, all types	90	9	2
Lite, 1 oz	60	4	4
Nalley's all flavors, average	120	12	3
Naturally Fresh, all flavors, 1 oz	80	0	19
Old Dutch Cheddar, Nacho	35	3	3
Old El Paso: Black Bean	25	0	5
Cheese'n Salsa: Mild; Medium	40	3	3
Lowfat, medium	30	1.5	3
Chunky Salsa varieties	15	0	3
Jalapeno Dip	30	1	4
Olys Bagel Spread: Berry	100	8	3
Honey Cinnamon; Raisin	100	8	6
Garden Veg; Garlic & Herb	90	9	1
Prices Orig. Pimiento Cheese Spr.	80	7	2
Rite Cream Cheese & Lox Spread	90	8	1
Ruffles French Onion; Ranch	70	6	4
Sealtest French Onion	50	4	2
Snyder's Mustard Pretzel	90	4	13
Stop & Shop: Veggie Dip, 2 Tbsp	110	10	3
Sour Crm French Onion, 2 T.	60	5	2
Supremo Chihuahua: Quéso Bianco	100	8	0
Quéso Fresco; Rancherito	80	6	0
TGI Fridays: Spinach,Chse,Artichoke	45	3.5	3
Black Bean & Cheese Dip	50	2.5	5
T. Marzetti: Blue Cheese	200	21	1
Light Ranch Veggie	70	6	3
Other flavors, average	130	13	2
Tostitos Dip: Con Quéso	40	2	5
Medium/Mild/Hot	15	0	3
Tzatziki (Cucumber/Yogurt Dip)	40	3	1
Wise: Jalapeno Bean	25	0	5
Taco	12	0	3

Salsa ~ See Page 91

Egg & Egg Dishes

Chicken Eggs

Fresh Eggs

Raw (weight with shell):	C	F	Cb
Small, 40g	65	4	0
Medium, 44g	70	4	0
Large, 50g	75	4.5	0
Extra Large, 56g	80	5	0
Jumbo, 63g	90	5.5	0
Egg Yolk, 1 extra large	63	5	0
Egg White, 1 extra large	16	0	0

Dried Egg Powder

Whole Egg: 1/4 cup, 1 oz	170	12	0
1 Tbsp	30	2	0
Egg White, 1/4 cup, 1 oz	105	0	0
Egg Yolk, 1/4 cup, 1 oz	195	18	0

Egg Substitutes

1/4 Cup (Equivalent to 1 Egg) ~ Zero Cholesterol.

Better 'n Eggs (Papetti), 1/4 cup, 2 oz	30	0	0
Egg Beaters (Fleischmann's):			
Regular/Flavors, 1/4 cup	30	0	1
Cheese Omelet, 1/2 cup	110	5	2
Vegetable Omelet, 1/2 cup	50	0	5
Egg Watchers (Tofutti), 2 oz	30	0	1
Eggstra, 1/2 envelope	50	2	0
Healthy Choice, 1/4 cup, 2 oz	25	0	0
Egg Substitute (Jewel), 1/4 cup	30	0	1
Scramblers (Morn Star), 1/4 cup	35	0	1
Second Nature: Regular, 1/4 cup	60	2	3
Fat Free, 1/4 cup, 60ml	30	0	1
Simply Eggs, 1/4 cup	35	1	1

Other Eggs

Duck, 1 large, 2 1/2 oz	130	9.5	0
Goose, 1 large, 5 oz	280	19	0
Quail, 3 eggs, 1 oz	42	3	0
Turkey, 1 large, 3 oz	135	9.5	0
Turtle, 1 egg, 1 3/4 oz	75	5	0

Omega-3 Fat Enriched

Eggs Land's Best, 1 large	70	4.5	0
Eggs Plus (Pilgrim's Pride), 1 large	70	4.5	0

Note: Cholesterol content same as regular eggs, but Omega-3 fats inhibit blood cholesterol increase.
(Also see Cholesterol ~ Page 253)

Cooked Eggs

Boiled Egg: Same as raw egg

Fried Egg:	C	F	Cb
With fat: 1 large egg	100	8	0.5
2 small eggs	175	13	1
No fat/nonstick pan, 1 large	80	5.5	0
Deviled Egg, 2 halves	145	13	0.5
Eggs Benedict (2) on toast			
or English muffin	860	56	25
Eggs Florentine (2) on toast			
or English muffin	890	59	25
Pickled Egg, 1 large	80	5.5	0
Poached Egg: 1 large	80	5.5	0
Scotch Egg, 1 egg	300	21	16
Scrambled Eggs: 1 large egg:			
w. 1 Tbsp milk + 1 tsp fat	120	9	1
w. 1 Tbsp skim milk/no fat	85	5.5	1
2 large eggs:			
w. 2 Tbsp milk + 2 tsp fat	260	20	2
w. 2 Tbsp skim milk/no fat	180	11	2

Omelets

1 Egg: Plain (w. 1 tsp fat)	125	10	0.5
with 1/2 oz cheese	175	15	0.5
w. 1/2 oz cheese +1/2 oz ham	200	16	0.5
2 Eggs: Plain (w. 2 tsp fat)	250	20	1
with 1 oz cheese	360	29	2
w. 1 oz cheese+1 oz ham	410	32	2
3 Eggs: Plain (w. 1 Tbsp fat)	360	29	1.5
w. 2 oz cheese	580	47	2.5
w. 2 oz cheese+2 oz ham	680	53	2.5
Extras: Tomato/Onion/Veges	20	0	4.5
Egg Substitute (Eggbeaters):			
2 eggs (1/2 cup) + 1 tsp fat	100	4	2
3 eggs (3/4 cup) + 2 tsp fat	160	8	3
Extras: 1 oz cheese	110	9	1
1 oz ham	50	3	1
Tom./Onion/Veges	20	0	4.5

Egg Nog ~ *Per 1/2 Cup (4 fl.oz)*

Regular: Borden	160	9	16
Crowley	190	9	23
Hood (Golden)	180	8	22
Light/Lowfat: Borden	120	2	23
Horizon; Hood	140	3	23
Fat Free: Hood	100	0	21

Breakfast Sides

	C	F	Cb
Toast: Plain, 1 thick slice	85	1	13
with 2 tsp butter/marg.	155	9	13
with 3 tsp/1Tbsp fat	190	13	13
English Muffin: Plain, 2 oz	130	1	26
with 3 tsp fat	230	12	26
Bacon, 2 strips	70	5	0
Ham: Lean, 2 oz	100	3	0
Hash Browns: 1/2 cup	125	6.5	14
1 cup serving	250	13	28
Sausages, 2 links (1 oz ea.)	180	16	1.5

Frozen Egg Breakfasts

	C	F	Cb
Jimmy Dean Breakfast Sandwiches			
Sausage Biscuit (2) 113g	400	28	27
Sausage, Egg & Cheese Muffin	380	25	26
Sausage, Egg & Cheese Biscuit	380	24	27
Bacon, Egg & Cheese Biscuit	290	15	26
Pillsbury Toaster Scrambles			
Cheese, Egg & Bacon/Ham	180	12	14
Cheese, Egg & Sausage	180	12	14
Swanson Great Starts: *Per Package*			
Egg, Bacon & Cheese Muffin	270	12	27
Egg, Chse & Bacon Biscuit	340	22	24
Sausage, Egg & Chse Biscuit	480	31	31
Sausage, Egg & Chse Croissant	470	33	27
Scrambled Eggs & Saus. Bkfst	370	27	17
French Toast & Sausage Bkfst	420	25	38
Pancakes & Sausage Breakfast	490	25	52
Uncle Ben's Breakfast Bowls: See Page 72			
Weight Watchers. Omelet	220	5	30

Frozen Egg Rolls

	C	F	Cb
Chun King/La Choy: *Average All Brands*			
Chicken Egg Rolls: Mini, 6 rolls	210	9	25
Restaurant Style, 1 roll, 3 oz	210	9	25
Pork & Shrimp Egg Rolls:			
Mini, 6 rolls, 3 oz	210	9	27
Shrimp Egg Rolls: Mini, 6 rolls	190	6	28
Restaurant Style, 1 roll, 3 oz	180	7	25
Lotus: Pork, 3 oz	180	7	18
Vegetable, 3 oz	70	1.5	13
Kahiki: Pork, 3 oz	190	6	25
Chicken, 3 oz	120	2	16
Vegetable, 3 oz	120	2	23

Fast Food/Restaurants

	C	F	Cb
Bojangles:			
Bacon/Egg/Chse S'wich	550	42	27
Burger King:			
Egg'wich Bacon/Egg/Cheese	420	23	36
Croissan'wich Saus./Egg/Chse	520	39	24
Carl's Jr: Scrambled Eggs	180	14	1
Denny's: Two Egg Breakfast	825	67	24
Omelette: Ham 'n Cheddar	605	47	5
Veggie-Cheese	510	39	11
Sirloin Steak & Eggs	655	45	1
Hardees: Bacon Egg, Chse Bisc.	520	30	45
Sausage & Egg Biscuit	620	40	45
Omelet	550	32	45
McDonald's: Egg McMuffin®	300	12	29
Bacon, Egg & Cheese Biscuit	480	31	31
Scrambled Eggs (2)	160	11	1
Perkins: Country Club Omelet	930	79	6
Roy Rogers: Ham & Egg Biscuit	470	26	44
Sausage & Egg Biscuit	560	35	44

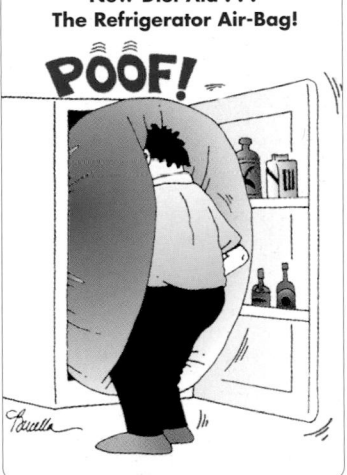

**New Diet Aid . . .
The Refrigerator Air-Bag!**

POOF!

Meat & Beef

Note: Cooking reduces weight of meat by 20-45% due to water and fat losses. Average weight loss is 30%. Actual loss depends on cooking method and cooking time. Examples:

4 oz raw wt. = approx. 3 oz cooked wt.
4 oz cooked wt. = approx. $5^1/2$ oz raw wt.

What 3 oz Cooked Meat Looks Like
- Half the size of this book ($4^1/4$" x 3" x $3/8$" thick)
- Rectangular piece (4" x $2^1/2$" x $1/2$" thick)
- Deck of cards ($3^1/2$" x $2^1/2$" x $5/8$" thick)

Quick Guide

Steak

Sirloin (Choice Grade)
External fat trimmed to $1/4$"
Broiled, Edible Portion (no bone)

Small Serving, 3 oz (cooked)	C	F	Cb
(3 oz cooked, from $4-4^1/2$ oz raw)			
Lean + fat ($1/4$"), 3 oz	230	14	0
Lean + marbling, 3 oz	195	10	0
(External fat trimmed **before** cooking)			
Lean only, 3 oz	170	7	0
(No external fat or marbling)			

Medium/Regular Serving, 5 oz (cooked wt)			
(from approx. 7 oz raw)			
Lean + fat ($1/4$"), 5 oz	470	29	0
Lean + marbling, 5 oz	400	20	0
Lean only, 5 oz	350	14	0

Large Serving, 8 oz (cooked wt)			
(from 11-12 oz raw)			
Lean + fat, 8 oz	610	38	0
Lean + marbling, 8 oz	520	26	0
Lean only, 8 oz	454	18	0

Extra Large Serving, 12 oz (cooked wt)			
(from approx. 16-17 oz raw)			
Lean + fat ($1/4$"), 12 oz	915	57	0
Lean + marbling, 12 oz	780	39	0
Lean only, 12 oz	680	27	0

Pan Fried			
Sirloin (choice), medium serving:			
Lean + fat ($1/4$"), 5 oz	450	32	0
Lean only, 5 oz	330	15	0

Other Steaks 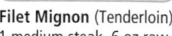 C F Cb

Filet Mignon (Tenderloin):
1 medium steak, 6 oz raw wt.
Broiled, with $1/4$" fat trim

Lean + fat ($1/4$"), 4 oz	340	24	0
Lean only, $3^1/2$ oz	210	10	0
Broiled, ($1/4$" fat removed before cooking)			
Lean + marbling, $3^1/2$ oz	220	12	0
Lean only, 3 oz	180	8	0

New York/Club Steak:
Top Loin/Short Loin
1 steak, regular ($9^1/4$ oz raw, $1/4$" fat)

Broiled: Lean + fat ($1/4$"), $6^1/4$ oz	510	35	0
Lean + marbling, $5^1/2$ oz	330	16	0
Lean only, $5^1/4$ oz	310	14	0

Porterhouse Steak:
1 medium, 6 oz raw wt. (no bone), broiled

Lean + fat ($1/4$"), $4^1/4$ oz	370	27	0
Lean only, $3^1/2$ oz	220	11	0
With Bone ~ See T-Bone Steak			

T-Bone Steak (Broiled/Grilled)
Medium, 8 oz raw wt.

Lean + fat ($1/4$")	380	27	0
Lean only	220	10	0
Large, 12 oz raw wt.	570	41	0
Supersize, 20 oz raw wt. ($1/4$" fat)	950	68	0

Also See Fast-Foods & Restaurants Section ~
Outback Steakhouse, WesterN SizzliN

Beef - Average All Cuts

Average All Retail Cuts
Edible weight (no bone)

Raw	C	F	Cb
(1 lb raw yields approx. 11-12 oz cooked)			
Lean + fat ($1/4$" trim), 1 oz	70	5.5	0
$1/2$ Pound, 8 oz	560	44	0
Lean only, 1 oz	40	2	0
$1/2$ Pound, 8 oz	320	16	0
Fat only, 1 oz	190	20	0

Cooked (No Added Fat)			
Lean + fat ($1/4$"), 1 oz	86	6	0
Small serving, 3 oz	260	18	0
Lean + marbling, (no ext. fat), 1 oz	78	5	0
Small serving, 3 oz	235	15	0
Lean only, 1 oz	60	3	0
Small serving, 3 oz	180	9	0
Fat only, 1 oz	193	20	0

Meat & Beef (Cont)

Beef - Individual Cuts

Average All Grades Edible Weight (no bone)	C	F	Cb
Brisket, whole, braised:			
Lean + fat (1/4"), 3 oz	330	27	0
Lean + marbling, 3 oz	250	17	0
Lean only, 3 oz	205	11	0
Chuck, blade, braised:			
Lean + fat (1/4"), 3 oz	290	22	0
Lean + marbling, 3 oz	285	20	0
Lean only, 3 oz	210	11	0
Flank: Raw, 4 oz	200	12	0
Braised, 3 oz	225	14	0
Broiled, 3 oz	190	11	0
Ribs, whole (ribs 6-12): Roasted			
(1 lb raw yields 10 1/4 oz roasted)			
Lean + fat (1/4")			
(3.6 oz w. bone, 3 oz no bone)	300	25	0
Lean only, 3 oz (no bone)	200	11	0
Round, bottom, braised:			
Lean + fat (1/4"), 3 oz	235	14	0
Lean only, 3 oz	180	7	0
Round, eye/tip, roasted:			
Lean + fat (1/4"), 3 oz	200	11	0
Lean, 3 oz	150	5	0
Round, top: Per 3 oz (cooked wt)			
Braised, Lean + fat	210	10	0
Lean only	175	5	0
Broiled, Lean + fat	185	8	0
Lean only	155	4	0
Pan-fried, Lean + fat	235	13	0
Lean only	190	7	0

Ground Beef

Ground Beef, Raw:	C	F	Cb
Regular: 70% lean (30% fat)	380	34	0
73% lean (27% fat)	350	30	0
80% lean (20% fat)	300	24	0
Reduced Fat, 85% lean (15% fat)	250	17	0
Lean, 90% lean (10% fat)	190	8	0
Extra Lean, 96% lean (4% fat)	150	4.5	0
Rinsed (boiled/skimmed): 4 oz	180	12	0
Healthy Choice (97% lean), 4 oz	130	4	0
Baked/Broiled: Reg., 3 oz	250	18	0
Lean, 3 oz	230	16	0
Extra lean, 3 oz	200	12	0
Pan-fried: Regular, 3 oz	260	19	0
Lean, 3 oz	230	16	0
Extra lean, 3 oz	200	12	0
Ground Beef Patties: Average (20% Fat)			
Frozen, raw, 4 oz	290	22	0
Broiled, 3 oz	240	17	0

Quick Guide
Roast Beef

Round (Eye/Tip, average) Average All Cuts	C	F	Cb
Small Serving, 3 oz			
(2 thin slices/1 thick slice)			
Lean + fat (1/4"), 3 oz	200	11	0
Lean only, 3 oz	150	5	0
Medium Serving, 5 oz, (3-4 thin slices)			
Lean + fat, 5 oz	330	18	0
Lean only, 5 oz	250	8	0
Large Serving, 8 oz, (3 thick slices)			
Lean + fat, 8 oz	530	29	0
Lean only, 8 oz	400	13	0

Roast Dinner Extras

	C	F	Cb
Gravy: Thin, 2 Tbsp	20	1	0.5
Thick, 2 Tbsp	50	2	0.5
1 Ladle/4 Tbsp	100	4	1
Veges: Beans, green, 1/2 cup	20	0	5
Cauliflower w. cheese sauce, 4 oz	135	9	15
Corn, kernels, 1/4 cup	35	0	9
Carrots, 1/4 cup	20	0	3
Peas, 1/4 cup	35	0	6
Pumpkin baked: w.fat, 4 oz	90	7	5
No added fat, 2 pces, 4 oz	25	0	5
Potato: Roasted w. fat, 1 small	155	8	30
Baked in Jacket, 1 large	220	0	50
with 1 Tbsp whipped butter	295	8	50
with Sour Cream, 2 Tbsp	270	6	51
Sweet Potato/Yam, 1 medium	80	0	50
Beef Kabobs: Beef & Veggies, 2 oz	160	10	4
If very lean meat	100	4	4

"347 ~ 348 ~ 349..."

49

Meat • Lamb, Veal, Pork

Lamb   C F Cb

Choice Grade

Leg (Whole), roasted:

	C	F	Cb
Lean + fat, 3 oz	220	14	0
Lean only, 3 oz	160	7	0

Leg (Sirloin Half), roasted:

Lean + fat, 3 oz	250	18	0
Lean only, 3 oz	175	8	0

Leg (Shank Half), roasted:

Lean + fat, 3 oz	190	11	0
Lean only, 3 oz	155	6	0

Loin Chop, broiled:

1 chop (raw wt., 4 1/4 oz):

Lean + fat (2 1/4 oz edible)	200	15	0
Lean only (1.6 oz edible)	100	5	0

Rib Chop, broiled/roasted:

1 chop (raw wt., 3 1/2 oz)

Lean + fat (2 1/2 oz edible)	255	21	0
Lean only (1 3/4 oz edible)	120	7	0

Shoulder (Arm/Blade):

Braised: Lean + fat, 3 oz	290	21	0
Lean only, 3 oz	240	14	0
Broiled: Lean + fat, 3 oz	240	16	0
Lean only, 3 oz	180	9	0
Roasted: Similar to Broiled			

Cubed Lamb (Leg/Shoulder):

For stew or kabob

Raw, lean only, 8 oz	310	12	0
Braised, lean only, 3 oz	190	8	0
Broiled, lean only, 3 oz	160	6	0

New Zealand Lamb (Imported):

Similar calories and fat to domestic.

Veal

Edible Weights   C F Cb

Leg (Top Round):

	C	F	Cb
Braised: Lean + fat, 3 oz	180	6	0
Lean only, 3 oz	170	5	0
Pan-fried, breaded:			
Lean + fat, 3 oz	195	8	9
Lean only, 3 oz	175	6	9
Pan-fried, not breaded:			
Lean + fat, 3 oz	180	7	0
Lean only, 3 oz	155	4	0
Roasted: Lean + fat, 3 oz	135	4	0
Lean only, 3 oz	130	3	0

Veal (Cont)   C F Cb

Loin Chop: 1 chop, 7 oz raw wt.

	C	F	Cb
Braised: Lean + fat	230	14	0
Lean only	155	6	0
Roasted: Lean + fat	175	10	0
Lean only	125	5	0

Rib, roasted: Lean + fat, 3 oz   195   12   0

Lean only, 3 oz	150	7	0

Shoulder, Arm/Blade, roasted:

Lean + fat, 3 oz	155	7	0
Lean only, 3 oz	145	6	0

Sirloin, roasted:

Lean + fat, 3 oz	170	9	0
Lean only, 3 oz	145	6	0

Cubed for Stew, braised:

Leg/Shoulder, lean only, 3 oz	160	4	0

(1 lb raw yields approx. 9 1/4 oz cooked)

Pork

Figures based on NLMB data (1990)

Fresh Pork (Cooked Wt., no bone)

(4 oz raw wt. = approx. 3 oz cooked wt.)

Blade Steak, broiled:

Lean + fat, 3 oz	220	15	0
Lean only, 3 oz	190	11	0

Country Style Ribs, broiled:

Lean + fat, 3 oz	270	22	0
Lean only, 3 oz	205	13	0

Spareribs, braised: lean & fat, 6 oz

(from 1 lb raw wt)	700	53	0

Leg (Ham), roasted:

Lean + fat, 3 oz	250	18	0
Lean only, 3 oz	180	9	0

(Ham, cured ~ See Cold Meats)

Loin Chops, broiled: Average

(From 1 chop. 5 oz raw wt. w.bone

or 4 oz raw wt., no bone)

Lean + fat, 3 oz	200	11	0
Lean only, 3 oz	165	7	0

Rib Chops, broiled:

Lean + fat, 3 oz	215	13	0
Lean only, 3 oz	180	7	0

Rib Roast, roasted:

Lean + fat, 3 oz	210	13	0
Lean only, 3 oz	175	9	0

Loin Roast, roasted:

Lean + fat, 3 oz	190	10	0
Lean only, 3 oz	160	7	0

Pork (Cont)

	C	F	Cb
Sirloin Chop, broiled:			
Lean + fat, 3 oz	175	8	0
Lean only, 3 oz	155	6	0
Sirloin Roast, roasted:			
Lean + fat, 3 oz	215	14	0
Lean only, 3 oz	180	9	0
Tenderloin, roasted:			
Lean + fat, 3 oz	147	5	0
Lean only, 3 oz	140	4	0
Ground Pork			
Raw: Average, 1/4 lb, 4 oz	300	24	0
Broiled, 3 oz	245	18	0
Pan-fried, drained, 3 oz	250	19	0

Bacon

	C	F	Cb
Raw: 1 med. slice (20 lb), 3/4 oz	125	13	0
1 thick slice (12 lb), 1 1/3 oz	210	22	0
(1 lb raw yields approx. 5 oz cooked)			
Broiled/Pan-Fried: 1 med. sl., 6 g	36	3	0
3 medium slices, 18g	110	9	0
2 thin slices, 1/2 oz	80	7	0
1 thick slice, 12g	70	6	0
Canadian-style: Cooked, 1 slice	43	4	0
As purchased, 1 slice, 1 oz	45	4	1
Bacon Bits, 1 Tbsp, 1/4 oz	20	1	0
Breakfast Strips: Broil, 1 sl., 12 g	50	4	0

Ham

	C	F	Cb
Boneless Ham, cooked:			
Regular, (approx. 11% fat):			
Unheated (as purch.), 1 oz	52	3	0
Roasted, 3 oz	150	8	0
Extra Lean (5% fat):			
Unheated, 1 oz	37	2	0
Roasted, 3 oz	125	5	0
Whole Ham, cooked:			
Lean + fat (as purchased)			
Unheated, 1 oz	70	5	0
Roasted, 3 oz	345	26	0
Lean only, unheated, 1 oz	40	2	0
Roasted, 3 oz	135	5	0
Canned Ham: Similar to boneless ham			
Chopped, canned, 3 oz	260	21	0
Ham Patties, ckd, 1 pty, 2 1/4 oz	205	18	1
Ham Steak, extra lean, 2 oz	70	2	0
Luncheon Slices: See Deli Meats, Page 53			

Game & Other Meats

	C	F	Cb
Bison Steak, lean, 6 oz (raw)	210	4	0
Boar (wild), roasted, 3 oz	140	4	0
Buffalo Steak *(New West Foods)*, 4 oz	70	3	0
Caribou, roasted, 3 oz	140	4	0
Deer/Venison, roasted 3 oz	135	3	0
Goat (Capretto): Raw, 3 oz	110	2.5	0
Roasted, 3 oz	150	3	0
Ostrich: *Blackwing Ostrich Meats,*			
Sport Jerky, 1/2 oz pce	25	0	0
Sausage Patties, (2) 2 oz	60	0.5	0
New West Foods:			
Ground Ostrich, 4 oz	110	2	0
Ostrich Steak, 4 oz steak	130	2.5	0
Rabbit: Roasted, 3 oz	130	6	0
Stewed, 1 cup, diced, 5 oz	300	14	0

Variety & Organ Meats

	C	F	Cb
Brains: Braised, 3 oz	130	9	0
Pan-fried, 3 oz	200	14	0
Chitterlings, pork, simmered, 3oz	260	25	0
Ears, pork, simmered, 1 ear	180	12	0
Feet, pork: Simmered, 3 oz	165	11	0
Cured, pickled, 3 oz	170	14	0
Hormel, 2 oz	80	6	0
Head Cheese (Pork Snouts/Ears/Vinegar/Spices):			
1 oz slice	50	4	0
Heart: Average, braised, 3 oz	140	5	0
Jowl, pork, raw, 4 oz	750	80	0
Kidneys, simmered, 3 oz	130	4	0
Liver: Raw, 4 oz	160	5	3
Braised, 3 oz	140	4	3
Pan-fried, 3 oz	200	9	3
Pancreas, braised, 3 oz	200	13	0
Pork Cracklins, 0.5 oz	80	6	0
Pork Hocks, 1 piece, 6 oz	340	23	0
Scrapple, pork, 1 oz	60	4	4
Spleen, braised, 3 oz	130	4	0
Stomach, pork, raw, 4 oz	180	11	0
Sweetbreads: Beef, ckd., 3 oz	270	20	0
Lamb, cooked, 3 oz	150	5	0
Tail, pork, simmered, 3 oz	340	31	0
Tongue, braised, 3 oz: Veal	170	9	0
Beef/Lamb/Pork, average	240	17	0
Tripe, beef, raw, 4 oz	110	5	0
Lean + fat	310	25	0

Sausages, Franks

Quick Guide
Franks & Weiners

Beef: *Average All Brands*
Regular/Smoked: *Per Frank*

	C	F	Cb
4 oz link	280	22	5
2.6 oz link	240	19	2
2 oz link (8/16 oz pkg)	180	17	2
1.6 oz link (10/16 oz pkg)	140	13	1
1.5 oz link (8/12 oz pkg)	135	12	1
1.2 oz link (10/12 oz pkg)	110	10	1
1 oz link (16/16 oz pkg)	90	8	0.5
Small/(Cocktail (50/lb), each	30	3	0.5

Beef Light/Reduced Fat Franks:

	C	F	Cb
Ball Park, 1 frank, 2 oz	100	7	3
Best's Kosher	50	1	5
Oscar Mayer, 2 oz link	110	8	2
Hebrew National: 97% Fat Free	50	1.5	2
Reduced Fat, 1	120	10	0
Healthy Choice, lowfat, 1.8 oz	60	2.5	7

Beef Fat-Free Franks: Oscar Mayer

	C	F	Cb
Oscar Mayer	40	0	3
Ball Park (1),1.76 oz	55	0	7

Pork Franks:

	C	F	Cb
Country Style, 2 oz panfried	240	22	1
Chorizo, 5 sausages, 2.5 oz	280	26	3
El Popular, 2 oz cooked	210	17	3
Jimmy Dean, cooked, 2 oz	240	21	0
Oscar Mayer (2), 1.7 oz, ckd	170	15	1
Light, 2 oz link	110	8	2

Turkey Franks:

	C	F	Cb
Butterball, 1 frank, 1.75 oz	45	5	7
Empire Kosher, 2 oz	90	6	1
Foster Farms, 2 oz	130	11	0
Jennie-O, 2 links, 2 oz	130	11	0
Louis Rich: Orig., Lower Fat (1)	100	8	2
Bun Length (1)	120	10	3
Mr Turkey, smoked, 2 oz	90	5	3
Shelton's, 1 frank, 1.2 oz	80	6	1

Chicken Franks:

	C	F	Cb
Empire Kosher, 2 oz	100	7	1
Foster Farms, 2 oz	140	12	0
Scott Petersen, 1.2 oz	80	6	1
Shelton's, 1.2 oz	95	6	1
Zacky Farms, 2 oz	150	13	0

Vegetarian Sausages
See Frozen/Canned & Packaged Meals

Quick Guide
Fresh Sausages

Pork/Beef: *Average All Types*

	C	F	Cb
Small: Raw, 4" link, 1 oz	120	12	1.5
Broiled/Pan-fried	50	4	1.5
Medium: Raw, 2 oz	235	23	2.5
Broiled/Pan-fried	100	8	2.5
Large: Raw, 3 oz	360	36	3.5
Broiled/Pan-fried	150	12	3.5
Italian: Raw, 3.2 oz	315	28	1.5
Cooked, 2.4 oz	215	17	1.5
Chorizo: Beef Chorizo, 2.5 oz pce	320	31	3
Pork Chorizo, 2.5 oz piece	250	22	4

Note: Fat is lost in broiling/pan frying.
(Cooked wt. = approx. 60-70% raw wt.)

Smoked Sausage

	C	F	Cb
Average All Brands: 2 oz link	180	16	4
3 oz link	270	24	6
Ball Park: Bun Size, 2 oz	190	17	4
Butterball (w. Turkey), 2 oz	60	0	4
Eckrich, 2 oz	180	16	4
Healthy Choice, Beef/Polska, 2 oz	70	2.5	6

Breakfast Sausages/Patties

	C	F	Cb
Butterball: Turkey Brkfast Pats (2)	100	7	2
Turkey Breakfast Links (3)	120	8	2
Healthy Choice: Patties/Links (3) 2 oz	70	3	1
Jimmy Dean: Pork Saus. Patties (2)	260	24	0
Pork Sausage Links: Original (3)	290	28	0
Country Maple (3)	230	20	3
Breakfast Sandwiches: See Page 47			
Jones/Golden Brown:			
Pork Sausage Patties: Original (1)	150	14	0
All Natural (1)	130	12	0
Sandwich Patties (1)	170	16	1
Pork Sausage Links: 2 links	190	18	1
Light, 2 links	100	8	1
Swanson 'Great Starts' ~ See Page 47			
Swift Premium Brown 'n Serve			
Pork/Turkey, 3 links, 2.1 oz	210	19	2
Lite Original, 3 links	120	8	3
Beef Sausage, 3 links, 2 oz	230	22	1

Vegetarian Patties:
Boca ~ See Page 62
Garden Burger ~ See Page 64

Hot Dogs ◆ Deli Meats

Bagel, Corn & Hot Dogs

	C	**F**	**Cb**
Hot Dogs, Ready-To-Go			
(Includes Ketchup/Relish; No Mayo)			
Small (1 oz frank/ 1 oz roll)	200	8	24
Regular (1½ oz frank/ 2 oz roll)	310	13	39
Large (2 oz frank/ 2 oz roll)	360	18	40
Super/Giant (3 oz frank/3 oz roll)	540	26	59
Weinerschnitzel: See Fast-Foods			

Corn Dogs

	C	**F**	**Cb**
Beef/Pork Frank: Average, 2.6 oz	170	10	16
Foster Farms Chicken Franks:			
1 dog, 2.6 oz (75g)	180	10	15
Chili Cheese, 1 dog, 2.6 oz (75g)	200	9	24
Mini Corn Dogs, (4) 2.68 oz	210	12	18
Oscar Mayer Turkey & Pork, 3.2 oz	260	15	25
State Fair w. Ball Park Franks,			
Corn Dogs, 1 dog, 2.7 oz (76g)	180	12	15
Mini Corn Dogs (4)	230	13	22
Turkey: *Gobblers! (Shelton's)*	220	11	27

Bagel Dogs

	C	**F**	**Cb**
Best's Kosher: 1 dog, 1 oz	320	11	43
Mini, 1 piece, 0.8 oz	60	2	8
Vienna Beef: 1 piece, 1 oz	85	3.5	7

Hot Dog Toppings/Extras:

	C	**F**	**Cb**
American Chse, 1 slice, 1 oz	110	9	1
Catsup, 1 Tbsp	16	0	4
Chili (w. Beans), ¼ cup	70	3.5	9
Mustard, 1 Tbsp	20	0	1
Pickle Relish, 1 Tbsp	20	0	5
Sauerkraut, ½ cup	20	0	5

WILL-POWER TONIC
~ RECIPE ~

- 1 Cup of Desire
- 1 Quart of Determination
- 1 Tbsp of Common Sense
- 1 Tbsp of Stick-to-itiveness
- 1 Tbsp of Foresight
- 1 Cup of Energy

Deli & Luncheon Meats

	C	**F**	**Cb**
Beef Jerky:			
Bridgeford Beef Jerky, 1 oz	50	1	3
Beef Stick (5.5 oz stick), 1 oz	140	12	0
Beef Steak, 1 oz	50	1	0
Beef & Cheese (Giant Size),			
½ pkg, 1.5 oz	170	14	1
Pepperoni Sticks, 2, 1 oz	140	12	1
Pepperoni (1" diam.), 1 oz	130	12	0
Teriyaki, 1.25 oz pkg	80	1	8
Original; Hot 'n Spicy	70	1	5
Berliner (pork/beef), 1 oz	65	4	0.5
Beerwurst (Beef):			
Small (2.75"diam), 1/16" slice	20	2	0
Large (4"diam), 1/8" slice	75	7	0.5
Beerwurst (Pork):			
Small (2.75"diam), 1/16" slice	15	1	0
Large (4"diam), 1/8" slice	55	4	0.5
Bologna, Beef & Pork:			
Regular: 1 thin slice, 1 oz	90	8	1
1 thick slice, 1.6 oz	145	13	1
Light *(Oscar Mayer),* 1 sl., 1 oz	60	4	2
Red. Fat *(Hebrew Nat.),* 1 oz	65	6	0
Fat Free *(Osc. M.),* 2 sl., 1.6 oz	40	0	1
Healthy Choice, 1 oz	35	1	3
Weight Watchers, 2 sl., ¾ oz	35	2	0
Turkey, average, 1 oz	60	5	0.5
Chicken *(Tyson),* 1 slice	45	4	0.5
Ring *(Boar's Head),* 2 oz	160	13	0.5
Blood Sausage, 1 oz	100	5	0.5
Bratwurst:			
Average, 1 oz	90	8	0.5
Boar's Head, cook., 1 wurst, 4 oz	300	25	0
Bob Evan's, Beer, 2.6 oz link	270	21	1
Braunschweiger (Pork/Liver/Sausage),			
Oscar Mayer, 1 oz slice	100	9	1
Chicken, Average All Brands			
1 thick or 2 thin slices, 1 oz	30	1	1
Chicken Roll, 1 slice, 1 oz	90	4	1.5
Corned Beef:			
Average, full fat, 1 oz	70	5	1.5
*Healthy Choice, Hillshire Farm,*1oz	30	1	0.5
Hebrew National, 4 slices, 2 oz	90	4.5	0
Loaf, jellied, 1 oz	45	2	0
Hash, canned, average, 1 oz	50	3	2
Dutch Brand Loaf, average, 1 oz	70	5	1.5

Continued Next Page

Deli & Luncheon Meats

Ham, Luncheon:	C	F	Cb
Baked/Boiled, sliced, 1 oz	30	1	0.5
Chopped: *Eckrich* (97% FF), 1 oz	25	1	1
Armour: Canned, 1 oz	35	1.5	0.5
97% Fat Free, 1 oz	25	1	1.5
Healthy Choice, 2 sl., 2 oz	60	1.5	2
Hormel (Black Label), 1 oz	70	6	0
Oscar Mayer, 1 oz slice	60	3	1
Honey/Brown Sugar, avg., 1 oz	30	1	0.5
Healthy Choice Deli Traditions:			
2 slices, 2 oz	60	1.5	2
Prosciutto, average, 1 oz	70	5	1
Ham & Cheese Loaf, avg., 1 oz	70	5	0.5
Head Cheese *(Osc. Mayer)*, 1 oz sl.	50	4	0
Honey Loaf *(Osc. Mayer)*, 1 oz sl.	35	1	2
Italian Sausage, 2.6 oz	270	21	1
Kielbasa *(Polish Sausage)*, 1 oz	85	7	0.5
Scott Petersen, 3.4 oz link	320	27	4
Beef, 2.8 oz link	290	25	4
Boar's Head, 1 oz	60	5	0
Kippered Beefsteak:			
(Hickory Farms), 3 slices, 0.75 oz	50	1	1
Knackwurst, 1 oz	90	8	0.5
Liverwurst, 1 oz	95	8	0.5
Liver Pate, fresh, average, 1 oz	110	10	3.5
Luncheon Loaf *(Foods Co)*, 1 oz	80	7	2
Mortadella, 1 oz	90	7	0.5
Olive Loaf, average, 1 oz	70	5	3
Oscar Mayer, 1 oz slice	70	6	2
Pastrami (Beef), average, 1 oz	40	2	0.5
Healthy Deli, 1 oz	34	1	0.5
Hillshire (DeliSelect), 6 sl., 2 oz	60	1	1
Turkey Pastrami, 1 slice, 1 oz	30	1	1
Peppered Beef, 1 oz slice	40	2	1
Pepperoni, 5 slices, 1 oz	135	12	0
Pickle Loaf, average, 1 oz	80	6	1
Pickle & Pimiento Loaf			
(Oscar Mayer), 1 oz	80	6	3
Polish Sausage: *See Kielbasa*			
Proscuitti, average, 1 oz	70	5	1
Hormel, 1 oz	90	7	1
Roast Beef: Lean, 1 oz	40	1	0.5
Healthy Choice, all types, 2 oz	60	1.5	4
Salami: Beef, average, 1 oz	80	7	1
Beer Salami, average, 1 oz	70	6	0.5
Cotto: *Oscar Mayer*, 1 slice, 1 oz	70	5	1
Dry: Hard, avg., 3 slices, 1 oz	110	10	0.5
Oscar Mayer, 2 slices, 1.6 oz	120	10	1

Salami: (Cont)	C	F	Cb
Genoa: Average, 1 oz	110	10	0
Stick *(Best's Kosher)*, 2, 1.75 oz	180	15	2
Italian *(Bridgeford)*, 1 oz	120	11	0
Turkey, average, 1 oz	55	4	1
Spam *(Hormel)*:			
Regular: 1/4" slice, 1 oz	90	8	0
1/2" slice, 2 oz	180	16	1
Lite: 1/4" slice, 1 oz	55	4	0
1/2" slice, 2 oz	110	8	1
Turkey: 1/4" slice, 1 oz	40	2	0.5
1/2" slice, 2 oz	80	4	1
Summer Sausage:			
Bridgeford, 1 oz	100	9	0
Oscar Mayer, 1 slice, 0.8 oz	70	7	0
Treet *(Armour)*, canned, 1 oz	100	9	1.5
Turkey: Average, 1 oz slice	30	1	0.5
3/4 oz slice	22	0.5	0.5
Turkey Breast:			
Butterball Fat Free, 4 sl., 2 oz	50	0	2
Deli Thin Smoked, 1 sl., 1 oz	30	5	1
Hillshire Deli Select, 6 sl., 2 oz	60	0.5	2
Louis Rich Carvery Board,			
2 slices, 1.8 oz (52g)	50	0	2
Free, 2 slices, 2 oz	50	0	2
Healthy Choice:			
Deli Thin: *Per 4 Slices, 52g (1.8 oz)*			
Oven-Roasted	60	1.5	2
Smoked/Rotisserie Seasoned	60	1.5	2
Honey Roasted & Smoked	60	1.5	3
Hearty Deli Sliced:			
Oven Rstd Turkey Brst. 1 sl., 1 oz	30	1	1
Turkey Ham, 1 slice, 1 oz	35	1.5	0.5
Turkey Pastrami, 1 oz	35	1.5	0.5
Turkey Roll, 1 oz	40	2	0.5
Turkey Loaf, 1 oz	30	1	0.5
Vegetarian Deli: *Worthington, Yves: Page 83*			

Meat Spreads	C	F	Cb
Average All Brands: Per 1/4 Cup (2 oz)			
Chicken	120	8	2
Ham, deviled	160	14	0
Liverwurst	170	14	3
Roast Beef	140	11	0
Sandwich Spread	140	10	8
Turkey	110	7	2

Paté

	C	F	Cb
Canned: *Average All Brands*			
Chicken Liver, 2 Tbsp, 1 oz	60	4	2
Paté de Foie Gras, goose liver, 1 oz	130	12	2
Fresh (Refrigerated):			
Average all types, 1 oz	110	10	1
Boar's Head Liverwurst Pate, 2 oz	150	12	0
Marcel Henri: 2 oz serving	220	20	2
Pate de Champagne, 2 oz	210	18	2
Chicken Liver w. Port Wine, 2 oz	210	18	2
Duck Truffle w. Port Wine, 2 oz	240	24	2
Old Wisconsin Pate, all types, 1 oz	105	9	1.5
Vegetable Pate: Spin/Mushr. 2 oz	110	7	10
Toby's Tofu Pate:			
Original/Jalapeno, 2 Tbsp, 1 oz	70	8	2
Lite, all flavors, 2 Tbsp, 1 oz	30	2	2
Trois Petit Cochons: Medit., 2 oz	140	11	3
Smoked Salmon, 2 oz	110	9	2
Wegmans: Alexian Wild, 2 oz	270	27	1
Cognac; Blk Peppercorn, 2 oz	160	17	4

Lunch Packs

	C	F	Cb
Funny Bagels: *Per Package w. Drink, Yogurt*			
Honey Ham; Cheese Pizza, avg.	435	9	72
PB & J	490	14	82
Cream Cheese and Jelly	470	14	77
Lunchables *(Oscar Mayer): Per Package*			
All-Star Burger/Juice/Candy	400	10	66
All-Star Hot Dogs/Choc Balls/Drink	450	19	64
Lean Ham/Chedd./Crackers/Cookie	420	21	39
Lean Ham/Turkey/Cheese, avg.	350	20	20
Lean Turkey Brst w. Ham, Cheese	370	20	20
Cracker Stackers: *Per Package w. Drink, Candy*			
Bologna & American Cheese	470	32	31
Ham/Turkey & American Cheese	430	19	52
Ham & Cheddar; Pizza, avg.	380	20	21
Ham & Swiss	350	9	52
Turkey & Cheddar	370	10	56
Fun Fuel: Chicken/Ham Wraps (2)	440	13	64
Ham/Turkey bagels, 2 bagels	420	10	64
Fun Packs: Pizza Dunks	490	13	64
Waffles and Sausage	460	16	66
Nachos: Cheese & Salsa	380	21	39
w. Capri Sun/Choc Fudge	540	26	70
w. Capri Sun/Nestle Crunch	570	29	70
Tacos: Beef Taco & Cheese	310	11	34
Beef Tortilla/Drink/Wonka Nerds	480	12	72
Mega Packs: Ultimate Nachos	780	32	113
2 Pepp. Pizza/Reese's P.B.Cup/Cola	760	28	105
2 Extra Cheesy Pizza/M&Ms/Drink	700	24	104
Mega Cracker Combo	770	32	102
Soft Pizzastix & Twix/Drink	680	16	118
Sandwiches: Ham, Turkey, Cheddar	470	22	47
Turkcy & Chcddar varieties	410	17	45
Smoked Ham & Cheddar Sub	380	14	44
Pizza: 3 Extra Cheesy	300	13	28
w. Fruit Punch, Crunch Bar	450	15	63
Pepperoni Flavored Sausage, 3	310	15	28
w. Capri Sun/Crunch	470	17	65
Lunchmakers *(Armour):* Loco Nachos	370	13	59
Cheese Pizza	310	13	36
CrackerCrunchers: Bologna	280	19	19
Other varieties, average	240	15	18
Fun Kits: Bologna	410	20	28
Turkey	360	14	48
Munch-A-Bunch *(Jewel): Per 4 oz Package*			
Bologna/Chse/Crackers/Cookies	430	29	27
Other varieties, average	350	19	29
Smuckers: Snackers, 3.3 oz pkg	410	20	47
Uncrustables, 1 sandwich	210	8	26

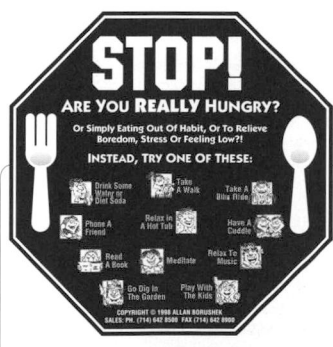

Chicken

Quick Guide

Chicken

	C	**F**	**Cb**
From 3lb ready-to-cook chicken			
Breast/Wing Quarter			
Roasted: With skin	300	15	0
Without skin	190	5	0
Fried, batter dipped	480	26	18
Leg Quarter: Thigh & Drumstick			
Roasted: With skin	265	15	0
Without skin	180	8	0
Fried, batter dipped	430	26	16
KFC ~ See Fast-Foods Section			

Average - All Meats

Average of Light & Dark Meats			
Per 4 oz Serving (no bone)			
Roasted: With skin	270	15	0
Without skin	215	8	0
Stewed: With skin	250	14	0
Without skin	200	8	0
Fried: Batter-dipped	330	20	11
Flour coated	305	17	3.5

Chicken Parts

Broilers or Fryers: Edible Weights (no bone)			
Breast: *Per 1/2 Breast*			
Raw: With skin, 5 oz	245	13	0
Without skin, 4 1/4 oz	130	2	0
Roasted: With skin, 3 1/2 oz	195	8	0
Without skin, 3 oz	140	3	0
Stewed: With skin, 4 oz	210	8	0
Without skin, 3 1/4 oz	140	3	0
Fried: Batter-dipped, 5 oz	370	19	12
Flour coated, w. skin, 3 1/2 oz	220	9	7
Drumstick: *Per Drumstick*			
Roasted: With skin, 2 oz	125	6	0
Without skin, 1 1/2 oz	75	2	0
Fried: Batter-dipped, 2 1/2 oz	195	11	7
Flour coated, 1 3/4 oz	120	7	1
Stewed: With skin, 2 oz	115	6	0
Without skin, 1 1/2 oz	80	3	0
Thigh Portion: Edible Wt. (no bone)			
Raw: With skin, 3.3 oz			
(4 1/4 oz with bone)	200	14	0
Without skin, 2.4 oz	80	3	0
Roasted: With skin, 2 1/4 oz	155	10	0
Without skin, 2 oz	110	6	0

Thigh Portion (Cont)	**C**	**F**	**Cb**
Stewed: With skin, 2 1/2 oz	160	10	0
Without skin, 2 oz	105	5	0
Fried: Batter-dipped, 3 oz	240	14	8
Flour coated, 2 1/4 oz	165	9	2
Wing: *Per Wing*			
Raw Weight 3.2 oz (with bone)			
Raw: With skin	110	8	0
Without skin	35	1	0
Roasted: With skin	105	7	0
Without skin	45	2	0
Fried: Batter-dipped	160	11	5
Flour coated	105	7	1
Stewed: With skin, 4 oz	100	7	0
Buffalo Wings ~ *See Fast-Foods Section*			
(Denny's, Domino's, O'Charleys, Pizza Hut)			
Neck: Simmered, with skin	95	7	0
Without skin	30	2	0
Skin Only: *Skin from 1/2 Chicken*			
Raw skin, 2 3/4 oz	275	26	0
Roasted skin, 2 oz	255	22	0
Stewed skin, 2 1/2 oz	260	24	0
Fried, Flour coated, 2 oz	280	24	5
Fried, Batter-dipped, 6 3/4 oz	750	55	45
Roasters			
Average of Light & Dark Meat:			
Roasted: With skin, 4 oz	250	15	0
Without skin, 4 oz	190	8	0
Light Meat: Without skin, roasted	175	5	0
Dark Meat: Without skin, roasted	206	10	0
Stewing Chicken			
Stewed: *Per 4 oz Serving*			
Average of Light & Dark Meat:			
With skin	325	21	0
Without skin	270	14	0
Light Meat: Without skin	240	9	0
Dark Meat: Without skin	295	17	0
Capon Chicken			
Roasted: With skin, 4 oz	260	13	0
1/2 Chicken, with skin	1460	74	0
Chicken Offal & Stuffing			
Giblets, simmered, 1 cup	230	7	1.5
Fried, flour-coated, 1 cup	400	20	6
Gizzard, simmered, 1 cup	220	5	1.5
Heart, simmered, 1 cup	270	12	0.5
Liver: Raw, 4 oz	140	5	3.5
Simmered, 1 cup	220	8	1
Liver Pate Fresh, 1 Tbsp, 1/2 oz	60	8	2
Stuffing: Average, 1/2 cup	200	2	22

Chicken Products

Shop Stop	C	F	Cb
Blazing Chicken Wings, 3 oz	200	12	1
Breaded Tenderloins, (3) 4 oz	240	12	15
Boneless Skinless Breasts, (1) 8 oz	210	5	3
Tyson: Chick. Chunks: Reg., (6)	280	20	19
Breast, (6)	220	19	11
Southern Fried, (6)	260	19	11
Breast Patties: Regular, each	190	12	11
Chick 'n Quick/Chedd., 74g ea.	220	14	12
Crispy Baked, each	80	0	9
Thick 'n Crispy, each	200	19	10
Southern Fried, each	180	12	8
Nuggets: Breaded White Mea, (6)	250	18	12
Wings: Flavored, average (3)	170	10	1
BBQ Style (3)	200	13	2
Stir Fry Kit: Chicken, 2³/4 c. froz.	430	4.5	73
M/wave S/wiches: Breast, 119g	320	15	33

Stove Top: Per Serving	C	F	Cb
Chicken Stuffing Mix: 1 oz	110	1	20
¹/2 cup prepared	170	9	20

Duck, Goose, Quail

	C	F	Cb
Duck: roasted, with skin, 3 oz	285	24	0
Without skin, 3 oz	170	10	0
¹/2 whole duck, with skin	1300	108	0
Goose: roast, with skin, 3 oz	260	19	0
Without skin, 3 oz	200	11	0
Pheasant: ¹/2 bird, raw	720	37	0
Quail: 1 whole, raw	210	13	0

Turkey

Fryer-Roasters: Per 3 oz Serving	C	F	Cb
Roasted: Light Meat, with skin	140	4	0
without skin	120	1	0
Dark Meat: with skin	155	6	0
without skin	140	4	0

¹/4 of Whole Turkey: (Approx. 3¹/4 lbs raw wt. w/out neck and giblets; 2 lb 6 oz cooked wt.)

	C	F	Cb
Roasted: With skin	1400	46	0
Without skin	1030	18	0
Ground Turkey, Raw: (4 oz raw wt. = 3 oz ckd wt.)			
Regular (85% lean), 4 oz	180	10	0
Lean (90% lean), 4 oz	160	8	0
Foster Farms, (94% lean), 4 oz	150	7	0
Jennie-o, (93% lean), 4 oz	160	8	0
Breast, no skin, 4 oz	115	1	0

Turkey Parts C F Cb

Roasted, Edible Weights (no bone)

	C	F	Cb
Breast (¹/4): (from 17¹/4 oz raw wt. w/bone)			
With skin, 12 oz (no bone)	525	11	0
Without skin, 10³/4 oz	415	2	0
Back (¹/2): With skin, 4¹/2 oz	265	13	0
Without skin, 3¹/2 oz	165	5	0
Leg (Thigh & Drumstick):			
(from 1 lb raw wt. w/bone)			
With skin, 8¹/2 oz (no bone)	420	13	0
Without skin, 7³/4 oz	355	8	0
Wing: (from 7¹/4 oz raw wt. w/bone)			
With skin, 3 oz (no bone)	185	9	0
Without skin, 2 oz	100	2	0
Neck: Simmered, 1 neck,			
(9 oz w. bone)	275	11	0
Giblets, simm., 1 cup, 5 oz	240	7	3

Young Hens (Roasted)

	C	F	Cb
Light Meat: With skin, 3 oz	175	8	0
Without skin, 3 oz	135	3	0
Dark Meat: With skin, 3 oz	200	11	0
Without skin, 3 oz	165	7	0
Young Toms — Similar to Young Hens			

Turkey Products

	C	F	Cb
Banquet: See Frozen Meals, Page 61, 62			
Circle L: Boneless Bacon, 3 oz	120	9	1
Jenny-O: Turkey Bacon, 2 slice	40	1.5	0
Louis Rich: Fat Free Breast of Turkey			
Rotiss'd/smoked/Rstd, 2 oz	60	0	1
Turkey Ham & Chunks, cooked:			
Breast & White Turkey, 2 oz	60	1	2
Turkey Ham/Pastrami, 2 oz	70	3	1
Turkey Salami, 2 oz	100	8	0
Luncheon Slices: See Deli Meats, Page 53			
Franks: Medium, 1¹/2 oz	80	6	2
Large, 2 oz	110	8	3
Smoked Sausage/Kielbasa, 1 oz	45	2	1
Turkey Bacon, 1 oz	35	2.5	0
Turkey Nuggets/Sticks, ckd, ea.	75	5	4.5
Turkey Patties, cooked, each	220	13	13
Swanson: Frozen Meals, Page 72			
Turkey Store			
Gobble Stix, Honey, each	25	0	1
Lean Burger Patties, 1 patty	180	8	5
Lean Italian Sausage, 1 link	190	8	2

Fish ~ Fresh & Canned

Quick Guide   **C F Cb**

Fresh Fish

Low Oil (Less than 2.5% fat)
White/pale colored flesh. Examples:
Cod, Flounder, Haddock, Halibut, Mahi Mahi
Perch, Pike, Pollock, Snapper, Sole, Whiting.

Per 4 oz Edible Portion	C	F	Cb
Raw, 4 oz (no bones)	90	1	0
Steamed, Broiled, Baked	130	1	0
Fried: Lightly Floured	210	8	3.5
Breaded	260	12	8
In Batter	320	16	27

Medium Oil (2.5-5% fat)   **C F Cb**
Pale colored flesh. Examples:
Bluefin Tuna, Catfish, Kingfish, Orange Roughy,
Salmon (Pink), Swordfish, Rainbow Trout,
Yellowtail.

	C	F	Cb
Raw, 4 oz (no bones)	140	5	0
Baked, Broiled, 4 oz	175	6	0
Fried, 4 oz	230	11	8

High Oil (Over 5% fat)   **C F Cb**
Darker colored flesh. Examples:
Albacore Tuna, Bluefish, Herring, Mackerel,
Salmon (Atl./Chinook/Sockeye), Sardines, Trout,
Whitefish.

	C	F	Cb
Raw, 4 oz (no bones)	230	16	0
Baked, Broiled, 4 oz	275	17	0
Fried, 4 oz	340	23	12

Cooking Yields (Fin Fish):
4 oz Raw wt. = 3$^1/_2$ oz Cooked wt.
4 oz Cooked wt. = 5 oz Raw wt.

Calorie & Fat Variations
The amount of fat/oil in fish varies with the
species, season and locality. Within the same fish,
fat/oil content is generally higher towards the
head.

Fish & Shellfish   **C F Cb**

Edible Weights: (no bones/shell)

	C	F	Cb
Abalone: Raw, 4 oz	120	1	7
Ahi Tuna: grilled, 6 oz fillet (no fat)	220	2	0
Anchovy: Paste, 1 Tbsp, $^1/_4$ oz	15	1	0.5
Cnd. in oil, drnd., 5 only, $^3/_4$ oz	40	2	0
Pickled, 1 oz	50	3	0
Barracuda (Pacific), raw, 4 oz	130	3	0
Bass: Black, raw, 4 oz	105	1	0
Striped: Raw, 1 fillet, 5$^1/_2$ oz	150	4	0
Baked, 3 oz	105	3	0
Blue Fish: Raw, 1 fillet, 5$^1/_2$ oz	185	6	0
Baked, 3 oz	130	5	0
Butterfish, raw, 4 oz	165	9	0
Cajun & Creole Dishes ~ *See Page 176*			
Calamari, breaded/fried, 1 serve	360	21	10
Carp, raw, 4 oz	145	6	0
Catfish: Raw Frozen, 4 oz	150	9	0
Fried, breaded, 1 fillet, 3 oz	200	12	7
Baked, 3 oz	120	5	0
Caviar: black/red, 1 Tbsp, 16g	40	3	0.5
Clams: Raw, 3 oz (4 lge/9 small)	65	1	2
Fried, breaded, $^3/_4$ cup, 4 oz	450	26	39
Canned, *(Snow's)* in clam jce 2 oz	25	0	2
Minced, $^1/_4$ cup, 2 oz	25	0	0.5
Clam Juice: *(Snow's)* 1 Tbsp	0	0	0
Cod, Atlantic/Pacific: Raw, 4 oz	95	1	0
Baked/Broiled, 1 fillet, 6$^1/_4$ oz	135	2	0
Canned, 3 oz	90	1	0
Minced, $^1/_4$ cup, 2 oz	25	0	0
Smoked, 3 oz	95	1	0
Crab: Alaska King, raw, 4 oz	95	1	0
1 leg, cooked, 4$^3/_4$ oz	130	2	0
Blue: Raw, 1 crab			
($^1/_3$ lb whole crab, $^3/_4$ oz flesh)	18	0.5	0
Steamed, 3 oz	85	1	0
Canned, $^1/_2$ cup, 2$^1/_2$ oz	65	0.5	0
Dungeness, 1 crab, 5$^3/_4$ oz edible			
(from 1$^1/_2$ lb whole crab)	140	2	2
Imitation Crab Legs/Stix, 3oz	80	1	8.5
Crab Cakes (Lowfat), (1), 2 oz	100	4	12
Crayfish, raw, 4 oz (edible)	100	1	0
Croaker, raw, 4 oz	120	3	0
Cuttlefish, raw, 3 oz	70	1	1
Dolphinfish, raw, 4 oz	95	1	0
Eel: Raw, 4 oz	210	13	0
Smoked, 2 oz	190	16	0
Fish & Chips, *Arthur Freachers*	1540	101	132
Denny's	955	57	77
Fish S'wich, w. Tartar Sce, 5$^1/_2$ oz	430	23	41
Fish Sticks, frozen ~ *See Brands, Page . . .*			

Edible Weights: (no bones/shell)

	C	F	Cb
Fish Oil, 1 Tbsp, 1/2 oz	125	14	0
Flounder/Sole: Raw, 4 oz	120	0.5	0
Baked, 3 oz	90	2	0
Frozen Fish & Entrees ~ See Page 60			
Gefilte Fish: See Kosher/Deli Foods, Page 179			
Grouper, raw, 4 oz	105	1	0
Haddock, raw, 4 oz	100	0.5	0
Broiled, 1 fillet, 5 1/4 oz	170	1	0
Smoked, 2 oz	22	0.5	0
Baked, 3 oz	90	1	0
Halibut: Raw, 4 oz	125	3	0
Baked, 3 oz	105	2	0
Herring: Atlantic, raw, 4 oz	180	10	0
Pickled, 2 pieces, 1 oz	60	4	2
In Sour Cream, 1 oz	75	5	1
Party Snacks, 1/4 cup, dr., 2 oz	120	5	0
Rollmops, 1 1/2 oz	110	8	6
Canned: Plain w. liq., 4 oz	235	15	0
in Tomato Sauce, 4 oz	200	12	1
Smoked, kippered, 4 oz	245	14	0
Jellyfish: Raw, 4 oz	30	0	0
Dried, Salted, 1 cup, 2 oz	20	1	0
Kingfish, raw, 4 oz	120	3.5	0
Ling, raw, 4 oz	100	0.5	0
Lobster, Northern: Raw, 4 oz	105	1	0.5
1 Lobster, 6 1/4 oz (from 1 1/2 lb whole lobster)	135	1.5	0.5
Cooked, 1 cup, 5 oz	140	1	2
Lobster Newberg, 3/4 cup	360	20	9
Lobster Thermidor, 1 serving	370	22	15
Lobster Salads, 1/2 cup	220	13	5
Lomi Salmon, 1/2 cup, 4 oz	20	1	3
Lomi Lomi Salmon, 1/2 cup, 4 oz	75	2	6
Lox, Regular/Nova, 2 oz	65	2.5	0
Mackerel: Atlantic, raw, 4 oz	235	16	0
Broiled, 3 oz	190	12	0
Jack, canned, 1/2 c., 3 1/3 oz	150	6	0
King, raw, 4 oz	120	2	0
Pacific/Jack: Raw, 4 oz	180	9	0
Broiled, 3 oz	190	12	0
Spanish, raw, 4 oz	160	7	0
Mahi-Mahi, raw, 4 oz fillet	100	1	1
Milkfish, raw, 4 oz	165	7.5	0
Monkfish: Raw, 4 oz	75	1	0
Baked, 3 oz	80	2	0
Mullet, striped, raw	135	4	0
Mussels: Raw, 4 oz (edible wt.)	100	2	4
1 cup, 5 1/4 oz (edible wt.)	130	3	5
Cooked, moist heat, 3 oz	150	4	6

	C	F	Cb
Ocean Perch: Raw, 4 oz	90	1.5	0
Baked, 3 oz	100	20	0
Octopus, common, raw, 4 oz	95	1	2
Orange Roughy, raw, 4 oz	145	9	0
Oysters: Common, raw, 3 oz	70	1	3.5
Eastern raw:			
6 medium, 3 oz	60	2	3
1 cup, 8 3/4 oz	170	6	8.5
Fried/breaded, 6 med., 3 oz	170	11	10
Pacific, raw, 1 med., 1 3/4 oz	40	1	2
Oysters Rockerfeller, 3 oysters	220	13	12
Perch, average, raw, 4 oz	105	2	0
Pike: Northern, raw, 4 oz	100	1	0
Walleye, raw, 4 oz	105	2.5	0
Pollock, raw, 4 oz	100	1	0
Pout, (Ocean), raw, 4 oz	90	1	0
Pompano, Florida, raw, 4 oz	190	10	0
Porgy/Scup, raw, 4 oz	130	4	0
Quahogs ~ See Clams			
Red-Snapper, raw, 4 oz	115	1.5	0
Rockfish, Pacific, raw, 4 oz	110	2	0
Roe, raw, 2 Tbsp, 1 oz	40	2	0.5
Sablefish: Raw, 4 oz	220	17	0
Smoked, 3 oz	220	17	0
Salmon:			
Raw: Chinook, 4 oz	205	7	0
Atlantic; Coho/Silver, 4 oz	160	7	0
Chum; Pink, 4 oz	135	4	0
Red/Sockeye, 4 oz	190	10	0
Baked: Atlantic/Coho, 3 oz	150	7	0
Smoked Salmon: Chinook, 3 oz	100	4	0
Pacific Supreme, 2 oz	100	4	0
Wild Oats, Pastrami Style, 2 oz	130	9	0
Canned Salmon: *Average All Brands*			
Pink: 1 oz	40	2	0
1/4 cup, 63g (2.2 oz)	90	5	0
3 3/4 oz can, whole	155	8.5	0
7 1/2 oz can, whole	300	17	0
Skinless/boneless, 1/4 c., 2 oz	70	2	0
Red Sockeye: 1 oz	50	3	0
1/4 cup, 63g (2.2 oz)	110	7	0
3 3/4 oz can, whole	190	12	0
Atlantic, 1/2 cup, 3 1/2 oz	230	14	0
Chinook/King, 1/2 cup	210	14	0
Chum, 1/2 cup, 3 1/2 oz	140	5	0
Coho/Silver, 1/2 cup	155	5	0
Atlantic Steaks: Small, 8 oz	320	14	0
Medium, 12 oz	480	21	0
Large, 16 oz	640	28	0
Salmon Cake, take-out, 3 oz	240	15	6

Fish ~ Fresh & Canned (Cont)

Fish (Cont)

	C	F	Cb
Sardines (Canned): *Average All Brands*			
In Oil, undrained, 1 oz	85	7	0
Drained of oil, 1 oz	60	3	0
3³/4 oz can, drained, (3¹/4 oz)	190	11	0
1 lrg/2 med. 3"/5 small, 0.8 oz	50	3	0
In Tom./ Mustard Sce, 1 oz	45	3	0
3³/4 oz can (8 sardines)	170	11	0
Sashimi: *See Japanese Foods, Page 178*			
Scallop: Raw, 6 lg./14 sm., 3 oz	75	0.5	2.5
Breaded/fried, 6 lge, 3 oz	200	10	9
Broiled, 3 oz	135	1	2
Seabass, raw, 4 oz	110	2	0
Seafood Salad, 1 scoop (#16)	140	10	8
Shark: Raw, 4 oz	150	6	0
Batter-dipped, fried, 4 oz	260	16	7
Baked, 3 oz	135	5	0
Shark Fin, dried, 1 oz	30	0	0
Shrimp: Raw, in shell, ¹/2 lb	140	2	1.5
Raw, shelled, 3 oz (12 lge)	90	1.5	0.5
Breaded/fried, 3 oz (11 lge)	210	11	10
Canned, 2 oz	45	0	0.5
Tiger, cooked, 1 shrimp, ¹/2 oz	15	0.5	0
Battered, fried, 1 shrimp	60	4	3
Smelt, Rainbow, raw, 4 oz	115	3	0
Snapper, raw, 3 oz	85	1	0
Cooked, 1 fillet, 6 oz	215	3	0
Sole, Lemon, raw, 4 oz	90	1	0
Squid: Raw, 4 oz	105	1	3.5
Fried, 4 oz	140	6	7
Surimi (Imitation Crab), 4 oz	110	1	7.5
Sweet & Sour Fish, ¹/2 dish, 10 oz	580	29	53
Swordfish: Raw, 4 oz	140	5	0
Broiled, 3 oz	120	4	0
Tilapia, Rain Forest Fillets, 3.5 oz	95	1	0
Trout, Rainbow: Raw, 4 oz	135	4	0
Broiled, 3 oz	125	4	0
Smoked, 2 oz	110	6	0
Tuna			
Raw: Albacore, 4 oz	190	8	0
Bluefin, 4 oz	160	5.5	0
Skipjack, Yellowfin, 4 oz	120	1	0
Broiled, 3 oz	110	1	0
Canned: *Average All Brands*			
In Water, drained:			
Chunk/Solid, 2 oz can	60	0.5	0
3 oz can	90	1	0
6 oz can	150	1.5	0
In Oil, drained:			
Chunk Light, 2 oz	110	5.5	0
6 oz can, drained	275	14	0

	C	F	Cb
Tuna (Cont)			
Solid White, 2 oz	90	2.5	0
6 oz can, drained	225	6.5	0
Tuna Salad: Deli Style, ¹/2 c., 4oz	300	24	15
Lower fat, 4 oz	210	10	11
Whitefish: Raw, 4 oz	150	6.5	0
Baked, 3 oz	140	6	1
Smoked, 3 oz	90	1	0
Whiting: Raw, 4 oz	100	1.5	0
Baked, 3 oz	85	1	0
Yellowtail: Raw, 3 oz	125	4.5	0
Grilled, 3 oz (from 4 oz raw)	160	6	0

Other Canned/Packaged Fish

	C	F	Cb
Bumble Bee			
Tuna Salad Kit (w. crackers), 3.5 oz	280	21	18
Fat-free Kit (w. crackers), 3.5 oz	150	2	24
Chicken of the Sea: *Per Pouch (7.1 oz)*			
Light Tuna, in water, 7.1 oz	210	1.5	0
Pink Salmon, boneless, 7.1 oz	210	7	0
Libby's: Crab Delights, 2 oz	30	0	5
Shrimp/Lobster Delight, 2 oz	35	0	4
Starkist:			
Pouch (3 oz):			
Tuna Chunk Light, in water	90	1	0
Albacore Tuna, in water	105	1.5	0
Lunch-To-Go: Chunk Light Tuna			
w. Mayo/Crackers, 4.5 oz	210	9	27
Tuna Creations: Chunk Light Tuna			
w. Moyo/Crackers, 4.5 oz	210	9	27

Frozen Fish Products

Fisher Boy: *See Page 64*
Gorton's: *See Page 64*
Kroger Fish Portions: *See Page 66*
Louis Kemp: *See Page 67*
Mrs Paul's: *See Page 68*
SeaPak: *See Page 70*
Van De Kamp's: *See Page 73*
Fast-Foods & Restaurant Chains ~ *See Page 183*
Captain D's Seafood ~ *See Page 94*
Long John Silvers ~ *See Page 220*
Shoney's ~ *See Page 243*

Amy's (Vegetarian)

Per Serving

	C	F	Cb
Bowls: Brown Rice & Vegs, 10 oz	240	8	42
Santa Fe Enchilada, 10 oz	340	9	47
Other varieties, average	300	12	35
Asian Meals: Thai Stir Fry, 9.5 oz	270	11	36
Asian Noodle Stir Fry, 10 oz	240	4.5	52
Entrees: Chse Enchilada, 4.75 oz	210	12	13
Blk Bean Vege. Enchilada, 4.75 oz	170	5	26
Cheese Lasagna, 10.25 oz	330	12	36
Macaroni & Cheese, 9 oz	410	16	47
Macaroni & Soy Cheeze, 9 oz	370	14	42
Pasta Prima.; Tofu Lasagne, avg.	300	11	37
Ravioli w. Sauce, 8 oz	340	12	43
Vegetable Lasagne, 9.5 oz	280	12	29
Whole Meals: Cannelloni, 9 oz	330	12	34
Black Bean Enchilada, 10 oz	320	6	55
Cheese Enchilada, 9 oz	330	14	38
Chili Cornbrd; Indian Mattar Paneer	320	6	59
Veggie Loaf, 10 oz	280	7	47
Skillet Meals: Country Ched., 1 c.	250	11	27
Pasta & Veges Alfredo, 1 cup	220	8	27
Teriyaki Stir Fry, 1 cup	320	2.5	64
Pot Pies: Country Vege, 7$^{1}/2$ oz	370	16	47
Mex. Tamale; Shepherd's Pie, avg.	160	4	27
Vegetable (Non Dairy), 7$^{1}/2$ oz	320	9	50
Burgers: Californian, 2$^{1}/2$ oz	130	3	19
Other varieties, avg., 2$^{1}/2$ oz	120	2.5	14
Burritos: Bean & Rice, 6 oz	280	6	44
Black Bean Vegetable, 6 oz	320	8	54
Breakfast Burrito, 6 oz	210	6	38
Non Dairy, 6 oz	270	6	48
Chili: Black Bean, 1 cup	160	1.5	25
Other varieties, avg., 1 cup	190	6	26
Pocket Sandwich: Cheese Pizza	300	9	42
Broccoli & Chse; Soy Cheeze	270	10	37
Other varieties, avg., 4.5 oz	230	7	35
Tofu Scramble: Vege Pie, 5 oz	300	9	45
Vegetarian Pizza	250	6	39
Toaster Pops: Apple; Strawberry	140	2.5	26
Cheese Pizza	150	4	23
Grilled Cheese	180	8	19
Snacks: Cheese Pizza, 5-6 pc, 3 oz	180	6	22
Spinach & Fetta Mini Pockets, 3 oz	170	6	24
Pizza: Cheese; Spinach; Pesto, $^{1}/3$	300	12	38
Mushr. & Olive; Vege Combo, $^{1}/3$	270	9	34
Roasted Vegetable, $^{1}/3$, 4 oz	270	8	43
Soy Cheese, $^{1}/3$ pizza	280	11	37

Astrochef

	C	F	Cb
Cheese Puffs (Tyropita) 1 pce, 1 oz	70	4	5
Mushroom Puffs, 1 pce, 1 oz	37	2	5
Spinach Puffs, 1 pce, 1 oz	58	2	8
Sth Western Bean Rolls, 1 pce, 1 oz	66	3	8

Atkins

	C	F	Cb
Enchiladas: Green Chili Chkn, 4.5 oz	190	9	11
Rstd & Shredded Pork, 4.5 oz	200	11	11
Spinach & Cheddar Chse, 4.5 oz	245	16	13
Crustless Quiche: Bacon & On. (1)	325	27	2
Other varieties, avg. (1)	300	24	2
Souffle: Broc., Cheddar & Bacon (1)	195	15	3
Crab & Cheddar (1)	285	25	2
Spinach, Tomato & Feta (1)	175	13	4
Fajitas: Grilled Chicken, 4.6 oz	255	13	16
Grilled Steak, 4.6 oz	305	18	16
Menu Classics: Beef Teriyaki, 8 oz	205	7	9
Chicken Marsala, 8 oz	240	6	9
Chicken Tetrazzini, 8 oz	355	16	9
Chicken Teriyaki, 8 oz	155	5	9
Pasta Entree: Baked Ziti, $^{1}/2$ tray	195	8	10
Chicken Cacciatore, $^{1}/2$ tray	95	1	10
Meatballs & Pasta, $^{1}/2$ tray	160	6	10

Banquet

	C	F	Cb
Pot Pies: *Per Serving*			
Beef, 7 oz	330	25	38
Chicken, 7 oz	195	23	35
Chicken & Broccoli, 7 oz	350	20	32
Macaroni & Cheese, 6.5 oz	210	5	34
Turkey, 7 oz	370	21	38
Sandwich Toppers: *Per Serving*			
Chipped Beef, 4 oz	105	6	6
Salisbury Steak, 5 oz	200	16	6
Sliced Beef, 4 oz	70	2	5
Turkey, 5 oz	155	11	6
The Hearty One: Beef Enchilada	520	16	73
Boneless Pork Rib Dinner	720	38	62
Fried Chicken Dinner	910	55	70
Salisbury Steak Dinner	780	54	47
Turkey Dinner	630	10	57
Chicken Fried Beef Steak	820	50	63
Veal Parmigiana Meal	360	19	35
Big Wings: Firehouse, 1.5 oz pce	100	7	0.5
Smokehouse BBQ, 1.5 oz pce	100	7	2

Banquet (Cont) | C | F | Cb

	C	F	Cb
Frozen Meals			
Beef Patty w. Country Style Veg	265	15	22
Beef Enchilada, 11 oz	380	12	54
Boneless Pork Rib	400	19	39
Chicken Finger	570	30	57
Chicken Fried Chicken, 10 oz	305	20	21
Chicken Primigiana	290	15	27
Corn Dog Meal, 7.5 oz	485	19	68
Country Chicken, 6 oz	380	13	55
Country Fried Pork	430	24	40
Fettuccine & Meatballs	280	7	42
Fish Stick Meal, 7.3 oz	300	20	58
Fried Rice w. Chicken & Egg Roll	315	9	46
Italian Pasta, 6 oz	370	16	46
Lasagna w. Meat Sauce, 11 oz	325	9	46
Macaroni & Cheese, 12 oz	415	14	57
Macaroni & Beef	310	8	44
Mexican Meal	445	20	56
Mexican Style Enchilada Combo	370	11	55
Our Original Fried Chicken	470	27	35
Pot Roast	215	8	21
Pork Cutlet, 10.25 oz	410	25	38
Roasted Honey Turkey Meal, 9 oz	270	12	29
Salisbury Steak Mea, 9.5 oz	400	25	28
Spaghetti & Meatballs, 10.5 oz	440	20	43
Swedish Meatballs, 10.25 oz	390	19	33
Turkey & Gravy w. Dressing Meal	280	10	34
Turkey Mostly White Meat	290	10	34
White Meat Fried Chicken	470	28	40
Homestyle Bakes			
Beef Chili w. Beans & Cornbread	385	11	57
Beef Stew & Biscuits, 9 oz	315	10	44
Cheesy Ham & Hashbrowns, 7 oz	60	2.5	8
Chicken & Dumplings, 8.3 oz	255	9	32
Creamy Turkey & Stuffing, 8.3 oz	260	17	29
Tuna Macaroni & Cheese, 8.5 oz	415	20	44
Turkey Tetrazzini, 5.6 oz	280	12	34

Birds Eye – Voila!

Per Cup, Cooked (2 Cups Frozen)

	C	F	Cb
Chicken Voila!: Garden Herb	310	15	28
Alfredo; 3-Cheese Chicken	230	8	26
Italian Pesto; Teriyaki	240	9	24
Zesty Garlic Chicken	270	11	28
Steak Voila! Beef Sirloin/Potato	240	9	26
Turkey Voila! Turkey w. Potato	200	6	24
Birds Eye Hearty Spoonfuls Soup Bowls: *See Page 84*			

Boca (Vegetarian) | C | F | Cb

	C	F	Cb
Breakfast: Links (2), 1.6 oz	80	4	6
Organic, Links (2), 1.6 oz	85	3	6
Burgers: Chseburger, patty, 2.5 oz	135	4.5	8
All American Flame Grilled, 2.5 oz	115	4	6
Grilled Vegetable, 2.5 oz	85	1	6
Meatless Ground, 1/2 cup, 2 oz	75	0.5	6
Roasted Garlic/Onion, 2.5 oz	100	2	7
Vegan, Original, 2.5 oz	80	1	6
Organic All Amer. Classic, 2.5 oz	140	5	9
Garden Vegetable, 2.5 oz	130	3.5	9
Meatless Ground, 1/2 cup, 2 oz	75	0.5	7
Roasted Garlic/Onion, 2.5 oz	125	3	10
Vegan, Original, 2.5 oz	105	2	9
Chik'n: Nuggets (4), 3.1 oz	190	7	16
Patties: Breakfast, 1.3 oz	70	4	5
Chik'n, 2.5 oz	155	6	12
Organic: Breakfast, 1.3 oz	75	2.5	5
Chik'n/Spicy Chik'n, 2.5 oz	155	6	12
Pizza: avg. all types, 1/3	260	8	30
Sausages: Bratwurst, 2.5 oz	120	7	3
Italian, 2.5 oz	125	6	6
Organic: Bratwurst, 2.5 oz	125	6	6
Italian, 2.5 oz	140	7	7
Meatless Ground, 2 oz	75	0.5	6
Smoked, 2.5 oz	120	5	7

Budget Gourmet

Classics: *Per Serving*

	C	F	Cb
Chinese Style Vege & White Chkn	250	6	40
Fettucini Alfredo w. Four Chses	310	11	49
Lasagna Mozzarella	280	8	39
Macaroni & Chse w. Cheddar	240	5	39
Pasta Primavera Parmesan, 8 oz	240	6	39
Spaghetti Marinara	280	5	49
Spicy Szechuan Vege & Chicken	280	9	41
Stir Fry Rice & Vegetables	350	16	45
Ziti Parmesano	230	7	36
Lean Gourmet: Cheese Lasagna	230	5	36
Macaroni & Cheese, 10 oz	305	5	51
Salisbury Steak w. Pot. & Gravy	205	7	23
Santa Fe Style Rice & Beans	340	9	56
Shrimp w. Pasta & Veges, 8 oz	255	6	37
Spaghetti & Meat Sauce, 9 oz	275	5	45
Swedish Meatballs, 9 oz	290	7	40
Premium: Beef Stroganoff	240	6	32
Beef Pepper Steak w. Rice	260	4	44
Chicken w. Fettuccine	340	14	40
Fettuccine Primavera w. Chkn	230	7	30
Glazed Turkey w. Stuff. & Pot.	250	10	33
Mandarin Chicken, 8.5 oz	270	6	4

Budget Gourmet (Cont)

	C	F	Cb
Premium (Cont):			
Orange Glazed Chicken	300	3.5	55
Pepper Steak w. Rice	260	4	44
Three Cheese Lasagna	450	16	53
Bowls: Cheese Stuffed Rigatoni	345	9	52
Grilled Chicken Caesar	300	4.5	45
Shrimp Fried Rice	430	7	76
Spicy Beef & Broccoli	380	3	78
Sweet & Sour/Teriyaki Chicken	420	4	82
Vegetables & White Chicken	370	9	59

Cascadian Farm

	C	F	Cb
Bowls: Pasta Primavera	280	8	41
Country Herb Chkn w. Veg Rice	250	3.5	38
Orange Dijon Veggie & Chicken	245	3	42
Schechuan Rice Veggie	210	1.5	45
Teriyaki Rice Veggie	270	7	44
Thai Style Veggie & Chicken	260	6	42
Entrees: Chicken Fettuccine	380	12	43
Chicken Enchiladas	395	15	44
Macaroni and Cheese	385	11	55
Penne Marinara	265	5	50
Spinach Lasagne, 11 oz	330	10	39

Celentano

See Rosina Presents Celentano ~ Page 70

Claim Jumper

	C	F	Cb
Meals: Baby Back Pork Ribs (3)	215	14	8
Buffalo Wings (2)	155	9	5
Chicken Pot Pie, 1/2 pie, 8 oz	565	39	37
Country Fried Beef Steak (1)	945	58	80
Country Fried Chicken, 19 oz	710	24	86
Lasagna w. Meat Sauce, 8 oz	275	13	22
Rst Turkey Brst w. Gravy & Dressing	540	23	51
Spicy Chicken Tenderloins, 3 oz	180	7	17
Turkey Pot Pie, 1/2 pie, 8 oz	575	41	35
Sauce: Hot Sauce, 15mL	0	0	0

Croissant Pockets

	C	F	Cb
Italian Style Chicken Melt	380	20	37
Egg, Sausage & Cheese	350	18	34
Ham & Cheddar	340	16	36
Pepperoni Pizza	370	19	40
Philly Steak & Cheese	360	20	34

Dwight Yoakam

	C	F	Cb
Bakersfield Biscuits: *Includes 1/4 Cup Gravy*			
Buttermilk Biscuits, 2.1 oz	190	9	22
and Beef/Chicken Stew	240	11	24
and Country Style Gravy	230	12	25
and Sausage Gravy	250	14	26
with Beef Chilli	260	14	24

El Monterey

	C	F	Cb
Family Classics: *Per Serving*			
Burritos: Chicken Fajita, 5 oz	250	6	40
Egg, Bacon, Chse & Salsa, 4.5 oz	270	12	33
Monterey Supreme, 5 oz	290	10	37
Sausage Breakfast, 4.5 oz	290	14	31
Steak Fajita, 5 oz	250	6	40
Ultimate Chicken, 5 oz	290	9	40
Chimichangas: Beef & Chse, 5 oz	310	13	35
Chicken & Cheese, 5 oz	320	13	38
Taquitos: Beef & Cheese, 4.5 oz	330	15	36
Chicken & Cheese, 4.5 oz	310	13	36
Egg, Bacon, Chse & Salsa, 4.5 oz	290	11	38
Tacos: Soft Beef & Cheese, 5.5 oz	440	23	42
Spicy Chicken, 5.5 oz	320	9	46
Spicy Beef & Cheese, 5.5 oz	420	21	40
Enchiladas: Beef w. Sce, 4.5 oz	180	9	17
Cheese w. Sauce, 4.5 oz	210	13	15
Chicken w. Sauce, 4.5 oz	190	10	18
Tamales: Beef, 4.5oz	230	10	26
Chicken, 4.5 oz	250	11	27
Regular Meals: *Per Serving*			
Burritos: Beef & Bean (Reg./Green Chili/Spicy Red),			
5 oz Size	370	17	42
8 oz Size	580	27	68
10 oz Size	730	34	85
Bean & Cheese, 8 oz Size	470	14	70
Chicken, 4 oz	210	6	32
Tamales: Chicken, 4.5 oz	250	11	27
Beef, 4.5 oz	300	19	24

Empire Kosher

	C	F	Cb
Express Meal: Chicken Fajita (1)	130	2.5	15
Chicken w. Pasta, 1 cup	140	2	17
Chicken Stir-Fry, 1 cup	160	2.5	20
Pierogies: Potato Cheese, 5.3 oz	250	4	44
Potato Onion, 5.3 oz	245	4	47
Pies: Chicken Pie, 8 oz	440	21	41
Turkey Pie, 8 oz	470	23	45
Blintzes: Cheese (2)	200	6	29
Blueberry (2)	190	4	36
Potato Pancakes: Mini (12), 3 oz	150	7	19

Frozen Entrees & Meals (Cont)

Ethnic Gourmet

	C	F	Cb
Meals: Chicken Biryani, 12 oz	340	9	52
Chicken Korma, 11 oz	335	10	38
Eggplant Bhartha, 12 oz	295	9	46
Kung Pao Chicken Rice Bowl, 12 oz	340	6	56
Palak Paneer, 12 oz	420	20	42
Shrimp Fried Rice, 11 oz	400	10	64
Teriyaki Chicken, 11 oz	360	5	66
Vegetable Korma, 12 oz	320	9	52
Vegetarian Teriyaki, 12 oz	350	3	73
Thai Chef: Peanut Satay Chicken	400	14	50
Thai Sweet & Sour Veges, 12 oz	340	5	70
Vegetarian Chicken, 11 oz	390	11	61
Lemongrass & Basil Chkn, 11 oz	390	10	55
Taj: Bean Masala; Channa Bhaji	360	10	57
Shahi Paneer, 12 oz	400	15	59
Tofu Samosa, 6 oz	160	5	23
Ethnic Wraps: Vege Paneer, 8 oz	320	10	50
Chicken Tikka Masala, 8 oz	320	7	47

Fisher Boy

	C	F	Cb
Quik Stix, 6 sticks, 3 oz	200	11	16
Quik Bake Crunchy Fish Portions, 2 portions, 3.2 oz	200	10	19
Fish Rings, 7 rings, 3.2 oz	230	12	20
Salmon Fillet, 1 piece, 3.8 oz	100	2.5	1

Foster Farms

	C	F	Cb
Corn Dogs (1), 2.6 oz	200	9	24

GardenBurger (Vegetarian)

	C	F	Cb
Breakfast Saus., 1 patty, 1.5 oz (43g)	50	3.5	2
Classic Hamburger Style, 2.5 oz	90	1	8
Garden Vegan, 1 patty	110	1	17
Classic Hamburger Style, 2.5 oz	90	1	8
Savory Portabello, 1 pce	120	2.5	18
The Original, 2.5 oz	110	3	16
Meatless: Meatballs, 6 balls (25g)	110	4.5	8
Riblets w. BBQ Sce., 5 oz (142g)	210	5	10
Flame Grilled: Hamburger Style	120	4	7
Chik'n Grill, 2.5 oz	100	2.5	5
Gourmet Style: Santa Fe, 2.5 oz	130	2.5	20
Fire Roasted Vege, 2.5 oz	120	2.5	18
Veggie Medley, 2.5 oz	90	0	18

Gorton's

	C	F	Cb
Crunchy Fish Fillets: *Per Fillet*			
Breaded: Lemon Pepper	135	9	9
Garlic & Herb; Hot & Spicy	125	7	10
Grilled: It. Herb; Lemon Pepper	130	6	2
Cajun Blackened; Lemon Butter	120	6	1
Battered: Parmesan, 1 fillet	130	7.5	10
Plain; Garlic & Herb, 1 fillet	125	6.5	11
Lemon Pepper, 1 fillet	135	9	9
Homestyle Baked: Au Gratin, 4.6 oz	230	12	14
Primavera, 1 fillet, 4.6 oz	120	5	4
Grilled Fillets: Garlic Butter (1)	100	3	1
Caesar Parmesan, 3.8 oz fillet	100	3	0.5
Cajun Blackened (1) 3.8 oz fillet	100	3	1
Lemon Butter/Pepper (1) 3.8 oz	100	3	0.5
Shrimp Bowl: Alfredo, 1 bowl	290	5	49
Fried Rice, 1 bowl	320	2	65
Garlic Butter, 1 bowl	280	5	46
Primavera, 1 bowl	270	6	41
Teriyaki, 1 bowl	320	6	57
Fish Portions, 1 portion, 2 1/2 oz	170	11	12
Fish Sticks, Breaded, 6, 3 oz	120	12	17
Popcorn Shrimp, 20 shrimp, 3 oz	240	12	26
Skillet Fillets, Traditional, 3.7 oz	200	11	14
Tenders: Extra Chunky, 3 1/2 pcs	260	12	29
Original, 3 1/2 pieces, 4 oz	260	15	22

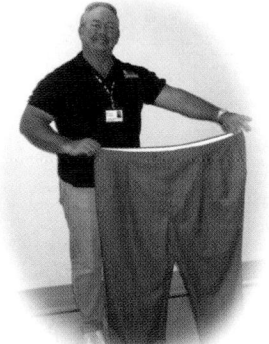

Butch Costello says:
"Take it one day at a time, inch by inch!"
Meet Butch online at: www.CalorieKing.com

Green Giant | C | F | Cb

Create A Meal: *Prepared with Meat & Oil (Prepared Wt. ~ Approx 10 oz)*
Oven Roasted:

	C	F	Cb
Garlic Herb Chicken, 1³/4 cup	350	9	35
Lemon Pepper Chicken, 1²/3 c.	310	8	30
Parmesan Herb Chicken, 1³/4 c.	340	11	29

Pasta Creations: *Per Cup (Prepared)*

	C	F	Cb
Creamy Cheddar	250	8	36
Garlic	260	10	36

Stir Fry: Beef & Broccoli, 1¹/3 cup

	C	F	Cb
Beef & Broccoli, 1¹/3 cup	290	13	15
Garlic & Ginger, 1¹/2 cup	270	7	25
Lo Mein, 1¹/4 cup	320	7	33
Sweet & Sour, 1¹/4 cup	340	7	43
Szechuan, 1¹/4 cup	310	14	20
Teriyaki, 1¹/4 cup	230	6	18

Complete Skillet Meal!:
Per 1¹/4 Cups (¹/4 Package, Prepared)

	C	F	Cb
Beef Stew	180	3.5	27
Chicken Alfredo/& Cheesy Pasta	270	7	39
Chicken Lo Mein; Garlic Chkn Pasta	250	7	30
Chicken Noodle	290	6	45
Chicken Teriyaki	250	1.5	45
Sweet & Sour Chicken	320	1.5	62

Health is Wealth

	C	F	Cb
Buffalo Wings, Meatless 2.2 oz	100	1.5	11
Chicken: Nuggets (4) 3 oz	150	6	9
Chicken Free (3) 2.25 oz	90	1	11
Patties (1) 3 oz	150	6	9
Chicken Free (1) 3 oz	120	1.5	15
Tenders (3) 3 oz	130	3	11
Munchies, average (2) 1 oz	60	1.5	10
Egg Rolls: Oriental Veg. (1) 3 oz	160	4	23
Oriental Chicken Free (1)	120	4	21
Spinach (1) 3 oz	180	8	20
Spring Rolls, 2 pce, 1.6 oz	70	2	10

Healthy Choice

Mixed Grills: *Per Serving*

	C	F	Cb
Chicken: w. Ginger Dipping Sce	450	9	59
w. BBQ/Honey Dipping Sce	390	9	46
w. Roasted Garlic Tomato Sce	420	9	47
w. Roasted Red Pepper	390	10	39
Steak: w. Teriyaki Dipping Sce	450	10	62
w. Zesty Dipping Sce	340	10	37

Bowl Creations: Beef Broccoli

	C	F	Cb
Beef Broccoli	300	8	50
Chicken Teriyaki w. Rice	300	6	45

Healthy Choice (Cont)

Duos: *Per Serving*

	C	F	Cb
Grilled Chick. Brst & Pasta	240	6	26
Grilled Chicken Breast w. Potato	200	7	21
Breaded Chicken & Mac. Chse	270	5	35
Sirloin Beef Tips & Mushr. Rice	270	6	35
Salisbury Steak & Mashed Pot.	210	6	21
Turkey Breast w. Potatoes	200	5	19

Medleys: Beef Teriyaki

	C	F	Cb
Beef Teriyaki	330	7	46
Chicken Breast w. Veg. & Pasta	230	5	29
Chicken Carbonara	310	7	39
Country Glazed Chicken	250	5	29
Mandarin Chicken	280	3.5	43
Oriental Style Chicken	240	5	28
Roast Turkey Breast	230	6	25
Sesame Chicken	240	6	35

Solos: Beef Macaroni

	C	F	Cb
Beef Macaroni	220	8	25
Cheese Rice & Chicken	230	4	33
Chicken Enchilada	310	7	46

Dinners: Beef Pot Roast

	C	F	Cb
Beef Pot Roast	330	9	40
Beef Tips Portabello	310	8	28
Blackened Chicken	310	6	36
Boneless Beef Ribs w. BBQ Sce	360	9	47
Chicken Enchilada	270	7	44
Chicken Parmigiana	310	9	40
Chicken Teriyaki w. Rice	270	6	37
Herb Baked Fish	360	8	55
Lemon Pepper Fish	320	7	50
Meatloaf	330	9	36
Mesquite Beef w. BBQ Sauce	320	9	47
Roasted Chicken Breast	230	8	32
Salisbury Steak	330	9	45
Sweet & Sour Chicken	350	7	54

Hot Pockets | *Per Pocket (¹/2 Pkg)*

	C	F	Cb
Barbecue Sce w. Beef; Chseburger	340	12	46
Beef Taco	320	13	37
Chkn Melt; Pepperoni & Saus. Pizza	360	18	39
Four Cheese Pizza, 1 pce	380	17	45
Italian Style Meat Trio	390	21	39
Pepperoni Pizza	360	17	41
Philly Steak & Cheese, 1 pce	280	7	42
3-Cheese & Chicken Quesadilla	300	10	38
Turkey & Ham w. Cheese	330	14	41
Croissant: 5 Cheese Pizza	400	23	36
Meatballs & Mozzarella	330	18	32
Pot Pie Express: Chicken	340	18	36
Chicken & Broccoli	350	17	40

Frozen Entrees & Meals (Cont)

José Olé

	C	F	Cb
Mexi Minis: *Per Serving*			
Beef & Cheese, 4 pce, 3 oz	200	10	23
Beef Steak Fajita Bowl, 12 oz	330	11	37
Cheese Mini Burrito, 3 pce, 3 oz	200	8	27
Chicken & Cheese, 4 pce, 3 oz	140	4.5	20
Chicken & Cheese Rolled Tacos	270	10	33
Chicken Monterey, 1 pce, 5 oz	320	7	47
Grilled Chkn Quesadilla (3) 3.4 oz	220	8	27
Shredded Beef Taquitos (3) 3 oz	160	5	24
Chimichanga: Chicken (1) 5 oz	330	12	45
Shredded Beef, 1 pce, 5 oz	400	19	43
Flour Tortilla Taquitos, avg.	200	8	24
Wraps: Chkn/Steak Fajita, 1 pce	340	10	46
Steak & Cheese, 1 pce, 5.3 oz	340	12	42
Chicken & Cheese, 1 pce, 5.3 oz	330	11	40

Kid Cuisine

	C	F	Cb
Cheese Pizza	410	10	70
Chicken Nuggets	500	24	54
Fried Chicken	600	38	41
Fun Nuggets	390	18	46
Macaroni & Cheese	380	13	54
Parachuting Pork Ribettes, 7.55 oz	380	15	43
Pepperoni Pizza	610	22	88
Taco Roll-Up, 7.35 oz	360	13	50

Kroger Fish Portions

	C	F	Cb
Batter Dipt, 2 pieces, 4 oz	260	14	22
Crispy Crunchy, 2 pieces, 4 oz	270	18	18

NOTICE
THIS IS AN
EQUAL
OPPORTUNITY
KITCHEN

Lean Cuisine

	C	F	Cb
Bowls: Chicken Teriyaki	330	2.5	59
Creamy Chicken & Vegetables	390	7	57
Grilled Chicken Caesar	290	7	36
Three Cheese Stuffed Rigatoni	300	8	44
Everyday Favorites:			
Cheese Ravioli	260	7	38
Angel Hair Pasta	240	4	43
Chicken Enchilada Suiza w. Rice	280	5	48
Fettucini Alfredo; Mac & Chse	280	7	41
Grilled Chicken w. Penne Pasta	250	5	29
Lasagna w. Meat Sauce	300	8	41
Macaroni & Beef, 9.5 oz	260	4	35
Rstd Chkn w. Lemon Fettucine	250	7	32
Santa Fe Rice; Spag. w. Meat Sce	300	5	52
Stuffed Cabbage, 9.5 oz	210	5	26
Swedish Meatballs w. Pasta	290	7	35
Teriyaki Stir-Fry, 10 oz	290	4	46
Cafe Classics:			
Baked Chicken	240	4.5	33
Baked Fish, 9 oz	290	6	40
Beef Portabello, 9 oz	220	7	24
Beef Pot Roast, 9 oz	190	6	19
Cheese Lasagna w. Chicken Brst	270	8	27
Chicken in Peanut Sauce	260	6	32
Chicken Piccata	270	7	40
Chicken & Vegetables	250	5	33
Chicken w. Basil Cream Sauce	290	7	37
Glazed Chicken w. Veg. Rice	230	5	25
Herb Roasted Chicken	200	3.5	24
Honey Roasted Pork, 9.5 oz	240	5	31
MeatLoaf w. Whipped Potatoes	260	7	28
Roasted Turkey Breast, 9.75 oz	270	2	49
Salisbury Steak	290	9	26
Sesame Chicken, 9 oz	355	8	55
Sweet & Sr/Teriyaki Chkn, avg.	320	3	54
Thai Style Chicken	270	5	39
Skillet Sensations: Chkn Alfredo	320	7	42
Chicken Primavera	310	4.5	49
Garlic Chicken	350	6	54
Herb Chicken & Rst. Potatoes	270	4.5	38
Other varieties, avg	290	4	50
Dinner Selections: Salisbury Steak	360	9	42
Beef Steak Tips Dijon, 12 oz	315	8	41
Grilled Chicken w. Penne Pasta	360	7	47
Roasted Chicken/w. Mushrooms	370	5	57

Lean Pockets
	C	**F**	**Cb**
BBQ Sauce w. Beef	290	7	48
Cheeseburger; Chicken Parmigiana	290	7	45
Chicken Fajita	260	7	38
Ham & Cheddar, 1 pce	280	7	42
Meatballs & Mozzarella	280	7	44
Pepperoni Pizza	290	7	42
Philly Steak & Cheese, 1 pce	280	7	42
Sausage & Pepperoni Pizza	280	7	41
Steak Fajita	240	7	22
Turkey/Broccoli/Cheese	270	7	39

Lightlife ~ Vegetarian
Meatless 'Lightburgers', 2.5 oz	120	2.5	12
Smart Deli Slices, 3 slices, 1 1/2 oz	50	0	2
Smart Dogs, 1 link, 1 1/2 oz	45	0	1
Tofu Pups, 1 link, 1 1/2 oz	60	2.5	2
Wonderdogs, 1 1/2 oz	55	1	1

Linda McCartney
Frozen Entrees: Per Serving
Southwestern Style Rice & Beans	340	12	46
Vegetable Burrito w. Spanish Rice	430	18	51
Vegetable Lasagna, 11.5 oz	350	13	42

Loma Linda (Vegetarian)
Chik Nuggets, 5 pieces, 3 oz	240	15	13
Corn Dogs, 1 link	150	4	22

"I got the idea while down at the bank."

ENGLEMAN.

Louis Kemp
	C	**F**	**Cb**
Crab Delights, Surimi, 1/2 c., 2.5 oz	80	0	10
Teriyaki Beef	240	2	5

Marie Callender's
Meals & Dinners: Per Serving
Beef Salsbury Steak & Gravy, 14 oz	480	23	40
Beef Stew w. Corn Bread	430	9	69
Beef Stroganoff	410	19	30
Beef Tips in Mushroom Sce, 13.6 oz	360	12	37
Breaded Fish w. Mac & Cheese	400	16	36
Cheesy Chicken w. Rice	470	20	39
Cheesy Rice Chick. Broccoli, 12 oz	390	13	44
Chicken Cordon Bleu, 1 dinner	490	23	38
Chicken Fried Beef Steak	640	41	46
Chicken Parmigiana, 1 dinner	680	34	63
Chicken Teriyaki	420	35	72
Chili/Cornbread	480	21	49
Chunky Chicken & Noodle, 1 meal	650	36	54
Country Fried Chick. & Gvy,1 din.	660	34	63
Country Fried Pork Chop, 1 dinner	620	36	50
Fettuccini w. Chkn & Broccoli, 13 oz	720	43	49
Grilled Chkn: & Mashed Pot., 15 oz	455	26	28
Tenderloins, 14 oz	425	19	36
S.W. Style w. Rice & Corn, 14 oz	430	11	50
Grilled Chicken Breast w. Pasta	570	21	64
Ham Steak w. Macar. & Chse, 1 din.	410	13	43
Herb Rstd Chicken & Mash. Pot.	530	35	19
Homestyle Chicken & Dumplings	540	30	46
Lasagna Bake	470	15	52
Lasagna w. Meat Sauce, 1 cup	270	12	25
Mac & Cheese	340	13	39
Meatloaf & Gravy w. Mashed Pot.	510	30	34
Roast Beef w. Mashed Potato	370	18	27
Spaghetti & Meat Sauce, 17 oz	680	22	90
Stuffed Pasta Medley	470	19	53
Swedish Meatballs	560	25	56
Sweet & Sour Chicken, 1 dinner	520	16	73
3 Cheese Ravioli, 16 oz	620	17	93
Turkey w. Gravy/dress., 1 dinner	390	16	33
Pot Pies: Beef	510	32	40
Cheesy Chicken, 8 oz	565	36	44
Chicken, 1 pie, 9.5 oz	630	38	53
Chicken Au Gratin, 1 cup	560	37	41
Creamy Mushroom & Chkn, 8 oz	550	35	43
Turkey, 1 cup	500	31	40

Frozen Entrees & Meals (Cont)

Michelina's

	C	F	Cb
Black Bean & Chili w. Rice, 8 oz	300	4	58
Chicken a la King	280	8	39
Fettucine Alfredo	390	16	45
Four Cheese Lasagna, 8 oz	290	7	42
Lasagna w. Meat Sce, 8 oz	240	7	29
Linguini w. Clams & Sauce	290	3	52
Macaroni Cheese	430	16	50
Meatloaf, Gravy, Mashed Potato	340	23	20
Noodles Stroganoff w. Beef, 8 oz	340	14	38
Noodles w. Chicken, 8 oz	300	10	40
Penne Pasta w. Mushroom Sce	280	8	41
Penne Pollo	290	8	39
Pepper Steak & Rice	260	4.5	46
Risotto Parmigiana	460	21	50
Salisbury Steak	330	21	21
Spaghetti & Meatballs	300	8	43
Spaghetti Marinara, 8 oz	250	2.5	46
Spaghetti w. Tomato Basil Sce	250	3	46
Standard Mac & Cheese	340	13	21
Swedish Meatball Egg Noodles	360	13	45
Yu Sing: Chicken Fried Rice	360	8	58
Chicken Lo Mein	220	3.5	34
Roasted Garlic Chicken	220	3.5	34
Sweet & Sour Chicken w. Rice	340	4	67
Teriyaki Beef	240	2	51

Mrs Paul's

	C	F	Cb
Battered: Fish Sticks, 6	240	11	13
Fish Portions, 2	280	17	22
Batter Dipped, Fish Sticks, 2	330	17	28
Crispy Crunchy: Fish Sticks, 5	200	14	20
Fish Fillets, 2	250	13	11
Breaded Fish Portions, 2	240	12	20
Crunchy Batter: Fish Fillets, 2	280	13	23
Flounder Fillets, 2	260	14	24
Haddock Fillets, 2	250	12	25
Healthy Treasures:			
Fish Sticks, breaded, 4 sticks	140	6	14
Fish Cakes (2) 4 oz	190	7	24
Light Seafood Entrees: Fish Dijon	200	5	17
Fish Florentine	220	8	10
Fish Mornay	230	10	12

Nancy's

	C	F	Cb
Quiche: Florentine (1)	440	26	35
Lorraine; Monterey (1) average	480	29	34

Natural Touch (Vegetarian)

Per Serving	C	F	Cb
Breakfast Pattie, 1	75	3	4
Classic Burger (2) 2 oz	160	7	10
Corn Dogs (1) 2½ oz	175	6	22
Lentil Rice Loaf, 1" slice, 3 oz	160	7	16
Nine Bean Loaf, 1" slice, 3 oz	155	8	13
Okara Pattie, 1 pattie, 2¼ oz	120	5	6
Roasted Herb Chik'n, 1 fillet	110	2.5	9
Tex Mex Burger, 1 pattie (67g)	120	1.5	17
Thai Burger, 1 pattie (67g)	100	3.5	7
Vegan Burger, 1 pattie, 2½ oz	100	2	8
Veggie Medley, 1 pattie (64g)	125	4	11
Zesty Tomato Basil Burger	130	6	7

Oberweis Dairy

Cafe Italia: *Per Serving*	C	F	Cb
Cheese Lasagna, 6.7 oz	330	14	34
Dip N Bread, 2 oz	190	7	19
Italian Beef w. Gravy, 6.9 oz	430	36	1
Italian Sausage & Green Peppers	265	18	7
Meat Lasagna	335	12	36
Ravioli w. Cheese	400	14	49
Veggie Rotolo, 1 slice	245	13	18
Chickadee Farms			
Boneless Chkn Brst Roast, 5 oz	255	9	12
Boneless Pork Chop	220	6	15
Boneless Turkey Brst Roast, 5 oz	210	4	10
Chicken Cordon Bleu	270	13	9
Italian Style Meatloaf	245	14	9

Old El Paso

Burrito: Bean & Cheese	C	F	Cb
Bean & Cheese	300	9	44
Beef & Bean	320	10	47
Pizza, all types	250	9	30
Chimichanga, all types	350	18	38

Ore-Ida | C | F | Cb

Bagel Bites: *Per 4 Pieces (3 oz)*
3 Cheese; Cheese & Pepperoni	200	6	28
5 Cheese	190	7	24
Cheese, Sausage & Pepperoni	200	6	27

Blasts: *Per 6 Pieces (3 oz)*
3 Cheese; Chse, Saus. & Pepperoni	200	5	25
Pepperoni & Cheese	220	7	25

Deep Dish Minis: *Per 2 Pieces*
Pepperoni & Cheese, 3.5 oz	280	12	26
Chse, Saus. & Pepperoni, 3.6 oz	260	10	27

Lil' Calzones: Sausage, Pepperoni
& Cheese, 2.8 oz	200	6	22
Tater Dogs, 4 pce, 2.8 oz	240	15	16

Ortega | | | |

Beef Taco Filling, 1/3 cup, 2 oz	100	6	4
Beef Enchilada, 9.3 oz pkt	430	21	45
Cheese Enchilada, 9 3/4 oz pkt	390	17	47
Chicken Enchilada, 9 1/2 oz pkt	380	16	46

Fiesta Dips: *Per 1/4 cup (11 oz Pkg)*
4 Layer Dip	80	3.5	8
Nacho Beef	60	7	4
Nacho Chicken	80	5	4
Salsa & Beef	50	2	4

Skillet Fajitas: Steak, 1/2 c., 2 oz
	35	1	3
Chicken, 3/4 cup, 2 1/2 oz	45	1	4
Nachos Ckn Supreme, 1/2 pkt	380	11	49

Bowls: Chicken Santa Fe, 1 bowl
	420	9	63
Pepper Jack Grilled Chicken (1)	480	16	60
Cheddar Rice & Grilled Chkn (1)	450	14	59

Pita | | | |

Broccoli & Cheese Pie, 1/4 pie	380	25	31
Cheese & Spinach Pie, 1/4 pie	370	23	32

Poppers | | | |

Cheese Sticks Mozzarella (1) 1 oz	90	4.5	8
Stuffed Jalapenos Cr. Chse (5) 5 oz	370	23	34

PopStickers | | | |

Chinese Dumplings: w. Vegetable Filling
13 Dumplings, 8 oz	330	45	61

w. Vegetable & Chicken Filling
13 Dumplings, 8 oz	320	5	51

Puck's | C | F | Cb

Breaded Chkn Parmagiana, 12 oz	540	21	58
Chicken & Spinach Pasta Wrap	460	11	68
Chicken Bolognese & Spaghetti	480	22	48
Chicken Pappardelle	460	18	47
Eggplant Parmesan	370	28	14
4 Cheese Lasagna; Meat Lasagna	490	22	51
4 Cheese Macaroni	610	33	51
Italian Sausage Pasta Wrap	700	29	67
Meatloaf in Wine Sauce	560	32	36
Mushroom & Spinach Ravioli	260	18	54
Mushroom Lasagna/Tortellini	440	17	53
Penne Pasta w. Beef & Vege	410	18	38
Radiatore Pasta Primavera	310	10	41
Spicy Chicken Lasagna	470	21	45

Quorn | | | |

Vegetarian Meals: *Per Serving*
Turkey Style Roast, 90g	115	2.5	8
Garlic & Herb Ckn-Style Cutlets (1)	190	8	20
Fettuccine Alfredo, 300g	370	16	40
Lasagna, 300g	370	12	43
Nuggets, 3-4 pieces, 85g	175	8	18
Patties, 75g each	145	7	12
Tenders, 1 cup, 85g	100	2	8
Grounds, 2/3 cup, 85g	100	2.5	5

Feedback Welcome

Please contact the author with comments and suggestions.

Write to: Allan Borushek
PO Box 1616 Costa Mesa CA 92627
email: allan@calorieking.com

Frozen Entrees & Meals (Cont)

Rosina | C | F | Cb
Meatballs: *Per Serving (3 oz)*

	C	F	Cb
Homestyle; Italian Style Sausage	280	23	5
Italian Style	245	19	5
Italian Style Turkey	170	9	7
Swedish Style	255	19	9

Rosina Presents Celentano
Entree: *Per Serving*

Eggplant Parmigiana, 10 oz	485	35	30
Eggplant Rolletts, 10 oz	340	17	38
Lasagna w. Cheese, 7 oz	270	12	29
Lasagna w. Light Cheese, 10 oz	275	5	45
Manicotti: 10 oz	320	14	35
Light Florentine, 10 oz	240	6	35
Light, 10 oz	260	6	39
Meatballs, regular, 2.3 oz	295	23	6
Pasta: Cavatelli, regular, 5.3 oz	270	1	55
Manicotti, Stuffed Cheese, 7 oz	300	11	32
Ravioli: Light, Stuffd Chse, 4.3 oz	240	3	42
Stuffed Beef Round, 5 oz	255	5	38
Stuffed Cheese, 4.3 oz	260	6	40
Stuffed Cheese, Mini, 4 oz	215	4	36
Stuffed Cheese, Round, 4.3 oz	235	4.5	38
Stuffed Shell: 10 oz	305	15	31
Light, 10 oz	225	6	32
Light Broccoli, 10 oz	230	5	30
Tortellini: Stuffed Cheese, 5 oz	285	4	59
Stuffed Meat, Round, 5 oz	300	6	48

Safeway Select
Gourmet Club Meals: *Per Serving*

Bacon Wrapped Sirloin Tip Fillets	350	27	0
Beef Meatloaf	180	9	9
Beef Sirloin Tip Fillets: w. Blk Pepper	210	8	5
w. Teriyaki Glaze	250	9	3
Beef Tamales w. Sauce	240	12	22
Beer Battered Cod Fillets	160	7	13
Boneless Pork Shoulder Ribs	180	7	9
Cheese Enchiladas w. Mole Sauce	200	11	22
Chicken Breasts	230	12	13
Chicken Enchiladas	180	12	13
Chicken Fried Steak w. Gravy	330	12	27
Chicken Strips	230	13	11
Chili Pot Roast	160	5	8
Deluxe Chicken Pot Pie	480	28	36
Extra Lean Steakhouse Beef Patties	130	5	1

Safeway Select (Cont)
Gourmet Club Meals (Cont):

	C	F	Cb
Fillet of Sole	190	10	18
Jumbo Chicken Wings BBQ Style	200	14	6
Low Fat Chicken Fillets, average	130	2	6
Low Fat Turkey Lasagna	300	3	48
Macaroni & Cheese	350	18	30
Meat Lasagna	290	11	30
Mexican Style Lasagna	390	22	26
Peppercorn Glazed Beef Kabobs	120	1	4
Pork Carnitas, Rice & Salsa	470	20	53
Pot Roast & Vegetables	210	6	15
Roasted Garlic Mashed Potatoes	190	10	22
Seasoned Boneless Beef Strips	120	2.5	13
Southwestern Quesadilla	280	15	21
Southwestern Wraps	260	12	26
Stuffed Baked Potatoes, 1 potato	280	11	35
St Louis Style Pork Spareribs	370	23	17
Tamale Bake	400	23	32
Vegetable Lasagna, 1 lasagna	310	17	27
Vegetable Quesadilla	330	15	33
w. Lemon Butter	120	2.5	5
Stir Fry: Chicken Fajita	130	2	14
Ginger Beef	310	17	22
Pork Fried Rice	330	17	32
Sesame Pork	410	21	28
Shrimp Fried Rice	300	13	33
Sweet & Sour Pork	250	3.5	42
Szechuan Chicken	250	11	28
Teriyaki Beef	190	3	28
Vegetable Potstickers	250	10	36

SeaPak

Crunchy Clam Strips, 5 oz pkt	410	2.5	41
Popcorn Fish, 7 pces, 3 oz	240	11	23
Popcorn Shrimp, 15 pces, 3 oz	210	12	18

Seeds of Change
Per Bowl (11 oz)

Bowtie Primavera	380	12	51
Creamy Spinach Lasagna	370	16	36
Macaroni & Cheese	420	16	52
Mushroom Wild Pilaf	350	16	40
Penne Marinara	290	7	44
Seven Grain Pilaf	390	14	52
Spicy Peanut Noodles	370	12	53
Teriyaki Stir-Fried Rice	340	8	56

Frozen Entrees & Meals (Cont)

Skyline Chili

	C	F	Cb
Original Chili, 1 cup	310	20	5
Chili & Beans, 1 cup	350	1	63
Chili & Spaghetti, 1 cup	340	13	37
Coney Calzonies (1)	340	17	33

SoyBoy (Vegetarian)

	C	F	Cb
Breakfast Links, 1 link, 1 oz	65	2.5	6
5-Grain Tempeh	135	6	9
Not Dogs, 1 link, 1.5 oz	95	3	10
Ravioli Rosa/Verde, 1 cup, 3.5 oz	180	3	29
Okra Courage Burgers, 1	130	5	8
Soy Tempeh, 3 oz	150	6	9
Tofu Ravioli, 1 cup, 3.5 oz	180	3	31

Stouffer's

	C	F	Cb
Entrees: Beef, Rst Pot. & Peppers	300	6	44
Creamed Chipped Beef	175	13	10
Lasagna w. Meat Sce, 10 1/2 oz	370	14	35
Macaroni & Beef w. Tomatoes	350	12	41
Macaroni & Cheese, 1 cup, 8 oz	335	16	33
Maxaroni, Macaroni & Cheese	395	17	44
Roasted Garlic Chicken	320	11	39
Spaghetti w. Meat Sauce	350	15	56
Stuffed Pepper, 10 oz	240	12	24
Swedish Meatballs w. Pasta	520	25	49
Tuna Noodle Casserole	360	16	36
Turkey Tetrazzini	400	19	36
Vegetable & Chicken Pasta Bake	380	17	40
Yankee Pot Roast	320	9	41
Family Style Recipes: Per Serving			
Chicken Cordon Bleu Pasta, 1/4	360	15	35
Grandma's Chkn & Vege Bake	360	15	36
Lasagna w. Meat Sce, 1/12 pkg	265	10	28
Macaroni & Cheese, 1 cup	370	18	37
Meatloaf in Gravy, 1 loaf, 5.5 oz	220	13	10
Oven Sensations			
Baked Chicken, 12 oz	415	14	46
Beef, Rstd Potatoes & Peppers	300	7	40
Chicken & Dumplings, 12 oz	370	13	40
Chkn, Stuffing & Gravy, 10.5 oz	395	13	47
Yankee Pot Roast, 12 oz	310	9	39
Italian Style: 3 Cheese Manicotti	335	13	39
Cheese Stuffed Rigatoni, 8.2 oz	475	22	51
Italian Sausage Stuffed Rigatoni	375	16	41
Rigatoni Pasta w. Chicken, 8.3 oz	430	16	47
Roasted Chicken Ravioli, 8.2 oz	360	13	42

Stouffer's (Cont)

	C	F	Cb
Homestyle Dinners: Per Serving			
Baked Chicken, 14 oz	260	8	55
Beef Pot Roast, 16 oz	250	14	43
Chicken Brst Tenders & Potatoes	465	24	40
Chicken Fettucini, 10.5 oz	350	14	34
Country Fried Beef Steak, 16 oz	675	37	60
Grilled Lime Chicken, 14 oz	485	13	67
Meatloaf, 17 oz	360	32	38
Monterey Chicken, 14.25 oz	575	21	68
Pork & Roasted Potatoes	400	14	62
Roast Turkey Breast, 16 oz	460	16	55
Roasted Beef & Gravy, 14 oz	405	16	41
Salisbury Steak, 16 oz	550	27	49
Veal Parmigiana, 17.5 oz	485	17	56
Hearty Portion: Fried Chkn, 15 oz	520	16	66
Pork w. Roast Potatoes, 15 oz	570	15	75
Homestyle: Per Serving			
Baked Chicken in Gravy w. Pot.	260	11	18
Beef Stroganoff, 9.75 oz	350	15	37
Breaded Boneless Pork Cutlet	370	20	34
Chkn Breast Tenders in BBQ Sauce	525	27	47
Chicken Monterey, 14.2 oz	575	21	68
Chicken Parmigiana, 12 oz	455	17	53
Fish Fillet w. Mac Cheese, 9 oz	410	16	44
Fried Chicken Breast	400	17	34
Green Pepper Steak, 10.5 oz	270	6	33
Roast Turkey Breast, 9.6 oz	310	14	27
Roasted Pork, 9.5 oz	400	18	46
Veal Parmigiana, 11.6 oz	410	17	49
Skillet Sensations: Per Bowl			
Beef Stroganoff, 10 oz	355	11	44
Broccoli & Beef	295	5	46
Homestyle Beef	360	15	37
Homestyle Chicken	390	9	43
Savory Chicken & Rice, 10 oz	285	4	44
Teriyaki Chicken, 12.5 oz	340	2.5	40
Slowfire Classics: Beef Stew, 11 oz	290	12	24
Cheesy Pizzatini, 12 oz	410	18	47
Chicken Minestrone Stew, 12 oz	260	6	30
Homestyle Chicken & Noodles	380	14	39
Steak & Mushroom, 11 oz	310	12	35
Side Dishes: Per Serving			
Corn Souffle	170	7	21
Cheddar Potato Bake, 1/2 cup	250	15	21
Creamed Spinach, 4.5 oz	135	20	8
Harvest Apples	210	4	43
Spinach Souffle	150	8	10

Frozen Entrees & Meals (Cont)

Swanson

	C	F	Cb
Standard Meal: Fish 'N Chips	470	22	52
Boneless White Meat Fr. Chkn	450	18	50
Breaded Fish fillet, 10 oz	405	15	51
Chicken Teriyaki (Original)	430	7	71
Chicken Teriyaki (Standard)	340	7	49
Classic Fried Chicken, 11 1/2 oz	640	36	41
Grilled Glazed Turkey Medallions	380	11	45
Grilled White Meat Chkn w.Penne	310	11	31
Mexican Style Fiesta, 13.25 oz	470	16	63
Rstd Carved Turkey Brst, 11 3/4 oz	420	18	44
Salisbury Steak	470	19	33
Turkey Breast w. Stuffing & Gravy	420	15	39
Hungry Man Dinners: Mexican	690	27	87
Boneless Pork Rib	840	39	99
Boneless White Meat Fried Chkn	640	24	72
Buffalo Chicken Strips	870	28	106
Classic Fried Chicken, 16 1/2 oz	790	40	75
Meatloaf Angus Beef	560	25	52
Mexican Style Fiesta	710	29	87
Salisbury Steak	470	19	33
Turkey Breast	630	20	82
Sports Grill: Per Serving			
Beer Battered Chkn & Fries	665	26	63
Chkn Quesadilla & Potato Skins	765	35	72
Pulled Pork w. BBQ Sauce			
in Flatbrd & Chse Fries, 16 oz	810	44	96
Steak House: Per Serving (20 oz)			
Grilled: BBQ Chicken	875	28	116
Beef Steak Strips	580	16	75
Smothered Chicken	595	24	56
Pot Pie: Per Serving			
Flaky Crust Chicken Pot Pie	380	21	38
Flaky Crust Turkey Pot Pie	370	20	36

TGI Friday's

	C	F	Cb
Buffalo Wings (3)	175	13	2
Honey BBQ Wings (3)	165	10	7
Chicken Quesadilla Rolls	250	11	26
Honey BBQ Wings	180	10	7
Mozzarella Sticks & Sce, 1 Serve	120	6	15
Potato Skins, 3 pc, 2.8 oz	210	11	19
South West. Egg Rolls, 1 pce 3 oz	190	9	20
Quesadilla Rolls: Chicken (2)	245	11	26
Steak (2)	215	11	21
Sides: Spinach, 2 Tbsp (1 oz)	50	3.5	2

Tyson

	C	F	Cb
Buffalo Style Chkn Strips (2), 3 oz	190	9	17

Uncle Ben's

	C	F	Cb
Breakfast Bowls: Bacon/Egg/Pot.	290	13	26
Egg, Cheese & Salsa, 7.5 oz	310	21	16
French Toast & Sausage, 6 oz	420	22	45
Pancakes: Apple Cinnamon, 6 oz	330	8	59
Blueberry Pancakes & Bacon	380	9	66
Buttermilk Pancakes & Sausage	375	9	63
Peach & Pecan, 6 oz	300	7	54
Sausage, Egg & Biscuit	350	20	31
Chef's Recipe: Per Cup (Prepared)			
Caribbean Black Beans & Rice	210	1	43
Chicken & Harvest Vege Pilaf	195	1	41
Fine Herb/Mushroom Risotto	190	0	44
Southwestern Pinto Beans & Rice	215	1	44
Spicy Cajun Beans & Rice	210	0.5	44
Traditional Red Beans & Rice	220	2	43
Chili Bowl: Chili w. Beans & Rice	360	7	48
Country Inn: Per Cup (Prepared)			
Broccoli Rice au Gratin	205	2	43
Chkn & Broc./Mexican Fiesta Rice	200	1	43
Chicken & Vegetable Rice	200	1.5	42
Three Cheese Rice	205	2.5	41
Other varieties, average	195	0.5	44
Mexican Style Bowl, avg., 12 oz	350	5	54
Mini Bowl: Sizzlin' Saus. Pizzeria	320	12	36
Natural Select: Per Cup (Cooked)			
Average all varieties, 2 oz	195	1	42
Noodle Bowls: Honey Ging. Chkn	430	5	69
Spicy Peanut Chicken	400	11	53
Spicy Thai Style Chicken	400	8	60
Pasta Bowls: Chicken & Bowties	295	7	35
Lasagna varieties, avg., 12 oz	330	7	42
Parmesan Shrimp Penne, 12 oz	390	7	58
Three Cheese Ravioli, 12 oz	365	7	55
Rice Bowls: Per 12 oz (340g)			
Cajun Style Chicken & Sausage	365	7	56
Chicken Fried Rice	420	7	65
Chicken & Vegetable	350	4.5	56
Honey Dijon Chicken	400	3.5	73
Spicy Beef & Broccoli	375	4.5	62
Sweet & Sour Chicken	355	3	61
Szechuan Chicken	360	4	58
Teriyaki Chicken	375	3.5	66
Turkey, Stir Fry Vegetable	355	3	74

Van De Kamp's

	C	F	Cb
Fish Sticks, Breaded, 6 stix, 4 oz	290	17	23
Battered Fillets, 2.6 oz fillet	180	11	12
Crispy Fish Fillets, 1 pce, 2.6 oz	160	8	15
Crisp & Healthy: Breaded,			
1 fillet, 1.8 oz	85	1.5	12
Grilled: Barbecue Tuna (1) 1.8 oz	100	0.5	5
Breaded Butterfly Shrimp (7) 4 oz	300	14	32
Creamy Dill Salmon (1)	90	2.5	1
Italian Herb (1) 4 oz	130	6	2
Lemon Pepper (1) 3.6 oz	130	6	0
Sesame Teriyaki Tuna (1)	110	1.5	4

Wampler Foods

Turkey Burger, Seasoned (1) 4 oz	230	12	0

White Castle

Cheese Burger, Microwaveable,			
1 pkg, 3.7 oz	310	17	23

Weight Watchers

Smart Ones: Per Meal

3 Cheese Ziti Marinara	290	7	47
Chicken Enchiladas Suiza, 9 oz	280	8	38
Chicken Mirabella	180	2	30
Chicken Oriental	230	4.5	34
Chicken Stir Fry Bowl	300	6	45
Fettucini Alfredo w. Broc., 9.25 oz	270	6	39
Fiesta Chicken, 8.5 oz	210	2	35
Grilled Salisbury Steak	260	6	25
Lasagna Bolognese	270	7	38
Lasagna Florentine, 10.5 oz	290	8	36
Lemon Herb Chicken Piccata	250	5	36
Mac. & Chse; Lasagna Bolognese	240	2.5	45
Ravioli Florentine, 8.5 oz	220	2	43
Santa Fe Style Rice & Beans, 10 oz	300	8	49
Southwestern Style Chkn Bowl	230	2.5	35
Spaghetti Marinara, 9 oz	280	7	46
Spicy Penne Mediterranean	260	6	40
Spicy Szechuan Veg. & Chicken	230	5	34
Swedish Meatballs, 9 oz	280	7	34
Teriyaki Chicken & Veg Bowl	280	3	48
Tuna Noodle Gratin	240	2.5	43
Smartwiches: Ham & Cheddar	260	7	36
Average other varieties	265	7	38

Weight Watchers (Cont)

Smart Ones Bistro Selections:

	C	F	Cb
Basil Chicken	270	6	34
Chicken Parmesan	300	5	32
Chicken Tenderloins w. BBQ Sce	300	8	30
Fajita Chicken Supreme	280	7	33
Fire-Grilled Chkn & Vegetables	280	5	40
Golden Baked Garlic Chicken	280	6	40
Meat Loaf w. Gravy & Potatoes	260	8	22
Peppercorn Beef Fillet	230	8	24
Rst Chkn w. Sour Crm & Chives	190	3.5	23
Slow Roasted Turkey Breast	220	7	20
Thai Style Chkn & Rice Noodles	290	4	39

Worthington (Vegetarian)

Bolono, 3 slices, 2 oz (57g)	80	3.5	2
Chicken Roll, 1 slices, 2 oz	90	4.5	2
Chicken, Diced, 1/4 cup, 2 oz	60	0	2
Chic-Ketts, 2 slices (3/8"), 55g	120	7	2
ChikStiks, 1 piece, 1 1/2 oz	110	7	3
Choplets, 2 slices, 92g	90	1.5	3
FriChik, 2 pieces, 3 oz	140	8	3
Low Fat FriChik, 2 pcs, 3 oz	80	3	2.5
FriPats, 1 pattie	130	6	4
Prosage Links, 2 links	60	2.5	2
Prosage Patties, 1 pattie, 38g	80	3	3
Stripples, 2 strips, 1/2 oz	60	4.5	2
Veja-Links, 1 link	40	1.5	1

ZonePerfect

Meals: Per Tray

Beef Jardiniere, 13.4 oz	340	10	36
Beef Lenti, 14.1 oz	375	12	39
Chicken Dijon, 14.1 oz	390	12	42
Chicken Gumbo, 14.5 oz	390	12	42
Salmon & Vegetables, 14.2 oz	430	17	41
Vegetarian Chili, 13.5 oz	390	12	42

> *In eating, one third of the stomach should be filled with food, one third with drink, and the rest left empty.*
>
> ~ Gitten, the Talmud

Frozen Pizzas

Frozen Pizzas	C	F	Cb
Amy's: Per $1/3$ Pizza			
Cheese; Spinach; Pesto	300	12	38
Roasted Vegetable, 4 oz	270	8	43
Soy Cheese; Veggie Combo, avg.	280	10	37
Mushroom & Olive	250	9	33
Bake to Rise			
Four Cheese, $1/6$	330	13	39
Pepperoni, $1/6$	350	15	39
Special Deluxe, $1/6$	360	15	40
California Pizza Kitchen			
Large: BBQ Chicken, $1/6$	310	9	38
Five Cheese, $1/6$, 4.5 oz	350	15	35
Thai Chicken, $1/6$, 4.5 oz	310	11	38
Small: BBQ Chicken, $1/3$	280	9	33
Garlic Chicken, $1/3$	290	12	30
Five Cheese & Tomato, $1/3$	320	15	29
Portobello Mixed Mushr., $1/2$	350	12	45
Rosemary Chicken Potato, $1/3$	290	11	35
Thai Chicken, $1/3$	290	10	33
Saus., Pepperoni & Mushr., $1/3$	290	13	30
Celeste			
Pizza For One: Cheese, 1 pizza	390	19	42
Deluxe	440	23	42
Original Four Cheese	430	21	40
Pepperoni	420	23	39
Sausage & Pepperoni; Suprema	500	28	44
Zesty Chicken Supreme	360	16	40
Connie's Pizza			
Super, $1/6$ pizza, 4.5 oz	260	14	22
Thin Crust, Sausage, $1/5$	290	15	24
Di Giorno			
Rising Crust (Large): Per $1/6$ Pizza			
Four Cheese	320	11	40
Pepperoni/& Sausage	360	16	40
Spicy Chicken Supreme	320	10	40
Spinach, Mushr. & Garlic; Vege	300	9	41
Supreme	370	15	41
Rising Crust (Small): Per $1/3$ Pizza			
Four Cheese	270	9	34
Pepperoni	310	14	35
Sausage & Pepperoni	320	14	35
Spicy Chicken Supreme	280	9	35
Spinach, Mushr. & Garlic; Vege	260	8	36
Supreme	330	14	35

Di Giorno (Cont)	C	F	Cb
Deep Dish: Four Cheese, $1/8$	320	11	40
Supreme, $1/8$	310	17	25
Pepperoni, $1/6$	390	22	32
Cheese Stuffed Crust: Chse, $1/6$	340	14	35
Pepperoni, $1/6$	390	20	35
Sausage & Pepperoni, $1/6$	360	16	39
Half & Half (Supreme/Pepperoni):			
Supreme, $1/6$ pizza, 5.8 oz	410	20	41
Pepperoni, $1/6$, 5.4 oz	400	19	40
Ellio's (McCain)			
Cheese, 1 slice	160	5	22
Freschetta			
Bake & Rise (Large): 4 Cheese, $1/5$	390	16	46
4 Meat, $1/6$	350	15	40
Pepperoni, $1/6$	360	17	38
Special Delux, $1/6$	370	16	40
Supreme, $1/6$	370	17	39
Vegetable Primavera, $1/6$	310	11	40
Brick Oven: Per $1/4$ Pizza			
3 Cheese & Bacon	320	14	35
5 Italian Cheese	330	14	36
Classic Supreme	370	17	38
Italian Style Pepperoni	410	22	37
Portabello Mushroom & Spinach	290	10	38
Southwest Style Chicken	340	14	38
Sauces Stuffed Crust: 4 Chse, $1/5$	320	11	41
Sausage & Pepperoni, $1/5$	350	15	41
Supreme, $1/5$	360	15	42
Supreme w. Grilled Vege, $1/6$	310	13	37
Small Pizzas: Pepperoni, $1/2$	440	20	47
Rstd Garlic Chicken, $1/2$	370	12	49
Mozzarella & Basil, $1/2$	370	15	46
Southwest Chkn Supreme, $1/2$	350	12	47
Healthy Choice: French Bread Pizza			
Solos: Cheese; Pepperoni, 6 oz	340	5	50
Sausage	345	5	55
Supreme, 6.35 oz	330	5	51
Vegetable, 6 oz	280	4	44
Heaven's Bistro: Per $1/3$ Pizza			
BBQ Chicken Pizza	270	2	48
Chicken Sausage Pizza	250	3	42
Pepperoni Pizza	250	2	42
Three Cheese Pizza	240	2	42
Veggie Pizza	230	1	42

	C	F	Cb
Home Run Inn			
Large: Cheese, 1/8 pizza	290	15	27
Sausage, 1/8 pizza	310	16	27
Small: Cheese, 1/6 pizza	260	13	26
Sausage, 1/6 pizza	280	14	26
Jack's (Kraft)			
Original: Cheese, 1/3 pizza	330	13	38
Sausage/Pepperoni, 1/4 pizza	310	16	29
Jaclyn's Not Even 1 Gram Fat Pizza			
1 slice, 4 oz	200	1	34
Jewel: Cheese, 1/3 pizza	310	11	40
Pepperoni, 1/4 pizza	290	13	32
Supreme, 1/4 pizza	320	15	32
Lean Cuisine: French Bread Pizza			
Cheese, 6 oz	340	8	46
Deluxe, 6 1/8 oz	330	9	44
Pepperoni, 5 1/4 oz	300	7	44
Mr. P's Pizza: Cheese Pizza	410	11	58
Combination (Saus./Pepp.), 1	460	17	58
Mystic: Cheese, 1/3 pizza	360	15	36
House Special, 1/3 pizza	375	17	36
Pepperoni, 1/3 pizza	380	18	36
Oberweis Pizzas (12"): *Per 1/6 Pizza*			
Cheese; Spinach	270	8	37
Pepperoni; Sausage	305	11	37
Single Pizzas: Cheese	270	8	37
Deluxe, 5 oz	315	12	37
Stuffed Sausage, 4 1/2 oz	305	11	37
Stuffed Spinach, 4 1/2 oz	270	8	37
Old Italian (Microwaveable Little Pizza)			
Party (1) 4.2 oz	340	15	40
Pepperoni (1) 4.2 oz	350	16	41
Puck (Wolfgang)			
Large: 4 Cheese & Pesto, 1/4	440	23	38
Barbecue Style Chicken, 1/5	310	13	30
Italian Sausage & Pepperoni, 1/4	410	20	36
Small: BBQ Chicken, 1/2	330	13	32
Primavera Vegetable, 1/2	300	13	30
Spicy Grilled Chicken, 1/2	380	18	35
Thai Style Chicken, 1/2	390	18	36
Vegetable Provencal, 1/2	270	8	36

	C	F	Cb
Ralphs			
Large (Self-Rising Crust):			
Four Cheese, 1/6 pizza	330	10	48
Pepperoni, 1/6	390	15	49
Supreme, 1/6	390	15	49
Small: Cheese, 1 pizza	440	11	62
Combination, 1 pizza	520	20	61
Pepperoni, 1 pizza	510	19	62
Red Baron			
Bacon Scramble, 1 pizza	400	22	33
Bake To Rise: 4 Cheese, 1/6	330	13	39
Pepperoni, Special Deluxe, 1/6	360	15	40
Classic (Large): 4 Cheese, 1/4	420	23	36
Pepperoni, 1/4 pizza	440	26	36
Sausage & Pepperoni, 1/5	360	21	29
Supreme, Special Deluxe, 1/5	350	20	30
Deep Dish Pan Style:			
4 Cheese, 1/3 pizza	370	17	39
Pepperoni; Meat Trio, avg., 1/3	400	21	39
Supreme, 1/3 pizza	410	21	40
Deep Dish Singles: 4 Cheese, 1	440	23	41
Pepperoni, 1 pizza	460	25	41
Cheese; Meat Trio, avg., 1 pizza	420	21	42
Special Deluxe, 1 pizza	430	24	40
Supreme, 1 pizza	470	27	40
Vegetable Supreme, 1 pizza	400	19	42
Deep Dish Mini Pizzas: Cheese, 8	380	15	44
Pepperoni, 8 pizzas	400	20	41
Sausage & Pepperoni, 8 pizzas	420	20	41
Supreme, 8 pizzas	430	23	43
Pizzeria Style, avg. all types, 1/3	380	16	44
Stuffed Pizza Slices: *Per Portion*			
Ital. Saus. & Pepperoni; Supreme	340	16	33
Rstd Garlic Chicken	290	10	35
5 Cheese & Tomato	320	15	34
Reggio's			
Family Size: Cheese, 1/6 pizza	320	12	38
Sausage, 1/6 pizza	330	12	38
Dinner Size: Cheese, 1/4 pizza	330	12	41
Pepperoni & Sausage, 1/4	400	18	41
Sausage, 1/4	380	16	41
Stop & Shop			
Single Serving: Cheese, 1	390	19	42
9 Slices: Cheese, 2 slices	350	10	49

Frozen Pizzas (Cont)

Stouffer's French Bread Pizzas	C	F	Cb
Cheese, 1 piece (1/2 pkg)	370	16	43
Deluxe, 1 piece	420	19	50
Extra Cheese, 1 piece	400	16	49
Pepperoni, 1 piece	410	20	47
Sausage, 1 piece	420	21	49
Three Meat, 1 piece	460	22	50
White Cheese/Garlic/Herbs, 1 pce	460	23	45

The Old City Cafe

	C	F	Cb
Mushroom Pizza, 1/4, 92g	165	3	28
Pizza De Deluxe, 1/4, 103g	195	3	29

Tombstone

Original Pizza, 12 inch: Per Serving

	C	F	Cb
Canadian Style Bacon, 1/4 pizza	350	14	36
Deluxe; Hamburger, 1/5 pizza	310	15	29
Extra Cheese, 1/4 pizza	350	15	35
Pepperoni, 1/4 pizza	380	19	37
Sausage& Mushroom, 1/5 pizza	300	14	29
Saus. & Pepperoni, Supreme, 1/5	320	16	29
Supreme, 1/4	300	12	38

Original Pizza, 9 inch: Per Serving

	C	F	Cb
Extra Cheese, 1/2 pizza	380	16	40
Deluxe; Hamburger; Sausage, 1/3	280	13	27
Pepperoni& Sausage, 1/3 pizza	300	15	27
Supreme, 1/3 pizza	310	16	27

Thin Crust Pizza: Per Slice

	C	F	Cb
Four Meat Combo, 1/4 pizza	380	23	26
Italian Sausage, 1/4 pizza	370	22	26
Pepperoni, 1/4 pizza	400	25	25
Supreme, 1/4 pizza	380	22	26
Supreme Taco, 1/4 pizza	370	23	27
Three Cheese, 1/4 pizza	360	21	25

Oven Rising Crust Pizza: Per Slice

	C	F	Cb
Italian Sausage; Supreme, 1/6 pizza	320	13	35
Pepperoni; Three Meat, 1/6 pizza	340	14	34
Three Cheese, 1/6 pizza	320	13	34

Mexican Style Pizza, Large: Per Serving

	C	F	Cb
Chse Quesadilla, 1/3 pizza	365	17	37
Chicken Fajita, 1/4 pizza	300	14	29
Nacho Grande, 1/4 pizza	380	17	37

For One Pizza: Per Whole Pizza

	C	F	Cb
Extra Cheese	520	28	41
Pepperoni; Supreme	550	32	41

Tombstone (Cont)

Double Top Pizza: Per Slice

	C	F	Cb
Pepperoni/& Sausage, 1/6 pizza	340	19	25
Sausage, slice, 1/6 pizza	320	17	25
Supreme, slice, 1/6 pizza	330	18	25
Two Cheese, slice, 1/5 pizza	380	19	29

For One, 1/2 Less Fat, Pizza: Per Whole Pizza

	C	F	Cb
Cheese; Vegetable, average	360	10	45

Tony's

Original: Cheese, 1/3 pizza

	C	F	Cb
Cheese, 1/3 pizza	390	22	33
Pepperoni, 1/3 pizza	410	22	37
Sausage & Pepperoni, 1/3 pizza	420	23	38
Sausage, 1/3 pizza	440	27	34
Supreme, 1/3 pizza	420	22	39

Thin Crust: Cheese, 1/3 pizza

	C	F	Cb
Cheese, 1/3 pizza	290	12	31
Sausage, 1/3 pizza	330	16	32
Sausage & Pepperoni, 1/3 pizza	350	18	33
Supreme, 1/3 pizza	340	17	33

Super Rise: 4 Cheese, 1/4 pizza

	C	F	Cb
4 Cheese, 1/4 pizza	340	13	40
Sausage, 1/4 pizza	380	18	41

Totino's

Crisp Crust Party Pizza: Per 1/2 Pizza

	C	F	Cb
Cheese	320	14	34
Pepperoni; Supreme	380	21	35

Verdi (Safeway Select)

Self-Rising Crust (Large): Per Serving

	C	F	Cb
Meat Magnifico, 1/6 pizza	370	15	41
Primo Pepperoni, 1/6	370	15	42
Quatro Formaggio, 1/6	300	9	41
Supremo Classico, 1/8 pizza	280	12	32

Self-Rising Crust (Small): Per Serving

	C	F	Cb
Rstd Mushr. & Garlic, 1/3 pizza	230	7	33
Primo Pepperoni, 1/3	300	13	32
Roasted Vegetable Speciale, 1/3	240	7	33
Supremo Classico, 1/3 pizza	300	13	33

Weight Watchers (Smart Ones): Per Pizza

	C	F	Cb
BBQ-Style Chicken, 7.5 oz	395	7	65
Four Cheese, 6.5 oz	400	7	65
Pepperoni, 7 oz	400	9	58
Veggie Ultimate, 7.7 oz	405	5	39

> '...and could you please cut the pizza into only 6 pieces - I couldn't possibly eat 8!'

B & M	C	F	Cb
Baked Beans: *Per 1/2 Cup (4 1/2 oz)*			
Bacon & Onion w. Brown Sugar	190	2	36
Baked Beans w. Pork	180	2	33
Barbeque	170	1	33
Maple Flavored Baked Beans	150	1	28

Banquet			
Homestyle Bakes: *Per Serving (Prepared)*			
BBQ Baked Beans & Chkn, 7.2 oz	350	7	58
Beef Chili w. Beans & Cornbrd	365	11	57
Beef & Sour Cream Sauce, 7 oz	380	11	54
Cheezy Ham & Hashbrns, 5.2 oz	290	15	30
Chicken & Dumplings, 7.8 oz	250	9	32
Chicken, Mashed Pot. & Biscuit	370	15	50
Creamy Chkn & Biscuits, 7.4 oz	340	16	40
Pizza Pasta, 6.1 oz	300	7	44
Tuna Mac & Cheese, 7.7 oz	420	20	44
Turkey Tetrazzini, 5.8 oz	280	12	34

Betty Crocker			
Potato Bakes: *Per Serving (Prepared As Directed)*			
Cheesy Scalloped; Au Gratin	150	6	21
Other varieties, average	125	4	22
Complete Meals: *Per Serving (1/5 Box)*			
Chicken & Buttermilk Biscuits	320	13	41
Chicken Fettuccini Alfredo	310	11	38
Ham & Au Gratin Potatoes	300	13	37
Herb Stuffing & Turkey	250	7	38
Homestyle Chkn & Dumplings	250	9	33
Lasagna Bake	240	8	35
Oven Favorites: *Per Serving (Prep. As Directed)*			
Chicken Helper: Pot. Au Gratin	280	10	29
Cheddar & Mozz; Crmy Chicken	320	12	30
Homestyle Chicken	310	8	38
Hamburger Helper: Lasagna	290	11	30
Italian Parmesan Bake	470	19	53
Meat Loaf & Mashed Potatoes	360	19	30
Pork Helper, Pork Chops & Potato	340	18	28
Tuna Helper, Classic Casserole	260	9	35
Hamburger Helper: *Per Serving (Prep. As Directed)*			
Cheesy Baked Potato	320	15	28
Four Cheese Lasagna	330	15	27
Cheeseburger Macaroni	350	16	31
Cheesy Enchilada	370	15	27
Other varieties, average	300	13	27
Tuna Helper: *Per Serving (Prep. As Directed)*			
Creamy Parmesan	260	9	32
Other varieties, average	300	13	33

Betty Crocker (Cont)	C	F	Cb
Pork Helper: *Per Serving (Prep. As Directed)*			
Pork Chops & Stuffing	320	2	23
Pork Fried Rice	340	0.5	24
Chicken Helper: *Per Serving (Prep. As Directed)*			
Homestyle Chicken & Dumpling	290	10	27
Chicken & Potatoes Au Gratin	270	7	25
Fettuccini Alfredo	300	8	27
Suddenly Salad: *Prepared*			
Caesar, 1/2 cup dry	170	1	34
Classic, 3/4 cup	250	8	38
Ranch & Bacon, 3/4 cup	330	20	30
Rstd Garlic & Parmesan, 3/4 cup	260	11	33

Bush's: *Per 1/2 Cup*			
Refried Beans: Traditional	150	3	24
Fat Free	130	0	24
Chili Beans	120	1	20
Baked Beans: Vegetarian	130	0	24
Other flavors, avg.	160	1	30

Campbell's: *Per 1/2 Cup (4 1/2 oz)*			
Barbecue; Old Fashioned Beans	170	2.5	29
Brown Sugar & Bacon Beans	170	3	29
New England Beans	180	3	32
Pork & Beans in Tomato Sauce	130	2	24
Supper Bakes: *Per 1/6 Box (Prepared As Directed)*			
Cheesy Chicken	310	10	26
Savory Pork Chops	380	18	31
Southwestern Style Chicken	280	7	29
Other varieties, avg.	340	7	43

Cedarlane (Vegetarian)			
Bruschetta, Pesto, Mozz., Tom., (1)	100	5	10
Burrito, Beans, Rice, Chse, (1) 6 oz	260	1	48
Eggplant Parmesan, 1/2 pkg, 5 oz	190	8	16
Enchilada: Garden Vege, (1) 4.8 oz	140	3	20
Three-Layer Pie, 1/2 pkg, 5.5 oz	215	7	27
Focaccia: Tomato & Basil, 1/3 loaf	275	9	33
Mediterranean Stuff., 1/3 loaf	296	10	37
Lasagne: Cheese, 1/2 ctn, 5 oz	190	6	22
Garden Vege, 1/2 ctn, 5 oz	180	3	26
Mini Bistro Pizza (3) 4 oz	280	15	27
Rice Bowl: Teriyaki Vege, 10 oz	460	6	86
Szechuan Vege, 10 oz pkg	440	6	80
Wrap: Vege "Ham" & Cheese, 6 oz	350	10	36

Canned & Packaged Meals (Cont)

Chef Boyardee	C	F	Cb
Beefaroni, all types, 1 cup	260	9	35
Cheesy Burger: Ravioli, 1 cup	300	7	48
Macaroni, 1 cup	220	6	32
Deep Dish Meals (Per 1/2 Package)			
Cheese Lover's Lasagna	290	14	38
5 Chse Ravioli; Chsy Burger Mac	270	12	39
Pepperoni & Sausage Rotini	250	9	41
Microwave Cups: Beef Ravioli	190	3.5	28
Beef Ravioli & Meatballs	240	9	32
Pasta Shells & Meatballs	240	11	27
Other varieties, average	220	6	33
Homestyle (15 oz Can): Per Cup (9 oz)			
Cannelloni	240	6	36
Cheese Tortellini in Tom. Sce	280	3	56
Chicken Alfredo w. Pasta	250	12	24
Dinosaurs w. M'balls in Tom. Sce	290	11	39
Rigatoni	250	10	31
Rotini in Tomato Sce	260	7	40
Mini Bites (14.75 oz Can): Per Cup			
Mini Beef Ravioli w. Meatballs	300	13	36
Mini Pasta Shells w. Meatballs	270	12	32
Mini Spaghetti w. Meatballs	280	13	31
Jumbo (15 oz Can): Per Cup			
99% Fat Free: Beef Ravioli	190	1.5	37
Cheese Ravioli	240	2.5	45
Lasagna	270	10	36
Mini Ravioli	240	7	35
Spaghetti w. Jumbo Meatballs	280	13	30
Overstuffed Ital. Sausage Ravioli	280	4	50
Twistaroni: Cheesy Nacho, 1 cup	250	6	40
Chili Cheese Dog, 1 cup	220	7	30
Tomato & Beef, 1 cup	280	13	31

Dennison's Chili (15 oz Can): Per Cup	C	F	Cb
Chili Con Carne With Beans:			
Original; Hot, 1 cup	350	15	36
Chunky, Hot & Chunky	320	12	32
Micro Cup, 7.5 oz bowl	290	13	26
99% Fat Free: Beef Chili w. Beans	220	2	27
Turkey Chili w. Beans	210	3	29

Dinty Moore (Hormel Foods)	C	F	Cb
1 1/2 lb Can: Beef Stew, 1 cup	230	14	16
7 1/2 oz Can: Beef Stew	190	10	15
American Classics: Per Microwave Bowl (10 oz)			
Beef Pot Roast	200	3	19
Beef Stew	250	11	22
Chicken w. Mashed Potatoes	230	5	27
Noodles & Chicken	250	8	28
Microwave Cup:			
Beef Stew, 1 cup	160	7	16
Corned Beef Hash, 1 cup	350	22	19
Chicken & Dumplings	190	6	24
Other varieties, average	240	13	19

Dr. McDougall's			
Per Cup			
Pasta w. Beans, Mediterranean	180	1	29
Pinto Beans & Rice, Sthwestern	190	2	38
Ramen Noodles; Chicken; Beef	140	1	39
Rice & Pasta Pilaf	210	1	36
Tamale Pie w. Baked Chips	200	1.5	39

Eden			
Per 1/2 Cup (4 1/2 oz)			
Baked Beans w. Sorghum, Mustard	150	0	27
Black Soy Beans	90	1.5	9
Lentils w. Onion, Bay Leaf	90	0	13
Refried Black/Pinto/Kid. Beans, avg.	110	1.5	18
Refried Black Soy & Black Beans	90	3	13
Other varieties, average	125	0	21

Fantastic			
Per Packet			
Cup Meals: Cajun Rice & Beans	230	3	46
Bombay Curry Rice & Beans	250	1.5	52
Cha-Cha Chili	220	1	37
Creamy Broccoli Cheese	160	3	26
Spicy Jamaican	250	1.5	52
Tex Mex Rice & Beans	240	2.5	48
Vegetarian Chili	160	1	27
Couscous: Black Bean Salsa	240	1.5	46
Creole Vegetable	220	1.5	41
Noodles, average	140	1	27

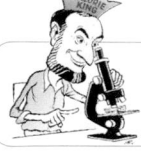

*F*or full nutritional data and product updates
check the database of the author's website
www.CalorieKing.com

Franco-American: *Per Cup*	C	F	Cb
Spaghetti in Tom. Sce w. Cheese	210	2	41
Spaghetti O's: w. Tom. Sce & Cheese			
A to Z's; Plus Calcium	180	1	36
w. Meat Sauce	170	2	31
w. Sliced Franks	240	10	30
Meatballs in Tomato Sce, avg.	265	9	33

Health Valley (Vegetarian)
Fat-Free Beans & Chili:

	C	F	Cb
Chili in a Cup, all types, 3/4 cup	120	1	21
Honey Baked Beans, 1/2 cup	110	0	25
Vegetarian/Chili, 1/2 cup	160	1	30
Turkey w. Chili Beans, 1/2 cup	220	3	34
Other varieties, 1/2 cup	80	0	15
Meal Cups, average all varieties	140	1	27

Hormel: *Per Cup*

	C	F	Cb
Kid's Kitchen: Beans 'N Wieners	310	13	37
Beefy Macaroni	190	6	23
Cheezy Mac 'N Beef	260	7	34
Cheezy Mac 'N Cheese	260	11	30
Cheezy Mac 'N Franks	300	16	26
Mini Beef Ravioli	240	7	34
Spaghetti & Mini Meatballs	230	9	26
Spaghetti Rings & Franks	240	9	32
Noodle Rings & Chicken	150	5	16
Microwave Cup: Chili w. Beans	220	6	27
Chili no Beans	190	8	15
Lasagna w. Meat Sauce	210	6	29
Scalloped Potatoes & Ham	240	14	20
Spaghetti w. Meat Sce	220	7	31
Chili (15 oz Can): *Per Cup*			
With Beans: Homestyle Chili	330	19	24
Reg./Hot/Chunky/Less sodium	270	7	34
Turkey (99% Fat Free)	200	3	26
Vegetarian (99% Fat Free)	200	1	38
Without Beans: Hot/Chili, 1 cup	210	9	17
Turkey No Beans	190	3	17
Tamales (15 oz Can), 2 Tamales	140	7	15

Hy Top: *Per Serving*

	C	F	Cb
Deluxe Shells & Ched. Chse Dinner	410	16	51
Refried Beans, 1/2 Cup	150	2.5	24
Cans: *Per Cup*			
Spagh. Rings & Tom. Meatballs	410	16	51
Spagh. Rings in Tomato Sce	190	0.5	40
Spaghetti w. Tomato Sce & Chse	180	0	39
11/2lb Can: Beef Stew, 247g	190	7	18
15oz Can: Corned Beef Hash	430	28	28
Chili w. Beans, 270g	510	32	34

Hungry Jack Potatoes	C	F	Cb
Instant Potato Flakes, 1/3 cup	80	0	18

Ken & Robert's: Veggie Burger	130	1	26
Veggie Pockets, average, 4.5 oz	250	8	39

Knorr

	C	F	Cb
Skillet Potatoes, 1/3 cup, dry	100	0.5	20
Hash Browns w. Chse Blend	120	3	22
Scalloped Potatoes, 1/2 cup, dry	110	2	18
Sliced Potatoes: in Crm Sce, 1/3 c., dry	100	0.5	20
w. Rstd Garlic, 2/3 cup, dry	120	1	23

Kraft
It's Pasta Anytime Meals: *Per Container*

	C	F	Cb
Spaghetti w. Tomato Sauce	495	5	97
Penne w. Tomato, avg all varieties	525	6	102
Spaghetti w. Sauteed On. & Garlic	480	6	91
Spaghetti w. Tom. Beef Flavor Sce	500	6	96
Dinners: *Per Serving (Prepared As Directed)*			
Macaroni & Cheese: Orig., 1/3 box	410	18	49
Scooby-Doo Spirals; Three Chse	418	18	49
Mac & Chse: Crazy Noodles, 1/2 box	290	4.5	48
Thick'n Creamy, 1/2 box	410	18	50
Easy Mac, avg. all variet., 1 pouch	250	8	38
Deluxe: Orig.; Sharp Chedd., 1/4 box	320	10	45
Rotini White Cheese Sce, 1/2 box	400	15	48
Velveeta Shells & Cheese, 1/3 box	360	13	47
Dinner Kits: *Per Serving (Prepared As Directed)*			
Chkn Parmesan w. Linguini	240	6	23
Three Cheese Chicken Enchilada	450	20	29
Cheesy Potatoes: *Per 1/2 Cup (Prep. As Directed)*			
Au Gratin Potatoes	200	7	27
Bacon Scalloped Potatoes	200	9	24
Mashed Potatoes	200	12	20

Lipton Packet Meals
Pasta Sides: *Per Cup (Prepared As Directed)*

	C	F	Cb
Alfredo; Parmesan	330	14	40
Butter	300	13	40
Stroganoff	290	11	40
Asian Sides: *Per Cup (Prepared As Directed)*			
Beef Lo Mein; Thai Ses. Noodles	230	2.5	43
Teriyaki/Swt & Sour Noodles, avg.	245	2	50
Rice Sides: *Per Cup (Prepared As Directed)*			
Chicken & Parmesan	260	7	43
Creamy Garlic Parmesan	320	11	47
Chicken Fried Rice	240	1.5	45
Other varieties, average	285	6	50

Canned & Packaged Meals (Cont)

Loma Linda (Vegetarian)	C	F	Cb
Big Franks: 1 link, 1.8 oz	110	7	2
Lowfat, 1 link, 1.8 oz	80	3	3
Chicken Supreme Mix, 1/3 cup mix	90	1	6
Dinner Cuts, 2 sl., 1.4 oz (41g)	90	1.5	3
Fried Chik'n/Gravy, 2 pcs, 3 oz	150	10	5
Gravy Quik, 1 Tbsp mix (1/4 pkt)	20	0	4
Linketts, (1), 1 1/4 oz	70	4.5	1
Little Links, 2 links, 1.6 oz	90	6	2
Nuteena, 3/8" slice, 2 oz	160	13	6
Ocean Platter, 1/3 c. dry mix, 1 oz	90	1	8
Patty Mix, 1/3 cup dry mix, 1 oz	90	1	7
Redi-Burger, 5/8" slice, 3 oz	120	2.5	7
Sandwich Spread, 1/4 cup, 2 oz	80	4.5	7
Savory Din. Loaf, 1/3 cup, dry mix	90	1.5	7
Soyagen, 1/4 c. (1 oz) dry (make 1 c.)	130	6	12
Swiss Stake, 1 piece, 3 1/4 oz	120	6	8
Tender Bits, 6 pieces, 3 oz	110	4.5	7
Tender Rounds, 6 pieces, 2 3/4 oz	120	5	6
Vege-Burger, 1/4 cup, 2 oz	70	1.5	2
Vita-Burger Granules, 3 T., 3/4 oz	70	1	6

Maruchan: *Per Cup*			
Instant Noodles, avg. all flavors	280	12	37
Instant Wonton, all flavors	200	12	19
Ramen flavors, 1/2 pkt, 1 1/2 oz	180	7	26

Morningstar Farms (Vegetarian)			
Better'n Burger, 1 pattie, 3 oz	80	0	6
Better'n Eggs, 1/4 cup, 2 oz	20	0	0
Breakfast Links, 2 links, 1 1/2 oz	80	3	3
Breakfast Strips, 2 strips	60	4.5	2
Buffalo Wings, 5 nuggets, 3 oz	200	9	18
Burger-Style Recipe Crumbles, 2/3 c.	80	2.5	4
Chik Patties, 1 pattie	150	6	16
Grillers: Original, 1 pattie, 2 1/4 oz	140	6	5
Prime (1) 2 1/2 oz	170	9	5
Grind Meatless Crumbles, 1/2 c., 2 oz	60	0	4
Mushroom & Pepper Burger, 1	120	4	9
Pot Pie: Hearty Chik'n, 269g	350	14	45
Homestyle Chili Pie, 255g	330	9	49
Saus. Recipe Crumbles, 2/3 c., 2 oz	90	3	5
Scramblers, 1/4 cup, 2 oz	35	0	2
Spicy Black Bean Burger, 1 pattie	150	4.5	16
Supreme Pizza, 1/2 pizza	300	9	38
Tom. & Basil Pizza Burger, 2.3 oz	130	6	7
Veggie Dog, 1 link, 2 oz	80	0.5	6
Breakfast Sandwiches:			
Muffin/Scramblers/Pattie/Chse	280	3	35
Muffin/Scramblers/Pattie	240	2.5	32

Natural Touch (Vegetarian)	C	F	Cb
Canned & Dry Products			
Gravy Mix, average all types,			
1 Tbsp (makes 1/4 cup)	20	0	4
Kaffree Roma, 1 rounded tsp, 2g	10	0	2
Roasted Soy Butter, 2 Tbsp, 1.1 oz	170	11	10
Vegetarian Tuno, 1/3 cup, dr., 2 oz	60	2	2
Vegetarian Chili, 1 cup, 8 oz	165	1	21

Near East: *Per Cup (Prepared as Directed)*			
Couscous: Original Plain	230	2	46
Chicken & Herbs	270	6	51
Toasted Pine Nut	230	6	40
Creamy Parmesan	280	7	48
Roasted Garlic; Broccoli	220	4	41
Roasted Pecan & Garlic	240	9	37
Rice Pilaf	190	0.5	42

New Menu (Vitasoy) Vegetarian			
VegiBurgers, 3 oz	110	1	12
VegiDogs, 1 link, 1.5 oz	45	0	1
Tofumate (Season. Mixes), 1/4 pkt	25	0	4

Nile Spice: *Per Cup*			
Couscous: Almondine	200	2.5	37
Lentil Curry	200	1.5	36
Minestrone	180	1.5	34
Parmesan	200	3	34

Nissan			
Cup Noodles, all types, average	300	14	38

Oberweis Dairy			
Sandwiches: Bessie's Beefeater	1275	27	92
Coley Club	655	29	67
Cowlifornian	665	28	76
Daisy's Delight	770	40	63
Holstein Hoagie	640	28	66
Save the Cow	800	38	85
Lowfat: Coley Club	450	8	65
Cowlifornian	425	5	70
Daisy's Delight	410	4	65

Old El Paso

Dinner Kits: *Per Serving (Prepared)*

Soft Taco	390	19	33
Burrito (1)	270	12	27
Hard & Soft Taco (2)	360	17	32
Shells, Taco Sce, Seasoning (2)	310	18	19
Fajita (2)	330	10	35
Taco Dinner (2)	300	17	19

Side Dishes: *Per Serving*

Boxed: Chsy Mexican Rice 1/3 pkt	250	2	55
Spanish Rice, 1/3 pkt	280	4.5	55
Canned, Chili Beans, 1 cup	240	11	19

Refried Beans: Regular, 1/2 cup

w. Green Chilies, 1/2 cup	100	0.5	17
w. Cheese, 1/2 cup	100	0.5	19
w. Sausage, 1/2 cup	130	3.5	18
Fat Free varieties, 1/2 cup	200	13	14
Mexe/Pinto Beans, 1/2 cup	100	0	18
	110	0.5	19

Pasta-Roni: *Per Cup (Prepared)*

Angel Hair Pasta varieties, avg.	320	14	40
Fettuccine Alfredo	460	25	48
Chicken (flavor)	310	13	41
Chicken; Shells & White Cheddar	310	13	41
Chicken & Broccoli	370	16	49
Homestyle Deluxe: Crmy Garlic	350	17	40
Four Cheese; Parmesano	390	17	50
Homestyle Chicken	310	13	31
Pritikin: Vegetarian Chili, 1 cup	160	1	27

Ragu

Express! Pasta Snacks: *Per 1/6 Box (4.2 oz)*

Classic Meat Flavor	205	3	37
Sweet Tomato & Garlic	200	2	39
Traditional Tomato	200	2.5	37

Ramen Noodles: *Per Serving*

Beef/Chicken/Shrimp Flavors,

1/2 block, 1 1/2 oz	190	7	26
Noodles: Fat Fried Shrimp, 1 1/2 oz	170	6	26
Other Flavors, 1 1/2 oz	160	6	26
Fried Cup Beef, 1 packet, 2.2 oz	290	11	41
Lowfat varieties, average, 2 oz	215	1.5	45

Rice Pride

Rice Bowls: Spicy Shrimp	230	0.5	48
Teriyaki Beef	260	1	56
Tex Mex Beef	250	2	52

Rice-A-Roni: *Per Cup (Prepared)*

Beef; Herb & Butter	310	9	52
Broccoli Au Gratin	370	17	47
1/3 Less Salt	320	11	50
Cajun Chicken	250	8	41
Chicken	310	9	52
1/3 Less Salt	280	5	53
Lowfat	210	3	41
Chicken & Broccoli	230	6	41
Chicken & Garlic; Chkn Teriyaki	260	9	41
Chicken & Mushroom	360	14	52
Four Cheese	280	12	37
Fried Rice	320	11	51
Long Grain & Wild Rice	240	6	43
Red Beans & Rice	290	7	51
Rice Pilaf; Risotto	310	9	51
Savory Chicken Vegetable	210	3	41
Spanish Rice	270	8	46
White Cheddar & Herbs	340	13	48

(Reduced Fat Recipe: If only 1 Tbsp fat is used instead of 2 Tbsp, deduct 35 calories and 4g fat.)

Rosarita

Refried Beans: *Per 1/2 Cup*

Traditional; Vegetarian; Spicy	100	2	18
Lowfat Black Bean	90	0.5	18
Fat Free varieties	90	0	18

Stagg Chili

15 oz Can: *Per Cup (8.7 oz)*

Chili w. Beans: Classic/Dynamite

Chili w. Beans: Classic/Dynamite	330	17	28
Country/Laredo	320	16	29
Fiesta Grille	240	9	25
Ranch House Chicken	290	9	32
Rio Blanco Chicken	250	12	19
No Beans: Steakhouse/Double	330	21	16
99% Fat Free: Veg. Gdn/4 Bean	200	1	37
Turkey Ranchers/Silverado Beef	240	3	31

Canned & Packaged Meals (Cont)

S & W: *Per 1/2 Cup*
Baked Beans, avg. all types	145	0.5	29
Caribbean Black Beans	90	0	18
San Antonio; Santa Fe Beans	90	0.5	20

Taco Bell: *Per 1/2 Cup*
Home Originals: Refried Beans	140	2.5	22
Fat Free Beans w. Green Chilles	120	0	23

Tasty Bite
Bread (Kontos): *Per 1/2 Loaf*
Handkerchief Bread, 1.6 oz	130	0	29
Kulcha Nan, 1.4 oz	125	1.5	23
Massala Nan, 1.4 oz	115	3	15
Other varieties, average, 1.4 oz	125	4	18

Meat: Beef Rogan Josh, 5 oz | 260 | 12 | 16
| Chicken Moglai, 5 oz | 325 | 15 | 18 |

Pilaf: Green Peas Pilaf, 4.5 oz | 205 | 4 | 36
| Curried Vegetable Pilaf, 5 oz | 180 | 6 | 26 |
| Vegetable Kofta Pilaf, 4.5 oz | 230 | 5 | 39 |

Vegetarian: *Per 1/2 Packet (5 oz)*
Agra Peas & Greens	140	10	9
Bengal Lentil	135	5	16
Bombay Potatoes; Jodhpur Lentils	110	4	13
Jaipur Vegetable	165	11	10
Madras Lentils	125	5	14
Mumbai Pav Bhaji	145	9	12
Simla Potatoes	120	7	12
Other varieties, average	115	8	5

Thai Meals: *Per 1/3 Packet (3.3 oz)*
Green Curry Vege. & Noodles	145	1.5	30
Pad Thai Sauce & Noodles	260	5	49
Peanut Sauce & Noodle	270	9	42
Stir Fry Sauce & Noodles	210	3.5	40
Red/Yellow Curry Veges & Noodles	170	3	33

Thai Kitchen
Bowls: avg. all types, 1.7 oz | 170 | 2 | 35
Rice Noodles: *Per Serving*
Thin/Stir Fry, 2 oz	195	0	46
Pad Thai varieties, 1/2 package	260	0	63
Savory Garlic, 1/2 package	270	6	51
Thai Peanut, 1/2 package	243	3	50

The Spice Hunter: *Per Package*
Risotto: Wild Mushroom	230	1	47
Three Cheese; Spinach, avg.	245	2.5	46
Stuffed Potato: Creamy Butter	140	3	25
Bacon & White Cheddar	160	3	28
Sour Cream & Chives	160	2	31

Trader Joe's: *Per Package*
Organic Beans, avg., 1/2 cup	110	0	21
Bean Medley, 1/2 cup	150	1	26
Refried Beans, avg., 1/2 cup	120	0	22
Beef/Turkey Chili w. Beans, 1 cup	230	3	33
Chicken Chili w. Beans, 1 cup	290	9	32
Black Bean Chili, 1 cup	230	1.5	37
Black Beans: Regular, 1/2 cup	130	0.5	22
Cuban Style, 1/2 cup	130	2	21
Premium: Beef Stew, 1 cup	130	2	21
Chicken Stew, 1 cup	230	14	16
Quiche: Broccoli & Cheddar, 6 oz	490	33	33
Mexicaine, 6 oz	510	36	29
Spinach & Mushroom, 6 oz	470	30	32

Tuna Helper ~ *See Betty Crocker, Page 77*

Valley Fresh
Chicken: *Per 1/2 Can*
White & Dark Chunk	80	2	0
Premium Chunk White	70	1	0

Turkey: *Per 1/4 Can*
Premium Chunk White	80	1.5	0

Westbrae
Vegetarian Chili, 1 cup	170	1	30
Lowfat Chili, 1 cup	220	2	42

White Wave (Vegetarian)
Tempeh: Five Grain, 1/3 pkg | 140 | 4 | 15
Original, 1/3 block, 2.7 oz	150	6	10
Sea Veggie, 1/3 block, 2.7 oz	120	3	11
Wild/Soy Rice, 1/3 block, 2.7 oz	140	5	13
Seitan: Chicken w. Broth, 5 oz	130	0	12
Traditional, 4 oz	140	0	4
Tofu: Baked, all flavors, 2 oz	120	6	3
Organic, Soft/Firm, 1/5 pkg, 3.2 oz	90	6	1
Fat-Reduced, 1/5 pkg, 3.2 oz	90	4	4
Extra Firm, 1/4 pkg, 3 oz	80	5	1
Soy Milks & Yogurts: *See Pages 27, 28*

Wolf
Chili w. Beans: 227g Can | 300 | 16 | 27
| 1 cup, 254g | 330 | 18 | 30 |
Chili No Beans: 227g Can | 390 | 27 | 18
| 1 cup, 248g | 420 | 30 | 20 |
Chunky Beef w. Beans:
| 1 cup, 254g | 300 | 15 | 28 |
| No Beans, 1 cup, 246g | 330 | 22 | 18 |

Worthington (Vegetarian)

	C	F	Cb
Chili, 1 cup, 8 oz	290	15	21
Chili (lowfat), 1 cup, 8 oz	170	1	21
Choplets, 2 slices	90	1.5	3
Corned Beef, 4 slices, 2 oz	140	9	5
Country Stew, 1 cup, 8 1/2 oz	210	9	20
Crispy Chic Patties, 1 pattie	150	6	16
Diced Chik, 1/4 cup, 2 oz	50	0	2
Dinner Roast, 3/4" slice, 3 oz	180	12	5
Fillets, 2 pces, 3 oz	180	9	8
Golden Croquettes, 4 pieces, 3 oz	210	11	14
Leanies, 1 link	100	7	2
Numete, 3/8" slice, 2 oz	130	10	5
Prime Stakes, 1 piece, 3 1/4 oz	120	7	4
Prosage Roll, 5/8" slice, 2 oz	140	10	2
Protose, 3/8" Slice, 2 oz	130	7	5
Salami, 3 slices, 2 oz	130	8	2
Savory Slices, 3 slices, 3 oz	150	9	7
Sliced Chik, 3 slices, 3.2 oz	80	0.5	2
Smoked Beef, 6 slices, 2 oz	130	7	7
Smoked Turkey, 3 slices, 2 oz	140	10	5
Super-Links, 1 link, 1 1/2 oz	110	8	2
Tuno, 1/2 cup (drained), 2 oz	80	6	2
Turkee Slices, 3 slices, 3.3 oz	180	12	5
Vega Links (1)	50	3	2
Vegetarian Burger, 1/4 c., 2 oz	60	2	2
Vegetarian Cutlets, 1 slice, 2.2 oz	70	1	3
Wham, 2 slices, 1 1/2 oz	90	5	2

Yves Veggie Cuisine (Vegetarian)

	C	F	Cb
Neatballs (1) 2 oz	75	2	9
Chick'n Nuggets (1) 2.7 oz	190	3	21
Breakfast: Brkfast Links (2) 1.8 oz	70	0	3
Breakfast Patties (1) 2 oz	70	2	4
Canadian Veg. Bacon, 1.3 oz	50	0.5	1
Burgers: Veggie (1) 2.6 oz	110	4	7
Garden Vege Patties (1) 3 oz	90	0	11
Veggie Chick'n Burger (1) 2.6 oz	120	3	6
Dogs: Jumbo Veggie Dog (1) 2.6 oz	105	1.5	5
Hot & Spicy Chili/Good (1) 1.8 oz	70	1	3
Veggie/Tofu Dog, avg. (1)	50	0.5	1
Veggie Ground Round: Orig., Ital.	60	0	4
Mexican, 1/3 cup, 1.93 oz	85	2.5	4
Veggie Meatballs (1) 75g	120	3	28
Slices: Bologna, 2 oz (62g)	80	1	4
Pizza Pepperoni, 1.7 oz (48g)	70	0	4
Veggie Ham/Salami, avg., 2 oz	80	0	6
Veggie Turkey, 2 oz (62g)	90	1.5	4
Veggie Entrees: Per Tray 300g (10.5 oz)			
Chili; Macaroni; Penne, average	230	2	38
Lasagne	300	3	51
Thai Lemongrass Veggie Crunch	320	8.5	49

Soybean Products

	C	F	Cb
Cheeses (Soy): See Page 44			
Miso: 1/2 cup, 5 oz	280	8	39
Cold Mountain: Red, 1 T., 0.5 oz	25	1	3
Mellow White, 1 Tbsp, 0.5 oz	35	0.5	6
Natto, 1/2 cup, 3 oz	190	10	13
Tempeh, 1 piece, 3 oz	170	6	14
Fried, 3 oz	250	14	14
White Wave: See Page 82			
Soybean Protein (TVP), 1 oz	90	0	7
Soy Bean Paste, 1 tsp	10	0	2
Soy Beans: See Page 151			
Soy Drinks: See Page 27			

Tofu

	C	F	Cb
Azumaya Tofu:			
Soft (Silken), 3 oz	45	2	4
Firm, 3 oz	60	2.5	3
Extra Firm, 3 oz	75	3.5	10
Age (Tofu Puff), 1/2 oz	40	1.5	2
Nama-Age (Fried Tofu), 3 oz	130	5	8
Calco: Tasty Tofu, 3 oz	50	3	2
Hinoichu Tofu:			
Soft, 3 oz, 1" slice	45	2.5	5
Reg. (Japanese), 3 oz, 1" slice	60	3	6
Firm (Chinese), 3 oz, 1" slice	60	3	6
Extra Firm, 3 oz	90	5	10
Mori-Nu Tofu (Silken):			
Soft, 4 oz	60	3	3
Firm, 4 oz	70	3	3
Extra Firm, 4 oz	70	3	2
Nasoya Tofu: Soft, 3 oz	60	3	2
Silken, 3 oz	50	3	2
Firm, 3 oz	80	4	2
Extra Firm, 3 oz	90	5	1
Chinese 5 Spice Tofu, 3 oz	80	4	2
Pulmuone Tofu: Soft, 3 oz	45	2	5.5
Silken, 3 oz	45	2	5.5
Firm, 3 oz	55	2.5	4
SoyBoy: Firm Organic, 3 oz	100	5	2
X-Firm Organic, 3 oz	120	6	2
X-Firm LowFu, 3 oz	90	2	6
TofuLin, 2 oz	100	5	4
Baked, Seasoned, Smoked, 2 oz	100	5	3
Carribean Tofu, 2 oz	100	5	3
Tree of Life: Firm Raw, 3 oz	100	5	2
Reduced Fat, 3 oz	90	4	4
Tofu Stir Fried, 4 oz	120	8	3

Soups

Homemade & Restaurant

Restaurant & Take-Out

Per 8 fl.oz	C	F	Cb
Bean Medley	200	3	34
Beef Consomme	30	0	2
Borscht (w. Cream)	130	8	14
Bouillabaisse	400	15	10
Chicken & Corn	290	14	20
Chicken & Wild Rice	80	4	9
Chicken Consomme	50	0	2
Chicken Curry	180	8	18
Chicken Jambalaya	160	7	8
Chicken Noodle	80	2	12
w. Chicken	160	4	12
Chicken Soup	80	2	6
Chili with Beans	250	12	25
Clam Chowder	240	15	17
Corn & Crab	120	3	18
Corn Chowder	150	8	16
Cream of Broccoli	200	12	20
Cream of Potato	220	12	25
Cream of Mushroom	290	21	20
Creamy Pumpkin	210	10	26
Fish Chowder	220	15	6
French Onion	420	15	25
Gazpacho	60	0	13
Lentil Soup	250	9	28
Lobster Bisque	320	15	14
Matzo Ball (w.1 large ball)	180	7	24
Minestrone	140	2	14
Mulligatawny	300	15	8
Pea & Ham	240	10	25
Potato & Bacon	170	7	19
Shark Fin Soup	220	6	4
Spicy Shrimp Soup, 1 bowl	160	7	10
Split Pea Soup	150	6	18
Vegetable (Fat Free)	75	0	18
Vegetable Beef	80	2	10
Vichyssoise	200	9	25
Watercress	90	4	13

● Ethnic & Restaurant Section: Pages 176-181
● Fast Foods/Restaurant Section: Pages 183
(Arby's, Au Bon Pain, Boston Market, Dunkin' Donuts, Denny's, Schlotzsky's, Sizzler, Souplantation, Sweet Tomatoes)

Homemade Soups: Calculate calories, fat and carbohydrates from ingredients.

Bouillon Cubes & Powders

Bouillon Cubes:	C	F	Cb
Average all types			
Regular, 1 cube	8	0	1
Low Sodium (LiteLine)	12	0	1
Powders: Average, 1 tsp	8	0	1
Herb-Ox: Instant Broth & Seasoning,			
Beef, 1 envelope	10	0	2
Chicken; Vegetarian	10	0	2
Herbs, Spices: 1 tsp	5	0	1
Soup Oyster Crackers			
40 small/20 large, 1/2 oz	60	2	8

Amy's

Per Cup (1/2 Can)	C	F	Cb
Black Bean Vegetable	110	1	22
Cream of Mushroom, 3/4 cup	120	9	10
Cream of Tomato, 1 cup	100	2	17
Lentil	130	4	19
No Chicken Noodle	90	3	12
Organic Vegetable Broth, 1 cup	30	0	6
Split Pea	100	0	19
Vegetable Barley	50	1	10

Andersen's

Per Cup	C	F	Cb
Split Pea	130	0	24
Split Pea w. Bacon	135	1	22
Tomato	130	3	24

Bean Cuisine

Per Cup (Made as Directed)	C	F	Cb
13 Bean Bouillabaisse	240	0	18
Island Black Bean	90	0	17
Soup Mix: Dry Mix Only			
Mesa Maize, 1 oz	95	0	18
White Bean Provencal, 1 oz	175	1	32

Birds Eye

Hearty Spoonfuls Soup Bowls (Frozen): *Per Bowl*

	C	F	Cb
Cheesy Cream of Broccoli	230	10	25
Chicken Noodle	140	1.5	19
Chicken, Rice & Vegetables	160	2	26
Italian Minestrone	240	4	37

Campbell's   **C** **F** **Cb**

Chunky (Red 19 oz Can): *Per 1/2 Can*

	C	F	Cb
Baked Potato: w. Chedd., Bacon	180	8	23
w. Steak & Cheese	215	10	20
Beef Rib Roasted w. Potato	110	1	17
Beef: w. White & Wild Rice	140	1.5	23
w. Country Vegetables	160	3	22
Cheese Tortellini	110	2	18
Chicken & Dumplings	190	10	16
Chicken Broccoli Cheese	200	12	14
Chicken Corn Chowder	250	15	18
Chicken Mushroom Chowder	230	17	12
Classic Chicken Noodle	130	3	16
Grilled Chicken Veg. & Pasta	110	2	17
Grilled Sirloin Steak & Vegies	120	2	20
Hearty Bean & Ham	180	3	30
Hearty Chicken & Vegetable	90	2	12
Herb Rstd Chicken w. Pot. Gravy	110	2	17
Honey Rstd Ham w. Potatoes	130	2	20
New England Clam Chowder	300	18	26
Old Fashioned Vegetable Beef	130	2.5	18
Potato Ham Chowder	220	14	16
Salisbury Steak w. Mushr. Onion	150	4.5	18
Savory Chkn & Rice; Pepper Stk	140	3	18
Sirloin Burger	180	7	20
Slow Rstd Beef w. Mushrooms	110	1.5	16
Split Pea & Ham	180	3.5	27
Steak & Potato	130	2	18
Vegetable	160	4	15

Fun Favorites: *Per Cup (Prepared)*

	C	F	Cb
Chick Stars/Noodles	80	2.5	11
Double Noodle	105	2.5	17
Funshaped	75	3	9
Goldfish Pasta in Tomato	115	0.5	25
Goldfish Pasta w. Chicken	70	2.5	9

Healthy Request: *Per Cup (Prepared)*

	C	F	Cb
Chicken Noodle/Rice	60	2	8
Cream of Chicken/Mushr., avg.	70	2	12
Minestrone	80	1	15
98% Fat Free, prepared, 1 cup	70	2	10

Soup At Hand: *Per Container (10 3/4 oz)*

	C	F	Cb
Blended Vege Medley	110	2	21
Classic Tomato	120	0	24
Crm of Broccoli; Crmy Chicken	160	9	17

Soup Bowls: *Per Bowl*

	C	F	Cb
Chunky, Chicken & Dumplings	190	8	19
Select: Chicken Egg Noodles	100	1.5	12.5
New England Clam Chowder	100	1.5	15

Campbell's (Cont)   **C** **F** **Cb**

Classics/Great for Cooking: *Per Cup (Prepared from 1/2 cup Condensed)*

	C	F	Cb
Bean & Bacon	180	5	25
Beef Broth	15	0	1
Beef w. Vegetable Barley	80	2	11
Cheddar Cheese	130	8	11
Chicken Gumbo	60	1	10
Chicken Broth	30	2	1
Chicken Vegetable	80	2	12
Chicken w. White & Wild Rice	60	1.5	10
Clam Chowder New England	100	2.5	15
Cream of Asparagus; Celery	110	7	9
Cream of Broccoli; Shrimp	100	6	9
Cream of Chicken Mushroom	120	8	9
Cream of Chicken w. Herbs	85	4	9
Cream of Mushr.; Broccoli Chse	110	7	9
Cream of Mushr. w. Rstd Garlic	70	2.5	10
Cream of Potato	90	3	14
Double Noodle in Chicken Broth	100	2.5	15
French Onion; Golden Mushroom	70	2.5	10
Mega Noodle	70	1.5	10
Minestrone	100	2	16
Split Pea w. Ham; Green Pea	180	3.5	28
Tomato	80	0	18
Tomato Noodle/Rice	120	1	25
Vegetable	90	1	16
Vegetable & Beef; Turkey Noodle	80	2	10
Vegetarian Vegetable	75	1	15

Ready to Serve: *Per Cup*

	C	F	Cb
Cream of Potato	170	8	22
Classic: Bean & Bacon; Crm Tom.	170	4	25
Tomato	115	0	27
Vegetable	85	0.5	17
Other varieties, avg.	80	2	12

Soup & Recipe Mixes (Dry): *Per Tablespoon*

	C	F	Cb
Chicken Noodle/w. Broth	30	0.5	5
Onion	20	0	5

Select (10 1/2 oz): *Per Cup*

	C	F	Cb
Beef w. Roasted Barley	130	1.5	21
Beef w. Portabello Mushrooms	120	3	14
Creamy Potato w. Garlic	180	9	21
Fiesta Vegetable	120	0.5	24
Herbed Chicken w. Rstd Veges	90	0.5	14
Ital. Style Wedding; Minestrone	120	2.5	18
New England Clam Chowder	190	13	14
Roast Chicken w. Rotini & Penne	110	2	17
Vegetable Beef	120	3	15
Avg. other varieties	100	1	20

Soup (Cont)

Dr McDougall's   C F Cb

Per Container (Mix)

Minestrone & Pasta	180	1	31
Ramen Noodles, all flavors	150	0.5	29
Split Pea w. Barley	200	2	36
Tamale Pie w. Baked Chips	200	1.5	39
Tortilla Soup w. Baked Chips	190	1.5	37

Fantastic Cup Soups

Per Container (Mix): Split Pea

Split Pea	190	1	35
Cha Cha Chili; Country Lentil	250	2	44
Corn & Potato Chowder	170	2	34
Couscous w. Lentils; Five Bean	245	1.5	45
Creamy Soups: Average	150	2.5	27
Split Pea	220	1	38

Big Soup Noodle Bowls: *Per Cup (1/2 Pkg)*

Hot & Sour	140	2.5	25
Miso w. Tofu; Spicy Thai, avg.	115	1	22
Sesame Miso	100	1	19

Goodman's

Soup Mixes (Prep.): Onion, 1 cup	30	1	5
Alphabet Vege; Noodle Soup, 1 c.	45	0.5	9

Hain

All Natural (canned): *Per Cup*

Black Bean	90	0	18
Chicken Broth	25	2	3
Chicken Noodle	150	3	24
Mushroom Barley	130	1.5	26
Vegetable Broth	25	0	6
Wild Rice	80	1.5	15

Healthy Choice

Per Cup

Bean & Ham	180	2.5	29
Beef and Potato; Chicken w. Pasta	110	1	19
Chicken & Dumplings	145	3	19
Chicken w. Rice Soup	100	3	12
Country Vegetable	110	0.5	22
Fiesta Chicken	90	2	17
Garden Vegetable; Vegetable Beef	120	1	25
Hearty Chicken	130	2	20
Hearty Chilli Beef	190	2	31
Italian Bean & Pasta; Crmy Tomato	100	1.5	18
New England Clam Chowder	120	1.5	21
Roasted Italian Chicken/ w. Garlic	135	2.5	19
Split Pea and Ham	170	2.5	30
Turkey w. Rice; Zesty Gumbo	100	1.5	16

Health Valley   C F Cb

Per Cup

Bean Vegetable	140	0	32
Beef Broth	20	0	0
Carotene varieties, average	70	0	17
Chicken Broth	45	1.5	0
Chicken Noodle/Rice	130	2	20
Corn & Vege; Super Broccoli	70	0	17
Garden/Tomato Vegetable	80	0	17
Italian Minestrone; Lentil & Carrots	90	0	25
Mushroom Broth	10	0	2
Real Minestrone; Italian Plus; Vege	80	0	20
Rotini & Vegetables	100	0	20
Split Pea	110	0	17
Pasta Soups, avg. all varieties	115	0	24
Organic: Black Bean; Split Pea	110	0	25
Mushroom Barley; Potato Leek	60	0	15
Lentil; Tomato; Minestrone	90	0	20
Dry Soups: 1/3 cup, average	120	0	24

Soup Cups: *Per Cup*

Chicken Broth	25	0	0
Corn Chowder w. Tomato	105	0	21
Creamy Potato w. Broccoli	85	0	17
Garden Split Pea; Zesty Blk Bean	115	0	22
Lentil w. Couscous	140	0	28
Pasta Marianara/Parmesan	100	0	20
Spicy Black Bean w. Couscous	135	0	29

Imagine

Per Cup

No Chicken/Vegetable Broth	30	0.5	5
Free Range Chicken Broth	20	0.5	2
Organic Creamy: Broccoli	70	1.5	10
Butternut Squash	120	2	23
Portobello Mushroom	80	3	10
Potato Leek; Sweet Corn	100	3	15
Tomato	90	1.5	17

Enjoy nutritious soup as part of a meal or as a snack.

Soup is an excellent filler - especially to beat the 4.30pm snack syndrome. Choose low fat varieties.

Knorr

	C	F	Cb
Kosher Soup Mix: *Per 3 Tablespoons*			
Chicken Vegetable w. Pasta	50	1	9
Potato Onion	85	1.5	16
Naturals Hearty Soup Mix:			
Potato Vegetable, 1 oz	105	1	21
Roast Vege w. Rice, 1 oz	85	1	17
Recipe Classics: *Dry Mix*			
Cream of Spinach; Leek, 2 Tbsp	70	2.5	10
French Onion; Vegetable, 2 Tbsp	35	1	6
Spring Vegetable, 2 Tbsp	25	0	5
Tomato & Basil, 3 Tbsp	85	2.5	13
Tomato Beef, 2 Tbsp	60	2	9
Savory Soups: *Per 3 Tbsp (Dry Mix)*			
Chicken Noodle	70	1.5	11
Cream of Vegetable	100	4.5	12
Creamy Chicken w. Rice	90	2.5	14
Minestrone	100	2	18

Lipton

	C	F	Cb
Cup-a-Soup: *Per Envelope*			
Cream of Chicken	70	2	12
Chicken Noodle	50	1	8
Recipe Secrets Mixes: *Per Serving*			
Beefy Onion; Onion Mushroom	25	0.5	5
Chicken Noodle	80	2	11
Onion	20	0	4
Savory Herb w. Garlic; Vegetable	30	0	7
Soup Secrets: *Per Cup (Prepared)*			
Chicken Noodle	65	1	11
Noodle Soup	60	2	9

Manischewitz

	C	F	Cb
Condensed: *Per 1/2 Cup (Unprepared)*			
Chicken	15	0.5	2
Chicken w. Kieplach	35	1	5
Chicken w. Matzo Balls	80	4	9
Four Bean	70	1	13
Lentil	140	2	24
Minestrone	90	1.5	16
Condensed: *Per 8 fl.oz (Prepared)*			
Borscht w. Beets	90	0	21
Borscht Low Calorie	25	0	6
Ready To Serve: Matzo Ball Soup	110	5	13
Matzo Balls in Broth	215	9	27
Whitefish & Pike in Broth	55	1.5	3
Dry Mixes: *Per Cup*			
Matzo Ball & Soup Mix	45	0.5	9
Split Pea Cello	140	0	25
Vegetable Soup Cello	115	0	22

Miso Cup

	C	F	Cb
Original; Golden Seaweed, 1 cup	30	1	3
Traditional, 1 pkg	35	1	4
Reduced Sodium, 1 pkg	25	1	3

Nile Spice

	C	F	Cb
Per Cup: Black Bean	170	1.5	36
Cheddar Broccoli	130	3	20
Chicken Flavored Vegetable	110	1.5	21
Country Mushroom	140	2.5	26
Lentil	180	1.5	31
Minestrone	140	1	30
Red Beans & Rice	170	1	36
Split Pea	200	1	35
Couscous: Parmesan	200	3	34
Other varieties, average	190	2	36

Pacific Foods

	C	F	Cb
Per Cup: Chicken Broth	5	0	0
Natural, Beef Broth	20	0	1
Organic: Creamy Broccoli	80	2	12
Creamy Butternut Squash	95	2	17
Creamy Tomato	105	2	17
French Onion	30	0	6
Roasted Red Pepper & Tomato	100	2	16
Vegetable Broth	0	0	0

Pritikin

	C	F	Cb
Per Cup: Black Bean w. Rice	200	1	37
Chicken Pasta	80	0	15
Fat Free Chicken Broth	10	0	0.5
Hearty Vegetable	90	0.5	16
Minestrone	130	0.5	25
Potato Broccoli	110	0	22
Split Pea	180	0.5	32
Vegetarian Vegetable	100	0	21

"He misses the way you used to bend over and pat him."

Soup (Cont)

Progresso

	C	F	Cb
Per Cup			
Beef Barley	130	4	13
Beef & Vegetable	125	2.5	16
Chickarina	130	5	12
Chicken Vegetable	95	1.5	13
Chicken with Wild Rice	100	1.5	15
Chicken Barley	110	1.5	16
Chicken Noodle	90	2	9
Chicken Rice w. Vegetable	90	2	13
Creamy Mushroom	180	14	12
French Onion	50	1.5	9
Green Split Pea	170	3	25
Grilled Chicken Italiano	110	2.5	14
Grilled Steak w. Veg. Penne	120	3.5	13
Hearty Black Bean	170	1.5	30
Hearty Chicken & Rotini	90	1.5	12
Hearty Tomato	110	1	23
Hearty Penne in Chicken Broth	80	1	14
Home Style Chicken w. Veges	90	1.5	11
Lentil	140	2	22
Macaroni & Bean	160	4	23
Manhattan Clam Chowder	110	2	11
Minestrone	120	2	21
New England Clam Chowder	190	10	21
Potato w.Broccoli & Cheese	160	6	21
Roasted Chicken Garden Herb	70	1.5	9
Roasted Chicken Italiano/Rotini	80	1.5	10
Southwestern Style Corn Chowder	200	7	29
Split Pea w. Ham	150	4	20
Steak & Baked Potato	130	2.5	18
Steak & Mushrooms/Vegetables	100	2	12
Tomato; Tomato Basil	100	2	19
Tomato Rotini	140	5	30
Turkey Noodle	90	1.5	11
Turkey Rice w. Vegetable	110	1	18
Vegetable	90	1	17
99% Fat Free: Chicken Noodle	90	1.5	13
Beef Barley; Lentil; Minestrone	130	2	20
New England Clam Chowder	110	1.5	18
White Cheddar Potato	100	1.5	20

Puck

	C	F	Cb
Canned: Per Cup			
Chicken & Egg Noodles/Vegetables	150	5	16
Chicken Parmesan	200	12	15
Chicken Pot Pie; Creamy Chicken	220	13	16
Chicken w. Broccoli	180	10	14
Chicken w. Rstd Potatoes & Garlic	180	8	16
Chicken w. Sweetcorn	200	10	20
Country Tom. w. Basil; Hearty Vege	140	6	20
Grilled Chicken w. Rice	115	5	12
Hearty Lentil & Vegetable	180	2.5	31
Hearty Vege Beef; Turkey & Noodle	140	6	13
New England Clam Chowder	240	13	18
Old Fashioned Beef Barley	140	5	16
Old Fashioned Beef Pot Pie	160	8	14
Minestrone; Rst Chicken & Veges	185	7	22
Rst Chkn w. Wild Rice; Steak & Pot.	150	5	18
Spicy 7 Bean w. Italian Sausage	230	11	22
Thick Country Potato	145	5	21
Thick Country Vegetable	170	7	23

Rokeach

	C	F	Cb
15 oz Can (Ready to Serve): Per Serving			
Barley & Mushroom; Vegetable	110	1	23
Chicken Consomme	50	4	0
Cream of Mushroom	120	7	13
Minestrone	170	1	32
Potato	100	1	20
Seven Bean	130	1	24
Split Pea & Egg Barley	190	1.5	35

Shari Ann's

	C	F	Cb
Per Cup			
Chicken/Vegetable Broth	20	1.5	1
Chicken Noodle/Rice	90	2.5	12
Cream of Tomato	80	0	17
Great Plains Split Pea	150	0	26
Indian Black Bean & Rice	150	1	30
Italian White Bean	170	1	32
Organic Minestrone	120	2.5	20
Chicken Vege; Potato & Cheddar	100	2.5	15
Savory Lentil	110	0	21
Spicy French Green Lentil	130	0	22
Spicy Mexican Bean	210	1	38
Tomato & Roasted Garlic	50	0	12
Vegetable Barley	100	1.5	18
Vegetarian French Onion	60	0	9

> **It's only fattening if you swallow it!**
> (Virginia Graham)

Shelton's

C F Cb

Per Cup

	C	F	Cb
Chicken Broth	35	2.5	0
Black Bean & Chicken	170	4	22
Chicken Noodle	120	3	17
Chicken Rice	95	1	0
Chicken Tortilla	110	1.5	16
Vegetable Chicken	150	2	28

Swanson

Per Cup

	C	F	Cb
100% Fat Free Chicken Broth	15	0	1
Beef Broth	20	1	1
Chicken Broth	30	2	1
Vegetable Broth	20	1	3

Tabatchnick

Frozen: *Per Bag (7¹/2 oz)*

	C	F	Cb
Pea	180	2	31
Barley Mushroom	70	0	13
Cream of Spinach	90	4	11
Old Fashioned Potato	70	0	16
Vegetable	110	1	20
Yankee Bean	160	2	27

Tasty Bite

Thai Soup: *Per ¹/2 Packet (3.3 oz)*

	C	F	Cb
Gang Pha	20	0	4
Tom Yum	80	6	5

Thai Kitchen

7 oz Can: *Per Serving*

	C	F	Cb
Coconut Ginger	190	15	11
Hot & Sour	40	0.5	7

Instant Rice Noodle: *Per Serving (1.6 oz)*

	C	F	Cb
Bangkok Curry	195	4.5	35
Garlic & Vegetable	170	2	35
Lemongrass & Chili	190	4	35
Spring Onion, 1.6 oz	170	2	35

Rice Noodle: *Per Serving*

	C	F	Cb
Curry, ¹/2 pkg., 2.5 oz	290	6	55
Hot & Sour, ¹/2 pkg., 2 oz	230	3.5	47
Lemongrass & Chili, ¹/2 pkg., 2.5 oz	240	3	51

Trader Joe's

C F Cb

Per Cup

	C	F	Cb
Barley w. Vegetables; Rich Onion	95	1	19
Chicken Broth	15	0.5	0
Chicken Noodle	90	1	14
Chunky Minestrone	100	2	16
Country Style Tomato	75	0.5	14
Creamy Corn Chowder	165	7	23
Lentil w. Vegetables	175	1.5	30
Mixed Vegetable	105	6	10
Mostly Unsplit Pea	175	0.5	32
Salmon Chowder	165	8	15
Spicy Bean	200	5	30
Spicy Black Bean	230	3	41
Split Pea, Low Fat	145	1	26
Condensed: Clam Chowder	150	4	22
Crab Bisque	150	6	18
Creamy Asparagus	195	13	16
Cups: Split Pea	210	0.5	37
Tortilla Salsa	175	1.5	33
Vegetarian Vegetable w. Pasta	160	1.5	31

Walnut Acres

Per Cup (250g)

	C	F	Cb
Autumn Harvest	100	2	19
Country Corn Chowder	150	3	28
Cuban Black Bean; Four Bean Chili	150	1	30
Ginger Carrot	100	1	22
Classic Minestrone	100	0	22
Mediterranean Lentil	130	0	26
Savory Tomato	120	2	23

Weight Watchers

	C	F	Cb
Chicken Noodle, 10¹/2 oz	150	2	25
Chicken & Rice, 10¹/2 oz	110	1.5	17
Minestrone; Vegetable, 10¹/2 oz	130	1	27
Instant Beef/Chicken Broth, 1 pkg	10	0	2

Westbrae

Canned: *Per Cup (240g) Unless Indicated*

	C	F	Cb
Alabama; Mediterranean Lentil	140	0	25
Instant Miso Soup, 1 pkt	35	1.5	3
New York UnChicken Noodle	60	1	10
Old World Split Pea	150	0	28
Santa Fe Vegetable	160	0	31
Other varieties, average	125	0	25

Condensed: *Per ³/4 Cup, Prepared*

	C	F	Cb
California UnChicken Broth, 180g	15	0.5	2
Monte Carlo Crmy Mushr., 180g	70	3	10
Tuscany Tomato, 180g	70	0	16

Herbs & Spices

Herbs & Spices | C | F | Cb

	C	F	Cb
Per Teaspoon: Average all types	5	0	1
Allspice, ground	5	0	1
Chili Powder	8	0	1
Cinnamon, ground	6	0	2
Curry Powder	6	0	1
Garlic Powder	9	0	2
Nutmeg, ground	12	0	1
Onion Powder	7	0	2
Parsley, dried	4	0	1
Pepper, black/red/white, avg.	6	0	1
Saffron	2	0	0
Tumeric, ground	8	0	1
Seeds: Fenugreek	12	1	2
Mustard, Poppyseed	15	1	1
Other types, average	7	0	1
Parsley Patch: Sesame, 1 tsp	16	1	1
Salt-free blends, average	10	0	2
All-purpose, 1 tsp	6	0	1

Seasonings & Flavorings

	C	F	Cb
Accent Flavor Enhancer, 1 tsp	10	0	0
Angostura Bitters, 1 tsp	12	0	3
Bacon Bits, average, 1 Tbsp	30	1	0
Bacon Chips *(Durkee)*, 1 Tbsp	45	1	2
Best O'Butter, 1 tsp	10	<1	2
Bragg Liquid Aminos, 1 tsp	5	0	0
Butter Buds, 1 tsp	8	<1	2
Garlic Bread Sprinkle, 1 tsp	8	<1	1
Garlic Salt, 1 tsp	2	0	0
Italian Seasoning, 1 tsp	4	0	1
Lemon Pepper Seasoning, 1 tsp	7	0	1
Meat Tenderizer, avg., 1 tsp	7	0	1
Molly McButter, 1 tsp	5	1	1
Mrs Dash Blends, 1 tsp	0	0	2
Perc Salt-free Seasoning, 1 tsp	8	0	2
Potato Toppings *(Knudsen)*, 1 Tbsp	30	2.5	1
Salad Sprinkles *(Lawry's)*, 1 tsp	16	<1	2
Salad Supreme *(McCormick)*, 1 tsp	10	<1	1
Salt: Regular, Sea Salt, Lite Salt	0	0	0
Seasoning Mixes, avg., 1/4 pkg	70	1	9
Taco Seasoning, avg., 1/4 pkg	30	<1	4
Old El Paso: Chili Season. Mix, 1 T.	15	0.5	3
Cheesy Taco Season. Mix, 1 Tbsp	15	0.5	3
Taco/Burrito Seasoning Mix, 2 tsp	15	0	4
Enchilada Seasoning Mix, 2 tsp	10	0	2
Fajita Seasoning Mix, 1 tsp	10	0	3
Vegit Seasoning Mix, 1 tsp	5	0	1

Condiments, Sauces

Average of Brands & Homemade

	C	F	Cb
Apple Sauce: (Also see Page 148)			
Sweetened, 1/4 cup, 2 1/4 oz	45	0	11
Unsweetened, 1/4 cup, 2 oz	27	0	6.5
Bac O's *(Betty Crocker)*, 1 tsp, 1/2 oz	60	3	4
Barbecue: Average, 1 Tbsp	25	0	6
Bearnaise Sce, 1/4 cup, 2 1/2 oz	190	19	5
Catsup (Ketchup): Reg., 1 Tbsp	15	0	4
Cheese, h/made, 1/4 cup, 2 1/2 oz	150	10	12
Chili Sauce: *Heinz*, 1 Tbsp	15	0	4
Del Monte, 1 Tbsp	20	0	5
Wolf Hot Dog, 1 Tbsp	15	1	2
Cocktail Sce: 1/4 cup	110	0	15
Cranberry, all types, 1/4 c., 2 1/2 oz	110	0	27
Escoffier Sauces, 1 Tbsp	20	0	4
Honey Mustard *(French's)* 1 tsp	5	0	1
Horseradish, 1 tsp	2	0	0
Sauceworks Sauce, 1 tsp	20	2	0
Ketchup: Regular, 1 Tbsp	16	0	4
Heinz Lite, 1 Tbsp	8	0	2
Heinz Kick'rs, 1 Tbsp	20	0	4
Mushroom Sauce, 1/2 cup, 2 oz	50	2	5
Mustard, average, 1 tsp	5	0	0.5
Pesto, 1/4 cup, 2 oz	35	3	2
Pizza Sauce, cnd., 1/4 cup, 2 oz	25	0	5
Seafood Cocktail Sce, 1/4 cup	60	0	14
Soy Sauce, all types, av., 1 Tbsp	10	0	0
Sour Cream Sce, 1/2 cup	250	15	22
Spaghetti Sce: 1/2 cup, 4 1/2 oz	135	6	19
Steak Sauce: *Heinz*, 1 Tbsp	15	0	3
Lea & Perrins, 1 Tbsp	25	0	6
Str'berry Puree Sce: Unsweet., 2 T.	9	0	2
Sweet & Sour Sauce:			
Contadina, 2 Tbsp	40	1	8
Kikkoman Lite Soy, 1 Tbsp	10	0	1
La Choy, 2 Tbsp, 34g	60	0	14
Tabasco Sauce, 1 tsp	2	0	0
Taco Sauce, average, 2 Tbsp	10	0	1
Tartar Sauce: *Heinz*, 2 Tbsp, 30g	140	14	4
America's Choice, 2 Tbsp, 27g	160	17	1
Hellman's: Regular, 2 Tbsp, 30g	80	7	3
Lowfat, 2 Tbsp, 30g	40	1.5	7
Teriyaki Sce: *Kikkoman*, 1 Tbsp	15	0	2
Vinegar, White or wine, 1 fl.oz	4	0	1
White Sauce, 1/2 cup, 5 oz	130	7	12
Worcestershire Sauce, 1 tsp	5	0	1

Pickles • Salsa • Gravy

Pickles & Relish

	C	F	Cb
Average All Brands			
Bread & Butter Pickles, 4 sl.,1 oz	20	0	5
Chutney, 2 Tbsp, 1¼ oz	40	0	12
Dill Pickle:			
Slices, 4 slices, 1 oz	3	0	0.5
1 large, (3¾" x 1¼" diam.), 2¼ oz	12	0	3
Extra lrg (4" x 1¾" diam.), 5 oz	30	0	6
Halves: Small, 1 oz	3	0	0.5
Large, 2½ oz	8	0	2
Sweet, small, ½ oz	22	0	6
Gherkins, sweet, 1 med., 1 oz	15	0	7
Green Chilies, chopped, 2 Tbsp	5	0	1
Horseradish, 1 Tbsp	10	0	2
Jalapenos, pickled, 2 whole	5	0	1
Jalapeno Relish, 1 Tbsp, ½ oz	5	0	1
Mustard, aver. all brands, 1 tsp	5	0	0.5
Peppers: Hot/Mild, 1 oz	8	0	2
Pickled: Beets, ½ cup, 4 oz	75	0	19
Onions, 1 medium, ¾ oz	10	0	2
Cocktail Onion, 1 onion	2	0	0
Red Cabbage, ½ cup, 3 oz	60	0	13
Pickles:			
Sweet, 2 Tbsp, 1 oz	35	0	0
Large (3" x ¾ diam.), 1¼ oz	40	0	10
Pickle in a Pouch, 1 large	12	0	3
Relishes: Sandwich Spread, 1 tsp	20	1	5
Cranberry-Orange, 1 Tbsp	30	0	7
Hot Dog (*Heinz*), 1 Tbsp	17	0	28
Sweet Pickle, 1 Tbsp	20	0	5
Sauerkraut, ½ cup, 3½ oz	25	0	5
Sweet Cauliflower	35	0	8

Salsa

	C	F	Cb
Average all Types: Per 2 Tablespoons			
Regular, no oil, 2 Tbsp	15	0	3.5
Homemade w. Oil, 2 Tbsp	40	3	8
Chef's Kitchen, 2 Tbsp	10	0	2
Del Monte, all flavors, 2 Tbsp	10	0	2
Kaukauma, 2 Tbsp	15	0	3
Wild Oats, 2 Tbsp, 1 oz	10	0	2

Gravy

	C	F	Cb
Homemade Gravy:			
Thin, little fat, 2 Tbsp, 1 oz	20	1	3
Thick, 2 Tbsp, 1¼ oz	50	2	9
¼ cup, 2½ oz	100	4	18
Franco-American (Canned)			
Au Jus Gravy, ¼ cup, 2 oz	10	0	2
Beef; Turkey Gravy, 2 oz	25	0.5	3
Chicken Gravy, ¼ cup, 2 oz	40	4	4
Franco-American (In Jars)			
99% Fat Free, ¼ cup, 2 oz	25	0.5	4
Pillsbury (Gravy Mixes)			
Brown; Homestyle, ¼ cup, 2 oz	15	0	3
Chicken, as prep., ¼ cup, 2 oz	20	0	4

Gravy-In-Jars-Homestyle

	C	F	Cb
Boston Market, ¼ cup, 2 oz	25	1	3
Heinz, reg., all types, ¼ c., 2 oz	25	1	3
Fat Free Rst. Turkey, ¼ c., 2 oz	10	0	2
Vons, all types, ¼ c., 2 oz	20	0.5	4

Tomato Products

	C	F	Cb
Whole/Chopped/Crushed/Diced			
1 cup, 8½ oz	50	0	10
In Aspic, ½ cup	50	0	12
w. Green Chili, 1 cup, 8½ oz	45	<1	11
Stewed, ½ cup	40	2.5	9
Wedges in Tom Juice, 1 cup	70	0.5	15
Salsa, average, 1 Tbsp	15	0	3.5
Tomato Ketchup:			
Regular, 1 Tbsp	16	0	4
Green (*Heinz*), 1 Tbsp	20	0	5
Tomato Paste, 2 Tbsp	25	0	5
Regular, 6 oz, ¾ cup	150	0	34
Tomato Puree, ½ cup	50	0	10
Tomato Sauce:			
Regular, ½ cup	40	0	9
Spanish Style, ½ cup	40	0	9
w. Mushrooms, ½ cup	40	0	9
w. Onions, ½ cup	50	0	11
Tomato Seasoning, 3 tsp	20	0	4
Sundried Tomatoes:			
Natural, 5-6 pces, 0.4 oz	22	0	5
In Oil, drained, 6 pces, ½ oz	60	4	5

Sauces ~ Pasta, Cooking

Brands	C	F	Cb
A-1			
Steak Sauce: *Per Tablespoon*			
Original	10	0	3
Bold & Spicy	20	0	5
Smoky Mesquite	30	0	8
Barilla: *Per 1/2 Cup*			
Marinara; Sweet Peppers & Garlic	90	3	11
Roasted Garlic & Onion	90	3.5	11
Tomato & Basil	80	2.5	12
Bertoli/Five Brothers: *Per 1/2 Cup*			
Alfredo w. Mushrooms	160	12	6
Creamy Alfredo	220	20	6
Grilled Summer Vegetable	80	5	12
Imported Romano & Garlic	90	4	10
Marinara w. Burgundy Wine	80	3	12
Mushroom & Garlic	90	3	13
Olive Oil & Garlic	90	4	9
Olive w. Sundried Tomato	100	4	13
Oven Roasted Garlic & Onion	70	1.5	10
Roasted Red Pepper	80	3	13
Tomato Basil	80	2	10
Best Foods			
Dippin' Sauce: *Per Tablespoon*			
Honey Mustard Madness	30	1	5
Rockin' Ranch	45	3	4
Totally BBQ	55	6	0.5
Bookbinders: *Per 1/2 Cup*			
White Clam Sauce	300	30	4
Bullseye: BBQ, 1 Tbsp	25	0	6
Classico: *Per 1/2 Cup*			
Alfredo	220	20	6
Italian Sausage w. Pepper & Onions	70	3	80
Mushroom & Olive	50	1	10
Portobello Mushroom	60	1	11
Roasted Garlic Alfredo	220	20	6
Roasted Peppers & Onions/Garlic	60	2	9
Spicy Red Pepper	60	2.5	9
Spicy Tomato & Pesto	90	5	9
Sun Dried Tomato; 4 Cheese	80	4	8
Sun Dried Tomato Alfredo	220	18	6
Sweet Basil Marinara	70	2	11
Tomato & Basil	50	1	9

Contadina	C	F	Cb
Pasta Sauces: *Per 1/2 Cup*			
Alfredo Sauce	360	32	10
Lite	160	10	10
Garden Vegetable Sauce	40	0	9
Marinara Sauce	80	4	9
Mushroom Alfredo	200	14	12
Mushroom Marinara Sauce	70	2.5	11
Pesto w. Basil, Red. Fat	460	26	22
Pesto w. Sundried Tomato	380	30	20
Roasted Garlic Marinara	60	2	10
Pizza Squeeze Sce, 1/4 cup	35	1.5	6
Del Monte			
Pasta Sauces: *Per 1/2 Cup*			
Chunky Sce, average all varieties	60	1.5	11
D'Italia Pasta: Four Cheese	60	2	8
Other varieties	50	1.5	9
Spaghetti Sauce: Traditional	60	0.5	15
Garlic & Onion	60	1.5	11
w. Mushroom/Meat	70	1.5	14
Sloppy Joe Sauce,1/4 cup, 67g	50	0	11
Dominick's: *Per 1/2 Cup*			
All Natural: Garl. & Onion; Marinara	80	4	10
Mushr. & Olive; Tomato & Basil	80	1	8
Italian Classics: Four Cheese	80	2.5	12
Portabella Mushroom	60	2	9
Puttanesca	70	3	8
Spicy Roasted Garlic	70	2	10
Sun Ripened Tomatoes	80	4	8
Tomato Basil	50	1	8
Estee			
Barbecue Sauce, 1 Tbsp	18	<1	3
Spaghetti Sauce, 1/4 cup, 4 oz	60	2	13
Steak Sauce, 1 Tbsp	14	<1	3
Enrico's			
Tomato Basil, 3.5 oz (100g)	65	2	10
Traditional Italian Style, 3.5 oz	55	0.5	11
Mushroom Onion, 1/2 cup (125g)	70	1	12
Other varieties, 1/2 cup (125g)	70	2	12
Emiril's: *Per 1/2 Cup (123g)*			
Puttanesca	80	5	9
Roasted Red Pepper	60	3	7
Vodka Sauce	130	8	13

Brands (Cont)

	C	F	Cb
Frank Sinatra: *Per 1/4 Cup*			
Alfredo; Pesto	160	14	4
French's Grill & Glaze			
Honey Mustard, 2 Tbsp	90	1	18
Teriyaki, 2 Tbsp	60	0	13
Garden Valley: *Per 1/2 Cup*			
Chunky Vege. Primavera	35	0.5	12
Four Cheese	35	1	8
Millina's Finest; Roasted Garlic	50	0	12
Sundried Tomato; Tomato Mushr.	50	0	11
Sweet Tomato Basil	60	0	13
Green Giant			
Sloppy Joe S'wich Sce, 1/4 c., 2.5 oz	50	0	11
Sloppy Joe Sauce & Meat	200	11	11
Hagerty Foods: *Per 4 oz*			
Artichoke	100	6	11
Asparagus Garlic	95	7	9
Healthy Choice: *Per Serving*			
Creamy Alfredo, 1/4 cup	45	3	3
Garlic & Herbs, 1/2 cup	50	0	13
Garlic Lovers, 1/2 cup	45	0	10
Mushroom Alfredo	45	3	3
Roasted Garlic & Romano	60	1	11
Sundried Tomato & Herb	60	0.5	12
Traditional Pasta Sauce, 1/2 cup	50	0	13
Super Chunky: Vege Primavera, 1/2 c.	60	0	13
Tomato, Mushroom Garlic, 1/2 c.	50	0	10
Heinz: *Per 1 Tbsp (Approx. 1/2 oz)*			
Barbecue Sauces, all flavors	35	0	9
Chili Sauce, 1 Tbsp	15	0	4
Horseradish Sauce	70	7	2
Mustard: Pourable/Mild, 1 Tbsp	8	0.5	0
Spicy Brown	13	1	1
Seafood Cocktail Sauce	20	0	3
Steak Sauce 57	15	0	4
Tartar Sauce, 1 Tbsp	70	7	2
Tomato Ketchup	16	0	4
Worcestershire Sauce, 1 Tbsp	8	0	1
Sloppy Joe Sauce, 1/2 cup, 125g	70	0.5	14
Hunt's			
BBQ Sauce: Original, 36g, 2 Tbsp	50	0	13
Hickory & Brown Sugar, 38g, 2 T.	70	0	18
Manwich Sloppy Joe Sce, 1/4 c., 64g	30	0	6
Hy Top: *Per 1/2 Cup (125g)*			
Spaghetti Sauce, all flavors	90	4	11

	C	F	Cb
KC Masterpiece: *Per Tablespoon*			
Marinades: Garlic & Herb	30	1.5	4
Honey & Teriyaki	35	0.5	7
Original BBQ	40	1.5	7
Knorr (Sauce Mix)			
Made As Directed: *Per 1/4 Cup (2 oz)*			
Au Jus	8	0.2	1
Bearnaise	170	17	5
Classic Brown Gravy	25	1	3
Demi-Glace	30	1	4
Hollandaise	170	18	5
Hunter; Lyonnaise	25	0.3	4
Mushroom Sauce	60	3	5
Napoli Sauce	100	3	17
Pepper Sauce	20	1	3
Knudsen: Potato Toppings, 2 T	50	4.5	2
Kraft			
Sauceworks: Cocktail, 2 Tbsp	30	0.3	6
Horseradish, 1 tsp	20	1.5	0
Sweet 'n Sour, 1 Tbsp	30	0	7
Tartar: 1 Tbsp	50	5	2
Lemon & Herb, 1 Tbsp	75	8	0
Nonfat Tartar, 1 Tbsp	12	0	5
Barbecue Sauces: Average, 2 T.	50	0.5	9
Other Sauces: Mustard, 1 Tbsp	10	0	0
Horseradish, Reg./Crm Style, 1 T.	10	0	0
Sandwich Spread & Burger, 1 T.	50	4	3
Sweet 'n Sour, 1 Tbsp	40	0.5	9
Las Palmas			
Red Chile Sauce, 1/4 cup, 2 oz	15	0.5	2
Enchilada Sauces: Green Chile	25	1.5	3
Hot/Original, 1/4 cup, 2 oz	15	0.5	3
Salsa: Mexicana, 2 Tbsp, 1 oz	5	0	1
Mexicana Hot/Medium, 2 Tbsp	10	0	2
Lawry's 30 Minute Marinade: *Per Tbsp*			
Carribean Jerk; Teriyaki	25	0	6
Hawaiian; Dijon & Honey	20	0	3.5
Mediterranean; Lemon Pepper	10	0	2
Mesquite	5	0	1
Thai Ginger; Herb & Garlic	10	0	2
Packet Seasonings: *Per Tablespoon (Dry)*			
Fajitas; Taco	30	0	6
Average other flavors	40	0	8
Libby's			
Sloppy Joe Sauce, 1/3 cup, 78g	45	0	10

Sauces ~ Pasta, Cooking

Brands (Cont)	C	F	Cb
McCormick Sauce Mixes			
Grillmates: Marinade, avg., 2 tsp	15	0	2
Sauce Blend Seasoning Mixes:			
Lemon Herb Chicken, 1 Tbsp	30	0	5
Chicken Fried Rice, 1 Tbsp	35	0	6
Stir Fry Chicken, 1 Tbsp	20	0	4
Chicken Teriyaki, 1^{1}/3 Tbsp	40	1	5
Mr Yoshida's			
Original Gourmet, 2 Tbsp, 30ml	90	0	20
Hawaiian Sweet & Sour, 2 Tbsp	35	0	9
Muir Glen: Per ^{1}/2 Cup (125g)			
Organic Pasta Sauce:			
Mushr. Marinara; Portobello Mushr.	50	0	11
Other varieties, average	50	1	11
Newman's Own: Per ^{1}/2 Cup			
Bombolina (Tomato & Basil)	100	5	15
Roasted Garlic & Peppers	70	2.5	11
Other flavors	60	2	9
Old El Paso			
Salsa: Thick 'n Chunky, 2 T., 1 oz	10	0	2
Homestyle; Green Chili; Verde 2 Tbsp, 1 oz	10	0	2
Taco Sce, all varieties, 2 Tbsp, 1 oz	10	0	2
Enchilada Sce, all types, ^{1}/4 c., 2 oz	20	1	3
Grilling Sauces, all types, ^{1}/4 c.	60	0	14
Tom. & Gr. Chiles/Jalapenos,^{1}/4 c., 2 oz	10	0	2
Pace			
Picante Sauce, ^{1}/4 cup, 2 oz	25	0	5
Chunky Salsa, avg. all types	10	0	2
Salsa Con Queso	45	3	4
Prego: Per ^{1}/2 Cup			
Extra Chunky: Garden Comb.	90	2	16
Garlic Supreme	120	3	23
Mushroom & Green Pepper	120	4.5	18
Mushroom Supreme	120	4.5	21
Pasta Bake: Per ^{1}/8 Jar			
Italian Sausage	90	3.5	12
3-Cheese Marinara	100	4.5	11
Hearty Meat Sauce	120	6	12
Tomato, Garlic & Basil	80	3.5	11
Mushroom w. Garlic & Onion	90	3	13
Pasta Bake: Per ^{1}/2 cup, ^{1}/2 c.	120	5	16
Meatball Parmesan, ^{1}/2 cup	160	7	15
Fresh Mushrooms, ^{1}/2 cup	130	5	15

Premier Japan (Organic)	C	F	Cb
Garlic/Ginger/Wasabi Tamari, 1 T.	10	0	2
Thai Soynut, 1 Tbsp	25	2	2
Ragu: Per ^{1}/2 Cup			
Meat Flavored Sauce	80	4	7
Traditional	70	3	8
Cheese Creations:			
Double Cheddar	200	18	6
Mushroom Green Pepper	110	3	16
Roasted Garlic Parmesan	240	22	6
Chunky Garden Style:			
Gard. Combo; Mushr. Gr. Pepper	100	3	16
Other varieties, average	110	3	18
Rich & Meaty: Classic Italian Style	150	10	9
Mama's Meat Sauce	130	8	8
Sausage, Peppers & Onions	160	11	9
Robusto!: Six Cheese	80	3	9
Italian Sausage & Cheese	100	4.5	11
Sauteed Onion & Mushr./Garlic	90	4	11
Tomato, Olive Oil, Garlic	90	4.5	9
Pizza Sauce: ^{1}/4 cup	30	1	4
Pizza Quick, average, ^{1}/4 cup	40	1.5	6
Rainforest Organic			
Ginger Curry, 1 Tbsp	15	1.5	1
Mango; Papaya Pepper, 1 Tbsp	5	0	1
Tamarind Spice, 1 Tbsp	5	0	1
Rinaldi: Per ^{1}/2 Cup			
3-Cheese	90	2	15
Original; Meat/Mushroom	90	4	11
Tomato & Basil	80	2.5	11
Tomato, Garlic, Onion	80	2	12
S & W: Per 1 Tbsp			
Mesquite Marinated Cooking	10	0	3
Teriyaki, Light/Marinade	25	0	5
Seeds of Change: Per ^{1}/2 Cup			
Average all varieties	50	0.5	9
Steel's Gourmet Sauce			
Barbeque Sce, Sweet & Spicy, 2 Tbsp.	15	0	2
Cocktail Sce w. Dill & Lemon, 4 Tbsp.	36	0	1
Hoisin, 2 Tbsp., 1 fl.oz	10	0	2
Rocky Mountain Ketchup, 1 oz	10	0	0
Spiced Cranberry Sce, 4 Tbsp.	16	0	4
Sweet & Sour, 2 Tbsp. 1 oz	10	0	2

Brands (Cont)   **C** **F** **Cb**

Sutter Home: *Per 1/2 Cup*

	C	F	Cb
Other varieties	80	2	12
Marinara Pasta Sauce	70	2	11

Taj: *Per 1/2 Cup*

Bombay Curry Simmer Sauce	90	5	10
Calcutta Masala Simmer Sauce	100	5	13
Kashmir Tandoori Marinade Sce	50	3	5
Seasoning Mixes: Chili, 1 tsp	40	1	6
Meat Loaf; Sloppy Joe's, 1 tsp	30	0	4
Beef Stew, 1 tsp	15	0	3
Chicken/Taco Seasoning, 1 tsp	25	0	4
Spaghetti Sauce: Italian Style, 1 T.	25	0	5

The Wizard's (Organic)

Hot Nutz, 1 Tbsp	30	2	2
Hot Stuff, 1 Teaspoon	0	0	0
Vegetarian Worcestershire, 1 Tbsp	10	0	2

Troy's Sauces (Organic)

Ginger Sauce, 1 Tbsp	5	0	1
Peanut Sauce, 1 Tbsp	30	2	1

Timpone's: *Per 1/2 Cup*

Spaghetti Sauce: Classic	50	2.5	8
Family Recipe	80	3	7
Mom's	70	3.5	8

Tomaso's: *Per 1/2 Cup*

Basil & Fresh Garlic; Spicy Eggplant	60	3	7
Black Olive Fresh Basil	40	2	5
Extra Garlic	55	2	8
Fresh Mushroom & Artichoke	50	2	7
Sugo Rosa	105	7.5	8

Tree of Life: *Per 1/2 Cup*

Pasta Sauce Plus, all varieties	45	0	9
Organic, average all varieties	35	0	8

Walnut Acres: *Per 1/2 Cup (125g)*

Organic Pasta Sauce, average	50	1	9

Wild Oats: *Per 2 Tbsp (1 oz)*

Wasabi; Seafood Marinade & Grilled	30	3	4
Korean Sesame Marinade & Grilled	30	0	8

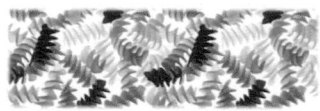

Quick Guide

Mayonnaise   **C** **F** **Cb**

Regular

	C	F	Cb
Average All Brands, 1 Tbsp	100	11	0
Bestfoods, Kraft, 1 Tbsp	100	11	0
1/2 cup, 4 oz	800	88	0

Light/Reduced Fat

Kraft, 1 Tbsp	50	5	1
Best Foods, 1 Tbsp	45	4	2
1/2 cup, 4 oz	360	32	4
Hain, Eggless, Tbsp	60	6	2
Hain, Safflower Oil, Tbsp	50	5	2
Hellman's, 1 Tbsp	50	5	1
Wild Oats Canola Oil, 1 Tbsp	100	12	0

Fat Free

Kraft, 1 Tbsp	10	0	3
1/2 cup, 4 oz	80	0	16
Smart Beat, 1 Tbsp	10	0	3
Sugar Free: *Dukes Mayo*, 1 Tbsp	10	12	0

Mayonnaise Style Dressing

BAMA Dressing, 1 Tbsp, 0.5 oz	50	4	3
Gourmayo (French's), 1 Tbsp, 0.5 oz	50	5	1
***Miracle Whip* Salad Dressing:**			
Regular, 1 Tbsp, 0.5 oz	70	7	2
Light, 1 Tbsp, 0.5 oz	40	3	3
Free, 1 Tbsp, 0.5 oz	15	0	3
Nayonaise (Nasoya)			
(Tofu Base/Dairy Free/Eggless)			
Regular, 1 Tbsp, 0.5 oz	35	3	1
Fat-Free, 1 Tbsp, 0.5 oz	10	0	2

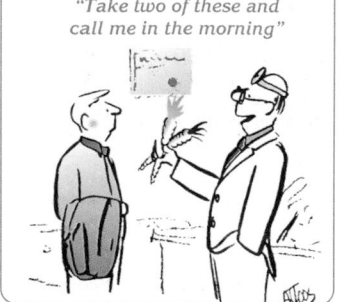

"Take two of these and call me in the morning"

Salad Dressings

Quick Guide

Salad Dressings

Average All Brands
Per 2 Tbsp (Approx 1 fl.oz)

	C	F	Cb
Blue Cheese: Regular	150	16	2
Light/Reduced Fat	80	8	1
Caesar: Regular	140	14	2
Light/Reduced Fat	50	5	0.5
French: Regular	130	11	5
Light/Reduced Fat	50	3	4
Fat/Oil-Free	40	0	4
Italian: Regular	130	11	3
Light/Reduced Fat	70	7	2
Fat/Oil-Free	10	0	2
Ranch: Regular	180	18	3
Light/Reduced Fat	90	8	3
Fat-Free	50	0	2
Russian: Regular	130	10	3
Light/Reduced Fat	50	5	3
Fat-Free	30	0	2
Thousand Island: Regular	130	12	5
Light/Reduced Fat	50	4	3
Fat-Free	35	0	3

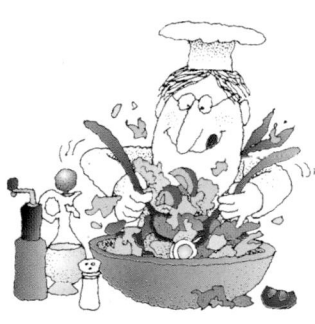

*Enjoy a healthy salad
but don't drown it
in high-fat salad dressings.*

Brands ~ Salad Dressings

Per 2 Tbsp (Approx 1 fl.oz)

	C	F	Cb
Annie's Naturals			
Cowgirl Ranch	120	11	3
French	90	9	3
Gardenstyle (vinegar free)	120	12	3
Goddess	90	8	3
Organic: Buttermilk	70	7	1
No Fat Yogurt	20	0	3
Red Wine & Olive Oil	160	17	1
Thousand Island	90	7	5
Tuscany Italian	80	7	5
Vinaigrette: Balsamic	100	10	3
Black Olives & Truffle	110	12	1
Cilantro & Lime	100	10	2
Low Fat: Honey Mustard	45	2	6
Gingerly	40	2	4
Raspberry	35	1.5	5
Roasted Red Pepper	70	6	3
Shiitake & Sesame	120	13	1
Yellow Pepper & Tomato	70	7	2
Bernstein's			
Balsamic Italian	110	11	2
Cheese: Garlic Italian; Fantastico	110	11	2
Creamy Caesar	120	13	2
Fat Free Cheese & Garlic Italian	10	0	1
Italian	110	12	1
Olive Oil Vinaigrette	90	9	3
Red Wine & Garlic Italian	110	11	2
Restaurant Recipe Italian	130	13	1
Light Fantastic: Cheese Fantastico	25	1.5	3
Roasted Garlic Balsamic	45	3.5	3
Bob's Famous			
Ranch Country	150	15	1
Roquefort; Thousand Isld; Blue Chse	140	14	1
Tartar Sauce	170	16	2
Brianna's			
Blue Cheese; Zesty French	130	13	4
Blush Vintage	100	6	12
French Vinaigrette, 2 Tbsp	150	17	0
Honey Mustard; Poppy Seed	130	12	6
Lemon Tarragon	35	8	8
Rich Santa Fe Blend	15	0	3

Per 2 Tbsp (Approx 1 fl.oz)	C	F	Cb
Cardini's			
Caesar, 2 Tbsp	160	17	1
Fat-Free Caesar	40	0	9
Light Caesar	80	7	5
Extra Virgin Olive Oil Ital.; Zesty Garl.	120	13	1
Honey Mustard	140	13	5
Kalamata Olive w. Romano Cheese	120	13	2
Lemon Herb	120	13	1
Parmesan Ranch	150	15	2
Poppyseed w. Shallots	160	14	8
Vintage White Wine	110	12	1
El Torito: Cilantro Pepita Caesar	140	14	2
Emirl's: *Per 2 Tbsp*			
House Herb Viniagrette	140	14	2
Kicked Up Gaaalic	150	15	3
Girards: *Per 2 Tbsp*			
Balsamic Basil	90	7	3
Blue Cheese Vinaigrette	100	10	3
Caesar	150	16	1
Lite	80	7	2
Champagne	150	16	2
Lite Champagne	60	5	2
Greek Feta Vinaigrette	110	11	1
Honey Dijon Peppercorn	120	13	7
Olde Venice Italian	120	13	2
Oriental Chicken Salad	120	11	6
Original French	120	13	0
Raspberry	90	10	9
Romano Cheese	130	13	2
Shiitake Chardonnay	100	9	4
Spinach Salad	80	2	14
Fat Free: Balsamic/Red Wine, avg.	25	0	6
Caesar	40	0	9
Raspberry	50	0	13
Good Seasons (Mix)			
Per 2 Tbsp (Prepared from 4g Dry Mix)			
Blue Cheese, Cheese Garlic	145	16	2
Cheese Italian, Garlic & Herbs	145	16	2
Classic Dill	30	0	5
Gourmet Caesar	150	16	3
Italian varieties	145	16	2
Lite Italian varieties	55	6	2
Ranch	115	12	2
Fat Free: Italian; Roasted Garlic	10	0	2
Gourmet Caesar	15	0	2

Hidden Valley: *Per 2 Tbsp*	C	F	Cb
Light Range			
Original Ranch w. Sour Cream	145	7	6
w. Garlic	130	13	2
w. Sundried Tomato	140	14	2
Regular Range: BBQ Ranch	120	12	3
B.L.T. Ranch; Coleslaw	150	15	5
B.L.T. Ranch Light	90	7	5
Caesar w. Garlic	120	11	4
French w. Honey & Bacon	150	12	10
Garden Vege; Garlic & Spice	130	13	3
Italian Herb & Cheese	30	0	6
Ranch: Caesar Creamy	110	11	1
Original Ranch	140	14	1
Light Ranch	80	7	3
w. Bacon	140	14	1
Fat Free: Caesar; Ranch	30	0	6
Honey & Bacon French	50	0	11
Honey Dijon	35	0	7
Italian Parmesan	20	0	4
Red Wine & Herb Vinaigrette	45	0	11
Roasted Garlic Italian	40	0	5
Ken's Steak House Dressings: *Per 2 Tbsp*			
3 Cheese Italian	110	10	4
Balsamic & Basil Vinaigrette	110	12	1
Chunky Blue Cheese	140	15	1
Country French	130	11	9
Creamy Caesar	170	19	0
Peppercorn Ranch	180	19	2
Ranch	180	20	1
Italian w. Aged Romano	110	12	1
Thousand Island	130	13	4
Lite: Chunky Blue Cheese	80	7	4
Caesar/Olive Oil Vinaigrette	70	6	3
Creamy Parmesan	90	8	3
Ranch	100	9	4
Knott's Berry Farm: *Per 2 Tbsp, 1 oz*			
Honey Dijon, 2 Tbsp	130	13	4
Honey Poppyseed	120	9	10
Oriental Chicken Salad	130	11	5
Parmesan & Peppercorn	160	17	1
Sun Dried Tomato	100	10	3
Low Fat: Raspberry	50	2	8
Tropical Fruit	45	1	9

Salad Dressings (Cont)

Per 2 Tbsp (Approx 1 fl.oz)

	C	F	Cb
Kraft			
Regular Dressings: *Per 2 Tbsp*			
3 Cheese Ranch	170	18	1
Buttermilk; Ranch w. Bacon	150	16	1
Caesar w. Bacon	150	15	1
Catalina	90	6	8
Classic Caesar	110	11	0.5
Coleslaw	150	12	8
Cucumber Ranch	140	15	2
Creamy Italian	110	11	3
French	120	12	4
Roka Brand Blue Cheese	90	7	5
Thousand Island, avg.	105	9	5
Thousand Island w. Bacon	100	8	6
Kraft Free (Fat Free): Italian	10	0	2
Blue Cheese, Catalina, French	50	0	12
Caesar Italian	25	0	4
Other varieties, avg.	45	0	11
Light Done Right!: Classic Caesar	70	6	3
Catalina	60	2	11
Ranch; Thousand Island	70	4.5	7
Roka Blue Cheese	70	6	3
3 Cheese Ranch	80	7	4
Special Collection: Caesar Italian	100	10	2
Balsamic Vinaigrette	90	8	4
Classic Italian Vinaigrette	50	4	4
Sun Dried Tomato	60	5	4
Sweet Honey Catalina	130	11	8
Seven Seas: Viva Italian	90	9	2
Red Wine Vinaigrette	90	9	2
Litehouse: Caesar	140	14	1
Chunky Bleu Cheese	150	16	1
Coleslaw	90	7	7
Honey Mustard	130	14	3
Jalapeno Ranch	120	12	1
Lite Bleu Cheese	70	6	2
Ranch; Thousand Island	120	13	3
Maple Grove: *Per 2 Tbsp (1 fl.oz)*			
Caesar	110	12	1
Greek	100	10	2
Shiitake w. Roasted Garlic	150	16	2
Sundried Tomato	35	1	7
Vermont Honey Mustard	120	9	9
Light: Presto Parmesan	70	5	5
Fat Free: Balsamic Vinaigrette	10	0	2
Poppyseed; Raspberry Vinaigrette	40	0	10

	C	F	Cb
Marie's: *Per 2 Tbsp*			
1000 Island	190	20	2
Blue Cheese	170	18	0
Caesar	150	13	8
Poppy Seed	190	20	1
Ranch (8 fl.oz ctn), 2 Tbsp	160	16	4
(15.5 fl.oz ctn), 2 Tbsp	170	19	1
Light: Blue Cheese	70	7	2
Ranch	70	7	2
Nasoya: *Per 2 Tbsp*			
Vegi-Dressing (Tofu Base/Dairy Free):			
Thousand Island	60	4	6
Other flavors	60	5	3
Nayonaise, Regular, 2 Tbsp, 1 oz	70	6	2
Fat-Free, 2 Tbsp, 1 oz	20	0	4
Newman's Own: *Per 2 Tbsp*			
Balsamic Vinaigrette, 2 Tbsp	90	9	3
Caesar; Olive Oil & Vinegar	150	16	1
Creamy Caesar	170	18	1
Family Recipe Italian	120	13	1
Parmesan & Roasted Garlic	110	11	2
Parmesan Italiano	140	14	2
Ranch	180	18	2
Two Thousand Island	140	14	4
Lighten Up: Light Italian	60	6	1
Light Raspberry & Walnut	70	5	7
Light Balsamic Vinaigrette	45	4	2
Pritikin: Honey Dijon	45	0	11
Dijon Balsamic; Zesty Italian	30	0	6
Honey French Style	40	0	10
Raspberry	35	0	11
San-J: Tamari Peanut	60	2	9
Tamari Sesame	45	2	5
Tamari Vinaigrette	45	3	4
Fat Free: Tamari Mustard	25	0	5
S & W: *Per 2 Tbsp, 1 oz*			
Light: Italian	35	0	8
Red/White Wine; Raspberry Blush	40	0	10
Seeds of Change: *Per 2 Tbsp, 1 oz*			
Balsamic/Greek Feta Vinaigrette	60	5	4
Italian Herb Vinaigrette	50	4	4
Spike Splashes!			
Original, 2 Tbsp	100	11	1
Salt Free	100	10	2
Fat Free	10	0	2

Per 2 Tbsp (Approx 1 fl.oz)

	C	F	Cb
Spectrum			
Fat Free: Creamy Dill/Garlic	25	0	4
Sweet On. & Garlic; Tstd Sesame	15	0	3
Lowfat: Blue Chse Style; Honey Dijon	35	2	3
Creamy Roasted Pepper	45	2	5
Mango Madness	50	2	7
Southwestern Caesar	40	2	3
Zesty Italian	30	2	1
Steel's (Sugar Free)			
Honey Mustard, 2 Tbsp	180	14	0
Sweet Ginger Lime, 2 Tbsp	140	14	2
Subway Select: *Per 2 Tbsp, 1 oz*			
Premium Collection: Caesar	170	16	1
Lite Blue Cheese; Lite Ranch	80	7	1
1000 Island	130	13	4
Jalapeno Ranch	100	10	1
The Spice Hunter: *Per 2 Tbsp (Mix Prepared)*			
Caesar Salad, 2 Tbsp	150	13	1
Chinese Salad; Garlic & Herb	140	13	2
T. Marzetti's: *Per 2 Tbsp, 1 oz*			
Regular: Balsam./Wild Berry Vinaig.	100	9	4
Buttermilk	180	19	1
Creamy Caesar	150	17	0
Caesar Lite	70	6	2
Italian	100	10	3
Original Slaw	170	16	6
Ranch	160	17	2
Red Wine Vinegar & Oil	130	14	2
Roasted Garlic	150	15	2
Roasted Garlic Vinaigrette	130	10	8
Sesame Oriental	110	9	8
Sour Cream Blue Cheese	170	16	0
Sun Dried Tomato Vinaigrette	130	11	6
Vinaigrette Blue Cheese	120	11	4
Light: Buttermilk Ranch	80	8	2
Chunky Blue Cheese	90	5	5
Original Slaw	100	7	10
Tree of Life: *Per 2 Tbsp, 1 oz*			
House Dressing: Cafe Venice	120	12	2
Maison Caesar	70	6	1
Shanghai Palace	80	7	3
Lowfat Free: Blue Cheese	15	1	2
Fat Free: Honey French	35	0	8
Italian Garlic	20	0	4
Oriental Ginger	15	0	3

	C	F	Cb
Walden Farms			
Fat Free, Calorie Free Range, 2 Tbsp	0	0	0
Weight Watchers			
Salad Celebrations Dressings			
Fat Free: Caesar (Single), 0.75 oz	5	0	1
Caesar, 2 Tbsp	10	0	1
Creamy Italian (8 oz), 2 Tbsp	30	0	7
French Style, 2 Tbsp	40	0	9
Honey Dijon, 2 Tbsp	45	0	11
Italian (8 oz), 2 Tbsp	10	0	2
Ranch Style, 2 Tbsp	35	0	7
Ranch (Single), 0.75 oz	25	0	6
Wild Oats: *Per 2 Tbsp, 1 oz*			
Balsamic Vinaigrette; Thousand Isle	80	7	5
Caesar Style	120	12	1
Creamy Peppercorn	100	10	1
Honey Toasted Sesame Ginger	100	10	3
Ranch	120	11	3
Thousand Isle	90	7	5
Wishbone: *Per 2 Tbsp, 1 oz*			
Regular: 5 Cheese Italian	120	10	6
Chunky Blue Cheese	170	17	2
Classic Caesar	110	10	2
Creamy Caesar	180	18	1
French: Deluxe French	120	11	5
Sweet 'N Spicy	140	12	6
Italian: Regular	80	8	3
House Italian	110	10	3
Robusto Italian	90	8	4
Ranch: Original	160	17	1
w. Garlic/Spring Onion	150	15	2
Red Wine; Balsamic Vinaigrette	60	5	3
Russian, regular	110	6	15
Thousand Island	130	12	7
Fat Free: Chunky Blue Cheese	35	0	7
Italian	15	0	2
Ranch	40	0	9
Dressing & Marinades: Asian	45	2	6
Balsamic Olive Oil & Herbs	40	2.5	4
Lemon Garlic & Herb	50	2.5	6
Tangy Honey Mustard	70	4	10
Ranch Up!	140	15	2
Just 2 Good!: Blue Cheese	45	2	6
Classic/Creamy Caesar; Ranch	40	2	5
Country Italian; Italian	30	2	5
Parmesan Peppercorn Ranch	45	2	6
Thousand Island	60	2	9

Breakfast Cereals

Quick Guide — Cooked Cereals

	C	F	Cb
Buckwheat Groats, roasted:			
Dry, 1/2 cup, 3 oz	280	2	60
Cooked, 1 cup, 7 oz	180	1	39
Bulgar: Dry, 1/2 cup, 2 1/2 oz	240	1	53
Cooked, 1 cup, 6 1/2 oz	150	<1	34
Corn/Hominy Grits:			
Dry, 1/4 cup, 1.4 oz	145	<1	33
3 Tbsp, 1 oz	110	<1	25
Cooked, 3/4 cup, 6 1/2 oz	110	<1	25
Instant, 1 pkt, 0.8 oz	80	<1	18
w. Imitation Bacon Bits, 1 oz	100	<1	22
Cream of Rice, ckd, 3/4 c, 6 oz	90	0	20
Cream of Wheat:			
Regular, ckd, 3/4 cup, 6 oz	180	<1	37
Quick, ckd, 3/4 cup, 6 oz	95	<1	20
Instant, ckd, 3/4 cup, 6 oz	110	<1	23
Farina: Cooked, 3/4 cup, 6 oz	85	0	18
Millet, dry, 1/4 cup, 1 oz	100	0	20
Oat Bran: Raw, 1/3 cup, 1 oz	75	2	14
Cooked, 1/2 cup	45	<1	8
Oatmeal: Dry, 1/3 cup, 1 oz	110	0	19
Regular, ckd, 3/4 cup, 6 oz	110	2	19
1 cup, 8 oz	145	3	25
Instant: Regular, avg., 1 oz	100	2	18
Flavored, average	150	2	32
Quaker: *See Brands*			
Wheat Hearts, 1 oz dry, 3/4 c. ckd	110	1	21

Brans, Wheatgerm, Add-Ons

	C	F	Cb
Bran: Wheat, unprocessed,			
1 Tbsp, 3g	10	0	3
Rice Bran, raw, 1 Tbsp, 5g	16	1	2.5
1/3 cup, 1 oz	90	6	14
Oat Bran, 1 Tbsp, 5g	15	<1	3
1/3 cup, 1 oz	75	2	15
Wheat Germ, 1 Tbsp, 1/4 oz	25	1	3.5
1/4 cup, 1 oz	105	3	15
Fruit: Dried, average, 1 oz	80	1	21
Banana, 1/2 medium	50	0	23
Prunes in Syrup, 5, 3 oz	90	0	24
Honey: 1 Tbsp, 3/4 oz	65	0	17
Lecithin Granules, 1 Tbsp, 10g	50	5	1
Nuts: Almonds, 6 (1/4 oz)	40	4	5
Bee Pollen Granules, 1 T., 8g	25	1	2
Psyllium Husks, 1 Tbsp, 5g	10	0	1

Quick Guide — Cold Cereals

Average All Brands

	C	F	Cb
Bran Flakes, 3/4 cup, 1 oz	90	<1	21
Corn Flakes, 1 cup, 1 oz	110	<1	24
Granola, 1/4 cup, 1 oz	130	4	21
Oat Bran Cereal, 1/3 cup, 1 oz	110	1	22
Puffed Rice, 1 cup, 1/2 oz	55	<1	12
Puffed Wheat, 1 cup, 1/2 oz	55	0	12
Raisin Bran, 1/2 cup, 1 oz	85	<1	20
Rice Crisps, 1 cup, 1 oz	110	1	25
Shredded Wheat, 1 bisc., 3/4 oz	80	<1	18
Sugar-frosted Flakes, 3/4 c, 1 oz	110	<1	26
Wheat Flakes, 1 cup, 1 oz	105	<1	23

Ready-To-Eat Cereal

	C	F	Cb
Arrowhead: Amaranth, 1 c., 1.2 oz	130	1	23
Bran Flakes, 1 cup, 1 oz	90	1	18
Corn Flakes, 1 cup, 1.2 oz	130	0	30
Kamut Flakes, 1 cup, 1.1 oz	110	1	25
Maple Buckwheat Flake, 1 c, 1.5 oz	160	1	35
Multi Grain Flakes, 1 cup, 1.2 oz	140	1.5	29
Nature O's, 1 cup, 1.1 oz	130	2	24
Oat Bran Flakes, 1 cup, 1.2 oz	140	2.5	24
Perfect Harvest, 1 cup, 1.2 oz	140	2	25
Puffed Corn/Rice, avg., 1 c., 0.8 oz	60	0.5	12
Puffed Kamut, 1 cup, 0.6 oz	50	0	11
Puffed Millet/Wheat, 1 cup, 0.5 oz	60	0.5	12
Raisin Bran, 1 cup, 2 oz	190	1.5	40
Rice Flakes, 1 cup, 1.7 oz	80	1	19
Shredded Wheat, 1 cup, 2 oz	200	1	44
Spelt Flakes, 1 cup, 1.1 oz	100	0.5	23
Sweetened Nature O's, 1 c., 1.5 oz	160	2.5	31
Wild Wheat Flakes, 1 cup, 1.5 oz	160	0.5	37

Barbara's Bakery

	C	F	Cb
Breakfast O's, 1 cup	120	1.5	22
Brown Rice Crisps, 1 cup, 1 oz	120	0.5	24
Corn Flakes, all types,1 cup, 1 oz	110	0	26
Crispy Wheats, 3/4 cup	115	0.5	25
Fruity Punch, 1 cup, 1.1 oz	110	0.5	26
Grain Shop, 1.6 oz	155	1.5	32
Honey Crunch 'n Oats, 1 cup, 1oz	115	1	24
Puffins, avg., 3/4 cup, 1 oz	120	1	24
Shredded Oats, 1 1/4 cup, 2 oz	230	2.5	46
Shredded Spoonfuls, 1.2 oz	125	1.5	24
Shredded Wheat, 2 bisc., 1.4 oz	150	1	31
Soy Essence, 1.4 oz	210	0.5	33
Toasted O's, average, 3/4 cup	120	2	24

Ready-To-Eat (Cont)

Breadshop

	C	F	Cb
Cranberry Crunch Muesli, 1 cup	200	3	44
Granola: Triple Berry Cr., 2/3 cup	220	7	36
Other varieties, 1/2 cup	210	7	34
Super Natural, 1/2 cup	210	9	31
Strawb., Blberry, Raspb., 1/2 cup	220	7.5	32
Kamut 'n Honey, 1 cup, 1 oz	120	3	22
Puffs 'n Honey, 3/4 cup, 1 oz	120	3	21
Sierra Crunch Muesli, 3/4 cup	190	3	38

Cap'n Crunch: All types, 3/4 cup   110   2   22

Cascadian Farms

	C	F	Cb
Honey Nut O's, 1 cup, 1 oz	120	1.5	25
Multi-Grain Squares, 3/4 c., 1 oz	110	0.5	25
Oats & Honey Granola, 3/4 c., 2 oz	240	6	42
Wheat Crunch, 3/4 cup, 1 oz	115	0.5	25

Chex: *See General Mills*

Dr McDougall's

	C	F	Cb
Oatmeal: 4 Grains, 2.2 oz	220	2	44
Barley, all varieties, 2.5 oz	270	3	51
Wheat, 2.4 oz	220	2.5	43
Muesli, 2.7 oz	260	3	51

Erewhon

	C	F	Cb
Apple Stroodles, 3/4 cup, 1 oz	110	0.5	25
Aztec, 1 oz	110	0	26
Banana O's, 3/4 cup, 1 oz	110	0	26
Barley Plus, 3/4 cup, 1.7 oz	170	1	37
Brown Rice Crm, 1/4 cup, 1.6 oz	170	1	36
Corn Flakes, 1 1/4 cups, 2 oz	210	2.5	45
Crispy Brown Rice, 1 cup, 1 oz	110	0	25
Fruit'n Wheat, 3/4 cup, 1.9 oz	170	1.5	39
Instant Oatmeal: *Per Packet*			
Apple Cinnamon, 1.2 oz	130	2	24
Apple Raisin, 1.3 oz	140	2	27
Maple Spice, 1.2 oz	130	2	25
Rasins, Dates & Walnuts, 1.2 oz	130	2.5	24
w. added Oat Bran, 1.2 oz	130	2.5	25
Kamut Flakes, 2/3 cup, 1.2 oz	110	0	25
Oat Bran, 1/3 cup, 1.8 oz	170	2.5	31
Raisin Bran, 1 cup, 1.8 oz	170	1	40
Whole Wheat Flakes, 1 cup, 2 oz	180	1	42

	C	F	Cb
Estee: Corn Flakes, 1 oz pkg	90	0	24
Raisin Bran, 1 oz pkg	90	1	21

	C	F	Cb
Familia: C.M.D., 2/3 cup	230	7	38
Muesli, 1/2 cup, 2.1 oz	210	3	45
No Added Sugar, 1/2 cup	200	3	41
Swiss Crunch, 2/3 cup	250	11	33

General Mills (Big G)

	C	F	Cb
Basic 4, 1/2 cup, 1 oz	100	1.5	22
Cheerios: Regular, 1 cup, 1 oz	110	1.5	21
Apple Cinnamon, 3/4 c., 1 oz	120	2	25
Berry Burst, 1 cup, 1 oz	110	1.5	24
Frosted; Team, 1 cup, 1 oz	120	1	25
Honey Nut, 1 cup, 1 oz	110	1.5	22
Multi-Grain, 1 cup, 1 oz	110	1	24
Chex: Corn, 1 cup, 1 oz	105	0.5	24
Frosted Mini Chex, 3/4 cup, 1 oz	110	0	27
Honey Nut, 1 cup	110	1.5	24
Morning Mix, 1 pouch, 1.15 oz	135	3.5	24
Multi-Bran, 1 cup, 2 oz	200	1.5	49
Rice, 1 1/4 cup, 1 oz	110	0.5	24
Wheat, 1 cup, 2 oz	180	1	41
Cinnamon Tst Crunch, 3/4 c., 1 oz	120	3	22
Cocoa Puffs: 1 cup, 1 oz	120	1	27
Milk & Cereal Bar, 1 bar, 1.4 oz	160	4	26
Cookie Crisp; Count Choc, 1 c., 1 oz	120	1	26
Fiber One, 1/2 cup, 1 oz	60	1	24
French Toast Crunch, 3/4 c., 1 oz	110	1.5	25
Green Slime, 1 cup, 1 oz	120	1	27
Golden Grahams, 3/4 cup, 1 oz	110	1	24
Honey Nut Clusters, 1 cup, 2 oz	210	2	47
Kix: 1 1/3 cup, 1 oz	110	0.5	24
Berry Berry, 3/4 cup, 1 oz	100	1	22
Lucky Charms, 1 cup, 1 oz	110	1	23
Oatmeal Crisp Almond, 1 c., 2 oz	220	5	41
Fruit & Cereal Bar, 1.4 oz	150	2	31
Raisin Nut Bran, 3/4 cup, 2 oz	215	4.5	43
Reese's P'nut Butter Puffs, 3/4 cup	130	3	24
Total Corn Flakes, 1 1/3 cup, 1 oz	110	0	26
TotalRaisin Bran, 1 cup, 2 oz	180	1	43
Total Whole Grain, 3/4 cup, 1 oz	110	1	24
Trix, 1 cup, 1 oz	115	1	25
Wheaties: 1 cup, 1 oz	110	1	24
Energy Crunch, 1 cup, 1.95 oz	210	3	42

Hansen's Natural *Per 1/2 Cup (2 oz)*

	C	F	Cb
Orange & Chocolate Cereal	230	9	35
Strawberry & Yogurt Cereal	230	9	30
Toasted Nut Crunch Cereal	230	6	39
Tropical Cluster Cereal	210	5	36

Healthy Choice

	C	F	Cb
Almond Crunch w. Raisins, 1 oz	200	2.5	43
Multi-Grain Flakes, 1 oz	105	0.5	25
Toasted Brown Sugar Squares, 2 oz	190	1	45

Breakfast Cereals (Cont)

Ready-To-Eat (Cont)

Health Valley	C	F	Cb
98% Fat Free Granola, 2/3 cup	180	1	43
Amaranth Flakes, 3/4 cup	100	0	24
Bran Cereal (w. Fruit), 3/4 cup	160	0	40
Corn Bran Flakes, 3/4 cup	100	0	24
Fiber 7 Flakes (100% Orig.), 3/4 c.	100	0	24
Golden Flax, 1/4 cup	190	3	38
Granola O's, all types, 3/4 cup	120	0	26
Healthy Crunches & Flakes, 3/4 c.	130	0	31
Healthy Fiber Flakes, 3/4 cup	100	0	23
Hot Cups: Apple; 10 Grain, 1 pkt	220	2.5	42
Maple; Banana, 1 pkt	240	2.5	46
Oat Bran Flakes, all types, 3/4 cup	105	0	26
Oat Bran/10 Bran O's, 3/4 cup	100	0	23
Orig. Soy Flakes, 1 1/4 cup, 1.9 oz	190	1.5	35
Puffed: Honey Sweetened, 1 cup	110	0	28
Raisin Soy Flakes, 1 cup, 2 oz	190	1	39
Real Oat Bran, 1/2 cup	200	3	34

Heartland Natural Cereal: *Per Cup*	C	F	Cb
Plain: w. Oats, Wheat Germ	500	18	79
w. Oats, Wheat Germ, Coconut	465	17	72
w. Oats, Wheat Germ, Raisins	470	16	76

Kashi: Breakfast Pilaf, 1/2 c., ckd	170	3	30
Cinna-Raisin Crunch, 1 c., 1.76 oz	150	1.5	39
GoLEAN Crunch!, 1 cup, 1.8 oz	190	3	36
Good Friends, 3/4 cup, 1 oz	90	1	24
Heart to Heart, 3/4 cup, 1.2 oz	110	1.5	25
Honey Puffed Kashi, 1 cup, 1 oz	120	1	25
Kashi GoLEAN, 3/4 cup, 1.4 oz	120	1	28
Kashi Medley, 1/2 cup, 1 oz	100	1	20
Kashi Pillows, 3/4 cup, 2 oz	200	1	45
Organic Promise: Cranberry, 1 oz	110	1	26
Strawberry Fields, 1 cup, 1.1 oz	120	0	28
Puffed Kashi, 1 cup, 0.9 oz	70	0.5	13

Kellogg's: Apple Jacks, 1 c., 1 oz	120	0	30
All-Bran: 1/2 cup, 1 oz	80	1	24
Bran Buds, 1/3 cup, 1 oz	80	0.5	16
with Extra Fiber, 1/2 cup, 1 oz	50	1	20
Apple Cinn. Rice Krispies, 3/4 c.	110	0	26
Apple Cinn. Squares, 3/4 c., 2 oz	180	1	44
Apple Raisin Crisp, 3/4 cup	90	0	23
Buzz Blasts,, 1 cup, 1/2 cup	120	2	24
Cinn. M'mallow Scooby-Doo, 1/2 cup	140	4	25
Cinn. Mini Buns, 3/4 cup	120	0.5	27
Complete Oatbran Flakes, 3/4 cup	110	0.5	23
Wheatbran Flakes, 3/4 cup	90	0.5	23

Kellogg's (Cont)	C	F	Cb
Cocoa Krispies, 3/4 cup	120	1	27
Common Sense O/Bran, 3/4 cup	110	1	23
Corn Flakes: 1 cup, 1 oz	110	0	24
Honey Crunch, 3/4 cup, 1 oz	120	1	26
Corn Pops, 1 cup, 1 oz	120	0	28
Cracklin' Oat Bran, 3/4 cup, 2 oz	190	7	35
Crispix: 1 cup, 1 oz	110	0	25
Cinnamon Crunch, 1.1 oz	120	1	26
Double Dip Crunch, 3 3/4 oz	120	1	26
Froot Loops: 1 cup	120	1	28
Other types, 1 cup, 1 oz	120	1	28
Frosted: Flakes, 1 cup, 1 oz	120	0	28
Mini-Wheats: 3/4 cup, 1.8 oz	180	1	42
Bite Size, 1 cup, 1 oz	200	1	48
Fruity Marshmallow Krispies, 3/4 c.	110	0	25
Fruit Harvest: Strawberry, 2/3 c.	110	1.5	24
Apple Cinnamon, 1 cup, 1.8 oz	190	2.5	42
Cinnamon Krunchers, 3/4 cup	130	3.5	23
Hunny B's, 1 cup	110	1	25
Just Right, 1 cup, 2 oz	210	2	48
Smorz, 1 cup, 1.1 oz	120	2	28
Healthy Choice: Müeslix, 2/3 c., 2 oz	200	3	41
Krave Bars, avg. all types (1)	200	7	30
Low Fat Granola: 1/2 cup, 2 oz	190	3	41
w. Raisins, 2/3 cup, 2 oz	220	3	47
Mickey's Magix, 1 cup, 1 oz	110	0.5	25
Mini Wheats: Frosted, 3/4 cup	180	1	41
Frosted Bite Size, 1 cup, 1 oz	200	1	48
Raisin Squares, 3/4 cup, 1.8 oz	180	1	42
Strawberry Squares, 3/4 c., 1.8 oz	170	1	40
Mud & Bugs, 1 cup, 1 oz	110	1	25
Müeslix: Apple & Almond, 3/4 c.	200	5	39
Raisin & Almond, 2/3 cup	200	3	40
Nut & Honey Crunch, 1 1/4 c., 2 oz	220	2.5	40
Nutri-Grain: Almond, 1 1/4 c., 2 oz	180	3	38
Cereal Bars, 1 bar, 1.3 oz	140	3	27
Golden Wheat, 3/4 cup, 1 oz	100	1	23
Minis, 1 pouch, 1.55 oz	160	3	32
Twists, 1 bar, 1.3 oz	140	3	26
Yogurt Bar, 1 bar, 1.3 oz	140	3	27
Pokèmon, 1 cup, 1 oz	110	0.5	25
Pop Tarts: Spider-Man	200	5	37
Fruit/Frosted, aver. all flavors	200	5	37
Low Fat, all flavors	190	3	39
Pastry Swirls, 2.2 oz	260	11	37
Snak Stix, 1 pastry, 1.8 oz	200	5	37
Product 19, 1 cup, 1 oz	100	0	25

Kellogg's (Cont)

	C	F	Cb
Raisin Bran, 1 cup, 2 oz	190	1.5	45
Raisin Bran Crunch, 1 cup, 1.9 oz	190	1	44
Rice Krispies: 1 1/4 cup	120	0	29
Treats, 3/4 cup	120	1.5	26
Original Bar (1)	90	2	18
Caramel/Peanut Butter (1)	110	4	19
Double Choc Chunk (1)	100	4.5	15
Scotcheroos (1)	120	5	18
Smacks, 3/4 cup, 1 oz	100	0	24
Smart Start: Soy Protein, 1 cup	200	1.5	40
Original, 1 cup, 1.8 oz	180	0.5	43
Special K: 1 cup, 1.1 oz	110	0	23
Cereal Bars, 1 bar	85	1.5	18
Plus, 1 cup	210	2	47
Red Berries, 1 cup, 1 oz	150	0	25
Wheat Chex, 1 cup	170	1	38

McCann's Instant Irish Oatmeal

	C	F	Cb
Apple & Cinnamon, 1.23 oz (35g)	130	1.5	26
Maple & Brown Sugar, 1.5 oz (43g)	160	2	32
Original, 1 oz pkg (28g)	100	2	18

Nature's Path

	C	F	Cb
Corn Flakes, all types, 3/4 cup, 1 oz	115	0	27
Granola: Apple Cinnamon, 2/3 cup	240	8	39
Ginger Zing; Hemp Plus, 2/3 cup	250	10	35
Avg. other varieties	250	7	40
Heritage, all types, 3/4 cup, 1 oz	115	0	24
Heritage Muesli w. Raspberry	215	3	41
Honeyed Raisin Bran, 3/4 cup, 1 oz	110	0	25
Instant Oatmeal: Apple Cinn.	190	2	37
Average other varieties	200	4	39
Multigrain & Rais. Muesli, 2/3 c., 1 oz	110	0.5	24
Optimum: Power Breakfast, 1 cup	190	2.5	41
Slim, 1/2 cup, 1 oz	100	1	21

New Morning

	C	F	Cb
Cocoa Crispy Rice, 3/4 cup, 1 oz	120	0.5	26
Cocomotion, 3/4 cup, 1 oz	100	0.5	22
Corn/Honey Frost. Flakes, 1 c., 1 oz	120	1	25
Cornfetti, 3/4 cup, 1 oz	110	1	24
Fruit-e-O's, 1 cup, 1 oz	120	1.5	25
Kamutios, 1 cup, 1 oz	120	1	25
Oatios: Cocoa, 1 cup, 1 oz	110	1	17
Apple Cinnamon, 1 cup, 1 oz	90	1.5	17
Honey Almond, 1 cup, 1 oz	120	1	17
Original, 1 cup, 1 oz	120	1	21
Ultimate Oat Bran, 1 c., 1 oz	110	2	22
Wafflers, 2/3 cup, 1 oz	110	1	26

Post

	C	F	Cb
100% Bran, 1/3 cup 1 oz	100	0.5	24
Alpha Bits, 1 cup	110	1	24
Banana Nut Crunch, 1/2 cup	240	6	44
Blueberry Morning, 1 cup	220	3	43
Bran Flakes, 3/4 cup	100	0.5	24
Cocoa Pebbles, 7/8 cup	115	1	25
Cranberry Almond Crunch, 1 cup	220	3	44
Fruit & Fibre, 2 oz	210	3	41
Fruity Pebbles, 1 1/4 cup	130	1.5	27
Golden Crisp, 1/2 cup	110	0	25
Grape Nut O's, 1 cup, 1.1 oz	120	1	28
Grape Nuts Flakes, 1/2 cup	110	1	24
Grape Nuts, 1/2 cup	210	1	47
Grape Nuts Raisin, 1/2 cup, 2 oz	200	1	47
Great Grains, 2/3 cup, 1.8 oz	200	6	38
Honey Bunches of Oats, 3/4 cup	120	2	26
Honeycomb, 1 cup	90	0.5	20
Maple Pecan Crunch, 3/4 cup	220	6	39
Marshmallow Alpha-Bits, 1 cup	130	1.5	27
Oreo O's, average, 3/4 cup	110	2.5	21
Raisin Bran, 2/3 cup, 1.4 oz	120	1	32
Shredded Wheat: Frosted, 1 cup	190	1	44
Wheat 'N Bran, 1 1/4 cup	200	1	47
Honey Nut, 1 cup, 1.8 oz	200	1.5	43
Strawb. Blasted Honey, 1 1/4 c., 1 oz	120	1	26
Toasties Corn Flakes, 1 cup	90	0	20
Waffle Crisp, 1 cup	130	3	24

Quaker

Ready to Eat Cereal:

	C	F	Cb
Oat Bran, 1 1/4 cup	210	3	41
100% Natural Granola: 1/2 cup	220	9	31
Lowfat, 2/3 cup	210	3	44
w. Raisins, 1/2 cup	230	9	34
Brown Sugar Bliss, 1cup, 1.7 oz	190	2.5	39
Cap'n Crunch: Regular, 3/4 c., 1 oz	110	2	23
Choco-Donuts, 3/4 cup	100	1	23
Fruit & Oatmeal Bites, 1 pouch	140	2.5	27
Honey Graham Oh's: 3/4 cup	110	2	23
Crunch Berries, 3/4 cup	110	2	23
Peanut Butter Crunch, 1 oz	110	3	21
Crunchy Corn Bran, 1 cup	90	1	23
Honey Nut Heaven, 1 cup, 1.7 oz	190	3.5	38
Life, all types, 3/4 cup	120	1.5	26
Oatmeal Squares, 1 cup, 1.8 oz	230	3	48
Puffed Rice, 1 cup, 1/2 oz	50	0	11
Puffed Wheat, 1 cup, 1/2 oz	55	0	13
Shredded Wheat, 3 biscuits	220	1.5	50
Unprocessed Bran, 1/3 cup	30	1	11

Breakfast Cereals • Grains & Flours

Quaker (Cont)	C	F	Cb
Bagged Cereal:			
Cocoa Blasts, 1 cup	130	1	29
Apple Zaps; Fruitany O's, 1 cup	120	1	27
Frosted Flakers, 3/4 cup	120	0	28
Frosted/Honey Nut Oats, 1 cup	110	1	24
Frosted Oats/ Sweet Crunch, 1 c.	110	1.5	23
Rice Crisps, 1 cup	110	0	26
Fruitany Oh's, 1 cup	120	1	27
Honey Crisp Corn Flakes, 3/4 cup	110	0	27
Honey Dipps, 1 1/4 cup	130	1.5	28
Grits: Regular, all types, 1 pkg	130	0.5	31
Instant: All types, 1 pkg	100	1	22
Quick'n Hearty *(Microwave Oatmeal): Per Pkt*			
Regular, 1 oz	110	2	19
Apple Spice; Cinn. Dble Raisin	170	2	35
Br. Sugar Cinnamon; Honey Bran	150	2	30
Instant Quaker Oatmeal: *Per Pkt*			
Oatmeal: Regular, 1 oz	100	2	19
Baked Apple; Banana Brd, 1.4 oz	150	2	31
Cinn. Roll/ Fr. Vanilla, 1 1/2 oz	160	3	33
Fruit & Cream, 1 1/4 oz	140	2.5	27
Honey Nut, 1 1/2 oz	170	3.5	31
Maple/Br.Sugar; Raisin/Spice	160	2	33
Raisin Cinnamon Swirl, 1 1/4 oz	170	2	36
Dinosaur Eggs, 1.76 oz pkt	200	4	38
Kid's Choice, 1 pkt, avg., 1 1/2 oz	160	2.5	32
Nutrition For Women, 1 pkt	170	2	33
Quaker/Hot: Multigrain, 1/2 cup	130	1.5	29
Oat Bran, 1/2 cup	150	3	25
Oats, all types, 1/2 cup	150	3	27
Whole Wheat Natural, 1/2 cup	130	1	30
Bars: Breakfast/Cereal, all types	130	3	26
"Oatmeal On The Go", 1.6 oz	195	6	34
Stone-Buhr: Bran, 1/4 c, 0.5 oz	65	0	14
7 Grain, 1/3 cup, 1 1/2 oz	140	2	31
Weetabix: 2 biscuits, 1.23 oz (35g)	120	1	28
Wild Oats			
CornFlakes, 3/4 cup, 1 oz	100	0	24
Honey Frosted Flakes, 1 c., 1 oz	100	0	24
Oat Bran O's, 1 cup, 1 oz	120	1.5	25
Zoe			
Almond & Oats, 2/3 cup	215	7	28
Apple & Cinnamon, 2/3 cup	190	6	25
Cranberries & Currants, 2/3 cup	205	6	29

Grains & Flours	C	F	Cb
Per 1/2 Cup (8 level Tbsp)			
Amaranth, 1/2 cup, 3 1/2 oz	350	6	60
Arrowroot, 1/2 cup, 2 1/4 oz	230	0	57
Atkins Bake Mix, low carb, 1 oz	115	2	6
Barley: Regular, 1/2 cup, 3 1/4 oz	325	2	56
Pearled, raw, 3 1/2 oz	350	1	78
Flakes, 1/2 cup, 1 1/2 oz	150	0.5	33
Buckwheat: Regular, 1/2 c., 3 oz	290	3	61
Groats, roasted, dry, 3 oz	285	2	60
Roasted, cooked, 3 1/2 oz	90	0.5	19
Flour, whole-groat	200	2	42
Bulgur: Dry, 1/2 cup, 2 1/2 oz	240	1	54
Cooked, 1/2 cup, 3 1/4 oz	75	0.5	17
Carob Flour, 1/2 cup, 1.8 oz	95	0.5	25
Corn Kernels (blue/yellow), 3 oz	300	4	66
Corn Bran, 1/2 cup, 1.4 oz	85	0.5	32
Corn Flour/Masa, 2 oz	210	2	44
Corn Grits: Dry, 1/2 cup, 2 3/4 oz	290	1	62
Cooked, 1/2 cup, 4 1/4 oz	75	0.5	16
Corn Germ, toasted	245	13	21
Cornmeal: Average All Types			
3 Tbsp, 1 oz	100	0.5	22
1/2 cup, 2.2 oz	220	2	46
Mixes: same as above	220	2	46
Cornstarch: 1 Tbsp, 8g	30	0	7
1/2 cup, 2 1/4 oz	230	0	57
Couscous: Dry, 3 1/4 oz	345	0	72
Cooked, 4.1 oz	60	0	12
Farina: Dry, 3 oz	325	0	70
Cooked, 4.1 oz	60	0	12
Flax Seeds, 2 oz	280	20	22
Flour ~ *See 'Wheat flour' Next Page*			
Garbanzo (Chick Pea), 1/2 c., 2 oz	200	3	35
Kuzu Root Starch, 1 Tbsp, 10g	35	0	8
Matzo Meal, 1/2 cup	260	1	55
Millet: Raw, 1/2 cup, 3 1/2 oz	375	4	76
Cooked, 1/2 cup, 4 1/4 oz	145	1	29
Oat Bran: Raw, 1/2 cup, 1.7 oz	115	2	31
Cooked, 1/2 cup, 4 oz	115	1	33
Oats, rolled/oatmeal:			
Dry/Groats, 1/2 cup, 1.5 oz	155	3	28
Cooked, 1/2 cup, 4.2 oz	75	1	13
Polenta: *See Cornmeal*			
Made Up, 1/2 cup, 5 oz	220	2	24
Potato flour, 1/2 cup, 3.2 oz	315	0	72
Psyllium Husks, 1 Tbsp (5g)	10	0	2
Quinoa: Dry 1/2 cup, 3 oz	320	5	53
Cooked, 1/2 cup	105	1.5	17

Grains & Flours (Cont)

Per 1/2 Cup (8 level Tbsp)

	C	**F**	**Cb**
Rice Bran, 1/3 cup, 1 oz	90	6	14
Rice Flour, 1/2 cup, 2 3/4 oz	290	2	63
Rice Polish, 1/2 cup	220	7	39
Rye Flour: Dark, 1 cup, 4 1/2 oz	415	3.5	88
Medium, 1 cup, 3 1/2 oz	360	2	79
Light, 1 cup, 3 1/2 oz	375	1.5	82
Rye Grain: 1/2 cup, 3 oz	280	2	59
Flakes, 1/2 cup, 1 1/2 oz	150	0.5	32
Semolina, 1/2 cup, 3 oz	305	1	61
Sorghum, 1/2 cup, 3.4 oz	325	3	72
Soybean Flakes, 1/2 cup, 1 1/2 oz	190	8	14
Soy Bean Flour:			
Defatted, 1 cup, 3 1/2 oz	330	1	34
Low-Fat, 1 cup, 3 oz	325	6	30
Full-Fat, 1 cup, 3 oz	370	18	27
Soy Meal, defatted, 1 cup, 4.3 oz	410	3	44
Spelt Flour, 1 cup, 3 oz	425	3.5	82
Tapioca, pearl, Dry: 1/2 c., 2. 7 oz	260	0	67
3 Tbsp, 1 oz	100	0	26
Teff (Seed) Flour, 2 oz	200	0.5	41
Tortilla Flour Mix, 1/2 cup, 2 oz	225	12	37
Triticale: 1/2 cup, 3.4 oz	325	2	70
Flour, whole-grain, 1/2 cup	220	1	47
Wheat: Average, 1/2 cup, 3 1/2 oz	320	2	28
Wheat Bran, unproc., 1/2 c., 1 oz	65	1	20
Wheat Flakes, 1/2 cup, 1 1/2 oz	160	0.5	32
Wheat Germ: 1/4 cup, 1 oz	105	3	15
Toasted, 1/4 cup, 1 oz	108	3	14
Wheat Flour:			
White, All Purpose/Self-Rising,			
1 level Tbsp, 0.6 oz	55	0	12
1/2 cup, 2.1 oz	225	0.5	47
1 cup, 4.4 oz	450	1	95
Whole Wheat, 1 cup, 4.2 oz	410	2	87

Also See Arrowhead Mills Cereals: Page 100

Eat it Today. . .
Wear it Tomorrow!

White Rice

	C	**F**	**Cb**
Raw: Short/Med. Grain, 1 c., 7 oz	720	1	156
Long Grain, 1 cup, 6 1/2 oz	670	1	144
Glutinous, 1 cup, 6 1/2 oz	680	1	150
Cooked Rice (Boiled/Steamed/Hot):			
Short/Medium Grain:			
1/2 cup, 3 1/4 oz	120	0	27
1 cup, 6 1/2 oz	240	0.5	54
Take-Out Rice: Small, 1 pint/13 oz	480	1	107
Large (1 1/2 pint), 21 oz	720	1.5	160
Long Grain: 1/2 cup, 2 3/4 oz	100	0	22
1 cup, 5 1/2 oz	200	0	44
Glutinous/Sticky, ckd, 1 c., 6 oz	170	0.5	36
Parboiled, cooked, 1/2 cup, 3 oz	90	0	20
Precook./Instant: Dry, 1/2 c., 3 1/2 oz	370	0	80
Cooked, 1/2 cup, 3 oz	90	0	20
Wild Rice: Raw, 1 cup, 5 1/2 oz	570	13	120
Cooked, 1 cup, 5 3/4 oz	165	0.5	35

Brown Rice

Average Short or Long Grain

	C	**F**	**Cb**
Raw/Dry: 1/2 cup, 3 1/2 oz	350	2.5	72
1 cup, 7 oz	700	5	144
Cooked: 1/2 cup, 3 1/2 oz	110	0.5	23
1 cup, 7 oz	220	1.5	46

Rice Dishes

	C	**F**	**Cb**
Chinese Fried Rice: 1/2 c., 2 1/2 oz	160	5	21
1 cup, 5 oz	320	13	42
2 cups, 10 oz	640	26	84
Mexican Rice: 1 cup	500	12	90
Taco Bell, 1 serving	190	10	21
Taco John's, 1 serving (6 oz)	250	5	44
Taco Time, 1 serving (4 oz)	150	2	30
Rice-A-Roni: See Page 81			
Rice Pilaf: Restaurant, 1 cup	270	7.5	43
Boston Market, 1 cup	140	4	24
Rice w. Raisins/Pinenuts, 1 cup	400	11	70
Risotto, 1 cup	420	18	65
Saffron Rice, 1 cup	370	12	66
Spanish Rice: 1 cup	390	9	72
El Pollo Loco, 1 serving	130	3	24
Sticky Thai Rice, plain, 1 cup	170	0.5	36
Sushi Rice, 1 Tbsp	25	0	6

Pasta ✦ Spaghetti ✦ Noodles

- Macaroni includes all shapes and sizes; (e.g. spaghetti, fettuccini, shells, tubes, ziti, twists, sheets, cannelloni, manicotti, elbows).
- All regular macaroni products have the same cals/fat/carb. on a weight basis.
- 1 oz Dry = approx. 2$\frac{1}{2}$ -3 oz cooked.

Dry Spaghetti/Macaroni

	C	F	Cb
1 oz quantity	105	0.5	21
1lb box/pkg., 16 oz	1680	7	336
Elbows, 1 cup, 3$\frac{3}{4}$ oz	395	2	77
Shells, small, 1 cup, 3$\frac{1}{4}$ oz	340	2	66
Spirals, 1 cup, 3 oz	315	2	61

Cooked Spaghetti/Macaroni

Plain, All Types (no added fat):

	C	F	Cb
Firm/Al Dente (8-10 mins.), 1 oz	42	0.5	8.5
Medium (11-13mins.), 1 oz	37	0.5	7.5
Tender (14-20mins.), 1 oz	32	0.5	7
(Longer cooking increases water absorbed)			
Spaghetti, $\frac{1}{2}$ cup, 2 $\frac{1}{2}$ oz	90	0.5	18
Medium serving, 1 cup, 5 oz	185	1	37
Large (restaurant), 2 c., 10 oz	370	2	74
Elbows/Spirals, 1 cup, 5 oz	185	1	38
Small Shells, 1 cup, 4 oz	150	0.5	31
Protein-fortified: Dry, 1 oz	107	0.5	21
Cooked, 1 cup, 5 oz	230	0.5	44
Spinach/Vegetable: Dry, 1 oz	105	0.5	21
Cooked, 1 cup, 5 oz	180	0.5	37
Whole-wheat: Dry, 1 oz	100	0.5	21
Cooked, 1 cup, 5 oz	175	0.5	37

Fresh Pasta (Refrigerated)

Plain/Spinach/Tomato, average:

	C	F	Cb
As purchased, 4 oz	325	2.5	64
Cooked, 1 cup, 5 oz	190	1	38
Home-made, without egg:			
Cooked, 1 cup, 5 oz	175	1	35

Buitoni

	C	F	Cb
Angel Hair, 1$\frac{1}{4}$ cup, 3 oz	230	2.5	43
Fettuccine/Linguini: 1$\frac{1}{4}$ cup, 3 oz	240	2.5	43
Spinach, 1$\frac{1}{4}$ cup, 3 oz	260	4	43
Ravioli: Beef, 1$\frac{1}{4}$ cup, 3.6 oz	330	9	46

Buitoni (Cont):

	C	F	Cb
Ravioli: Chk., Herb Parm., 1$\frac{1}{4}$ c., 3.6oz	310	9	44
Dblestuff. Mozz. Herb, 1$\frac{1}{2}$ c., 4 oz	360	12	44
Four Cheese, 1 cup, 3 oz	290	9	38
Light, 1 cup, 3 oz	230	4	37
Garden Vegetable, 1 cup, 3 oz	250	5	39
Mini Beef, 1 cup, 3.5 oz	270	5	44
Rst Chick. & Garlic, 1 c., 4.5 oz	330	11	45
Tortellini: Chse & Rst Garlic 1 c., 3 oz	270	8	38
Chkn & Prosciutto, 1 c., 3.6 oz	360	13	45
Herb Chicken, $\frac{3}{4}$ cup, 3 oz	260	7	40
Mozzarella & Herb, 1 c., 3.6 oz	320	9	45
Mushroom & Chse, 1 c., 3.6 oz	290	6	46
Sundried Tomato, 1 cup, 3.6 oz	320	10	46
Sweet Italian Saus., 1 c., 3.6 oz	320	8	49
Three Cheese, $\frac{3}{4}$ cup, 3 oz	250	6	39

Noodles

	C	F	Cb
Plain/Egg: Dry, 1 oz	108	1	20
1 cup, 1$\frac{1}{3}$ oz	145	1.5	28
Cooked, 1 oz	38	0.5	7
$\frac{1}{2}$ cup, 2$\frac{3}{4}$ oz	105	1	20
1 cup, 5$\frac{1}{2}$ oz	210	2	40
Stir-Fried: 1 cup, 5$\frac{1}{2}$ oz	270	9	40
2 cup serving, 11 oz	540	18	80
Yolk Free (Cooked): Per Cup			
'No Yolks' (Foulds)	210	2	40
Passover Gold (Manischewitz)	200	0	42
Chinese: Cellophane/Rice, dry, 1 oz	100	0	25
Chow Mein/hard, dry, 1 oz	150	5	17
Ramen Noodles: See Page 81			
Japanese: Soba, dry, 1 oz	95	0.5	21
cooked, 1 cup, 4 oz	110	0.5	21
Somen, dry, 1 oz	100	0.5	22
cooked, 1 cup, 6 oz	225	0.5	49
Japanese Style Pan Fried:			
Maruchan's Yaki-Sobu, 5.6 oz cup	260	3	50
Udon (Chikara), avg., 7.5 oz pkt	250	1	52
Stir Fry/Yakisoba, 3.5 oz serving	220	2	44
Thai Kitchen: See Page 82, 89			

Egg Roll Skins/Won Ton

	C	F	Cb
Egg Roll Skins:			
(Golden Dragon) 1 pce, 1 oz	80	0	18
(Wung Hung) 4 skins, 4 oz	300	0	64
Won Ton Wrappers:			
(Dynasty) 10 wrappers, 2.1 oz	170	1	36
Egg Roll/Spring Roll Wrapper:			
(Dynasty) 3 wrappers, 2.1 oz	170	1	36

Bread

Note: All breads have similar calories on a weight basis. However, volume may vary. For example, 1 oz of bread may equal 1 slice regular bread or 2 slices of a lighter bread. It is best to weigh bread used and calculate on 1 oz bread = 70 calories.

Quick Guide

Bread

Average All Varieties:

	C	F	Cb
Thin slice (1/4") 1 oz	70	1	13
Extra thin slice 3/4 oz	55	0.5	10
Light thin slice, 0.6 oz	40	0.5	7.5
Toasting slice, 1.2 oz	85	1	16
Thick slice (3/8"), 1.5 oz	105	1.5	20
Large slice (1/2"), 2 oz	140	2	26
1-lb Loaf, 16 oz	1120	6	208

Toast has same calories as bread used.

1 thin slice + 1 tsp of fat	105	5	13
1 thick slice (3/8") +2 tsp fat	175	10	20

Breads

	C	F	Cb
Batard (8 oz), 1/4, 2 oz slice	140	0.5	28
Boule, 1/2" thick, 2 oz slice	130	0	29
Bran style/Dark, 1 oz slice	70	1	14
Buttermilk, average, 1 1/2 oz slice	120	1.5	24
Caraway Rye, 1 oz slice	70	0	15
Challah, 1 oz slice	85	2	14
Corn Bread, avg., 1 pce, 3 oz	180	7	30
Cracked Wheat Sourdough, 1 1/2 oz	130	0.5	27
Croutons, 2 Tbsp	35	1	6
Date & Nut, 1 oz slice	90	1	14
'Enriched' Breads, avg., 1 oz sl.	75	1	18
12-Grain, 1 1/2 oz slice	120	1.5	23
Foccacia: Plain, 2 oz portion	150	4	23
Cheese & Garlic; Pesto, 2 oz	170	8	21
Tomato & Olive, 2 oz	120	2	20
French Stick/Baguette, 1 oz slice	70	1	15
French Toast, 1 slice, 2 1/4 oz	160	7	18
Sticks (Aunt Jemima), 1 pce, 1 oz	75	3	12
Garlic Bread, 1 pce. w. fat, 1 oz	125	6	14
Garlic Toast (Pepp.Farm), 1.4 oz sl.	160	10	15
Italian Bread, 1 oz slice	75	1	15
Light Bread, avg., 0.8 oz slice	40	0.5	7.5
Melba Toast, 2 pces	25	0	6
MultiGrain: 1 slice, 1 oz	75	1	14
Nut/Health Nut, 1 oz slice	85	2	15

Breads (Cont)

	C	F	Cb
Oatmeal/Oatbran Bread, 1 oz sl.	70	1	13
Party Breads (Pepp. Farm): Rye, 1 sl.	15	0.5	3
Dijon; Pumpernickel, 1 sl.	18	0.5	3.5
Pita Bread, avg. all types, 2 oz	150	2	30
Mini/Pocket, 1 oz	75	1	15
Pizza & Bread Mix, (Zone Perfect) 2 oz slice	100	4.5	15
Poppyseed (Vienna), 0.8 oz sl.	55	1	10
Pumpernickel, 1 oz slice	75	1	15
Cocktail size, 0.4 oz	30	0.5	6
Raisin Bread, 1 oz slice	80	1.5	15
Raisin Walnut, 2 oz slice	160	3.5	29
Roman Meal, 1 oz slice	70	1	14
Country Potato & Oat, 1 1/2 oz	110	1.5	20
Rye: Average, 1 thin slice, 1 oz	75	1	13
1 thick slice, 2 oz	150	2	25
Cocktail size, 0.4 oz	25	0.5	4
Sandwich Bread, 1 oz slice	70	1	13
Sandwich Pockets: Reg., 2 oz	150	1	30
Sara Lee: H/Style Wheat, 1 1/2 oz	100	1	20
Sourdough, 1 1/2 oz slice	100	1	20
Sprouted 7-Grain, 1.5 oz slice	110	1.5	18
Squaw, (33g) 1.1 oz slice	85	0.5	13
Turkish/Middle Eastern, 1 oz sl.	80	1.5	16
Wonder Light (Red'd Cal), 1 sl. 3/4 oz	40	0	9

Bread Rolls & Buns

	C	F	Cb
Brown 'n Serve, average, 1 oz	80	2	15
Concha, (Mexican Sweet Bread), 3 oz	400	19	50
Dinner Rolls: 1 small, 1 oz	85	2	15
1 medium (3" diam),1 1/2 oz	130	3	23
English Muffins, avg., 2 oz	140	2	27
Frankfurter/Hot Dog: 1 1/2 oz	100	2	19
1 1/2 oz size	120	2	23
French: 1 medium, 1.3 oz	110	1	24
1 large, 3 oz	240	2	52
Hamburger: Regular, 1 1/2 oz	120	2	23
Large, 3 oz	240	4	46
Hoagie/Submarine, 4 3/4 oz	400	8	77
Kaiser Roll, 2 oz size	170	3	18
Onion Roll, 2 oz size	170	2	20
Parker House Roll, 0.7 oz size	65	1	12
Party Roll, 0.6 oz	55	1	10
Sandwich Roll, 1.6 oz size	120	2	23
Soft Pretzel Roll (J & J), 3 oz	235	3	50
Sourdough Roll, 1 1/4 oz	100	1	18
Sweet Rolls, 1 oz	100	2	20
w. Icing, average	160	6	20
Wheat Roll: Small, 1 oz	75	0.5	14
Medium, 1 1/2 oz	110	1	20

107

Bagels ◆ Tacos ◆ Rice Cakes

Quick Guide

Bagels

	C	F	Cb
Average All Brands			
Plain/Onion:			
1 mini/bagelette, 1 oz	80	<1	15
1 small bagel, 2 oz	160	1.5	30
1 medium bagel, 3 oz	240	2	45
1 large bagel, 4 oz	320	3	60
Bagel Chips (New York Style),			
4 slices, 3/4 oz	90	2	17
Pizza Bagel, 6 oz each	380	7	60
Bagel Bites (Ore-Ida), 4 pces	190	7	25
Bagel Crisps (Burns Ricker), 1 oz	150	9	28

Bagel Brands

	C	F	Cb
Amy's Kitchen, average, 3 1/2 oz	235	2	50
Awrey's, 2.7 oz each	190	0.5	42
Cosco Bakery: Plain, 4 oz	300	1	61
Everything, 4 oz	330	3.5	62
Lenders, all flavors, 3.6 oz	280	3	55
Oroweat: Oatmeal, 3.4 oz	270	4	49
Multi-Grain, 3.4 oz	260	1.5	51
Sara Lee: Mini, average, 1 oz	80	0	15
Toaster Size, all types, 2.2 oz	160	0.5	33
3.4 oz Size (95g): Egg	260	2	50
Other flavors, 3.4 oz	260	1	55
4 oz Size (113g):			
Apple Cinnamon	310	1.5	64
Banana Walnut	350	7	61
Chocolate Chip	320	3.5	61
Cranberry Orange	310	1.5	64
Honey & Oat	310	2	61
New York Style, 4 1/2 oz	330	1	69
Sun Dried Tomato Basil	300	1.5	61
The Works	330	3.5	62
Western: All flavors, avg., 3 oz	230	1	47
Bagels: See Einstein Bros Bagels, Page 206			
Bagel Sandwiches: See Page 175			

Bagel Spreads

	C	F	Cb
Cream Cheese: Plain, 1 oz	80	8	2
Reduced Fat, 1 oz	60	5	2
Flavors: Lox, 1 oz	75	6	1
Raisin Walnut, 1 oz	90	6	8
Strawberry, 1 oz	60	3	7
Sundried Tomato, 1 oz	80	7	2
Vegetable, 1 oz	60	6	1

Bread Products

	C	F	Cb
Bread Crumbs, dry:			
Plain or seasoned, 1 slice	110	1	20
1 rounded Tbsp, 10g	35	<1	6
1 cup, 3 1/2 oz	390	5	73
Corn Flake Crumbs, 1 oz	110	1	20
Graham Cracker Crumbs, 1 oz	115	1	21
Keebler, 1 cup, 4 1/4 oz	520	14	84
Bread Dough: Frozen, 1 slice	75	<1	14
Refrigerated, French, 1" slice	60	1	13
Wheat/White, 1" slice	80	2	14
Breadsticks: Boboli, 1.75 oz	130	2	22
Stella D'oro: Sesame (1)	50	2	7
Plain/Onion/Wheat, 1 pce	40	1	7
Keebler/Lance, 2 sticks	30	<1	5
Salt Sticks, plain, 1 oz	110	1	20
Croutons: Avg. all brands, 1 oz	100	3	17
2 Tbsp, 10g	35	1	6
Coating Mixes:			
Seasoned, average, 1 oz	110	3	20
Featherweight, 1.4 oz pkg	72	<1	17
Pretzels: See Snacks ~ Page 126			
Stuffing: Average, dry mix, 1 oz	110	1	10
Made-up, 1/2 cup, 4 oz	180	9	11

Croissants ~ See Page 117, 175

Rice Cakes

	C	F	Cb
Average All Types/Brands:			
Regular size, 1 cake, 9g	35	0	7.5
Hain, Mini, average, 3g each	12	<1	2
Lundberg, all types, 15g each	60	1	14
Quaker: Large, all flavors, 13g each	50	0	11
Crispy Mini's, average, 15g	70	2	12
Westbrae, 1 cake, 7g	25	0	5

Taco Shells

	C	F	Cb
Regular size, all types, each	55	3	6
Super Size, each	90	4	11
Mini Size, 1 taco	25	1.5	2
Salad Shell, flour (Azteca), 1.4 oz	180	11	19
Tortilla (Soft Taco), each	85	2	15
Corn Tortilla: 6", 1.2 oz each	45	0.5	9
Flour Tortilla: each, 1.75 oz	160	3	28
Lowfat	110	1.5	22
Burritos, 1 tortilla, 2.3 oz	190	5	32
Lowfat	110	1.5	22
Tostada Shells, each	55	3	6

Crispbreads ◆ Crackers, Cookies

Crispbreads — C F Cb

Per Crispbread/Cracker

	C	F	Cb
Ak-Mak: Sesame, 5 crackers, 1 oz	35	0	7
Finn Crisp: Original, rye,1	35	0	7
Other types,1	19	0	3
Kavli Norwegian: Thin,1	17	0	3
Thick,1	20	0	3
Malsovit Meal Wafers.1	75	4	7
New York Flatbread Crisps, 1	35	0	7
Ry-Krisp: Natural, 1 crispbread	20	0	3
Seasoned,1	30	0	5
Sesame,1	25	1	3
Ryvita: Dark/Light, 1 piece	26	0	4
WASA: Breakfast; Sesame	50	0	9
Extra Crisp; Light Rye	25	0	5
Hearty Rye	45	0	9
Organic Rye	25	0	7
Sourdough Flatbread, 3	50	0	11
Sourdough Rye	35	0	7
Westbrae Rice Wafers (7), 15g	50	0	11

Matzos

Manischewitz

	C	F	Cb
American Matzos, 1 board, 1 oz	115	2	22
Passover Matzos, 1 board, 1.1 oz	130	0	27
Passover Egg Matzos, 1.1 oz	130	2	27
Egg 'n Onion Matzo, 1 oz	112	1	23
Thin Salted Tea Matzos, 0.9 oz	100	1	21
Unsalted; Whole Wheat, 1 oz	110	0	24
Dietetic Matzo Thins, 0.83 oz	90	0	19
Crackers: Miniatures, 1 cracker	9	0	20
Passover Egg Matzo, 1 cracker	11	0	20
Matzo Meal, 1 cup, 4³/₄ oz	515	2	110
Matzo Farfel, 1 cup, 2.7 oz	180	0.5	60
Grape Matzo, 1 oz each	110	0	25

Quick Guide — Crackers — C F Cb

Average All Brands: Per Cracker

	C	F	Cb
Cheese Crackers: Plain, 1" square	5	0	0.5
Small, octagonal	10	0	1
Round (2" diam.)	15	0	1.5
Sandwich (Peanut Butter)	35	1	4
Graham, 2¹/₂" square,1 cracker	30	0.5	5
Melba Toast, plain, 1 piece	20	0	4
Oyster & Soup Crackers, 1/4 oz	60	2	10
(40 small oysters/20 lge hexagons)			
Rice Crackers: 1 small	9	0	2
Rice Snax *(Amsnack)*, 1/2 oz	60	1	12
Saltines, 2 crackers	25	1	4.5
Snack-type, 1 round cracker	15	0	3
Soda, 1 cracker, 1/2 oz	60	2	10
Water Cracker *(Carr's),* regular, 1	32	0	7
Small, 1 cracker	14	0	4
Wheat, thin, 1 cracker	9	0	2
Zweiback Toast, 1 piece	30	0	5

Quick Guide — Cookies — C F Cb

Average All Brands: Per Cookie

	C	F	Cb
Biscotti: Small, 0.5 oz	65	2.5	10
Regular, 1 oz	130	5	20
Chocolate Chip Cookies:			
Small/Thin 0.5 oz	55	3	7
Regular, 1 oz	110	6	15
Large, 2.3 oz *(Mrs Field's)*	280	13	38
Jumbo, 4 oz	450	22	64
Oatmeal/Oatmeal Raisin:			
Small/Thin 0.5 oz	50	1.5	8
Regular, 1 oz	95	3.5	15
Large, 2.3 oz *(Mrs Field's)*	280	12	39
Jumbo, 4 oz	380	14	62
Peanut Butter:			
Small/Thin 0.5 oz	60	3	7
Regular, 1 oz	125	6.5	14
Large, 2.3 oz *(Mrs Field's)*	310	16	34
Jumbo, 4 oz	500	25	54
Lowfat Cookies			
Choc Chip (Lowfat), 1 oz (1)	100	1	21
Oatmeal Raisin (Fat-free), 1 oz (1)	90	0	20
Peanut Butter (Lowfat), 1 oz (1)	105	2	14

Crackers ◆ Cookies (Cont)

Brands

Per Cookie/Cracker (Unless Indicated)

	C	F	Cb
Archway: Coconut Macaroon	100	6	12
Apple/Date-filled Oatmeal	100	3	16
Apricot/Strawb. filled Oatmeal	100	3.5	16
Aunt Bea's Pound Cake Cookie	100	4	16
Chocolate Chip: Drop	100	3.5	15
Ice Box	120	6	15
N' Toffee	130	6	18
Fat-Free: Oatmeal Raisin (1)	110	0	25
Cinnamon Honey Heart (3)	110	0	25
Devil's Food Cookie (1)	70	0	16
Frosty Lemon/Orange	110	4.5	17
Fruit & Honey Bar; Molasses	100	3	18
Ginger Snaps: Regular/Iced (5)	150	5	23
Reduced Fat (5)	140	3.5	25
Lemon Snaps (5)	150	7	20
Oatmeal: Regular; Raisin	110	3.5	17
Iced	120	5	19
Ol' Fashioned Peanut Butter	120	6	15
Old Fashioned Windmill	90	3.5	14
Peanut Butter Choc	150	7	17
Peanut Jumble	110	6	13
Pecan Icebox	120	6	15
Ruth's Golden Oatmeal	120	5	18
Sugar Cookies (1)	100	3	16
Atkins			
Cookies; Crackers, avg. all	140	9	10
Meringue Cookies, avg. all flav. (1)	5	0	1
Sesame; Whole Wheat, crackers (2)	45	3	4
Austin: Sandwich Cookies	240	2	36
Big Munch Wafer Bar, each	200	2.5	24
Cheese/Toast/Wheat Crackers, w. filling			
All types, average	200	2.5	29
Reduced Fat	170	1.5	25
Smackers Crackers, all types	130	1	32
Zoo Animal Crackers, all types	125	1	20
Zoo Animal Pretzels	200	0	40
Barbara's Bakery: Fig Bars, avg.	60	1	15
Animal Cookies (1)	16	0.6	2
Cheese Bites, all types (26)	120	1.5	24
Coconut Almond, 1 bar, 1 oz	120	4.5	20
Crisp Cookies, all types (1)	80	4	11
Espresso Bean; Lemon Yog., 1 bar	120	3.5	22
Fat Free: Mini, all types, each	18	0	4
Rite Lite Rounds, 5 crackers	55	0.5	12
Roasted Peanut, 1 bar, 1 oz	130	4.5	20
Snackimals (1)	15	0.5	2
Wafer Crisps (3)	60	1	12
Wheatines, all types, 1 large square	50	1.5	10

	C	F	Cb
Burns & Ricker			
Biscotti, average all types, (1)	70	2.5	10
Carr's			
Crackers: Table Water (5)	70	1.5	13
Monterey: Hearty Wheat (3)	60	2	9
Savory/Sesame (3)	70	3	9
Entertainer; Whole Wheat (2)	80	3.5	11
Cocktail, Croissant Orig. Gold (22)	140	3	21
Cookies: Bisc. for Tea (2)	140	6	20
Milk Choc Bisc for Tea (2)	130	6	16
Choccines (3)	150	9	16
Ginger Lemon Cremes (2)	140	7	19
Hob Nobs (2)	140	6	19
Imperials: Milk Chocolate (2)	140	7	18
Dark Choc (2)	150	7	19
Petites Bijoux (4)	140	5	21
Dominick's			
Pecan Shortbread	100	6	11
Grahams: Cinnamon (8)	140	5	22
Fudge (3)	140	7	19
Honey (8)	150	6	22
Lowfat (9)	120	1.5	25
Saltine Crackers (5)	60	2	11
Sugar Wafers (5)	140	7	25
Unsalted Tops (5)	70	2	11
Cookies: Choc Chip Chewy (1)	100	5	14
Choc Chip Reduced Fat (3)	150	6	23
Old Fashioned: Assort.; Oatmeal	80	3.5	11
Sandwich Cremes, Chocolate	70	2.5	11
Striped Shortbread (3)	160	4	21
Vanilla Wafers (6)	160	6	23
Dr Soy: Average (2)	85	2	5
Entenmann's			
Orig. Choc Chip (3)	150	7	20
Chocolate Brownie (2)	150	2	21
No Fat, 2 cookies	100	0	24
Soft Baked: Choc Chip	100	5	13
Gourmet English Toffee	100	5	13
Milk Choc Chip	100	5	13
Oatmeal Raisin, Fat Free (2)	100	0	23
White Choc Macadamia Nut (1)	100	6	12

Real women don't have hot flashes. . . . They have power surges!

Per Cookie/Cracker (Unless Indicated)

Estee

	C	F	Cb
Chocolate Chip; Fudge Cookies	40	2	5
Coconut Cookies, Oatmeal Raisin	35	1.5	5
Fig Bars, each	50	0.5	11
Sandwich Cookies	55	2	6
Shortbread: Vanilla; Lemon	35	1.5	5

Famous Amos

	C	F	Cb
Butter Shorties	80	4.5	10
Chocolate Chip Cookie (1)	37	1.5	5
4 cookies, 1 oz	150	7	20
Belgian Style (4)	150	7	20
Choc Chip & Pecans (4), 1 oz	150	8	19
Chocolate Chunk	80	4	10
Oatmeal Choc Chip & Walnut (4)	150	7	19
Oatmeal Raisin (4), 1 oz	140	5	21
Pecan Shorties (1)	90	5	10
Lowfat: Iced varieties (7), 1.1 oz	130	1.5	25

Frookie

	C	F	Cb
Cookies, average all types	45	2	7
Animal Frackers	10	0.3	1.5
Apple Cinnamon Oatbran	45	2	7
Fruitins: Apple; Fig	60	1	12
Large Frooks, all types	120	4	18

Grandma's

	C	F	Cb
Choc Chip; Nutty Fudge	190	9	25
Fudge Choc Chip; Oatmeal Raisin	170	7	26
Old Time Molasses	160	4	29
Peanut Butter varieties, avg.	190	9	23
Cookie Bits, average (9)	150	7	22
Sandwich: Fudge (3)	180	5	31
Fudge Vanilla (3)	120	4	21
Vanilla (3)	180	5	32
Peanut Butter (5)	210	10	28
Rich & Chewy, 1 pkt	270	12	39
Sugar Wafers (3)	160	7	23
Tiny Bites (12)	280	12	39

Hain

	C	F	Cb
98% Fat-Free, all types (11)	110	0	23
Cheese Bites (22)	120	1.5	23
Cookie Jar Bits (Rice Cakes), 17 bits	60	0.5	12
Mini Rice Cakes: Plain (8)	60	0	13
Oyster Crackers, Fat-Free (36)	60	0	13
Veg/Rice/Sesame Crackers (11)	140	6	19

Harvest Bakery

	C	F	Cb
Crackers, average all types (2)	75	3.5	10

Health Valley

	C	F	Cb
Graham: Amaranth; Oat Bran	15	0	3
Original Amaranth/Oat Bran	20	0.5	4
Healthy Pizza, all flavors (6)	50	0	11
Lowfat, all flavors (6)	60	1.5	10
Original Rice Bran	18	0.5	3
Whole Wheat, all flavors	10	0	2
Cookies: Jumbo, all flavors (1)	80	0	19
Healthy Biscotti, all flavors (1)	60	1.5	12
Raspberry Fruit Center (1)	70	0	18
Avg. other varieties (1)	70	0	18
Tarts: All types, 1 tart	35	0	8

Hy-Top

	C	F	Cb
Assorted Cookies (5), 1 oz	120	4	19
Assorted Sandwich Creme, avg.	80	3	12
Chewy-a-riffic	90	3.5	12
Chip-a-riffic (3)	170	9	23
Chocolate Chip (5), 1 oz	110	5	16
Honey Cinnamon Grahams (2)	120	4	21
Oatmeal	80	3.5	11
Iced Oatmeal	70	3	11
Pecan-a-riffic	100	5	11
Sugar	80	3	12
Vanilla Wafers (8), 1 oz	130	5	21

Jewel

	C	F	Cb
Animal Crackers (9)	140	3.5	25
Chip-A-Riffic (3)	180	9	24
Choc/Vanilla Sandwich Creme (2)	130	5	20
Chocolate Chip: Regular (3)	170	9	23
Chewy (1)	90	3.5	12
Chunky (1)	80	4.5	10
Choc Chunk, 1½ oz	200	9	26
Chocolate Sandwich Creme (2)	120	5	19
Cinnamon Grahams (8)	140	5	22
Cookie Jar Assortment (3)	150	9	23
Duplex Sandwich Creme (2)	120	5	19
Fudge Creme Wafer (3)	150	8	18
Fudge Marshmallow	110	4	18
Oatmeal; Oatmeal Old Fashioned	80	3.5	11
Peanut Butter (2)	140	5	21
Peanut Butter Chip, 1½ oz	210	12	21
P'nut Butter Fudge Wafer (2)	180	8	14
Saltine Crackers; Unsalted Tops (5)	60	1.5	11
Striped Shortbread (3)	170	8	20
Sugar Wafers (5)	140	7	20
Unsalted Top Crackers (5)	70	2	10
White Choc Macadamia, 1½ oz	200	10	26

Crackers • Cookies (Cont)

Per Cookie/Cracker (Unless Indicated)

Joseph's Cookies	C	F	Cb
Sugar-Free (Bite Size):			
Almond; Choc. Chip; Lemon (4)	100	5	13
Coconut (2)	105	5	14
Oatmeal: Pecan Shortbread (2)	100	5	14
Peanut Butter (2)	95	5	13
Lite: Choc Pecan B-Fit (2)	100	1	20
Peanut Butter Choc Chip (2)	120	4	20
Other varieties, average (2)	100	3	18

Kalahari
	C	F	Cb
Rusks: Avg. all types (1)	110	3	18

Keebler
	C	F	Cb
Crackers: Sandwich, 1 pkt, 1.3 oz	190	10	23
Club: Orig.; 50% Red. Sodium (4)	70	3	9
33% Reduced Fat (5)	70	2	11
Grahams: Regular (8), 1 oz	130	3.5	22
Lowfat varieties (9), 1 oz	115	1.5	24
Munch'ems, average (40), 1 oz	140	5	20
Snax Stix, average (20)	130	5	18
Toasted: Reduced Fat (5)	60	2	10
Regular varieties (5)	80	3.5	10
Town House: Regular (5)	80	4.5	9
Reduced Fat (6)	70	2	11
Wheatables: Reduced Fat (13)	130	4	22
Other varieties, average (12)	140	6	20
Cookies: Classic Collection (1)	80	3.5	12
Chips Deluxe: Soft & Chewy (1)	80	3.5	11
Peanut Butter Cup; Rainbow (1)	80	4.5	9
Chocolate Lovers; Coconut (1)	90	5	11
Crunchy Walnut; Chips Deluxe (1)	90	6	9
Mini's, all types (4)	150	8	19
Cookie Stix (5)	140	6	22
Country Style Oatmeal w. Rais. (2)	140	6	21
E.L. Fudge Sandwich (2)	120	6	17
Mini Butter S'wich (7)	130	6	21
Double stuffed (2)	170	9	23
S'mores Blasted (2), avg.	170	9	23
Fudge Shoppe: S'mores (3)	160	8	22
Deluxe Grahams, Reg. (3)	140	7	19
Double Fudge 'n Caramel (2)	140	7	20
Fudge Sticks (3)	150	8	20
Fudge Stripes (3)	160	8	21
Mini, 1 pkg (3)	270	13	38
Reduced Fat (3)	140	5	21
Mini's (4); Grasshopper (4)	150	7	20
Mini Grahams (10)	160	8	22

Keebler (Cont)	C	F	Cb
Ginger Snaps (5)	150	6	24
Golden Fruit (1)	80	2	14
Iced Animal, (6)	150	5	24
Krisp Kreem, (5)	140	7	19
Lemon Coolers (5)	140	5	23
Rainbow Chips Deluxe S'wich (1)	90	4.5	11
Sandies Swirl: 25% Red. Fat (2)	80	3	11
Choc Chip Pecan (2)	80	5	9
Cookies (1) avg. all flavors	80	5	9
Soft Batch, 0.5 oz all types, each	80	3.5	10
Choc Chunk types, 1 oz	130	7	17
Homestyle Oatmeal Raisin, 1 oz	130	4.5	20
Vienna Fingers: Regular (2)	140	6	21
Reduced Fat (2)	130	4.5	22
Wafers: Golden Vanilla Wafers (8)	150	7	20
Reduced Fat (8)	130	3.5	25
Rainbow (artif. flavored) (8)	130	5	20
Sugar: Vanilla (4)	150	8	18
Peanut Butter (4)	160	9	18
Sugar Free: Vanilla Creme (3)	130	6	19

Kraft
	C	F	Cb
White Cheddar Chse Nips (27), 1 oz	150	7	19
Teddy Graham Bearwiches (1)	150	7	21

Lance:	C	F	Cb
Lance: Big Town, 1 pkg	250	11	38
Chocolate Chip, each	130	6	18
Dunking Sticks, each	180	10	22
Fig Bar, each	180	3.5	34
Fat Free: Apple/Cranberry, ea.	160	0	38
Oatmeal, each	130	6	18
Creme, each	240	10	35
Apple Bar, each	190	6	32
Peanut Butter, each	140	8	14
Peanut Butter Creme Wafer, 1 pkg	230	12	26

Little Debbie:	C	F	Cb
Little Debbie: Apple Flips	150	5	24
Chse Crackers w. P'nut Butter (4)	140	8	16
Fudge Brownies (1)	270	13	39
German Choc Cookie Rings	140	8	17
Ginger Cookies	90	3	15
Marshmallow Pies, each	160	6	27
Nutty Bar (2), 2 oz	310	18	32
Oatmeal Creme Pies (1)	170	7	26
Toasty Crackers w. P'nut Butter (4)	140	7	16
Yo-Yo's	130	6	21
Peanut Clusters, each	190	11	21
Figaroos, each, 1.5 oz	150	3.5	31
Peanut Butter & Jelly Sandwich	130	5	22

Per Cookie/Cracker (Unless Indicated)

	C	**F**	**Cb**
Lotte			
Chocolate (13), 1 oz	**190**	10	13
Koala Vanilla (13)	**190**	11	15
Koala Yummies (13), 1 oz	**200**	11	13
Peanut Butter (13)	**190**	10	11
Strawberry (13)	**190**	10	14
Lu Marie Lu			
Le Choclateur (3)	**150**	8	17
Le Petit Beurre (4)	**150**	4	25
Le Petit Ecolier (2)	**130**	6	17
Pim's: Orange; Raspberry (2)	**90**	3	17
Manischewitz			
Matzo Boards: See Page 104			
Biscotti: Toffee Crunch Macaroons	**50**	2.5	7
Choc. Chip Cappuccino	**70**	2.5	10
Chocolate Macaroons, each	**45**	2	5
Matzo Cracker, Miniatures	**9**	0	2
Whole Wheat Crackers	**9**	0	2
M&M/Mars Co: *Per Bar*			
Cookie Bars, average, 1.2 oz	**180**	11	21

Mrs Fields' Cookies ~ See Page 224

	C	**F**	**Cb**
Mother's			
ABC Cinnamon Grahams (1)	**12**	0.5	1.5
ABC Sugar Cookies (1)	**12**	0.5	1.5
Blasters (2)	**120**	6	17
Candy Chip (4)	**150**	7	21
Checkerboard Wafers	**20**	1	4
Chocolate Chip: Cookies	**80**	4	10
Cookies (bag) (1)	**30**	1	5
Cookie Parade Assortment, each	**35**	1.5	5
Chocolate Chip Parade	**35**	1.5	5
Angel Cookies	**60**	3	7
Circus Animal Cookies (1)	**25**	1	3
Cocodas Coconut	**30**	2	4
Coffee Creme S/wich (2)	**180**	7	26
Dinosaur Grrrahams	**65**	1.5	12
Double Fudge	**90**	4.5	12
English Tea/Taffy Sandwich	**90**	3.5	13
Flaky Flix Fudge/Vanilla	**70**	3.5	8
Fudge & Mint (2)	**150**	8	21
Fudge Circus (6)	**140**	7	20
Fudge Gauchos (2)	**190**	8	26
Gaucho Peanut Butter S'wich	**95**	5	11
Iced Raisin; Macaroon	**80**	4	9

	C	**F**	**Cb**
Mother's (Cont)			
Oatmeal Cookies: Regular	**55**	2.5	9
Butterscotch Chip	**60**	2.5	9
Iced; Chocolate Chip	**65**	2	11
Oatmeal Raisin Cookies	**30**	2	4
Oatmeal Walnut Choc. Chip	**65**	3	9
Peanut Butter	**75**	4.5	8
Striped Shortbread Cookies	**55**	2.5	7
Sugar Free: Shortbread (4)			
Choc & Lemon Sandwich			
Sugar Cookies	**70**	3	10
Sugared Lemon	**75**	4	9
Taffy	**90**	4	13
Murray SugarFree Cookies			
Choc Chip& Pecan (3)	**160**	9	19
Double Fudge (3)	**140**	6	23
Fudge-Dipped Wafer, Vanilla (4)	**140**	10	19
Lemon/Choc Cremes (3)	**120**	7	18
Lemon Crisp (4)	**140**	4.5	22
Peanut Butter (3)	**150**	7	18
Shortbread (8)	**120**	4.5	20
Vanilla Sugar Wafers (6)	**160**	9	21
Newman's Own			
Fig Newmans (2)	**120**	0	28
Snack Pack, 1.6 oz	**140**	0	33

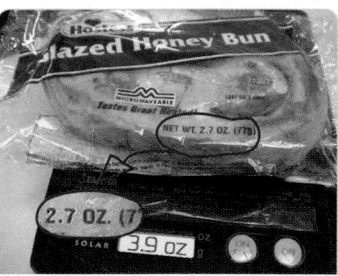

Weigh packaged foods for actual weight. It can be up to 50% more than the label net weight (the minimum legal weight). Allow extra calories.

Crackers ◆ Cookies (Cont)

Per Cookie/Cracker (Unless Indicated)

Nabisco	C	F	Cb
Crackers:			
Air Crisps: Ritz (24), 1 oz	140	5	22
Cheese Nips (24), 1 oz	130	4	21
Potato varieties (24), 1 oz	120	3.5	21
Pretzel Original (24), 1 oz	110	1	22
Tortilla (25)	130	5	21
Wheat Thins (24), 1 oz	130	4.5	21
Bacon Flavored Thins (7), 1/2 oz	80	4	9
Barnum's Animal Cracker	15	0.5	3
Better Cheddars, Reg; Low Salt	5	0.5	1
Cheese Nips, avg. (29), 1 oz	155	7	17
Chicken in a Biskit (12), 1.1 oz	160	9	19
Garden Crisps (7), 1/2 oz	60	2	10
Graham Crackers (4)	130	3	23
Honey Maid Graham, sticks (13)	120	2.5	24
Oysterettes (19), 1/2 oz	60	2.5	10
Ritz; Wheatsworth; Stoneground (1)	15	1	2
Mini Ritz (33), 1 oz	150	8	18
Ritz Bits S'wiches, Chse 1.5 oz pkt	230	14	23
Ritz Chips, avg. all varieties (15)	140	5	23
Peanut Butter (4), 1 oz	160	8	18
Xtreme Cheese (13), 1 oz	160	10	16
Premium Saltine, avg. (1), 1 oz	10	0.5	2
Royal Lunch (1)	60	2	8
Sociables Crisps (7)	80	4	9
Swiss Crisps (7), 1/2 oz	70	3.5	10
Teddy Cheddy (23), 1 oz	140	6	19
Tid Bit Cheese (16), 1/2 oz	80	4	8
Triscuit Thin Crisps (15)	130	5	20
Triscuit Wafers, all types (1)	20	1	1
Uneeda, Unsalted Tops	30	.5	3
Vegetable Thins (7), 1/2 oz	80	4.5	9
Waverly (5)	70	3.5	10
Wheat/Oat Thins: Orig., (8) 1/2 oz	70	3	10
Big Wheat Thins (10)	140	6	20
Ranch (14)	150	7	19
Zings! 1 pkg, 1.8 oz	240	11	34
Cookies: Biscos: Sugar Wafers	20	1	2
Waffle Cremes	35	2	4
Brown Edge Wafers	30	1	4
Bugs Bunny Graham Cookies	10	0.5	5
Café Creme: Vanilla Fudge (2)	200	10	27
Vanilla; Cappuccino (2)	160	8	22
Cameo Creme Sandwich	65	2.5	10
Choc Cherry Bar, 1 bar	130	2	26
Chocolate Chip Bite Size	10	0.3	2
Chocolate Chip Honey Grahams	5	0.2	1
Chocolate Snaps	17	0.5	3
Chocolate Wafers (Red. Fat)	14	0.2	3
Candy Blasts (1)	80	4	10

Nabisco (Cont):	C	F	Cb
Chips Ahoy!: Chocolate Chip (1)	80	4	10
Mini (1)	30	1.5	4
Snack Pack (4), 1.4 oz	200	10	27
Chewy Chocolate/Fudge	55	2.5	8
Chunky Choc Chip; Cremewiches	80	4	10
Mini Chips Ahoy! (5)	160	8	20
Snack Pack, 1.5 oz (43g)	220	11	28
Peanut Butter (1)	80	4	9
Reduced Fat (1)	50	1.5	8
Warm 'n Chewy, avg. (2)	245	10	38
Famous Chocolate Wafers	28	1	5
Fig Newtons: 1 cookie	110	2.5	22
Snack Pack, 2 pces, 2 oz	200	4	39
Snackable Dessert, (2)	125	3	25
Fat-Free Fig (1)	90	0	22
Apple/Fruit Newtons (2)	90	0	22
Cobblers, Apple/Peach	70	0	17
Grahams	15	0.5	3
Honey Maid: Grahams, all types (2)	30	0.5	6
Low Fat Cinnamon Grahams (2)	28	0.4	6
Ideal Bars: Chocolate & Peanut	90	5	10
Lorna Doone Shortbread	35	1.5	4
Marshmallow Puffs; Mystic Mint	90	4	14
Marshmallow Twirls	140	6	20
Nilla Wafers: Original	15	0.5	3
Reduced Fat	15	0.3	3
Chocolate	110	2	23
Nutter Butter: Bites, each	15	0.5	2
P'nut Butter S'wich, 2 oz pkg	470	20	65
Oatmeal Crunch	80	3	12
Old Fashioned Ginger Snaps	30	0.5	5
Oreo: Original, 3 cookies	160	7	23
Snack pkg, 2 oz	270	12	40
Cookie Barz, 1 bar	180	10	23
Reduced Fat, 3 cookies	130	3.5	25
Choc. Creme; Coffee 'n Creme (2)	150	7	20
Double Delight: Mint 'n Creme (2)	140	7	20
P'nut Butter & Choc Creme (2)	140	7	20
Double Stuf, 2 cookies	140	7	20
Fudge-Covered, 1 cookie	90	5	13
Mini Oreo: 9 pieces, 1 oz	140	3	21
Snack Pack, 1.5 oz (43g)	200	9	31
Uh-Oh!, 3 cookies	170	7	24
Pecanz	90	5	9
Pinwheels, Choc./Marshmallow	130	5	21
Teddy Cheddy Crackers (23), 1.1 oz	150	6	19
Teddy Grahams Snacks, all types (1)	5	0.1	1

Per Cookie/Cracker (Unless Indicated)

	C	**F**	**Cb**
Parmalat ~ Bed & Breakfast			
Chocolate Chunk Pecan	130	8	14
Chunky Chocolate Chip	120	6	16
White Chocolate & Macadamia	130	7	15
Cranberry Raisin	110	5	17
Key Lime/Raspb. Fruit Center	140	6	22
Peak Freans: Trad. O'meal (2) 20g	90	3	15
Pepperidge Farm			
American Collection: Sante Fe	120	4.5	18
Sausalito, Choc Macadamia (4)	160	10	20
Average other flavors	140	7	16
Biscotti: Figaro	110	4	14
Caruso; La Scala; Tosca	90	3	13
Fruit Cookies: Cherry Cobbler	70	2.5	11
Average other flavors	50	2	7
Dessert Bliss: Choc. Alm.; Mint Choc. (3)	160	8	22
Distinctive: Bordeaux; Pirouette	45	1.5	7
Brussels, 1 pkt, 0.7 oz	100	2	13
Brussels Mint; Milano (1)	65	3.5	7
Chantilly Raspberry (2)	160	6	23
Chessman	40	1.5	7
Double Choc. Milano	75	4	9
Geneva	55	3	7
Hazelnut Milano	65	3.5	8
Lido	90	4.5	11
Linzer Strawberry Filled	100	4	15
Milk Choc. Bordeaux	60	3	7
Milk Choc. Milano	60	3.5	7
Mint/Orange Milano	70	4	8
Goldfish: Plain, 55 pces, 30g	140	6	19
Flavor Blasted (51) 30g	150	8	19
Giant: Wheat (14)	140	5	21
Flavor Blasted, average (31)	145	7	19
Graham Snacks: Average (38)	140	5	22
Cookie varieties (4)	20	0	14
Nantucket: Choc Chunk Minis (4)	150	8	20
Double Choc Chunk (1)	140	7	18
Old Fashioned: Hazelnut	55	2.5	7
Brownie; Butterscotch Oatmeal	55	3	6
Chocolate Chip; Irish Oatmeal	45	2.5	6
Gingerman; Molasses Crisps	45	2	7
Lemon Nut Crunch	60	3	6
Oatmeal Raisin	55	2	7
Pecan Shortbread	70	4.5	7
Shortbread	70	3.5	8
Sugar	45	2	7
Pepperidge Farm (Cont)			
Soft Baked: Oatmeal Raisin	110	4	17
Other varieties	130	7	16
Spritzers, all flavors (5)	140	7	21
Vanilla Raspberry Tart	60	1.5	12
Pirouline: 8 rolls, 1 oz	130	3.5	17
Salerno: Almond Windmill (2)	120	4.5	17
Bonnie Shortbread (4)	160	7	22
Butter Cookies: Original (6)	160	7	22
Reduced Fat (6)	150	5	22
Coconut Bar (4)	150	8	18
Creme Wafer Sugar-free (5)	190	13	18
Dinosaur Graham	70	2.5	11
Farm Animal Crackers (13)	140	5	22
Grahams: Cinnamon (2)	130	3.5	22
Chocolate (2)	130	3	24
Iced Oatmeal (2)	120	5	18
Mini Butter: Flavored (25)	150	6	20
Angel/Chocolate Creme (9)	140	6	20
Mini Dinosaur (15)	140	5	21
Mint Creme Patties (2)	130	7	16
Oyster Crackers: Regular (42)	60	1.5	11
Fat-Free (42)	60	0	11
Royal Crispy Stix (3)	150	8	18
Royal Stripes (3)	180	8	24
Saltine Crackers: Reg./Unsalted (5)	60	1.5	11
Fat-Free (5)	50	0	11
Santa's Favorites, Aniseed (6)	150	5	22
Scooter Pie Choc Marshmallow	140	5	23
Sugar Wafers, assorted (5)	180	11	20
Vanilla Wafers (7)	130	5	21
Santa Fe Farms			
Fat Free, average, 1 pkg	120	0	26
Sinful: Chocolate Chip (2)	150	7	19
All Butter Raisin & Oatmeal (2)	130	6	20
Butter w. Soft Creme Raspberry (1)	70	3	12
Choc w. Vanilla Creme (2)	120	5	16
Snackwell's (Nabisco)			
Choc Chip (3)	150	8	23
Coconut Creme (2)	110	4	19
Creme Sandwich, 1 pkg (4)	210	5	38
Double Choc Chip Bite Size (13)	130	4	22
Lemon Creme Sugar Free (3)	130	6	24
Mint Creme (2)	110	4	19
Oatmeal (1)	90	2.5	17
Peanut Butter Chip, 1 oz	120	4	20
Shortbread (3)	130	5	22
Crackers: Cracked Pepper (5)	60	1.5	10
Wheat (5)	70	1.5	11

Cookies (Cont) ◆ Refrigerated

	C	F	Cb
Stella D'Oro: Angel Wings	70	4.5	7
Almond Delight Chinese (1)	85	1	11
Angelica (1)	100	4	15
Anginetti (4)	140	4	23
Anisette Sponge (2)	90	1	19
Anisette Toast (3)	130	1	27
Banana Walnut Toast (1)	100	2	19
Blueberry Toast (1)	100	1	20
Breakfast Treats, Chocolate (1)	100	4	15
Biscotti (Hazelnut) (1)	100	3.5	15
Castelets, regular/chocolate (1)	70	3	9
Como Delight (1)	70	3.5	9
Fruit Delight Apple Cinnamon (1)	70	0	17
Golden Bars; Love Cookies (1)	110	4	16
Lady Stella Assortment (3)	130	5	19
Margherite, Reg./Low Sodium (1)	70	3	11
Swiss Fudge (1)	70	3	9
Sunshine: Cheez-It Crackers (1)	5	0.5	0.5
Big Cheez-It (1)	10	1	1
Cheez-It Cheddar Jack (26), 1 oz	165	10	16
Cheez-It Juniors (44), 1 oz	140	7	13
Grab Bags Crackers (1)	5	0.5	0.5
Heads & Tails, 1 pkt, 1.5 oz	210	9	28
Hi-Ho Crackers: Original (1)	17	0.5	2
Reduced Fat (1)	15	0.5	2
Krispy: Original (1)	10	0.3	2
Oyster & Soup, 17 crackers	60	1.5	11
Reduced Fat (1)	10	0	2
Party Mix: 1 pkt, 1.7 oz	230	9	32
Reduced Fat, 1/2 cup, 1 oz	130	3	21
Snack Mix: *Per 1/2 Cup*			
Big Crunch; Dble Cheese, avg.	70	4	14
Get Nutty	150	9	16
Original	130	4.5	21
Trader Joe's: Oatmeal Raisins (1)	250	11	37
Choc Chip Cookies (1)	270	13	36
Joe-Joe's Choc s/wich (1)	65	2.5	9
Weight Watchers: O'meal Rais. (2)	120	2	22
Apple Raisin Bars, each	70	2	14
Chocolate Chip (2)	140	5	22
Choc. S'wich Cookies (2)	140	3.5	23
Fruit Filled, 1 bar	70	0	16
Vanilla Sandwich Cookies(2)	140	3	25
Wild Oats: Ginger Snaps (5) 1 oz	130	5	20
Crunchy P'nut Butter (5) 1 oz	150	8	16
Oatmeal Raisin (5) 1 oz	130	5	20
Oat Choc Chip (5) 1 oz	130	5	20
Water Crackers (4) 0.5 oz	63	1.5	11

Zesta	C	F	Cb
Saltine: Export Sodas (3)	60	1.5	10
Fat Free, 5 crackers	50	0	13
Original, 5 crackers	60	1.5	11
Red. Sodium; Unsalted tops (5)	70	1.5	11
Soup & Oyster, 45 crackers	70	3	9
Unsalted Tops, 5 crackers	70	1.5	11

Thaw, Bake & Serve

	C	F	Cb
Big Country: Avg. all types (1)	100	4	15
Cookietree: *Per Cookie*			
Buttersugar; Cinn. Apple Oatmeal	120	5	17
Choc. varieties; Pecan/Macadam.	130	7	17
Cookie w. M&M's; Dble Fudge	120	6	17
Fat Free varieties, average	125	0	28
Peanut Butter/Chocolate	130	7	17
Raisin Oatmeal	110	3.5	18
Guiltless Indulgence (1.3 oz Cookie)			
Fat Free varieties, avg.	120	0	28
Lowfat Fudge/Choc., avg.	130	2	18
Grands!, *Per Biscuit:* Extra Rich	220	12	25
Blueberry; Golden Corn	210	9	28
Butter Tastin'; Buttermilk	200	10	24
Reduced Fat	190	7	27
Cinn. Raisin; Extra Fluffy; Wheat	200	8	22
Flaky; Homestyle	200	10	25
Southern Style	200	10	24
Hungry Jack: Avg. all types (1)	100	4.5	14
Jewel: Buttermilk Biscuits (2)	100	1.5	20
Old Fashioned Biscuits (2)	100	1.5	20
Pillsbury Cookies: *Per 1 oz*			
Buttermilk; Country, each	50	1	3
Choc. Chip/Dbl Choc Chip Chunk	140	7	17
Choc. Chip. Reduced Fat	110	4	18
Chocolate Chip w. Walnuts	130	7	16
Holiday, all types (2)	130	7	16
M&Ms	130	6	17
Oatmeal Choc. Chip; Reeses	125	6	19
One Step Pan Cookies	130	6	19
Peanut Butter	120	6	19
SnackWells; Choc. Chip Red. Fat	110	3	18
Chocolate Fudge	90	1.5	18
Sugar (2), 1 oz	130	5	20
Tender Layer Buttermilk	160	4.5	18
Toll House *(Nestlé):* Choc Chip	140	6	20
Reduced Fat Choc Chip	130	3.5	23
Choc. Chip White; Chunk	150	6	22
Peanut Butter Choc Chip	150	7	20
Sugar	120	5	18

Cakes, Pastries, Croissants

Ready-to-Eat

	C	F	Cb
Angel Food: Plain, no oil, 2 oz	120	0	25
Plain with oil, 2 oz	160	1.5	25
w. Cream Frosting	230	7	37
Apple Fritters, 3 oz	360	22	38
Apple Pie: See Pies/Tarts Page 120			
Baklava, 1^1/$_2$" square, 1^1/$_2$ oz	110	6	13
Banana w. Butter Cream, 3 oz	300	13	40
Black Forest, 3 oz	230	10	34
Brownie, 3.5 oz	420	25	52
Bundt, 3 oz	300	17	35
Carrot Cake: Plain, 3 oz	230	8	41
w. Cream Cheese Frosting	380	21	42
Cheesecake: Small serving, 3 oz	260	18	24
Large serving, 5 oz	430	30	40
w. Lowfat Cheese/fruit, 3 oz	150	8	30
Cheesecake Factory: See Page 195			
Denny's Cheesecake, 1 slice	470	27	48
Cherry Cobbler, 5 oz	350	10	62
Chocolate Cake: Plain, 2 oz	220	11	40
w. Chocolate Frosting, 4 oz	320	15	42
& Cream Filling, 3^1/$_2$ oz	360	21	43
Churros, 1 stick, 1^1/$_2$ oz	150	8	18
Cinnamon Crumb Cake, 4 oz	450	23	57
Cinnamon Roll, Large, 6 oz	630	27	87
Coffee Cake, 2^1/$_2$ oz	230	7	38
Concha: Medium size, 3 oz	400	19	50
Large (5" diameter), 5^1/$_2$ oz	720	35	92
Cream Cheese Crumb, 4 oz	410	20	52
Cream Puff (custard fill), 4^1/$_2$ oz	300	18	26
Creme Horns, each	190	13	19
Croissants: See Next Column			
Cupcake: Plain, 1^1/$_2$ oz	140	6	25
w. Frosting	170	7	30
Danish Pastry: Small, 2 oz	220	10	25
Large, 4 oz	440	20	51
Date Nut Roll, ^{1}/$_2$" slice	80	2	12
Devil's Food, w. Frosting, 3 oz	460	25	55
Donut Holes, 1^1/$_4$" balls, 2 oz (5)	220	10	30
Donuts: See Page 119			
Eclair, Choc., Cust. Fill, 3^1/$_2$ oz	240	14	23
Fig Bars, average, each	150	3	30
Fig Cake, ^{1}/$_2$ piece	110	2	21
Fruit Cake, Dark/Light, 1^1/$_2$ oz	165	7	29
Fudge Nut Brownie, each	340	13	56
Gingerbread: From mix, 3" sq.	200	6	37
Honey Bun, each	330	13	47
Key Lime Pie, 4.5 oz	440	22	54
Kolacky, Apricot/Rasp., ^{1}/$_2$ oz (1)	60	3.5	8

Ready-to-Eat (Cont)

	C	F	Cb
Lemon Cake,			
2^1/$_2$ oz piece	220	9	40
Lemon Poppy Seed Creme, 3 oz	310	15	40
Marble Cake, 1 slice, 4 oz	380	14	60
Mississippi Mud Pie, 4 oz	380	24	37
Mud Cake, 1 piece, 3^1/$_2$ oz	350	16	48
Muffins ~ See Next Page			
Orange Creme (Ring), 3 oz	300	15	40
Pineapple Upside Down, 2^1/$_2$ oz	230	9	37
Peach Melba, 3^1/$_2$ oz	300	8	52
Strawberry Creme, 3 oz	290	14	40
Strudel Bites, ^{3}/$_4$ oz	85	4	12
Pecan Twirls, 1 piece	110	5	16
Pecan Pie, 3 oz	330	13	51
Pies & Tarts: See Page 120			
Pound Cake, 3 oz	420	27	42
Sponge: Plain, 2^1/$_2$ oz	190	3	36
w. Cream & Strawberry	325	8	38
w. Chocolate Icing	300	12	38
Raisin Bun, 1 bun, 2^1/$_4$ oz	180	2	37
Strudel, fruit, average, 3 oz	280	8	45
Sweet Roll, average, 1^1/$_2$ oz	155	7	24
Swiss Rolls, each	170	9	23
Tarts: See Page 109			
Tiramisu, 1 piece, 5 oz	400	29	30
Toaster Strudel, 2 oz	190	10	26
Turnovers, fruit, average, 3 oz	270	12	36

Croissants

Average All Brands	C	F	Cb
Plain/All Butter:			
Petite, 1 oz	120	7	14
1 Medium, 1^1/$_2$ oz	180	10	21
1 Large, 2^1/$_2$ oz	300	18	35
Sweet: Per Croissant (3^1/$_2$ oz)			
Almond Croissant	420	25	39
Apple Croissant	250	10	30
Chocolate Croissant	400	24	36
Sandwiches: See Page 175			
Au Bon Pain: See Page 187			
Burger King: Croissan'wich, See Page 193			
Dunkin' Donuts: Plain Croissant	330	18	37
Sandwiches, See Page 204			
Sara Lee: All Butter, 1^1/$_2$ oz	180	9	19
All Butter Petite, 1 oz	120	6	13

Muffins, Sweet Rolls

Quick Guide | C | F | Cb

Muffins: Ready-To-Eat

Average All Types:

	C	F	Cb
Small, 1 oz	80	3	12
Medium, 2 oz	160	6	24
Large, 3 oz	240	9	36
Extra Large, 4 oz	320	12	48
Giant, 6 oz	480	18	60
Super Size, 8 oz	640	24	96
English Muffin, 2 oz	150	2	29

Brands ~ Ready-To-Eat

	C	F	Cb
Au Bon Pain ~ *See Page 187*			
Awreys: Blueberry, 2.25 oz	210	9	29
Raisin Bran, 2.5 muffin	190	7	30
Carl's: Blueberry Muffin	340	14	49
Bran Raisin Muffin	370	14	61
Dunkin' Donuts: *See Page 204*			
Hostess: Mini, average, each	55	3	7
Fruit Pie, avg., 4.5 oz	480	21	70
Krispy Kreme ~ *See Page 216*			
McDonald's: Apple Bran, 4 oz	300	3	61
My Favorite Muffin: Plain, 6 oz	600	30	75
Chocolate, 6 oz	510	24	69
Fat Free, avg., 6 oz	380	0	88
Oroweat: Cinnamon Rais., 2.4 oz	170	1	35
Extra Crisp; Sourdough, 2 oz	130	0.5	26
Health Nut, 2.3 oz	170	3	30
Otis Spunkmeyer: *Per Whole Muffin (4 oz)*			
Banana Nut, 4 oz	480	24	60
Cheese Streudel	440	20	60
Wild Blueberry	420	22	48
Our Daily Muffin: Each, 3 oz	120	0	31
Pepperidge Farm: Average	150	3	28
Ralphs: Banana, 4.5 oz muffin	470	21	62
Blueberry, 4.5 oz	410	16	60
Bran & Raisin, 5 oz	380	8	78
Sara Lee: Blueberry	220	11	27
Corn	260	14	30
Snackwell's: Blueberry, 1/6 pkt	120	0	28
Starbucks ~ *See Page 250*			
Weight Watchers: *Per Muffin*			
Chocolate Chocolate Chip	190	2	39
English Muffin Sandwich	210	5	28
Fat Free, average, all flavors	165	0	39
Low Fat, average, all flavors	175	3	37
Winchell's ~ *See Page 263*			

Muffin Mixes | C | F | Cb

Prepared: Per Muffin

	C	F	Cb
Atkins: Blueberry Muffin	65	0.5	9
Betty Crocker: Apple Streusel	210	8	33
Blueberry	160	6	25
Choc Chip; Cinn. Streusel	170	8	23
Fat Free, all flavors	120	0	26
Duncan Hines: Blueberry, reg.	120	3	21
Bakery Style: Pecan Crunch	220	11	27
Avg. all other flavors	200	7	32
Oat Bran Blueberry	110	4	17
Oatmeal & Apples/Walnuts	210	9	30
Gold Medal: Apple; Blueberry	250	8	41
Chocolate Chip w. Glaze	330	12	51
Cornbread varieties	140	3.5	25
Variety	105	7	9
Average other flavors	280	8	46
Oberweis Dairy Newberry: *Per Muffin (3 oz)*			
Banana Nut	260	9	39
Carrot Walnut	340	20	36
Avg. other varieties	225	8	36
Sweet Rewards: Low Fat	230	1.5	51

Sweet Rolls & Buns

Note: Weigh for actual weight as can be 10-50% higher than label weight.

	C	F	Cb
Cinnabon: Classic	730	24	114
Caramel Pecanbon, 1 serving	1100	56	141
Minibon, 1 serving	300	11	45
Entenmann's: Cinn. Bun, 2.15 oz	230	10	32
Reduced Fat, 2.15 oz	160	3	32
Swirl Buns, average (1)	330	15	44
Pecan/Walnut Danish Ring, 2 oz	250	15	25
Twists: Raspberry, 1/8, 2 oz	220	11	27
Nonfat, 1/8, 2 oz	140	0	32
Cinnamon Danish, 1/8, 2 oz	240	13	29
Lemon Danish, 1/8, 2 oz	210	11	26
Hostess: Honey Bun, Glazed, 2.7 oz	320	19	34
Actual weight up to 3.9 oz	460	27	49
Iced/Frosted, 3.5 oz	410	24	42
Little Debbie: Pecan Spinwheels, 1 oz	110	4	16
Mickey: Cinnamon Pastry, 4 oz	200	5.5	35
Cinnamon Nut, 2 1/2 oz	230	8	37
Raisin Cinnamon, 2 1/2oz	200	4.5	35
Pillsbury: Cinnamon Roll, 1.5 oz	150	5	23
Reduced Fat, 1.5 oz	140	3.5	24
Svenhard's: Viking Size Cinn. Bun, 4 oz			
Actual weight up to 5.6 oz	650	35	79
Label data based on 4.8 oz	560	30	68

Quick Guide   **C** **F** **Cb**

Donuts
Average All Brands

	C	F	Cb
Plain, 1³/4 oz	210	12	25
Sugared, 1³/4 oz	220	11	27
Glazed, 2 oz	250	12	34
Chocolate Iced, 2 oz	260	14	29

Brands   **C** **F** **Cb**

Buttercrumb
	C	F	Cb
Cinnamon, 1 cake, 1.6 oz	170	6	28

Dolly Madison Donuts
	C	F	Cb
Regular, 1³/4 oz	270	12	40
Gem varieties, 1/2 oz each	65	3	8
Powdered Mini, 1/2 oz each	60	3	8

Dunkin' Donuts: See Fast-Foods, Page 204

Dutch Mill: Plain, 1³/4 oz
	C	F	Cb
Dutch Mill: Plain, 1³/4 oz	210	12	25
Sugared, 1³/4 oz	220	11	27
Glazed, 2 oz	250	12	34
Double-Dipped Chocolate, 2 oz	280	17	31

Entenmann's Donuts
	C	F	Cb
Powdered, 1³/4 oz	230	14	25
Glazed Buttermilk, 2¹/4 oz	270	13	35
Light, 2 oz	190	7	31
Light Fantastic Fudge, 2 oz	210	9	40
Milk Chocolate Frosted, 2.4 oz	310	19	35
Dark Choc. Frosted, 2 oz	280	19	27

Hostess Donuts
	C	F	Cb
Cinnamon Sweet Rolls, 2.3 oz	210	7	34
Regular: Plain, 1 oz	140	7	15
Chocolate Frosted, 1¹/2 oz	180	11	19
Powdered, 1¹/2 oz	150	8	19
Old Fashioned Glazed, 1¹/2oz	260	13	33
Blueberry, 1¹/2 oz	210	13	21
Hostess O's, Raspberry, 2 oz	230	10	34
Donettes: Plain, 1/2 oz	70	4	8
Frosted, 0.5 oz ea	65	4	7
Crumb, 0.7 oz ea	80	3.5	10
Powdered, 1/2 oz ea	60	3	8

Jewel: Cinnamon Spiced, 2 oz
	C	F	Cb
Jewel: Cinnamon Spiced, 2 oz	230	15	24

Krispy Kreme: See Fast-Foods, Page 216

Little Debbie Donuts
	C	F	Cb
Donut Sticks, 1.6 oz pkg	210	13	21
3 oz pkg	390	23	39

Brands (Cont)   **C** **F** **Cb**

Mickey
	C	F	Cb
Egg Fluff (2) 1.65 oz	210	11	25
French Twirl (2) 1.65 oz	240	16	21
Jumbo, avg. all types (1) 1.5 oz	190	11	21
Mini (2) 1 oz	130	8	15

Sara Lee Donuts
	C	F	Cb
Choc. Frosted Mini, 3/4 oz each	100	5.5	13
Powdered Mini, 1/2 oz each	85	4.5	9
Glazed, 1/2 oz each	110	5	14
Reduced Fat, 1/2 oz each	55	2.5	8

Tastykake Donuts
	C	F	Cb
Plain, 1¹/2 oz	190	10	22
Cinnamon, 1¹/2 oz	180	8	26
Frosted Rich, 2 oz	260	16	28
Glazed, Mini (6) 2¹/2 oz	270	12	38
Honey Wheat, 2 oz	210	8	32
Powdered Sugar, Mini (6) 2¹/2 oz	280	13	38

Van De Kamp's Donuts
	C	F	Cb
Old Fashioned: Plain	270	11	40
Chocolate, 2.4 oz	340	22	34
Powdered, 2 oz	240	11	35
Assorted, 2¹/4 oz	280	17	32
Mini Donuts: Chocolate (4) 2 oz	290	17	32
Crumb (4)	220	8	35
Powdered (4)	250	12	33
Lowfat: Maple Buttermilk (1)	200	2	43
Chocolate Buttermilk (1)	200	2	43
Double Chocolate (1)	190	2.5	41
Powdered (1)	150	1.5	32

Zingers
	C	F	Cb
Devil's/Vanilla Food, 2 cakes	280	8	50

"Now cut that out!"

Pies & Tarts

Quick Guide   **C** **F** **Cb**

Pies ~ *Average All Brands*
1/8 of 9" Pie, 4 oz Serving

	C	F	Cb
Apple; Blueberry; Cherry	290	13	46
Boston Cream Pie	330	14	55
Chocolate Pie	300	18	35
Custard; Coconut Custard	250	13	27
Lemon Chiffon Pie	360	14	50
Lemon Meringue	270	11	42
Mince Pie	300	13	46
Pecan Pie	470	24	52
Pumpkin Pie	240	13	28
Strawberry Pie	230	9	37

Brands ~ *Per Serving*

	C	F	Cb
Denny's: Apple Pie	485	24	64
Chocolate Peanut Butter	665	39	64
Chocolate Silk Pie	650	43	60
Dutch Apple Pie	440	19	55
Hershey's Choc Chunks N' Chips	600	36	58
Oreo® Cookies & Creme	650	40	67
Pumpkin Pie	235	7	38
Entenmann's			
Homestyle Apple, 1/6 pie, 4.3 oz	340	12	56
Hostess: Fruit; Cherry, 4.5 oz pie	470	22	65
Lemon, 4.5 oz pie	500	24	66
Long John Silver's: *Per Serving*			
Chocolate Cream Pie	310	22	24
Pecan Pie	370	15	55
Pineapple Cream Pie	290	13	39
Marie Callender's			
Per 1/5 Pie: Apple	865	49	92
Blueberry	885	57	76
Boysenberry	860	57	82
Cherry	900	58	87
Banana Cream	630	28	67
Chocolate Cream	535	29	66
Coconut Cream	650	32	64
Per 1/4 Pie: Fresh Strawberry	615	28	89
Mince	885	59	97
Lemon Meringue	550	23	76
Pumpkin	615	28	80
Tastykake: Fruit, average	310	11	50
French Apple	360	12	61
Coconut Creme	390	20	47
Lemon Pie	300	13	44

Pastry & Pie Crusts

Pie Crust: Baked, 9" diameter shell	C	F	Cb
1 Pie Shell, 6 1/2 oz	900	60	79
2-crust Pie, 9", 11 1/4 oz	1500	93	137
Betty Crocker, 9", 1/8 shell	110	8	9
Boboli, thin Pizza Crust, 1/5, 2 oz	170	4	28
Hershey's Choc Crust, 1/8	110	5	14
Jewel, 1/8 of 9" crust	130	8	13
Keebler Graham Cracker, 1/8 of 9"	110	5	14
Reduced Fat, 1/8	90	3.5	14
Shortbread Crust, 1/8	110	5	14
Mrs Smith's Deep Dish, 9" (1/8)	110	7	11
Nabisco Oreo, 1/6 of 9" crust	140	7	18
Honey Maid Graham, 1/6, 1 oz	140	7	18
Nilla Pie Crust, 1/6, 1 oz	140	8	18
Pet-Ritz, all types, 1/8, 3/4 oz	90	5	10
Pillsbury (All Ready), 1/8 pie, 1 oz	120	7	13
Piecrust Sticks, 8 oz	960	64	90
Choux Pastry, raw, 1 oz	60	4	3
Filo Pastry: 4 sheets, 2 1/2 oz	210	2.5	40
Athens: 5 sheets, 2 oz	180	1	35
Mini Dough Shells, 2, 8g	45	2	1
Pepp. Farm, 2 sheets, 1 1/2oz	120	1	25
Flaky Pastry, 1 sheet, 6 oz	780	72	18
Puff (Pepp.Farm), 1/2 sheet, 4.5 oz	510	33	42
1/6 sheet, 1 1/2 oz	170	11	14
Bake & Fill Shell, 1.7 oz	190	13	16
Pizza Crust, 1/8 whole	90	1	16
Bisquick Baking Mix:			
Original, 1/3 cup, 1 1/2 oz	160	6	25
Reduced Fat, 1/3 cup, 1 1/2 oz	140	3	27

Pie Filling

Canned: Average All Brands *Per 4 oz*	C	F	Cb
Apple: 4 oz	120	0	28
21 oz Can	600	0	145
Apricot, 4 oz	150	0	36
Blackberry, Blueberry, Cherry	120	0	28
Chocolate, Coconut, 4 oz	140	3	33
Lemon, 4 oz	200	2	47
Mincemeat, 4 oz	190	1	45
Peach, Strawberry	120	0	28
Pumpkin, 4 oz	170	0	40
Raisin, 4 oz	130	0	30
Raspberry, Black/Red, 4 oz	190	0	45
Strawberry, 4 oz	120	0	28

Cakes & Pastries – Packaged

Cakes & Pastries	C	F	Cb
Atkins			
Cheesecake, 3 oz slice	250	24	3
Dessert Cake Roll: *Per 1/6 Whole*			
Carrot, 2.6 oz slice	220	18	5
Chocolate, 2.6 oz slice	240	20	6
Mini Cheesecake. avg. all flavors	250	24	3
Banquet: Crm Pies, avg., 1/3 pie	350	21	42
Cheesecake Factory: *See Page 195*			
Dolly Madison: Honey Bun, 3.75 oz	440	25	49
Cinnamon Sweet Rolls (1)	210	7	34
Dunkin' Stix, 1 stix	170	9	20
Eli's Frozen Cheesecakes: *Per 1/8 Pkg (3 oz)*			
Cookies N Creme; Choc. Caramel	320	23	11
Keylime; Original, average	320	22	26
Entenmann's			
All Butter Loaf, 1/6 loaf, 2 oz	210	9	30
Banana Cake, 1/8 cake, 2.5 oz	290	15	39
Cheese-Topped Coffee, 1/8, 2 oz	200	9	26
Cheese-Filled Crumb Coffee, 2 oz	210	10	25
Chocolate Fudge, 1/6 cake, 3 oz	280	12	42
Chocolate Loaf, Light, 1/8, 2 oz	120	0	27
Creme-Filled: Choc Cupcakes, 1	160	0	39
Golden Cakes, 1 cake, 2.3 oz	280	15	34
Golden Loaf (Light) 1/8, 1.7 oz	130	0	28
Louisiana Crunch, 1/9, 3 oz	330	14	48
Mocha Cake, 1/6 cake, 3 oz	340	17	45
New York Crumb Coffee, 1/10, 2 oz	250	12	33
Ultimate Crumb, 1/10, 2 oz	250	13	33
Brownie: Ultimate Fudge, 1	220	13	27
Light: Fudge, 1/10 strip, 1.4 oz	110	0	27
Lemon; Coffee, 1/8 strip, 1.9 oz	130	0	29
Buns/Twists: *See Page 118*			
Grands!			
Blueberry Biscuits, 2 oz	210	9	29
Cinnamon Rolls, 3.5 oz each	300	7	54
Hostess: *Per Cake Unless Indicated*			
Angel Food Cake, 1/8 cake	160	1.5	33
Brownie Bites, each	57	3	7
Carrot Cake, 2 pces, 3.5 oz	300	7	55
Chocodiles	240	11	33
Coconut Cakes, Creme (1) 1 oz	260	13	32
Crumb Coffee	130	5	19
Cup Cake, each	160	6	30

Hostess (Cont)	C	F	Cb
Dessert Cups, each	100	2	17
Ding Dongs	190	10	23
Fudge Brownie	330	11	54
Hearty Muffin, avg.	620	33	73
Ho Ho's, each	125	6	17
Honey Bun: Glazed, 2.7 oz	320	19	34
Actual weight up to 3.9 oz	460	27	49
Muffin Loaf, avg.	440	19	63
Mini Muffins (3)	160	9	16
Snoballs	180	5	31
Suzy Q's, 1 cake, 2 oz	230	9	35
Twinkies, 1 cake, 1.5 oz	150	5	25
Low Fat Cupcakes; Twinkies, avg.	135	1.5	28
Jewel Bake Shop			
Choc Mini Cupcakes, 1 cake	100	12	30
Cinnamon Swirl Bread, 1 oz slice	160	2.5	30
Creme Horns, 1 horn	190	13	19
Elephant Ears, 2.5 oz	340	22	34
Fancy Jelly Roll, 1/6 roll, 2.7 oz	190	2.5	38
French Torpedo Roll, 2.7 oz	170	1	35
Gourmet Cinn. Rolls, 6 oz roll	640	29	88
Key Lime Meringue Pie, 1/6, 5 oz	340	12	55
Little Debbie			
Cakes: Coffee (2) 2 oz	230	7	39
Choc Chip Snack (2), 2.4 oz	290	14	42
Creme-filled Strawb. Cupcake (1)	200	9	29
Devil Cremes, 1.65 oz cake	190	8	29
Devil Squares, 2 cakes, 2.2 oz	270	13	37
Frosted Fudge , 1.5 oz cake	200	10	25
Swiss Cake Rolls, 2 cakes	260	12	39
Zebra Cakes, 2 cakes, 2.6 oz	330	16	45
Honey Buns, 1.75 oz bun	220	13	24
Manischewitz: Cheesecake, 3 oz	250	19	16
Marie Callendar (Frozen)			
Cobbler, all types, 1/4 pie, 4.25 oz	390	19	45
Mrs Smith's			
Cream Pies: *Per 1/6 Pie*			
Choc Chip Delight, 4.9 oz	410	18	59
Moose Tracks, 4.5 oz	495	29	51
Oreo, 4.3 oz	380	17	54
Flip it Cake Frozen Desserts: *Per 1/2 Cake (5 oz)*			
Apple Caramel	490	13	90
Chocolate Carame	580	25	84
Strawberry Delight	385	9	73

Cakes & Pastries (Cont)

Pepperidge Farm	C	F	Cb
Cakes Supreme: *Per 3 oz Slice*			
Lemon Mousse	290	12	35
Chocolate Mousse	250	10	35
Boston Creme	260	9	32
Cream Cakes Supreme:			
Cream Cheese Carrot, 1/9, 3 oz	320	20	38
Pineap./Strawb. Crm., 2.7 oz sl.	240	10	38
Old Fashioned Cakes: *Per 3 oz Slice*			
Butter Pound	290	13	39
Deluxe Carrot	310	16	39
Turnovers (Frozen): Apple, 3.2 oz	290	15	36
Raspberry, 3.2 oz	290	15	35
3-Layer Cakes: Coconut, 1/8, 2.5 oz	250	11	35
Golden, 1/8 cake, 2.5 oz	250	12	33
Fruit Squares: Apple/Blueb./Cherry	210	10	27
Rich's: Chocolate Eclairs (Frozen)	190	9	24

Sara Lee	C	F	Cb
Cakes: *Per Serving*			
All Butter Pound, 1/6, 2.7 oz	320	16	38
Reduced Fat, 1/4, 2.7 oz	280	11	42
All Butter; Chocolate, 1/4, 2.7 oz	320	16	40
Banana Sundae, 1/10, 3 oz	270	14	32
Butter Streusel Coffee, 1/6, 2 oz	220	12	25
Choc Layer, 1/8, 3 oz slice	340	17	46
Dble Choc Layer, 1/8, 2.8 oz	260	13	33
Free & Light, 1/4, 2.7 oz	200	4	39
Golden Butter, 1/4, 2.7 oz	300	13	41
Pecan Coffee, 1/6, 2 oz	230	12	24
Red, White, Blueb. 1/10, 3 oz	210	8	31
Strawberry, 1/4, 2.7 oz	290	11	44
Dessert Cakes: Carrot, 1/6, 3.2 oz	320	17	39
Banana, 1/6, 2.3 oz	230	8	37
Layer Cakes: *Per 1/8 Whole*			
Strawberry Shortcake, 2.5 oz	180	7	27
Other flavors, average, 3 oz	260	13	32
Bars: 1 bar, 2.75 oz	190	14	14
Cheesecake: *Per Serving*			
Cherry/Strawberry, avg, 4.75 oz	340	12	53
Chocolate Chip, 4.3 oz	410	21	47
Peanut Butter Cup, 3.5 oz	380	22	3i4
New York Cheesecake: Classic, 1/6	500	30	50
Mixed Berry Swirl, 1/6	490	28	52
Choc Chip Cookie Crumble, 1/6	520	27	61
Classic Cheesecakes:			
Original Cream, 1/4 cake, 4.3 oz	340	18	38
Orig. Strawb., 1/4 cake, 4.8 oz	330	12	49
French, 1/5 cake, 4.7 oz	410	25	41

Sara Lee (Cont)	C	F	Cb
Cheesecake Singles: *Per Slice*			
Caramel Choc Pecan, 110g	400	25	37
Strawberry Drizzle, 113g	380	20	46
Bites: Carrot Cake Bites, 5 pces	370	25	32
Choc-Dipped Orig., 5 pces	480	33	40
Choc Praline Pecan, 5 pces	470	30	42
Toasted Almond, 5 pces	450	29	42
Triple Choc Fudge, 2 pces	170	8	24
Cream Pies (9"): *Per Serving (5 oz)*			
Choc. Silk; Coconut Cream, 1/5	500	32	49
Lemon Meringue, 1/6	350	11	59
Oven Fresh Pies (9"): *Per 41/2 oz (1/8 of Pie)*			
Apple; Cherry, average	340	16	46
Blueberry; Dutch Apple	355	15	53
Mince/Raspberry, average	380	19	48
Pecan	520	24	70
Pumpkin	260	11	37
Southern Sweet Potato	280	10	45
Deep Dish Pies: *Per 1/10 Pie (4.7 oz)*			
Cinnamon French Apple	360	15	48
Golden Peach	340	16	48
Orchard Apple	400	24	43
Individual Slices: *Per Slice*			
Apple/Cherry Pie, 4 oz	300	11	47
Carrot; Cookies N Cream, 3.5 oz	335	20	40
Lemon Icebox Pie, 3.5 oz	260	10	41
Southern Pecan Pie, 4 oz	470	23	62
Strawberry Swirl Ch'cake, 3.5 oz	300	17	31
Round Danish: Cheese, 1/6 whole	180	6	28
Butter Streusel/Pecan, 1/6	225	12	24
Raspberry, 1/6 whole	200	8	27
Deluxe Cinnamon Roll, 1/6	320	15	41
TastyKake: Chocolate Jnr, 3.4 oz	320	12	52
Creme Filled Koffee Kakes, 3 oz	360	14	54
Koffee Kake Junior, 21/2 oz	250	8	40
Weight Watchers: *Per Serving*			
Brownie à la Mode	190	4	33
Chocolate Mousse	190	5	31
Chocolate Eclair	150	4	25
Choc. Chip Cookie Dough Sundae	190	4.5	35
Choc. Raspberry Royale	190	3	39
Double Fudge Brownie Parfait	190	2.5	39
Double Fudge Cake	190	4.5	36
French Style Cheesecake	170	4	28
Mississippi Mud Pie	160	5	24
New York Style Cheesecake	150	5	21
Strawberry Parfait Royale	180	2	35

Cakes, Cookies & Dessert Mixes

Made As Directed	C	F	Cb
Aitkens			
Quick Cuisine: *Per Serving*			
Blueberry Muffin	160	9	10
Chocolate Chip Muffin	190	8	18
Orange Cranberry	160	10	6
Arrowhead Mills: *Per Serving (Prep'd)*			
Cookie (1), avg. all types	90	2.5	16
Perfect Harvest Muffin, 1/12 pkg	270	12	40
Wheat Free Brownie, 1/20 pkg	160	7.5	21
Aunt Jemima			
Coffee Cake, 1/8 cake, prep.	180	6	27
Banquet			
Dessert Bakes: *Per Serving (Prep'd)*			
Apple Crisp, 1/6	210	3.5	42
Choc. Cherry Decadence, 1/6	310	5	62
Chocolate Lava Cake, 1/7	370	7	73
Peach/Cherry Cobbler, 1/6	230	3.5	46
Betty Crocker			
Cakes (Super Moist): *Per 1/12 Cake (Prep'd)*			
Butter Recipe Yellow	260	11	36
Chocolate Chip	250	11	35
Chocolate varieties	270	13	36
Cinnamon Swirl	280	11	42
Devil's Food	270	13	35
White	230	10	34
Other flavors, average	250	10	35
Per 1/10 Cake (Prepared): Carrot	320	15	42
Sour Cream	280	12	43
If using *No Cholesterol Recipe*, deduct 40 cals and 4g fat.			
Other Cakes: Pound Cake, 1/8	260	8	35
Angel Food Cake, 1/12 mix	140	0	32
Gingerbread Cake, 1/8	230	6	39
Pineapple Upside Down, 1/6	400	14	64
Sunkist Lemon Bar (1)	140	4.5	24
Brownie Mixes: *Per 1/20 Pkg (Prep'd)*			
Chocolate Chunk varieties	180	9	25
Dark Chocolate	170	7	25
Fudge	170	7	24
Original Supreme	160	6	27
Peanut Butter; Walnut	180	9	24
Turtle (Caramel & Pecan)	170	8	23
Cookie Mix: *Per 2 Cookies (Prep'd)*			
Rainbow Chocolate Candy	150	7	33
Other varieties, average	160	8	21

Made As Directed	C	F	Cb
Betty Crocker (Cont)			
Muffin Mix: *Per Muffin (6.5 oz)*			
Apple Streusel	210	8	33
Blueberry; Golden Corn	160	6	25
Triple Berry	120	3	23
Twice the Blueberries	140	4	25
Wild Blueberry	170	5	28
Other varieties, average	175	7	24
Snackin' Cake: *Per 1/9 Pkg*			
Banana Walnut	180	6	31
Cinnamon Swirl	190	5	34
Chocolate varieties	180	5	32
Dr Oetker: *Per Serving (Prep'd)*			
Chocolate Chip Cookie Mix, 1/12	170	7.5	24
Muffin Mix, 1/12 pkg, average	170	2	30
Simple Organic Cake Mix, 1/12	255	11	32
Duncan Hines			
Angel Food, 1/12 whole	140	0	30
Brownie Mix (lowfat recipe)			
1/16 pkg, avg. all types	140	3.5	22
Cookies, all flavors, 1 cookie	65	3	8
Moist Deluxe Cake Mix:			
Average, 1/12 pkg, prepared	250	11	36
Lower Fat Recipe, 1/12 pkg, prep.	200	5	36
Estee: Brownie, 1 pce, 2"x 2"	50	2	12
All cakes, 1/5 cake	200	4	38
Choc. Chip Cookie, 1 cookie	45	2.5	6
Ghirardelli: *Per Serving (Prepared)*			
Brownie, 1/16 pkg	200	10	27
Chocolate Chip Cookie (1)	280	13	38
Dble Choc Muffin (1)	250	10	37
Jell-O-No Bake Cheesecakes: *Prep'd As Directed*			
Cherry/Strawberry, 1/9 pkg	300	13	42
Chips-Ahoy!, 1/16 pkg	360	17	46
Chocolate Silk Dessert, 1/6 pkg	280	15	34
Oreo, 1/6 pkg	360	16	48
Peanut Butter Cup, 1/8 pkg	360	23	38
Real, 1/6 pkg	360	17	42
Krusteaz: Cinn. Crumb Cake, 1"	230	7	38
Lemon/Key Lime Bar, 2" bar	160	4.5	29
Muffins: Blueberry (1)	150	4	26
Oat Bran (1)	180	4	32
Fat Free varieties (1)	140	0	33

Frostings • Baking Ingredients

Cakes & Dessert Mixes (Cont)

Made As Directed

	C	**F**	**Cb**
No Pudge			
Fudge Brownie, 1/12 pkg, prep'd.	100	0	21
Pamela's			
Ultra Chocolate Brownie, 1/16	170	8	23
Oil Free, 1/16	110	1.5	24
Pillsbury			
Moist Supreme: *Per 1/12 Cake (Prepared)*			
Angel Food Cake	140	0	31
Devil's Food Cake	270	14	33
French Vanilla; German Choc.	250	11	34
Funfetti	250	9	36
Streusel Coffee, 1/16 cake	260	11	37
Other flavors, average 1/12	255	12	35
Thick 'n Fudgy Deluxe Brownie (Prepared):			
Caramel Swirl, 1/20 pkg	190	8	27
Cheesecake Swirl, 1/18 pkg	150	8	19
Choc./Vanilla Frosted, 1/16 pkg	200	9	27
Double Choc, 1/16 pkg	160	7	23
Fudge, 1/20 pkg	170	8	33
Fudge Toffee, 1/20 pkg	170	8	23
White Chunk, 1/16 pkg	160	8	21
w. Walnuts, 1/12 pkg	200	11	24
Muffins, avg. all types (1)	185	6	30
Robin Hood: Yellow 1/5 cake	280	13	37
Devil's Food, 1/5 cake	310	17	36
Fudge Brownie (1)	170	7	24
Muffin, 1/6 pkg	150	6	25

Cake Frostings

	C	**F**	**Cb**
Betty Crocker Rich & Creamy,			
Average all flavors, 2 Tbsp	130	5	24
Whipped, all flavors, 2 Tbsp	100	5	15
Easy Flow Icing, 1 Tbsp	25	1	4
Duncan Hines: *Per 2 Tbsp (1.2 oz)*			
Creamy Homestyle, avg all flavors	140	5	23
Pillsbury: *Per 2 Tbsp (approx.1/12 Tub)*			
Caramel Pecan	150	8	19
Chocolate Cream Cheese	140	6	21
Chocolate Walnut	150	7	20
Coconut Pecan	160	10	17
Cream Cheese; Lemon	150	6	24
French Vanilla	160	6	26
Milk/Chocolate; Choc. Fudge	140	6	21
Rainbow Chip	140	5	23
All other flavors	150	6	23
Decorators, Choc., 1 Tbsp	70	2	11

Baking Ingredients

	C	**F**	**Cb**
Almond Paste:			
(Marzipan), 1 oz	125	7	12
Baking Powder: Regular, 1 tsp	3	0	0.5
Cream of Tartar, 1 tsp	2	0	0.5
Bisquick Baking Mix:			
Original, 1/3 cup, 1 1/2 oz	170	6	25
Reduced Fat, 1/3 cup, 1 1/2 oz	150	2.5	28
Butter/Margarine: 1/2 cup, 4 oz	820	91	0
Carob Flour, 1/2 cup	90	0.5	26
Chocolate Baking Bars: *Average All Brands*			
Unsweetened, 1 oz	150	15	8
Grated, 1 cup, 4 1/2 oz	680	68	36
Semi-sweet, 1 oz	160	8	20
Bitter-sweet/White Baking 1 oz	160	8	20
Chocolate Baking Chips: *Average All Brands*			
Milk Choc./Semi Sweet 1 oz	160	9	18
1/4 cup, 1 1/2 oz	240	12	30
1 cup, 6 oz	960	48	120
Mini Kisses *(Hershey),* 1 pce	5	0.5	1
Cocoa Powder, Baking: *Nestle,* 1 T.	15	1	3
1/3 cup, 1 oz	80	4	12
Hershey's, 1 Tbsp	20	0.5	3
1/3 cup, 1 oz	115	3.5	21
Coconut, dried: Unsweet., 1 oz	190	18	7
Sweetened/flaked, 1 oz	135	9	14
1/2 cup, 1.3 oz	175	12	18
Toasted *(Baker's),* 1 oz	170	13	17
Coconut Cream/Milk: *See Page 39*			
Cornstarch, 1 Tbsp	30	0	7
Flour, white: 1 Tbsp, 0.6 oz	55	0	12
1 cup, 4.4 oz	450	1	95
Whole Wheat, 1 cup, 4.2 oz	410	2	87
Flavor Extracts: *Average All Brands*			
Imitation, 1 tsp	15	0	3.5
Pure Extract, 1 tsp	20	0	4
Almond, Vanilla, 1 tsp	10	0	3
Fruit Pectin: Swtnd 1 Tbsp, 1/2 oz	35	0	10
Unsweetened, 1 Tbsp	2	0	0.5
Gelatin, dry, 1/4 oz pkg	30	0	0
Lemon/Orange Peel, 1/4 cup	30	0	4
Rennin, 1 pkg (11g)	12	0	3
Sprinkles: All types, 1 Tbsp, 1/2 oz	70	3	10
Vinegar, aver. all types, 1 oz	4	0	2
Whey, sweet, dry, 1 oz	90	0.5	20
Yeast: Active, dry, 1/4 oz pkg	15	0	2
Fleischmann's, 0.6 oz pkg	15	0	2
Bakers, compressed, 1 oz	25	0	3
Brewers; Torula, 1 oz	80	0.5	11

Puddings, Desserts, Gelatin

Ready-To-Serve	C	F	Cb
Instant Pudding, Reg., 1/2 cup	170	4	30
Reduced Calorie: D-Zerta; Estee	70	0	12
Jell-O, sugar-free, 1/2 cup	80	2	11
Royal, sugar-free, 1/2 cup	100	2	17
Del Monte Pudding Snacks	130	4	24
Fat Free Vanilla	90	0	20
Dr McDougall's Rice Pudd., 3 oz	310	1.5	69
Hershey's Portable Pud., 2.25 oz	100	3	16
Hunt's Snack Pack: Per 3.5 oz Cup			
Puddin' Cakes: Choc Brownie	180	7	27
German Choc Cake	160	3.5	30
Puddin Pie: Lemon Meringue	130	2.5	24
Apple; Choc Mud	170	7	26
Dessert Favorites, avg. all flavors	140	5	22
Imagine Foods: Natural Pudding (Cups)			
Average all flavors, 1/2 cup, 3.7 oz	150	3	32
Jell-O: Pudding, Choc., 1/5 pkg	190	5	33
Pudding Bites, average 1 pouch	90	1.5	18
No Bake Mix: Oreo, 1/6 pkg	270	8	48
Peanut Butter Cup, 1/8 pkg	290	15	38
Real Cheesecake, 1/6 pkg	220	6	40
Other flavors, avg.	200	3	42
Pudding & Pie Filling: Per 1/4 Pkg			
Cook & Serve, average	150	0	22
Instant, regular, avg.	100	0	25
Fat & Sugar Free, avg.	30	0	8
Pudding Snacks: Fat Free, 4 oz	100	0	23
Cheesecake Snack; Oreo, avg.	150	4	26
Chocolate; Creme Savers, 4 oz	160	5	28
Smoothie Snacks, 4 oz	100	2.5	18
Jewel: Chef's Kitchen			
Rice Pudding, 1/2 cup, 4.5 oz	230	8	35
Tapioca Pudding, 1/2 cup, 4.5 oz	170	8	35
Jolly Rancher: Reg., 3.5 oz cup	100	0	25
Sugar-Free, all flavors, 3.5 oz cup	10	0	2
Kozy Shack: Avg. all types, 4 oz	140	4	25
Lite	110	1	22
Creme Caramel Flan, 1 cup, 4 oz	160	4	28
Kraft Handi Snacks: Per Cup (3.5 oz)			
"Doubles", avg. all flavors	125	3.5	22
Chocolate Pudding Fat Free	85	0	21
Rice Pudding	140	6	19
Tapioca; Vanilla Pudding	115	3.5	20
Manischewitz			
Choc., 1/2 cup	110	0.5	26
Passover Gold Noodle, 1/2 cup	140	2	28
President's Choice			
Key Lime Pie (36oz) 1/8 pie, 4.5 oz	440	22	54
Mississippi Mud Pie (36oz) 1/9, 4 oz	380	24	37

Swiss Miss Pudding Snacks	C	F	Cb
Swirls, Choc. Pudd. Snacks, 31/2 oz	150	5	23
Tapioca: 1 pudding cup, 31/2 oz	120	3.5	21
Fat Free varieties, 31/2 oz	90	0	20
Weight Watchers (Frozen)			
Chocolate Mousse, 23/4 oz	190	5	31
Zone Perfect Mix, 1/2 cup	160	4.5	18

Homemade Puddings			
Apple Tapioca, 1/2 cup	150	0	32
Bread Pudding, 1/2 cup	250	8	40
Blancmange, 1/2 cup	140	5	19
Chocolate, 1/2 cup	190	6	30
Corn Pudding, 1/2 cup	135	4	21
Crème Brûlée, 1/2 cup	400	35	16
Plum Pudding, 2 oz	170	3	32
Rennin Dessert, 1/2 cup	115	4	16
Rice with Raisins, 1/2 cup	200	4	38
Sponge Pudding, 31/2 oz	340	16	45
Tapioca Cream, 1/2 cup	110	4	15
Trifle, 1/2 cup	180	7	26

Custards			
Custard Mix			
Jell-O (Americana) Golden Egg:			
Dry, 1/6 pkg	80	0	19
Prep. w. 2% milk, 1/2 cup	140	2.5	19
Jello Flan, w. 2% milk, 1/2 cup	140	2.5	20
Royal-Flan: Prep. w. 2% milk, 1/2 c.	130	2.5	18
Homemade Custard			
Baked: Plain, 1/2 cup, 41/2 oz	150	7	16
w. skim milk, artif. sweetened	70	3	4
Boiled, 1/2 cup	165	7	18

Meringues			
Meringue Swirl, 1/2 cup	50	0	8
Meringue Shell, 1 oz shell	100	0	16
(Add extra calories/fat/carbohydrate for fillings)			

Jell-O • Cups • Parfait			
Gelatin Mix: Jell-O, Royal ~ Made Up			
Regular, all flavors, 1/2 cup	80	0	18
Sugar Free/Low Calorie, 1/2 cup	8	0	0
Creme Gelatin/Parfait: Per 1/2 Cup			
Ida Mae, 1/2 cup	60	2	10
Winky: Strawberry (109g)	110	1.5	22
Rainbow (130g)	100	0	24
Reser's, Dessert Parfait (110g)	100	2	19
Mrs Crockett's Kitchen, Str. Parfait	160	4	26
Gel Snacks (Jell-O): Regular, 3.5 oz	70	0	17
Sugar Free, 3.2 oz	10	0	1
X-Treme Cups, 2.5 oz	100	0	24
X-Treme Sticks, 2.2 oz	60	0	16

Pancakes & Waffles

Quick Guide

Pancakes

Plain: *Average All Types*	C	F	Cb
Small (3" diam.), 3/4 oz	50	2.5	6
Medium (4" diam.), 1 1/4 oz	80	3	11
Large (5" diam.), 2 1/2 oz	160	6	21
Add Extra for Syrups/Butter			
Pancake Syrup: Regular, 1 Tbsp	50	0	13
1/4 cup	200	0	52
Lite, 1 Tbsp	25	0	6
1/4 cup	100	0	24
Butter/Margarine: Regular, 1 T.	100	11	0
Whipped, 1 Tbsp	70	7.5	0

Restaurant Style Pancakes

Denny's			
Buttermilk Hot Cakes: Plain, 3	675	23	47
w. Syrup & Margarine	905	33	83
Original Grand Slam Breakfast	795	50	65
w. Syrup & Margarine	1030	60	101
Maple Flavor Syrup, 1 serving	145	0	36
Whipped Margarine, 1/2 oz	90	10	0

Hardees			
3 Pancakes (no fat)	280	2	56
w. Sausage Pattie	430	16	56
w. 2 Bacon Strips	350	10	56

IHOP (International House of Pancakes)			
Pancakes (Syrup/Butter extra):			
Buttermilk, 1 (2 oz)	110	3	17
Short Stack, 3	330	9	51
Full Stack, 5	550	15	85
Buckwheat, 1 (2 oz)	110	4	15
Country Griddle, 1 (2 oz)	120	3.5	19
Harvest Grain 'N Nut, (2 1/4 oz)	180	9	20
Crepes (Egg Pancakes), 1 (2 oz)	120	6	14
Waffles (Plain): Regular, 1 (3 oz)	310	15	37
Belgian: Regular, 1 (4 oz)	390	19	48

McDonalds			
Hotcakes: Plain (3)	340	8	58
w. Marg. (2 pats) & Syrup (1)	600	17	104

Perkins			
Buttermilk, 3, plain	440	12	70
Harvest Grain: Short Stack, Plain (3)	270	2	56
w. Lowcal Syrup	295	2	63
5-Stack w. Lowcal Syrup	475	3.5	93

Brands

Atkins:	C	F	Cb
All-Purpose, 2 tsp. dry mix	30	0	5
Pancake & Waffle, 1/4 cup dry mix	90	1.5	6
Aunt Jemima			
Frozen: Lowfat (3)	130	2	33
Original; Blueberry (3)	200	3	40
Pancake & Waffle Mix:			
Original, 1/3 cup, prepared	240	6.5	38
Complete, 1/3 cup	160	2.5	32
Mini Pancakes (13)	240	4	46
Thaw & Pour B'milk Pancake Batter:			
1/2 cup, 4 x 4" pancakes	260	3.5	51
Betty Crocker Pancake Mixes			
Complete Original/Buttermilk, 3	200	2.5	40
Bisquick (Shake 'N Pour), 3	200	3	38
Hungry Jack Pancakes			
Mixes: Per 1/3 Cup (Prepared)			
Buttermilk: Complete, 1/3 cup	160	1.5	32
Original, w. 2% Milk, Oil, Egg	290	13	32
w. Skim Milk, Oil, Egg Whites	220	6	32
Extra Lights: Complete	150	2	30
Microwave: Buttermilk (3)	270	4.5	51
Original, 3 pancakes	270	4.5	51
Northern Pines: Complete Gourmet			
3 x 4" pancakes, 3.5 oz	380	7	71
Zone Perfect Mix, 1/7 box prep.	110	6	117

Waffles

	C	F	Cb
Homemade: 7" waffle, 2 1/2 oz	245	13	26
From Mix: 7" waffle, 2 1/2 oz	205	8	28

Frozen Waffles

	C	F	Cb
Aunt Jemima: Blueberry (1)	95	3	15
Buttermilk (1)	100	3	17
Eggo (Kelloggs): Banana Bread (1)	95	3	16
Chocolate Chip, 1 waffle	100	3.5	16
Cinnamon Toast/Homestyle (1)	95	3.5	15
Nut & Honey (1)	110	4.5	15
Nutri-Grain (1)	85	2.5	14
Special K (fat free), 1	60	0	13
Waf-fulls, all types (1) 2 oz	160	5	26
GO-LEAN (Kashi): Average, 1	90	1.5	16
Hungry Jack: Blueberry, 1 waffle	105	4	17
Buttermilk; Homestyle (1)	95	3	15
Mini Funfetti (1)	65	2	11
Nature's Path: Optimum Power, 1	90	2	20
Average other types (1)	125	4	16
Pilsbury Waffle Sticks:			
6 sticks & syrup, avg.	325	6	62

Sugar, Syrup, Jam, Honey

Sugar

	C	F	Cb
White Sugar, granulated:			
1 level teaspoon, 4g	15	0	4
1 heaping teaspoon, 6g	25	0	6.5
1 cube, 1/2"	24	0	6.5
Single portion, 1 packet	25	0	6.5
1 Tablespoon, 12g	48	0	12
1 ounce, 1 oz	110	0	20
1 cup, 7 oz	770	0	203
1 pound	1760	0	464
Brown Sugar:			
1 Tbsp, 13g	50	0	13
1 ounce, 1 oz	109	0	28
1 cup, not packed, 5 oz	540	0	140
1 cup, packed, 7 3/4 oz	845	0	218
Powdered/Confectioners:			
Sifted, 1 cup, 3 1/2 oz	385	0	98
Unsifted, 1 cup, 4 1/4 oz	460	0	117
Other Sugars: Glucose, 1 oz	110	0	27
Tablets (Dex 4), 1	15	0	4
Barley/Wheat/Rye Malt,			
1 Tbsp, 3/4 oz	60	0	14
Cinnamon Sugar, 1 tsp	15	0	4
Dextrose, 1 oz	110	0	27
Fructose: 1 tsp	15	0	4
3 Tbsp, 1 oz	110	0	27
FruitSource, 1 oz (powder)	110	0	27
Palm Sugar, 3 Tbsp, 12g	45	0	11
Piloncillo (Brown Sugar), 3oz Cone	325	0	81
Sorbitol, 1 oz	110	0	27
Turbinado Sugar, 2 Tbsp, 1 oz	110	0	27
Unrefined Cane Sugar, 1 oz	110	0	27

Sugar Substitutes

	C	F	Cb
DiabetiSweet, 1 teaspoon	9	0	4
(Carbohydrate as Sugar Alcohol)			
Equal: Tablet/Liquid	0	0	0
Granulated, 1 pkg	4	0	1
Powdered, sachet, 0.04 oz	0	0	0.5
NutraSweet Spoonful, 1 tsp	2	0	0.5
Nutra Taste; Sweet One, 1 pkt	0	0	0
PerfectSweet, 1 tsp	15	0.5	1
Splenda: Powder, cup	96	0	24
Sachet, sachet	0	0	0.5
Granular, 1 tsp	5	0	1
Sprinkle Sweet, 1 tsp	2	0	0.5
Stevia; Walgreens Wal-Sweet, 1 pkt	0	0	0
Sugar Delight, 1 pkt	8	0	2
Sugar Like (Bateman's), 1 tsp	4	0	1
Sugar Twin: 1 pkt	3	0	0
Sugar Substitute, 1 tsp	2	0	1
Sweet 'N Low, 1 pkt	0	0	1
Weight Watchers Sweetener, 1 tsp	4	0	1

Honey, Jam, Preserves

Average All Brands	C	F	Cb
Honey: 1 tsp, 1/4 oz	22	0	5.5
1 Tbsp, 3/4 oz	65	0	17
1 ounce, 1 oz	86	0	23
1 cup, 12 oz	1030	0	269
Single Portion, 1/2 oz pkg	43	0	11
Jams/Jellies/Marmalade/Preserves			
Regular, 1 tsp, 1/4 oz	18	0	5
1 Tbsp, 3/4 oz	65	0	16
1 ounce	90	0	22
Single Portion, 1/2 oz pkg	38	0	11
Apple/Fruit Butters, 1 T., 0.6 oz	20	0	6
Fruit Spreads: Regular, 1 tsp	16	0	4
Low Sugar, 1 tsp	8	0	2
Low Cal. (Featherweight), 1 tsp	4	0	1
Jelly: Regular, average, 1 tsp	18	0	4.5
Imitation, Low Calorie, 1 tsp	4	0	1

Syrups, Molasses

	C	F	Cb
Syrups: *Average All Types & Brands*			
(Corn/Rice/Maple/Pancake/Sundae/Waffle)			
Includes *Aunt Jemima, Cary's, Karo, Hershey's,*			
Hungry Jack, Log Cabin, Mrs Butterworth's			
Regular/Dark/Light Color:			
1 Tbsp, 1/2 fl.oz	55	0	14
1/4 cup (4 Tbsp)	220	0	55
Single Portion: 1 1/2 oz pkg	170	0	42
Lite: 1 Tbsp	25	0	6
1/4 cup (4 Tbsp)	100	0	25
Sugar-Free: *Atkins,* all types	0	0	0
Cary's, 2 Tbsp, 1 oz	18	0	5
Cozy Cottage, 2 Tbsp	10	0	3
Da Vinci, 2 Tbsp, 1 oz	5	0	1
Molasses: Dark/Light, 1 T., 3/4 oz	55	0	14
1 cup, 11 1/2 oz	880	0	224
Blackstrap: 1 Tbsp, 3/4 oz	47	0	13
1 cup, 11 1/2 oz	750	0	208

Icecream Toppings

Average All Types & Brands	C	F	Cb
(Hershey's, Kraft, Smuckers)			
Butterscotch, Caramel, 2 Tbsp	140	1	30
Chocolate, Hot Fudge, 2 Tbsp	140	4	22
Fat Free Chocolate (Hershey's), 2 Tbsp	100	0	23
Pineapple, Strawberry, 2 Tbsp	110	0	28
Smuckers: Guilt-Free, all flavors	100	0	24
Magic Shell, 2 Tbsp	210	15	18
Milky Way, 2 Tbsp	130	3.5	24
Lite Hot Fudge, 2 Tbsp	90	0	23

Candy, Chocolate

Quick Guide

Chocolate

	C	F	Cb
Average All Brands			
Milk Chocolate, regular:			
Plain/Nuts/Fruit, average, 1 oz	150	10	13
1½ oz Bar	225	15	23
2 oz Bar	300	20	30
4 oz Block	600	40	60
8 oz Block	1200	80	120
1 Pound, 16 oz	2400	160	240
Dark/White Chocolate, 1 oz	150	10	16
Sugar Free, *(Hershey's)* 1 pce, 0.3 oz	225	14	23
Chocolate-coated:			
Almonds, 5-6, 1 oz	160	11	11
Clusters, nut, 2, 1 oz	160	11	15
Coffee Beans, 1.4 oz	180	10	23
Creme/Cordial Centers, 1 oz	120	4	21
Fudge, 1 oz	125	5	18
Macadamias, 2-3 pces., 1 oz	180	13	11
Mints, 1 med., 11g	45	1	9
Nougat & Caramel, 1 oz	120	4	21
Peanuts, 12 med., 1 oz	160	11	15
Raisins, 30 med., 1 oz	120	4	21
Cooking Chocolate:			
Sweet/Semi-sweet, 1 oz	160	8	20
Chips, ¼ cup, 2½ oz	210	12	24
Unsweetened, 1 oz	150	15	8
Carob: Plain, 1 oz	160	11	9

Brands & Generic

Per Piece/Serving

	C	F	Cb
Abba Zaba, 2 oz bar	250	5	48
Absolutely Almond, 2.5 oz bar	380	23	40
Aero Bar *(Nestlé),* 1.45 oz bar	210	13	26
After Dinner Mints, 1 small	45	1	9
After Eight Mint, each	35	1.2	6
Air Head, 2 bars, 1 oz	120	1	30
Allen Wertz: Simply Sugar Free			
Coffee Time (decaf), 4	45	1.5	8
Coffee Toffee, 6	120	3	23
Other types, 4	120	2.5	24
Almond Joy: 1.76 oz bar	230	13	29
King Size, 2 pces, 1.7 oz	230	13	29
Snack, 1, 0.68 oz bar	90	5	11
Bites (8)	90	6	9
Almond Roca, 3 pces	220	15	19
Sugar Free, 3 pces	205	15	16

Brands & Generic (Cont)

Per Piece/Serving

	C	F	Cb
Almonds, sugar-coated, 7, 1 oz	130	5	20
Almond Clusters *(Trader Joe's),*			
2 pce, 1.2 oz	210	14	5
Altoids *(C & B),* each	3	0	1
Amazin' Fruit, 1 bag, 1.9 oz	180	0	41
Andes: Creme de Menthe; Cherry Jubilee			
Choc covered Patty, (3), 1½ oz	180	3	35
Thins, avg. all flav., (8), 1.4 oz	210	13	22
Anthon Berg: Cognac, each	180	8	25
After Dinner Sweet:			
Marzipan w. Madeira, 1.4 oz	175	7.5	26
Marzipan Brod	120	7	13
Asteroid *(Nestlé),* 54g	260	10	40
Atkins Endulge: Caramel Nut Chew	175	9	17
Caramel Nut Clusters, 2 pieces	220	14	21
Choc.; Chocolate Crunch	150	12	2
Fruit Gum, 2 pieces	5	0	1.5
Jelly Beans, 35 jelly beans	145	0	36
Mints, 2 pieces	5	0	1
Peanut Butter Cups, 3 cups	195	13	17
Salt Water Taffy assorted (6)	140	2.5	29
Wafers, 2 bars, avg. all flavors	155	9	15
Baby Ruth: King Size, 3.7 oz bar	480	24	66
2.1 oz bar	280	13	34
Fun size, each	100	4.5	17
Snack, 1 bar, ¾ oz	100	5	12
Baci *(Perugino),* each	85	5	8
Bar, 1.58 oz	230	15	27
Bar None, 1.5 oz bar	240	14	23
Barley Sugar, 1 pce, 0.2 oz	23	0	6
Baskin-Robbins, 3 pce, 0.5 oz	60	1	13
Big Hunt, 2 oz	230	3	47
Bit-O-Honey, 1.7 oz	200	3.5	41
Chews, 6 pces, 1.4 oz	170	3	34
Blow Pops, each	50	0	14
Bonus Bar, 2.1 oz bar	290	16	34
Boston Baked Beans, 30 pces, 1 oz	135	5	20
Brach's: Almond Supremes,11	220	15	18
Butterscotch Disks (3) 0.6 oz	70	0	16
Choc Bridge Mix (16) 1.4 oz	190	9	25
Circus Peanuts, each	25	0.6	3
Clusters (3)	220	14	19

Brands & Generic (Cont)

Per Piece/Serving

Brach's (Cont):	C	F	Cb
Double Dip Choc Peanuts (15)	220	14	19
Golden Butter/Internation. Toffee	25	0.6	5
Lemon Drops (4), 0.6 oz	50	0	13
Malted Milk Balls (15)	190	9	27
Milk Maid Caramel (4)	160	4.5	30
Orange Slices Hi-C, each	50	0	13
Breath Savers, all types, each	10	0	2
Brite Crackers, 1 bag, 1.5 oz	140	0	32
Brock: Candy Corn (10) 0.7 oz	75	0	18
Gummy Bears; Sour Balls, each	26	0	6
Lemon Drops, each	20	0	5
Orange Slices, each	35	0	9
Spice Drops, each	12	0	3
Starlight Mints, each	20	0	5
Toffee, each	25	0.8	5
Bubble Gum: *See 'Gum'*			
Buncha Crunch, 1/2 cup, 1.4 oz	200	10	26
Burnt Peanuts, 40 pces, 40g	190	8	32
Butterfinger:			
Huge Size, 3.7 oz bar	480	18	75
2.1 oz bar	270	11	41
Fun size, each	100	3.5	15
Mini, each	20	1	7
Snack (2) 1.3 oz	170	7	27
Butterfinger B.B's, 1.7 oz bag	220	9	34
Buttermints, 18 pces, 1 1/2 oz	160	0	40
Butterscotch: 5 pces	120	2.5	20
Buttons (*Walgreens*), 3, 18g	70	0	16
Chips (*Hershey's*), 1 oz	160	8	20
Discs (*Sathers*), 3, 0.6 oz	110	0	16
Candy Apple, medium, 6.5 oz	260	4	54
Candy Cane, medium, 5", 1/2 oz	50	0	12
Candy Corn, 1 oz	110	0	27
4 oz Pkt: 24 pces, 1 1/2 oz	150	0	37
Candy Jar Mix (*Jewel*), 3, 17g	70	0	17
Candy Necklaces, 20g each	80	0.5	20
Caramels: each	30	1	6
Chocolate, each	25	0.3	6
Creams, 3 pces, 1 1/4 oz	130	3	23
2.75 oz pkt, 5 pces, 1 1/2 oz	160	3.5	30
Hershey's Classic Caramels:			
Soft 'n Chewy, 3 pces	80	2.5	13
Choc Creme Filled, 3 pces	80	3	13
Caramel Nips, each	30	1	6
Caramel Popcorn, 1 cup, 1 oz	120	1.5	26

Per Piece/Serving

	C	F	Cb
Caramel Truffles (*Godiva*), 1 pce	110	6.5	11
Caramello (*Hershey's*): 1.6 oz bar	220	10	29
Snack, 0.66 oz	90	4	12
Cadbury: 1.6 oz bar	210	9	29
Kingsize, 2.7 oz bar	360	16	49
Certs: Breath Mints, 1 pce	6	0	2
Sugar-free, 1 piece	7	0	2
Charleston Chew, 1 bar, 53g	230	7	40
Cherry Sours (*Sathers*), 11, 1 1/2 oz	150	0	38
Chews, all types, 1 oz	110	1	25
Chocolate Mints (*Hershey's*), each	20	0.5	4
Chocolate Parfait Nips, each	30	1	5
Chuckles Jelly: each	35	0	9
Jujubes (*Hershey's*), each	10	0	3
Chunky Bar (*Nestlé*), 1.4 oz	210	11	24
Chupa Chups, 1 pce, 0.42 oz	50	0	11
Cinnamon Bears (*Walgreens*), 5	150	0	38
Cinn. Buttons (*Walgreens*), 3 pce	70	0	17
Cinnamon Drops (*Sathers*), 19 pce	150	0	36
Coconut Stacks, 4, 41g	190	6	33
Coffee Go Coffee/Cappuccino, ea.	18	0.4	4
Coffee Rio-Gold, each	15	0.5	3
Collard & Bowser, Eng. Toffee (2)	80	4	12
Conversation Hearts (*Necco*), 1 lge	16	0	4
Corn Nuts, 1/3 cup, 1 oz	130	4	20
Cote d'Or: Bouchee, each	130	8	12
Chokotoff, each	210	9	30
Nougatti	150	8	19
Bar & Nuts, 1.3 oz	220	18	12
Cotton Candy, 1 oz	70	0	17
Cough Drops: *See Page 135*			
Cracker Jack, 1.25 oz box	150	2.5	29
Crisped Rice: Almond, 1 bar	130	6	18
Choc Chip, 1 bar	115	4	18
Crispy Rice Snacks (*Hershey's*), 1 bar	70	2	10
Crows, 7 oz pkg	150	0	37
Crunch: 5 oz bar	725	38	90
King Munch, 2.75 oz bar	400	20	51
1.55 oz bar	230	12	29
Fun size, each	50	2.5	7
Snack (3), 1 1/2 oz	220	11	28
Pieces, 1/4 cup, 38g	190	10	25
White Bar, 1.4 oz bar	220	13	23
Crunch Berries Treats, 1.6 oz bar	190	4.5	36
Decadence (*NuBar*) Bar, 1.3 oz	140	2.5	30
Dots, 12 dots	150	0	37
Double Dip Stick, 1 stick	16	0.5	3

Candy, Chocolate (Cont)

Brands & Generic (Cont)

Per Piece/Serving

	C	F	Cb
Dove: Dark/Milk, 1.3 oz bar	200	12	22
Bar, 6 oz	920	56	104
Miniatures, each	30	2	3
Drops Candy (Hershey's), 9 pces	100	0	24
Dum Dum Pops (Spangler), 1 pop	25	0	6
English Toffee, 1 pce	48	3	5
Eda's Sugar Free, all flav., 5, 1/2 oz	40	0	15
Estee Dietetic Candies:			
Caramels, all flavors, 1 pce	30	1	5
Chocolate, Dark/ Mint, 1/2 bar	200	14	23
Gummy Bears; Gum Drops, 1 pce	7	0	1.5
Hard Candies: Butterscotch (2)	25	0	6
Assorted Fruit Lollipops (5)	60	0	15
Peppermint (3)	30	0	7
Mint/Toffee (5)	60	0	15
Lollipop	30	0	8
Milk Chocolate, 1/2 bar, 4 oz	230	17	17
Peanut Butter Cups, 1 cup	40	3	3
Fructose Sweetened, 1 cup	40	2	3
Peanut Brittle, 1/3 box, 1.5 oz	240	9	28
5th Avenue: 2 oz bar	280	12	38
King Size bar	460	20	64
Snack Size, 0.58 oz	80	3.5	10
Fanny May: Single Wrapped Pieces			
Mint Meltaway Patty, 1.5 oz	250	17	22
Pixie, 1.5 oz	215	12	24
Trinidad, 1.5 oz	205	11	24
Fast Break, 2 oz	270	13	34
Ferrero Rocher: each	75	5	6
3 pces, 1.3 oz	220	15	17
Fifty 50 Snack Bars:			
Peanut Butter, 2	200	14	16
Almond Choc., 7 pce, 1 1/2 oz	210	15	20
Crunch Choc., 7 pce, 1.1 oz	160	11	19
Fruit & Nut Choc., 7 pce, 1 1/2 oz	200	14	21
Milk Choc., 3 pce, 1/2 bar, 43g	210	14	25
Mini Bars, 8 bars, 1 oz	140	9	16
Fluffy Stuff (Harms), 0.6 oz bag	70	0	17
Fondant: Choc-coated, 1.2 oz	130	3	28
Mint, 1 oz	105	0	27
Franklin Crunch 'N Munch:			
all varieties, average, 1.25 oz	170	7	30
Fran's: Gold Bar, 1.75 oz	260	14	34
Gold Bites (Almonds), 1	130	7	17
Fruit Crystals (Walgreens), 3 pces	70	0	17
Fruit Drops, each	6	0	1
Fruit Gems (Sunkist), 3, 1.1 oz	105	0	26

Per Piece/Serving

	C	F	Cb
Fruit Leathers, average, 0.5 oz	45	0	12
Fruit Pastilles, 1 roll, 1.4 oz	100	0	26
Fruit Rolls, 1 roll	80	0	20
Fruit Roll-Ups, 1/2 oz	50	0	12
Fruit Runts (Walgreens), 1T., 1/4 pkt	60	0	14
Fruit Shapes (Fruitfield), 1 oz (10)	100	0.5	23
Fruit Waves, 0.5 oz	50	0	12
Fudge: Chocolate/Vanilla, 1 oz	115	3	20
with Nuts, 1 oz	120	4	21
Choco. Marshmallow, 1 oz	120	5	18
w. Nuts, 1 oz	125	5.5	18
Peanut Butter, 1 oz	105	2	21
Ghirardelli: Milk/Dark Chocolate,			
1.25 oz bar	185	12	20
w. almonds, 1.5 oz bar	220	14	25
Choc Nuts & Chews, 1 pce	55	3.5	4
Godiva: Hearts, each	45	2	4
Almond Butter Dome, 1 pce	80	6	6
Bouchee au Chocolate, 1 pce	220	13	23
Cordial Assortment, each	60	2.5	9
Gold Ballotin, 1 pce	70	3.5	9
Milk/Dark/Ivory Assortment, each	75	4	8
Nut & Caramel, each	75	4	9
Truffle Amaretto, 1 pce	110	6.5	12
Golden Almond Bar, 1 bar	520	34	40
Golden 111 Bar, 1 bar	500	30	52
Go Lightly: Box Candies, 4	60	0	15
Bags: Assorted Taffy, 6	140	3	36
Vanilla Caramels, 5	150	6	31
Super Free Choc Crunch (7) 1 1/2 oz	180	13	23
Goobers Peanuts, 1 pkg, 1.4 oz	210	13	20
Good 'N Fruity: 1 box, 1.8 oz	140	1	35
Snack Size, 1 box, 17g	60	0	15
Good & Plenty (Hershey's), 1.8 oz box	160	0	40
Snack Size, 1 box, 17g	60	0	14
GooGoo Cluster, 1 bar, 1.75 oz	240	11	32

Rev. Dr Robert Schuller

*Inch by inch
Life's a cinch*

*You'll never win
If you don't begin!*

Per Piece/Serving

GUM: *Per Piece*	**C**	**F**	**Cb**
Bazooka, each	30	0	7
Beechies	6	0	1
Big League Chew	10	0	2
Bubble Gum Balls *(Hershey's)*	10	0	2
Bubble Yum	25	0	6
Sugarless	10	0	3
Candilicious	30	0	2
Carefree (Sugarless/Regular)	5	0	2
Chiclets	5	0	1
Clorets, stick	10	0	2
Dentyne	6	0	2
Estee, bubble/regular	5	0	2
Extra *(Wrigley's)*,			
Sugar-Free Bubble Gum (1)	5	0	2
Freshen-Up	13	0	2
Hubba Bubba: Regular	23	0	6
Sugar-free, average	14	0	0.5
Ice Breakers, 1 stick	5	0	2
Sonic Boom Bubble Gum	15	0	3
Sticklets	7	0	2
Super Bubble	15	0	4
Trident: Slab	5	0	1
Soft Bubble Gum	9	0	1
Wrigley's, all flavors	10	0	2
Gum Drops: 1 small	15	0	3
1 large, 0.4 oz	40	0	7
6 oz pkt: 4 pces, 1.4 oz	130	0	31
Gummi Bears: 1 bear	17	0	4
8 bears, 1¹/₂ oz	140	0	32
Gummi Novelties *(Walgreens)*, 6	150	0	22
Gummi Savers, each	12	0	3
Gummi Sweet Tarts, 1 bug, 1.5 oz	150	0	34
Gummi Watch, 1, 2 oz	105	0	24
Gummi Worms, each	25	0	5
Guylian: No Sugar Added			
Milk Chocolate, 8 squares, 1 oz	126	9	15
Dark Chocolate, 8 squares, 1 oz	117	9	14
Halvah *(Joyvah)*:			
Plain/Marble, ¹/₂ bar, 2 oz	390	25	18
Choc.coated Sesame, ¹/₂ bar, 2 oz	380	23	20
Hard Candy: All flavors, 1 oz	110	0	28
1 regular piece	18	0	5
Heath: Original, 1.4 oz bar	210	12	24
Bites, 1.4 oz	210	12	25
Snack, 0.33 oz	50	3	6

Per Piece/Serving

Hershey's:	**C**	**F**	**Cb**
Bar: 1.55 oz bar	240	14	25
King Size bar, 2.6 oz	410	25	38
w. Almonds, 1.45 oz bar	230	14	20
Cookies 'n' Creme, 1.55oz bar	230	12	26
Bites: Almond Joy (8)	100	6	10
Cookies 'n' Creme (8)	90	5	10
York (9)	90	1.5	19
Milk Choc w. Almond (7)	90	6	8
Cookies 'N Mint: 1.55 oz bar	230	12	27
Snack, 0.6 oz	90	4.5	11
Crunchy Cookie Cups, 1.4 oz	210	12	23
Hugs: Regular (1), 4.5g	25	1.5	3
Regular (9), 40g	220	13	23
w. Almonds (9), 40g	230	13	22
Kisses: Milk Choc./Almond (1)	25	1.5	3
Milk Chocolate: 1.55 oz bar	230	13	25
Eggs, candy coated (4)	90	4	12
Snack, 0.6 oz	90	5	10
Kingsize, 2.6 oz bar	400	23	42
7 oz bar, ¹/₅ bar	200	12	21
w. Almonds Snack, 0.6 oz	100	6	9
w. Almonds, 1.45 oz bar	230	14	20
Miniatures: 5 pces, 1.5 oz	230	13	25
Nuggets: Snack, avg. all bars (1)	50	3	6
P'nut Butter Crispy Rice, (1)	230	13	25
Special Dark Choc., 1.45 oz bar	230	13	25
Sweet Escapes: 1.4 oz bar, avg.	180	7	27
Snack, avg. (1) 0.7 oz	80	3.5	12
Whoppers, 10 pces	100	4	16
Candy-Coated Eggs:			
Milk Choc (4), 0.6 oz	90	4	12
w. Almonds (4) 0.6 oz	100	6	9
Honeycomb: Plain, 1 oz	115	0	27
Choc-coated, 1 oz	125	1	28
Hot Tamales: 1 box, 60g, 2.1 oz	220	0	55
Sathers, 19 pces, 1.4 oz	150	0	36
Ice Blue Mints *(Walgreens)*, 3, 17g	70	0	17
Jawbreakers *(Sathers)*, 3, 17g	70	0	17
Jellies, 3 medium, 1 oz	120	0	30
Jells Raspberry *(Joyva)*, each	70	1	8
Jelly Beans: Small, 22 beans, 1 oz	100	0	24
Regular, 12 beans, 1 oz	100	0	24
1 bean	8	0	2
Jumbo, 1 bean	20	0	5
Jewel, 13 beans, 1.4 oz	140	0	36
Sathers/Walgreens, (17) 40g	150	0	37
Wonderbeans, 33 beans	100	0	24
Jelly Bellys: each	4	0	1
32 pces, 1.4 oz	150	0	37
1 tin, 2.5 oz	250	0	65
Jelly Rings *(Jewel)*, (3) 1.5 oz	160	0	39

Candy, Chocolate (Cont)

Per Piece/Serving	C	F	Cb
Jolly Rancher: Candy (1)	40	0	9
Fruit Chews (6), 1.4 oz	150	1.5	33
Hard Candy (3), 18g	70	0	17
Jolly Jellies, 7 oz	120	0	30
Lollipops, 1 pce, 0.6 oz	60	0	16
Sugar Free, 4 pces, 0.5 oz	35	0	14
Junior Mints: 1.84 oz box	210	3.5	40
16 pces, 1.4 oz	160	2.5	34
Juicefuls: Red Raspb., (3), 0.6 oz	60	0	15
Assorted Fruits, 1 pce	20	0	5
Jujubes, all types (6), 1.4 oz	5	0	3
Juju Mix *(Sathers),* 11 pce, 1½ oz	150	0	36
Juju Toys: 6 pce, 1.5 oz	150	0	37
Jujyfruits, 1 box, 0.2 oz	40	0	10
Kit Kat: 1.5 oz bar	220	11	27
2.8 oz bar	400	20	50
Big Kat, 1.94 oz	290	15	35
Bites (15), 1.4 oz	200	10	25
King Size, 3 oz bar	495	25	62
Miniature, 0.35 oz	50	2.5	6.5
Multipack/Snack Bar each	80	4	10
Krackel: 2.6 oz bar	330	18	38
Snack size, 0.6 oz	90	4	12
Kraft: Caramels, (5), 40g	160	3.5	30
Kudos: 1 oz bar, avg. all types	120	5	20
M&M's Milk Choc Minis, 0.8 oz	90	2.5	17
Snickers, 0.8 oz	100	3.5	16
Lance: Popscotch, 1.2 oz pkg	160	6	24
Chocolaty Peanut Bar, 2 oz bar	320	18	30
Peanut Bar, 1.8 oz pkg	260	14	24
Lemon Drops (3) ½ oz	50	0	12
Sugar Free *(Walgreens),* 5, ½ oz	35	0	14
Lemonhead, 10, ½ oz	60	0	14
Licorice:			
Average all types, 1oz	100	0	25
Bites *(Switzer),* each	10	0	1
Chews *(Panda),* each	10	0	2
Tid Bits, each	5	0	1
Twists: Black/Red, avg. 1 pce	30	0	7
American Licorice Co.: Laces, 1	35	0	8
Stick, (1) 0.5 oz	45	0	11
Choco Sticks, (4) 1.4 oz	145	0	35
Red Bites, 1.4 oz	140	0	34
Super Red Ropes, 1 rope, 2 oz	200	0	46
Vines, 1 pce	70	0	17

Per Piece/Serving	C	F	Cb
Lifesavers: Large size, 1 candy	15	0	4
Regular, all flavors, 1 candy	10	0	2
1 Roll (14 candies), 1.14 oz	130	0	32
Creme Savers (1)	25	0.5	4
Sugar-Free Delites: *Per Candy*			
Orchard Fruits; Summer Blend	5	0	2
Butter Toffee; European Collect.	10	0.5	3
Gummi Savers, 1.5 oz roll	140	0	32
Lollipops Fruit, 1 pce, 0.4 oz	45	0	11
Pepomint, 4 mints	60	0	15
Lik-m-aid *(Nestlé),* 1.7 oz	60	0	15
Lindt: Lindor, Balls, average	75	4	8
Dark Choc Truffles, each	70	6	4
Lollipops, each, 0.2 oz	20	0	5
Lollipops C Pops *(Glenny's),* each	35	0	8
Mamba, 9 pces, 1½ oz	160	2	36
M&M's: Plain, 1.7 oz pkg	240	10	34
Milk Chocolate, 1 pce	5	0.2	0.5
20 pces, 1.5 oz	80	4	10
¼ cup, 1.5 oz	210	9	30
Almond Choc., 1.3 oz pkg	200	11	21
1.5 oz pkg	230	13	25
Caramel, ¼ cup, 1.5 oz	220	11	28
Crispy, 1.65 oz	220	9	34
King Size, ½ pkg, 1.6 oz	220	9	32
1.5 oz pkg	220	11	26
Minis, Mega Tube, 1.94 oz tube	270	11	37
Peanut, 1.7 oz pkg	250	13	30
Fun Size, 0.7 oz pkg	110	5	13
Peanut Butter, 1.6 oz pkg	240	13	27
Fun Size, 0.7 oz pkg	110	6	12
Mars Bar: All varieties, 1.76 oz	240	13	31
Fun size, 1 bar	95	5	12
Marshmallows: Firm/Soft, 1 oz	90	0	23
Regular size, 6 pce, 33g	110	0	26
Mini-Marshmallow, ½ c., 30g	100	0	24
Choc-coat. Twists *(Joyva),* each	95	2	10
Kraft: Mini, ½ cup	80	0	21
Creme, 2 Tbsp	40	0	10
Jet-Puffed, 5 pces	90	0	23
Funmallows, each	25	0	6
Miniature, ½ cup	100	0	25
Teddy Bear, ½ cup	50	0	12
Marshmallow Egg, 1 egg	110	0	26
Marzipan, 1 oz	140	7	16
Mauna Loa: Choc., 2.5 oz bar	420	29	36
Choc. coated Macadamias (9)	230	17	19

Per Piece/Serving	C	F	Cb
Mega Fruit Gummi, each	10	0	2
Mexican Hats, (9)	100	0	24
Mentos, each	10	0	2
Mike & Ike: 1 pkg, 2.1 oz	220	0	55
19 pce, 1.4 oz	150	0	36
Milkfulls *(Storck),* 6 pces, 1.4 oz	170	3	35
Milk Chocolate: See *Hershey's*			
Milk Choc. Crisp, 1.45 oz bar	205	11	22
Milk Duds, 7 pces	240	9	37
Milk Shake Bar, 1.8 oz bar	220	7	37
Milky Way: Midnight Bar, 1.75 oz	220	8	36
Regular bar, 2 oz	270	10	41
Fun size, 2 bars, 1.4 oz	180	7	28
King Size, 3.63 oz bar	480	18	72
Midnight, 1.76 oz bar	220	4.5	36
Miniatures, 3	190	7	30
Milky Way Lite, 1.57 oz	170	5	34
Miniatures, 1.4 oz pkg (5)	150	4.5	29
Mints: Uncoated, 1 oz	100	0	23
1 small mint (³/4" diam.)	7	0	2
1 large mint (1¹/2" diam.)	30	0	7
Mon Cheri *(Ferrero),* 4 pces, 45g	260	18	20
Mounds: 1.75 oz bar	240	13	29
Snack, 0.68 oz	90	5	11
Mr Goodbar:			
King Size, 2.6 oz bar	420	26	38
1.75 oz bar	280	18	26
Snack, 0.6 oz	100	6	9
Necco Candy Wafers (3) 57g	15	0	4
Neuhaus, average all types	80	5	7
Newman's Own: Pepp. Cups, 1 pkg	170	11	20
P'Nut B. Cups (Milk/Dark), 3, 1 pkg	180	12	17
Nibs, all types, 1 pouch, 0.5 oz	45	0	10
Nips *(Pearson),* all flavors, 2, 14g	60	2	10
Nite Bite *(Glucose Bar)*	100	3.5	15
Nothing But Nuts Butter Toffee			
3 Tbsp, 1 oz	200	15	9
Nougat, 2 pces, 1 oz	115	1	25
Chocolate Covered, 1 oz	120	4	20
Nougat Nut Cream, 3.5 oz	340	31	50
Now & Later *(Nabisco),* 1 pkg	270	2.5	63
Nutrageous Bar *(Reese's),* 3.4 oz	500	30	46
Snack, 0.6 oz	90	5	9
Oh Henry! 1.8 oz bar	240	10	32

Per Piece/Serving	C	F	Cb
100 Grand, 1.5 oz bar	190	8	30
Orange *(Lindt),* 6 block, 40g	190	10	24
Orange Slices: *(Jewel)* 3, 41g	140	0	36
(Walgreens) 3, 43g	150	0	36
Pastel Mints *(Walgreens),* 33 pce	150	0	36
Patteez *(Sweet n' Low),* ¹/2 ctn, 5	120	2.5	32
PayDay Bar: 1.85 oz bar	260	13	27
King Size, 3.4 oz	480	26	50
Snack, 0.7 oz	100	5.5	10
Peanut Bar, 1.6 oz bar	210	14	20
Peanut Butter Bars, 3 pces, 18g	80	1.5	15
Peanut Butter Cups: See *Reese's; Newman's Own*			
Peanut Brittle, 1 oz	130	5	20
Peanut Chews *(Goldenberg's),* ea.	60	3	21
Peanut Riesen (5), 41g	190	7	28
Peanuts, choc-covered, each	25	1.5	2
Pearson's Mint Patties, (5), 38g	150	2.5	31
Pecan Roll, ¹/3 bar, 40g	200	10	26
Peppermints, 7 small, 0.5 oz	50	0	12
Hershey's, 3 pces	60	0	15
Peppermint Twists (2), 13g	60	0	12
Pez, 1 roll	30	0	6
Planters: Choc. Peanuts (25) 7 oz	220	13	20
Orig. Peanut Bar, 1.6 oz	230	14	22
Popcorn: See *Snacks, Page 136*			
Positively Pecan, 2.5 oz bar	390	24	38
Pralines: Small, 0.3 oz	38	2	5
1 large piece, 1.4 oz	180	10	24
Pretzels: Choc-covered,			
3 minisize, 1.15 oz	150	5.5	23
1 regular, 1 oz	130	4.5	20
Pretzel Flipz *(Nestlé),* 8, 1 oz	130	5	19
Raisinets, 1 pkg, 1.7 oz	210	8	33
Raspberry Cream, each	80	2.5	5
Red Hot Dollars, 7 pce	100	0	24
Reese's: Chocolate Bar, 2.8 oz	420	24	43
Candy (Multipack), each	95	5.5	9
Miniatures, each	40	2.5	4
Peanut Butter Bites (7)	90	5	10
Mini, 1 pce	42	2.5	5
Peanut Butter Cups, 1.6 oz pkg	250	14	25
Kingsize, 2.8 oz	420	24	43
Mini, 1 pce, 0.27 oz	40	2.5	4
Peanut Butter Eggs (1), 0.6 oz	90	5	9
Reese's Pieces (25), 1.6 oz	225	10	28
Snack Size, (2), 1.2 oz (34g)	190	11	19
ReeseSticks, Kingsize, (2), 1.5 oz	230	13	23

Candy, Chocolate (Cont)

Per Piece/Serving

	C	F	Cb
Rice Crunchy Bars, 19g bar	60	0	14
Rice Krispies Treats: 1.3 oz bar	150	3.5	29
Chocolate Chip, 1.3 oz bar	160	5	28
Riesen Choc. Chew, (5) 1.4 oz	180	7	29
Peanut & Milk Choc, (5)	190	7	28
Ritter Sport: Plain Choc, 50g	260	16	26
w. Hazelnuts, 1/2 pkg, 50g	290	19	24
Rocky Road, 1.8 oz bar	240	11	34
Robin Eggs: Large, 2 pces	70	2	14
Medium, 4 pces	90	2.5	16
Mini, 10 pces	70	2.5	13
Rolo, all types (3), 0.64 oz	90	2.5	12
Root Beer Barrels (3) 0.5 oz	60	0	16
Russell Stover Candy: Creams (1)	60	2	10
Almond Delight, 2 oz	290	17	32
Caramel Bar, 46g	230	11	20
Jelly Cups (P/Nut Butter), 2, 34g	140	9	14
Mint Dream	160	8	19
Pecan Delight (Sugar Free), 2 oz	260	18	27
Pecan Delight, 2 oz bar	310	20	27
Pecan Roll, 50g	260	18	23
Salt Water Taffy (Sathers), 5, 43g	150	2.5	34
Seashells (Guylian) 1 shell	65	4	6
See's Candies: *Average all Flavors*			
Bon Bons, 2 pieces	155	4	30
Brittles (2), 1.3 oz	220	15	18
Caramels & Chews, 2 pieces	175	6	19
Creams, 2 pieces	180	9	24
Little Pops, 4 pieces	60	2	11
Lollypops (1)	80	2.5	14
Nut Clusters, 3 pieces	225	16	16
White Coating, 2 pieces	187	11	20
Sesame Crunch, 3 pces	80	4	7
Simply Lite, 1/2 ctn, 36 pieces	130	5	18
Simply Sugar Free: *See Allen Wertz*			
Sixlets (Hershey), 24 pces	90	3.5	14
Skittles: Sour, 1.8 oz bag	200	2	44
Orig./Trop./Wild Berry, 2.1 / oz bag	240	2.5	54
Fun size, 1 bag, 0.7 oz (20g)	80	1	18
King Size, 4 oz bag	440	4.5	100
Large bag (16 oz): 1/4 cup, 1.5 oz	170	2	37
Mint (Pepp./Sprmint), 1.6 oz pkg	180	2	40
Skor Toffee Bar, 1.4 oz	220	13	24
Smarties Candy Rolls, 1 roll	25	0	5
Snackwell's Raisin Dips, 5 oz	160	5	34
Snickers: 2.07 oz bar	280	14	35
3.7 oz bar	510	24	63
Cruncher, 2.54 oz	370	21	44
King Size, 1/2 bar, 1.2 oz	170	8	21
Munch Bar, 1.4 oz bar	230	15	17
Fun size, each	95	5	12

	C	F	Cb
Snickers (Cont):			
Miniatures, each	42	2.5	5
Creme Egg, each	170	10	19
Snack (2), 40g	190	10	24
Sno Caps, 2.3 oz pkg	300	13	48
Soft Chews (Maalox), 1 chew	20	0.5	4
Soft 'N Chewy Butter Toffee, ea.	32	0.5	7
Soft Drops (9)	100	0	24
Soft Hot Dollars (11)	90	0	23
Sonic Boom Pops (Walgreens), ea.	60	0	14
Sour Brite Crawlers, 13 pces	140	0	31
Sour Punch: All types, 2 oz	190	1	45
1 straw	20	0	5
Spearmint Leaves: (Jewel), 5, 40g	140	0	35
(Walgreens), 5, 11/2 oz	150	0	38
Spice Drops, 10 pces, 11/2 oz	130	0	33
Spree Candies: Original, 8 pces	60	0	14
Chewy Spree, 8 pces	50	0	12
Starburst: Candy Canes, 0.5 oz	70	0	18
Fruit Chews, each	20	0.4	4
2 oz pkg	240	4.5	48
Fruit Twist	35	0	8
Fruit Twist, 2 oz pkg	190	1	45
Jellybeans, 1.5 oz	150	0	38
Jellybean Egg, 2 oz	200	0	51
Tropical Fruit, 2.07 oz pack	240	4.5	48
Starlight Mints: 3 pces, 1/2 oz	60	0	16
Suckers (Walgreens), 1 sucker, 11g	45	0	11
Sugar Babies, 1.7 oz	190	2	43
Sugar Coated Peanuts, 1 oz	120	8	10
Sweet 'N Low: Chews, each	14	0	1
Sugar-Free Hard Candy, each	8	0	2
Peanut Butter Wafer Bars (1)	52	3	7
Sweet Escapes: *See Hershey's*			
Sweet Success Bars, 1 bar	120	4	23
Sweet Tarts (Nestlé), 7, 1/2 oz	50	0	13
Symphony: 1.5 oz bar	240	15	22
Snack: Chocolate (1), 0.6 oz	90	5	10
w. Almds & Toffee (1), 0.5 oz	80	5	7
Taffy, 1 pce. 1/2 oz	55	0.5	12
3 Musketeers: 2.13 oz bar	260	8	46
Fun size, each	70	2	13
Miniatures, each	25	0.5	5
Snack (2), 33g	140	4.5	26
Tang-a-Roos: 1 roll	24	0	6
Tarts (Walgreens), 4 pce, 15g	60	0	15
Tails (Walgreens), 8 pce, 15g	60	0	15
Tastetations (Hershey's),			
avg. all varieties (3)	60	1.5	12
Terry's Choc Orange, (5), 1.5 oz	230	12	27
Tic Tac, all varieties, each	1.5	0	0
Toblerone: 50g (1.76 oz) bar	270	15	32
1 bar, 100g (3.5 oz)	540	30	63
1/3 bar, 33g	180	10	21

Candy, Chocolate (Cont)

Per Piece/Serving	C	F	Cb
Toffees: Regular, 1 oz	150	9	15
Tongue Torchers *(Walgreens)*, 3	70	0	17
Tootsie Roll Midgies *(Walgreens)*, 6	160	3	33
Tootsie Roll, 2.25 oz roll	260	4	54
Treasures *(Nestlé)*: (4), 1.6 oz	240	16	26
Nestlé Crunch (3)	160	8.5	20
Butterfinger Pieces (3)	180	9	23
Creamy Caramel (3)	180	9	22
Peanut Butter Miniatures (3)	180	12	17
Trolli Gumm Candy, avg., 5 pces	120	0	29
Truffles: Regular, 1 pce 0.4 oz	60	4	5
Large *(Godiva)*, 0.75 oz	110	6.5	12
Extra Large *(J.Schmidt)*, 1¹/₂ oz	220	13	24
Turtles *(Nestlé)*, each	85	4.5	10
Twists (Sugar Free): Licorice; Strawberry, 6 twists, 40g	140	0	32
Twix: Caramel 2 oz pkg	280	14	37
King Size, 3.35 oz pkg	480	24	64
Fun Size: 0.5 oz	80	4	10
2 oz pkg, 2 bars	280	14	37
Peanut Butter, 0.9 oz	140	8.5	14
Snack, 1 cookie, 0.5 oz	80	5	8
Twizzlers: Candy, avg., 1 pce, 9g	30	0	8
Pull 'n' Peel Cherry (1), 1 oz	100	0	25
Velamints Sugar Free, 1 pce	10	0	2
Werther's: Original, 3 pce, 15g	60	1	13
Chocolates (5), 20g	110	6	13
Whatchamacallit Bar, 1.6 oz	230	11	28
Snack (1), 0.57 oz	80	4	10
Whitman's:			
Pecan Roll, 2 oz roll	300	20	26
Sampler, 3 pces, 1.4 oz	200	11	25
Assorted; Dark Chocolate, 1 pce	65	3	9
Snoopy Treats, 2 pces	190	10	24
Whoppers, 9 pce	100	3.5	15
Yogurt Candy: Plain, 1 oz	120	6	15
Coated Raisins, 1 oz	120	4	21
York Mints: 1.5 oz patty	145	5	34
Snack size, 0.5 oz	50	1	11
Peppermint Patties, 3	150	2.5	30
York Peppermint Pattie: 1.4 oz	150	3	31
Snack size, 0.49 oz	50	1	11
Zachary Old Fash. Creme Drops (3)	170	3	36
Zagnut: 1.75 oz bar	230	10	31
Snack size (1), 0.5 oz	70	3	9
Zero Bar, 1 pce, 0.6 oz	70	2.5	12
Zingos, 3 pce, 2g	5	0	2

Carob Candy

Per Piece/Serving	C	F	Cb
Carob: Plain/Natural, 1 oz	160	11	9
Carob Coated: Raisins, 1 oz	130	8	15
Almonds/Peanuts, 1 oz	150	10	14
Malt Balls, 1 oz	135	8	15
Caramels, 1 oz	110	4	18
Dates, 1 oz	125	5	20
Soybeans	145	9	16
Trail/Party Mix, 1 oz	140	9	15
Carob Chips, unsweetened, 1 oz	140	7	19
Carob Bars: Plain/Nut, 1 oz	160	11	13
Fruit & Nut, 1 oz	155	10	13
Mint/Orange, 1 oz	160	11	14
Carafection: Cashew Coconut Crunch, ¹/₂ Bar, (42g) 1.5 oz	250	14	5
Caroby Natural Touch, 3 oz	450	27	36

Cough Drops

	C	F	Cb
Beech Nut, 1 drop	10	0	2
Diabetic Tussin, 1 drop	0	0	0
Halls Defense Vit. C, 1 drop	15	0	4
Halls Fruit Breezers, 1 drop	14	0	4
Halls Menthol Drops, 1 drop	15	0	4
Sugar Free, 1 drop	6	0	4
Halls Plus, 1 drop	18	0	5
Helps Cough, all flavors, 1	14	0	3
Listerine Lozenge (Amer. Chicle)	9	0	2
Luden's Throat Drops, all flavors, 1	10	0	3
Sugar Free, 1 drop	10	0	2
Pine Bros, 1 cough drop	10	0	2
Ricola: Cough Drops, 1 drop	12	0	3
Sugar-Free Lemon Mint, 2 mints	0	0	1
Rite Aid, Menthol Cough, 1 drop	12	0	3
Robitussin: Regular, 1 drop	14	0	3
Honey Cough, 1 drop	40	0	10
Sugar Free Throat, 1 drop	10	0	3
Sunny Orange Vit. C, 1 drop	12	0	3
Rolaids/Sodium Free, 1	4	0	1
Sathers Peppermint Lozenges, 1	13	0	3
Squibb Cough/Throat Loz.'s, 1	16	0	4
Sucrets (Beecham) Lozenges, 1	36	0	2
Wintergreen Loz. (Walgreens), 1	13	0	3
Cough Suppresant Liquids: *See Page 144*

Popcorn

Home-Popped Popcorn

	C	F	Cb
Popping Corn Kernels:			
2 Tbsp, 1 oz	100	1	22
(makes approx. 3½ cups)			
Air-popped (no oil), plain, 1 oz	100	0	22
1 cup (6g)	20	0	4
Oil-popped, plain, 1 oz	140	8	10
1 cup (11g)	55	5	4
Popcorn Oil, 1 Tbsp	120	14	0

Microwave Popcorn

Average All Brands (Popped)

	C	F	Cb
Butter: Regular, 1 cup	35	2	4
Light, 1 cup	25	1	4
Act II Popcorn:			
Butter, 1 cup, 0.3 oz	35	2	4
4 cups, popped, 1 oz	140	8	16
Light Butter, 1 cup, 0.2 oz	25	1	4
5 cups, popped, 1 oz	125	4	20
Butter Lovers,1 cup, 0.3 oz	45	3	4
3.5 cups, 1 oz	160	10	14
Butter Lovers (Reduced Fat), 1 c.	30	1.5	4.5
4.5 cups, 1 oz	130	6	20
American Fare (K-Mart):			
Butter, 1 cup, 0.3 oz	37	2.5	4
3.5 cups, 1 oz	130	9	14
Light Butter, 1 cup, 0.3 oz	28	1	5
3.5 cups, 1 oz	100	4	17
Healthy Choice			
Butter, 6 cups	100	2.5	22
Natural, 6 cups, 1 oz	100	2	22
Newman's Own: Butter, 1 oz	170	11	16
Light Butter Flavor, 3½ cups	110	3	22
Orville Redenbacher's: *Per Cup, Popped*			
Corn on the Cob, 1 cup, popped	35	2.5	3
Movie Theater Butter, 1 cup	30	2	3
4 cups, popped, 1 oz	120	8	12
Light Movie Theater Butter, 1 cup	20	1	2
4 cups, 1 oz	80	4	8
Double Feature Jumbo, 1 cup	30	2	3
Smart Pop!:			
94% Fat Free Butter, 1 cup	20	0.5	4
Butter Light, 1 cup	20	0.5	3
Sweet 'n Buttery, 1 cup	45	3.5	4
Butter, 1 cup	35	2	4

Bagged Popcorn   C F Cb

Average All Brands (Ready-to-Eat)

	C	F	Cb
Regular: Plain, ½ oz pkg	80	5	7
1 oz pkg	160	10	14
4 oz pkg	640	40	56
Box (store/airport), 2 oz	320	20	28
Bag (9" high x 5" wide), 3 oz	480	30	42

Brands ~ Bagged Popcorn

	C	F	Cb
Act II Popcorn: Supreme, ¾ cup	130	5	22
Butter Toffee: ¾ cup, 1 oz	110	1	27
w. Peanuts, ¾ cup, 1 oz	120	2.5	24
Boston's: Fat Free, ⅔ cup, 1 oz	100	0	23
Lite, 2 cup, 1 oz	140	6	19
Gourmet Super Prem., 2 c., 1 oz	160	11	13
40% Less Fat, 2¾ cup, 1 oz	140	6	17
Cracker Jack: Original, ½ cup, 1 oz	120	2	23
Fat Free varieties, ¾ cup, 1 oz	110	0	26
Crunch 'N Munch: ½ cup, 1 oz	140	5	22
Buttery Toffee, ⅔ cup, 1 oz	150	6	22
Caramel w. P'nuts, ⅔ c., 1.2 oz	140	3.5	25
Fiddle Faddle: Skippy ¾ c., 1 oz	130	3	23
Honey Nut, ½ cup, 1 oz	130	3.5	24
w. Real Planters Peanuts, ⅔ cup	130	3	24
Hixon's: Caramel Corn, 1 oz	125	4.5	20
Cheese Corn, 1 oz	160	11	15
Korn Krunch: *(Kornfections Treasures):*			
Almond Pecan (Sugar Free), 1 oz	150	8	19
Orville Redenbacher:			
Butter Toffee, ⅔ cup, 1.1 oz	140	4.5	24
Skippy P'nut Butter, ¾ c., 1 oz	130	3	23
Choc. Lovers Poppycock,½ c., 1 oz	140	5	21
Heath Toffee Candy, ½ c., 1 oz	100	1.5	23
Pizza Hut Cheese Pizza, 2 oz bag	360	26	26
Poppycock: Pecan Delight, 1 oz	300	14	40
Just Be Nuts!, ¼ cup, 1.3 oz	205	15	13
Slimmons (Fat Free): ¾ c., 1 oz	110	0	25
Weight Watchers Butter, ⅔ cup	90	2.5	14
Wild Oats, all types, 2.5 cup, 1 oz	160	10	15

Movie Theater Popcorn

	C	F	Cb
Small (7 cups): Plain	400	27	30
with Butter	580	47	30
Medium (16 cups): Plain	900	60	70
with Butter	1170	90	70
Large (20 cups): Plain	1150	76	90
with Butter	1500	116	90

Potato Chips/Crisps

Average All Brands

	C	F	Cb
Regular:			
Plain or flavored, 1 chip	9	1	1
17 chips, 1 oz pkg	150	10	15
4 oz quantity	600	40	60
Lay's Stax, avg. all, 1 oz	150	10	15
Pringles, 14 crisps, 1 oz	160	11	15
Large, 5.75 oz can	920	63	86
Snack Stack, 23g tub	140	9	12
Ruffles, 14 chips, 1 oz	160	10	14
Reduced Fat: *Pringles,* 1 oz	140	7	20
Crunch Tators, 1 oz	140	7	19
Kettle Fry (Eagle), 1 oz	150	8	16
Sun Chips, 1 oz	140	6	19
Terra, average, 1 oz	140	7	19
Lowfat/Baked varieties, 1 oz	110	1.5	23
Atkins Crunchers, avg., 1 oz	110	3	8
Fat Free:			
Childer's/Louise's, 1oz	100	0	22
Pringles (Fat Free), 1 oz	70	0	15
Lay's Wow!, 20 chips, 1 oz	75	0	17
Ruffles Wow!, 17 chips, 1 oz	70	0	17
Cheddar Sour Crm (15) 1 oz	70	0	16

Corn & Tortilla Chips

Corn Chips:	C	F	Cb
Average all types, 1 oz	160	10	15
8 oz bag	1280	80	120
Doritos: (12), 1 oz	150	7	20
Nachos; 4-Cheese, 1 oz	140	8	17
3D's Nacho Cheesier (32) 1 oz	130	5	19
Fritos (Sabrositas), 1 oz	150	9	17
Pringles, Torengos (13), 1 oz	140	9	15
Tortilla Chips: Average, 1 oz	150	8	22
(1 oz = approx. 12 chips or 13 strips)			
Boston, Baked, 13 chips, 1 oz	110	1.5	20
Doritos: 18 chips, 1 oz	140	6	20
Light, 13 chips, 1 oz	130	5	20
Wow! Nacho Cheesier, 1 oz	90	0.5	16
Frito Lay, Baked, (15) 1 oz	120	3.5	21
Garden of Eatin', 1 oz	140	7	28
Keebler Suncheros Light, 1 oz	150	8	18
Kettle, average, 1 oz	140	6	18
Padrino Reduced Fat, 1 oz	130	4	22
Torengos, 13 chips, 1 oz	140	9	15
Utz Lowfat Baked, 8 chips, 1 oz	120	1.5	23
Wild Oats, 14 chips, 1 oz	150	7	18

Pretzels C F Cb

Average All Brands

Hard Baked Pretzels: *Per Pretzel*	C	F	Cb
1 oz	110	2	22
Sticks, thin, 2¼" (9/oz), each	12	0	3
Twists, thin, ¼" thick, (5/oz), 1	25	0.2	5
Dutch (2¾"x 2⅝") ½ oz, 1	55	1	11
Sourdough *(Shultz),* ¾ oz, each	80	0	17
Fat Free Pretzels:			
Snyders (1), 1 oz	100	0	22
Mini (20), 1 oz	110	0	25
Utz Wheels/Nuggets, 1 oz	100	0	22
Rold Gold: Sticks (48), 1 oz	100	0	23
Sourdough Nuggets (12), 1 oz	100	0	23
Sourdough Hards (1), ¾ oz	80	0	17
Thins (12), 1 oz	110	0	24
Twists (16), 1 oz	110	1	22
Tiny Twists/Sticks (18), 1 oz	100	0	23
Low Fat Pretzels:			
American Fare Mini Twists, 1oz	120	1	23
Frito Lay, Rold Gold:			
Butter Checkers 20 pcs., 1 oz	110	1.5	22
Braided Twists (8) , 1 oz	110	1	23
Choc-coated *(Nestlé),* 1 oz	130	6	20
White Fudge covered *(Nestlé),*			
1 oz, 7 pieces	140	6	19
Yogurt *(Wild Oats)* 8 pcs., 1.4 oz	210	10	27
Soft Pretzels (Twists) average:			
Plain: Regular, 2.5 oz	190	0	41
King Size, 5 oz	390	0	83
Big Cheese, 5 oz	380	7	61
Peanut Butter filled *(Tr. Joe's)* 1 oz	160	7	18
Frito Lay Pretzels			
Flavor Twists, 23 pces, 1 oz,	160	10	16
Rold Gold Flavor Rush, ⅓ c. 1 oz	150	7	20
Braided Twists, 8 sticks, 1 oz	110	1	23

Auntie Anne's: See Fast-Foods Page 188

Snyder's of Hanover Pretzels	C	F	Cb
Logs (7), 1 oz	120	1	21
Homestyle (15), 1 oz	120	1	24
Mini (20), 1 oz	110	0	25
Super Pretzel: Jalapeno, 5 oz	360	0	78
Bavarian Twist, 3 oz	210	3	41
Cinnamon Raisin w. Icing, 5 oz	420	4	76
Sweet Dough Twist, 3.7 oz	300	3	60

Snacks

138

Snacks | C | F | Cb

Note: Actual weight of packaged snacks is usually 5-10% more than label Net Wt. For accuracy, weigh snack and allow extra calories for any extra weight.

Item	C	F	Cb
Bacon Cheese Crackers, 1 oz	140	6	14
Banana Chips, 1/4 cup, 1 oz	150	8	20
Beef Jerky, average, 1 oz	70	1	3
Beef Sticks (Frito-Lay's) 0.3 oz	50	4	1
Bugles: Original, 1 1/3 cup, 1 oz	160	9	18
Baked Bugles, 1 1/2 cup, 1.1 oz	130	3.5	23
Cajun Jerky, 1 1/2 oz	150	6	6
Carrot Chips (Hain)	160	9	26
Cheddar Lites (Health Valley) 1 oz	120	3	21
Cheese Crackers, 1 oz	130	6	18
Cheese Filled (Frito-Lay's)	210	11	24
Cheese Curls, 1 1/4 cup, 1 oz	160	9	19
Reduced Fat (Utz), 1 oz	140	6	21
American Fare, 1 1/4 cup, 1 oz	140	5	22
Cheese Nips (Nabisco), 29, 1 oz	150	6	19
Cheese Puffs: Average, 1 oz	150	10	15
Lowfat, 1 oz	140	5	20
Health Valley, 1 1/2 cup	110	3	21
No Fries, 1 oz	110	0	23
Cheese Straws, 4 pieces	110	7	8
Cheese Twists, 23 twists, 1 oz	150	8	15
Cheetos: Regular all flavors, 1 oz	160	10	15
Light, cheese flavored, 1 oz	140	6	19
Cheez Balls: 45 balls, 1 oz	150	10	15
Reduced Fat, 45 balls, 0.73 oz	100	4.5	15
Cheez Bopps (Boston's), (28) 1 oz	130	6	17
Cheez Curls/Doodles, 1 oz	160	12	15
Cheez Mania (Planters), 35, 1 oz	160	10	15
Cheez It: White Cheddar, 1 pkt	210	11	26
Cheese Sandwiches, 1 pkt	220	13	21
100% Real Cheese, 1 pkt	220	12	23
Chex Mix: General Mills, 1.1 oz	150	10	15
Bold 'N Zesty (40% less fat), 1/2 c.	140	6	24
Chedder (50% less fat), 1/2 oz	130	5	20
Traditional (60% less fat), 2/3 c.	130	4	22
Churros (Mex. Pastry) 10", 1.2 oz	140	9	12
Cinna Chips (T.J. Cinn.) 3, 1 oz	110	4	19
Combos: (Oven Baked):			
Crackers, 1/3 cup, 1 oz	140	7	18
1 cup, 3 oz	420	21	54
Pretzels, 1/3 cup, 1 oz	130	4.5	19
1 cup, 3 oz	390	14	57
Cookies: See Pages 109-116			
Corn Chips: See Page 137			

Snacks (Cont) | C | F | Cb

Item	C	F	Cb
Corn Crunchies/Spirals, 1 oz	160	10	15
Corn Crisps (Pringle), 1 oz	140	7	18
Corn Nuts, 1/3 cup, 1 oz	130	4	20
Corn Puffs (Health Valley) 2 c., 1 oz	120	1.5	25
(Pirate's Booty) 1 oz	130	5	18
Dunkaroos, 1 tray, 1 oz	130	4.5	20
Flavor Twists (Fritos), 1 oz	160	10	16
French's Potato Sticks 3/4 c., 1 oz	180	12	16
Fruit Snack Cups: See Page 148			
Funyun's Onion flavor, 1 oz	140	7	18
Goldfish (Pepperidge Farm) 1 oz	140	7	18
Gold-N-Chees (Lance), 1 3/8 oz	180	7	25
Handi Snacks (Kraft), Bearwiches	150	7	21
Honey Mustard Onion Pieces			
(Snyder's) 1 pkg, 2 oz	280	13	35
Hot Peanuts (F.'o Lay), 1 3/4 oz pkg	310	25	10
Keebler: Wheatables Snack Mix,			
Toasted Honey, 1/2 cup, 1 oz	130	5	20
Peanut Butter Crunch, 1/2 c., 1 oz	160	7	20
Chse & P'nut Butter			
Sandwich Cookies, 1 pkg	250	12	30
Koolstuf: All flavors, 1 bar, 1.3 oz	130	3	27
Lance Sandwich: Bonnie, 1 pkg	160	7	23
Capt. Wafers; Choc-O-Mint, pkg	190	10	23
Sour Dough w. Cheddar, 1 pkg	240	15	23
Other varieties, average, 1 pkg	200	10	22
Lunchables: Fudge Brownie	250	9	42
'S'Mores	200	6	35
Munchos, 16 pieces, 1 oz	160	10	16
Nabisco: Chips Ahoy, 1.3 oz	150	7	20
Chips Ahoy! Cookie Barz, 35g	180	10	23
Nutter Butter Bites (10)	150	6	20
Oreo, 1.3 oz	160	7	24
Ureo Cookie Barz, 1 bar	180	10	23
S'Mores	200	6	35
Sportz, Cheese Nips (38), 1 oz	150	7	19
Sweet Crispers (18), 1 oz	135	3	25
Nibblers (Snyder's): Regular (13)	130	3	23
Sourdough Fat Free (16)	120	0	25
Onion Rings (Lance), 1 pkg	120	6	16
Oriental Mix (Rice Snacks), 1 oz	155	7.5	15
Rice Snacks (Wild Oats) 2/3 c. 1 oz	110	0	25
Oyster Crackers (Bradshaw's), 1 oz	140	5	14
Party Mix (Flavor Tree) 1/4 c., 1 oz	160	11	14
Pirate's Booty w. White Ched., 1 oz	130	5	18
Popcorn: See Page 136			

Snacks (Cont) | C | F | Cb

	C	F	Cb
Pork Skins/Rind: Baken-ets,1 oz	160	10	0
Gram's Crunchies, avg., 1 oz	150	10	4
Grande, 2/3 cup	80	5	0
Lance, 1 pkg	65	4	1
Potato Chips: See Pages 137			
Potato Puffs (Health Valley), 1 oz	110	3	21
Potato Skins (TGI Friday's), 1 oz	150	9	14
Potato Sticks (French's), 3/4 c., 1.1oz	180	12	16
Puffs: 1 2/3 cup, 1 oz	140	8	17
8 oz pkg	1120	64	136
Quakes Rice Snacks (Quaker)			
Apple Cinnamon (8) 16g	60	0	15
BBQ, Ranch, Sour Crm (10) 16g	70	2.5	12
Caramel Corn (7) 15g	60	0	13
Cheddar/Nacho Cheese (9) 15g	70	2.5	11
Chocolate (7) 15g	60	1	13
Ranch Puffs (No Fries), 1 oz	110	0	23
Rice Chips, Bar-B-Q/Onion, 1/2 oz	70	3	9
Santitas (Frito Lay), 1 oz	140	6	20
Sesame Sticks (Cityfarm), 1 oz	160	11	13
Snack Crackers (No Fries), 1 oz	110	0	24
Soy Nuts: Dry Roasted, 1 oz	130	6	9
Choc-coated, 12-15 pces, 1/2 oz	70	4	7
Spicers Wheat Snacks, 1 1/2 oz	150	7.5	18
Sport Jerky Ostrich,			
(Wild Oats), 1/2 oz	25	0	0
Sun Chips (Frito Lay), 1 oz pkg	140	6	19
TastyKake: Koffee Kake Jnr	250	8	40
Chocolate Jnr	320	12	50
Creme Filled Koffee Kakes	360	14	54
Toast/Cheese Crackers, 1 pkg	205	10	24
Tortilla Chips: See Pages 137			
Tostitos: Regular, average, 1 oz	140	8	18
Fat Free, 1 oz	90	0	20
Trail Mix (Nuts/Seeds/Dried Fruit):			
Regular, 3 Tbsp, 1 oz	130	8	13
Tropical, 3 Tbsp, 1 oz	120	5	19
w. Chocolate Chips, 1 oz	140	9	13
Turkey Jerky Teriyaki (Oberto)	80	0.5	0
Vegetable Snacks/Chips, 1 oz	130	4	24
Veggie Chips, 1 oz	130	5	18
Veggie Stix, 1 oz	140	7	18
Wahoos, 1 oz, 23 pces.	140	8	18
Weight Watchers: Chse Curls, 1/2 oz	70	2.5	10
Apple Chips, 3/4 oz pkg	70	0	18
Yogurt Raisins, 1 oz	130	6	20

Fruit Snacks | C | F | Cb

	C	F	Cb
Betty Crocker:			
String Things, 1 pouch, 0.75 oz	80	1	17
Lucky Charms Fruit Shapes,			
1 pouch, 0.9 oz (25g)	80	0	20
Squeezit, average, 1 bottle	100	0	25
Nabisco: Rugrats; Wacky Faces (1)	80	0	18
Blues Clues; Dora the Explorer (1)	60	0	14
Fruit Rolls, 1 roll, 0.74 oz	80	2	16
Sunkist: All flavors, 1 pch, 0.9 oz	80	0	21
Fruit Snack Cups: See Page 148			

Vending Machines

	C	F	Cb
Brownie, frosted	180	9	24
Cheese Balls, 1 oz	150	8	16
Choc Chip Cookies, 4	130	7	19
Choc Milk, 8 fl.oz	225	9	26
Coca Cola Classic, 12 fl.oz	140	0	35
Diet Coke, 12 fl.oz	1	0	0
Corn Chips, 1 oz	160	10	15
Danish Pastry, 2 oz	220	10	25
Donut, plain, 1 3/4 oz	210	12	25
Fruit Pie, 4 oz	290	13	46
Granola/Cereal Bars	130	3	26
Hershey's, 1.55 oz bar	240	14	25
Hot Fries, 1 oz	140	10	11
Kellogg's Rice Krispies Treat	120	1.5	26
Lance: Captain's Wafers, 1 pkg	230	12	26
Big Town, 1 pkg	250	11	38
M & M's: Plain, 1.7 oz	240	10	34
Peanuts, 1.7 oz	250	13	30
Milk: Whole, 8 fl.oz	150	8	12
Reduced Fat, 2%, 8 fl.oz	120	5	12
Milky Way, 2 oz	270	10	41
Onion Rings, 1 oz	120	6	16
Orange Juice, 8.75 fl.oz	120	0	28
Peanuts, roasted, 1 oz	165	14	6
Popcorn, plain, 1 oz	160	10	14
Pork Skins, 1 oz	160	10	0
Potato Chips: 1 oz	150	10	15
Reduced Fat, 1 oz	140	7	20
Pretzels, 1 oz	110	2	22
Raisins, 1/2oz pkg	40	0	9
Reece's Peanut Butter Cups, 1.8 oz	280	17	28
Snickers, 2.1 oz bar	280	14	35
Tortilla Chips, 1 oz	150	8	22

Granola, Sports & Diet Bars

Note: Actual weight of bars is usually 5-10% more than label Net Wt. Weigh bar and allow extra calories.

Per Bar	C	F	Cb
AllGoode Organics: *Per 1.73 oz Bar*			
Cashew Almond Passion	190	8	24
Chocolate flavors, average	200	8	29
Honey Nut Harvest	160	3.5	32
Nutty Choc Apricot	200	10	26
Amway (Trim Advantage):			
Protein Bars, average	250	9	22
Meal Replacements, average	230	8	30
Animal Parade, 30g bar	110	3	15
Arbonne Balanced Nutr., 1 bar	190	4.5	24
Atkins: *Per Bar*			
Advantage Bar: Smores	260	10	26
Average other varieties	230	11	22
Morning Starts Breakfast Bar (1)	175	9	13
Endulge: *See Confectionery, Page 128*			
Balance Bar: Oasis, avg., 1.7 oz	185	4	26
High Protein, average, 1.76 oz	200	6	23
Gold, average, 1.76 oz	210	7	22
Satisfaction, average, 2.64 oz	280	6	47
Kid Sport Bar, 1.8 oz	200	6	27
Baker's: *Per Cookie (3.5 oz)*			
Apple Pie; Pumpkin Spice	280	3.5	54
Peanut Butter	355	10	55
Peanut Butter & Jelly	345	8	60
Vegan Peanut Butter Choc. Chunk	380	10	60
Avg. other varieties	320	6	58
Barbara's Bakery: Real Fruit	50	0	13
Cereal Bars, fruit filled	110	0	27
Granola Bars, average, $^3/_4$ oz	90	2	15
Bariatrix Proti-Bar (15g Protein):			
Caramel Nut, 40g	150	5	10
Blueberry; CookitCrunch, 35g	130	4	6
Biochem: Ultimate Lo Carb, 2.1 oz	240	6	25
Protein Bar, Caramel Nougat	250	9	26
Ultimate Protein Bar, 78g	290	4.5	19
Ideal For Her, avg., 1.7 oz	200	7	20
Strive, average	190	9	24
Bio-Tech: Bio-Protein, 81g	300	7	39
Body Smarts: Choc. P'nut Crunch	210	6	34
Yogurt Berry Crunch	200	5	35
Boost: Choc./Strawb. Crunch	190	6	30
Boulder Bar Endurance, 2.5 oz	220	4	13
Burn-IT, 50g bar	180	3	13
Cap'N Crunch, all types, 0.8 oz	90	2	17
Carb Solutions Taste Sensations (2.1 oz):			
Choc. Peanut Butter	250	12	14
Choc. Toffee Hazelnut	260	13	15
Other flavors, average	240	10	16
Carb Watchers Lean Body, 2.5 oz	260	8	18

Per Bar	C	F	Cb
Carbolite: Choc Almond, 1.75 oz	230	17	25
Choc Crisp Bar, 1.75 oz	250	17	27
Milk/Dairy Choc, avg., 1.75 oz	250	19	28
CarboRite Bars, 1.06 oz	120	5	13
CarbRite Diet (Doctor's), 2 oz	180	3	25
Carnation Breakfast Bars, 35g (1.2 oz):			
Granola (Honey/Choc), average	130	2.5	26
Choc Chip/P.nut Butter, chewy	150	5	24
Champion Nutrition: SnacBar	180	3	25
UltraProtein Bar, average	300	4.5	32
Cheetah (NutraFig), 2.25 oz bar	210	2	43
Choice, all types, 1.23 oz bar	140	4.5	19
Clif Bars: Luna Bar, average, 1.5 oz	180	4.5	27
Ice Series (w. Caffeine), 2.4 oz	250	5	43
Mojo Bar, average, 1.6 oz	200	7	29
Nutrition Sustained Energy (68g)			
Apricot; Cranb. Apple Cherry	220	2.5	44
Other varieties, average	250	5	44
Energy Gel, 1.1 oz	95	0	24
Coach's Iced Energy Bars, 2 oz	220	3	35
Designer Whey Gourmet Bars: *Per Bar (2.7 oz)*			
Choc Malted Muscles	250	5	7
Choc Triplement/Espresso	250	7	7
Dble Chocolats; Lemon Crunches	260	4.5	7
Peanut Better Body	270	7	6
Perfect Absberry	260	6	9
Detour, 2.8 oz bar	310	10	25
Dr Soy: Protein Bar, Lemon, 1.76 oz	180	2.5	28
Chocolate/Peanut, 1.76 oz	185	4	27
Healthy Snacker, avg., 1.7 oz bar	190	6	23
EAS Advantage Edge:			
Carb Control, average, 2.12 oz	200	5	21
HP Energy bar, avg., 2.46 oz	260	5	37
Extreme Outdoor, avg., 2.5 oz	250	6	42
Complete Nutrition, 2.12 oz Bar:			
Choc Caramel	240	7	32
Iced Oatmeal Raisin Crisp	220	5	31
EAS Myoplex:			
Deluxe Bar, average, 3.2 oz	340	7	44
Lite Bar, average, 1.97 oz	190	3.5	28
Carb Sense, average, 2.5 oz	250	7	20
EAS Results for Women:			
Weight Management Bar, 1.94 oz	190	5	17
Complete Energy Bar, 1.67 oz	200	6	28
Eclipse 2000 Deluxe Protein, 78g	290	6	29
ELEV8 Protein & Fruit Trail:			
All Fruit Blend, 66g bar	250	4.5	34
Cocoa & Coconut, 66g	255	7	29
Ensure Chewy Choc P'nut, 2.12 oz	230	6	35
Entenmann's Multi-Grain, 1.3 oz	140	3	25

Note: Actual weight of bars is usually 5-10% more than label Net Wt. Weigh bar and allow extra calories.

Per Bar	C	F	Cb
Especially Yours, 1.76 oz bar	190	4	32
Extreme Body, 3 oz bar	340	8	24
Extreme Ripped Force, 45g	160	3	33
Fi-Bar Nectar Granola Bars, 1 oz	100	0	22
Chewy & Nutty Bar, 1.2 oz	140	4.5	23
Fi-Pro-Tein (R-Kane), 1.2 oz bar	107	1	16
Figurines Diet Bar, avg., 1 bar	110	6	12
Fit! (Medifast), 1.5 oz bar	160	4	20
Fruitein Energy Bar, 1.3 oz	130	3	18
General Mills: *Milk 'n Cereal*			
Chex; Cheerios, Cocoa Puffs 1.4 oz	160	4	26
Cinnamon Toast Crunch, 1.6 oz	180	4	31
GeniSoy: Average all bars, 2.2 oz	230	5	33
Extreme, average, 1.6 oz	170	4	27
Glucerna Meal Replacement, 2 oz	220	7	32
Grove Organic Energy Bars, 2 oz	250	10	30
Hain Mini Munchies Rice	90	1.5	2
Hansen's (1.4 oz): Active Nutr., avg.	140	3.5	20
Natural Crunch, avg. all flavors	185	3	37
Natural Functional, avg. all flav.	190	5	25
Health Valley: Fruit/Granola Bars	140	0	34
Cereal: Strawberry Cobbler	130	2	27
Healthy Recipes (Novartis)	150	4	21
HeartBar, Orig., Cranberry, 50g	190	3	29
HMR Benefit Bar, 1.1 oz	160	5	22
Iron-Tek: Vanilla Fudge, 2.73 oz	290	5	21
Triple Decker Protein, 2.3 oz	250	10	27
Jenny Craig: Meal Bars, 1.97 oz			
Milk Choc; Lemon Meringue	210	5	32
Choc Peanut; Yogurt Peanut	220	5	33
Oatmeal Raisin	210	3	35
Jewel Granola Bars: Cereal	140	3	27
Choc Chip/P'nut Butter	130	4.5	20
Lowfat varieties	110	2	22
Joyva Sesame Crunch, 1.1 oz	190	8	15
Kashi Golean Bars, avg, 2.7 oz	290	5	53
Kid Sport Bars, avg, 1.76 oz	200	6	29
Kudos: Bar (1)	90	2.5	17
Granola: M&M's; Snickers	105	4	16
Snack: M&M's	90	2.5	17
Snickers	100	3	16
Avg., other varieties	125	4.5	19
Lean Body, 76g	300	6	15
Luna Bars, average, 48g	180	4.5	27
Medifast Fit! 1.5 oz bar	160	4	20
Metabolife, average, 2 oz bar	230	6	36

Per Bar

	C	F	Cb
Met-Rx: "Big 100", avg., 100g	340	3.5	52
Protein Plus, 3 oz bar	310	8	25
MightyBite Choc. Bar, 25g	100	4	11
MLO Bio Protein, 2.85 oz	300	7	39
Muscle Tech: Nitro-Tech, average	290	6	33
Meso-Tech, avg., 3.11 oz	340	8	44
Meso-Tech Lite, avg., 2.12 oz	220	6	16
Myoplex: *See EAS*			
Natrol Prolab, 1.76 oz bar	190	6	12
Naturade, Total Soy, 2.1 oz	250	8	32
Nature Valley Granola: Average	145	4	24
Lowfat varieties	110	2	21
Nature's Best: Solid Protein, 2.75 oz			
Blueberry Cheesecake	280	4	14
Choc. Peanut Butter; S'Mores	290	7	12
Chocolate Mint	290	7	12
Cookie Dough Chip; Dble Choc	270	4	10
Other varieties, average	290	4	11
Nature's Plus: Energy Bar, 1.45 oz	140	4.5	24
Chi Chinese Herbal, 1.5 oz	150	4	20
Calcium Almond Blitz, 1.5 oz	150	2.5	29
Spiru-tein, all flavors, 1.4 oz	150	4	20
New You: Peanut Butter, 1.65 oz	185	5	25
Choc Chip; Lemon Crisp, 1.65 oz	170	3	26
Next Proteins: Designer Whey, 78g	290	9	23
Detour, 2.8 oz	310	10	25
U-Turn Protein, 2.8 oz	300	8	26
NiteBite (Time-release Glucose Bar)			
Choc. Fudge; P'nut Butter, 25g	100	3.5	15
NuBar Decadence, 1.3 oz	140	2.5	30
NuSkin (Pharmanex) Body Design			
Meal Replacement Bars	250	6	34
Nutiva: Hempseed, 1.4 oz	210	14	11
Flax Chocolate, 1.4 oz	200	12	19
Nutri-Grain Bars: Twists Bar	140	3	28
Cereal Yog. Bars, 1.3 oz	370	3	27
Granola Bar, Mini's, 1.5 oz pouch	165	3	32
Low Fat Granola Bar	80	1.5	17
Squares Bar Chocolate Chip	190	6	33
Muffin Bars	168	4	30
NutriSystem Sweet Success, 2.1 oz	220	3	33
100% Bar, 50g	190	6	31
Odwalla Energy Bars: Chocolate	240	6	40
Choc. Chip Peanut/Crunch, avg.	250	7	39
Carrot; Cranberry C Monster	225	2.5	47
Super Protein	235	5	31
Superfood	225	5	41

Granola, Sports & Diet Bars (Cont)

Note: Actual weight of bars is usually 5-10% more than label Net Wt. Weigh bar and allow extra calories.

Per Bar	C	F	Cb
Perfect Rx Nutrition Bar, 100g	340	3	50
Planters Peanut Bar, 1.6 oz	230	11	24
Power Bar: Pria, average 1 oz	110	3	17
Dipped Harvest, avg., 2.3 oz	260	5	45
Energy Bites, avg., 1.76 oz bag	210	5	33
Harvest; Performance, avg 2.3 oz	240	3	45
Power Crunch Bar, average, 1.3 oz	185	9	13
Protein Plus: Average, 2.75 oz	290	5	38
Layered: Strawberry Creme	220	5	30
Choc Caramel Nut	220	6	26
Sugar Free, average	170	4	20
PR Bar Ironman, 49.6g	200	6	22
Precision, all flavors, 50g	200	7	18
Premier: Protein Eight, 2.4 oz	260	8	23
Protein Meal Replacement, 2.5 oz	280	8	20
Complete Nutrition, 48g	190	4.5	28
Odyssey Protein, 80g	310	11	29
Pro 42, average, 3.7 oz bar	380	8	33
Promax, average, 2.7 oz bar	290	6	40
Protein Complete, avg., 1.97 oz	220	6	28
Prozone Nutrition Bar, 50g	195	6	18
Pure Protein High Protein, 1.76 oz	180	4.5	18
Pure Fit, average, 2 oz bar	235	6	27
Quaker: Fruit & Oatmeal Bites (3)	140	2.5	28
Fruit & Oatmeal Breakfast Bar	130	2.5	24
Chewy Dipps Granola Bars:			
Caramel Nut	145	6	21
Chocolate Fudge	165	8	21
Peanut Butter	155	8	19
Chewy Granola Bars: Low Fat	110	2	22
Baby Ruth; Butterfinger	120	3	22
Choc. Chip; Nestle Crunch	120	3.5	21
Peanut Butter	110	3.5	19
Peanut Butter & Choc. Chunk	120	3.5	20
Fruit & Oatmeal Bars: Apple Crisp	90	3	15
Average other flavors	140	3	26
Real Protein, 2.75 oz bar	290	5	28
Restart: Peanut Butter, 1.25 oz	140	4	10
Strawb. Banana; Chocolate	130	2.5	21
Revival Soy Bars (Direct): Per Bar			
Cool Krispy Protein:			
Choc. Temptation	220	3.5	30
Apple Cinnamon; Marsh.Krunch	220	3	33
Peanut Butter/Choc Pal, avg.	240	6	32
Low Carb, average all flavors	200	5	28

Per Bar	C	F	Cb
Rice Krispies Treats (Kellogg's): Per Bar			
Caramel Chocolate	110	3.5	19
Double Choc Chunk	100	4.5	15
Other varieties, average	110	4	16
SCAN Diet, 45g	160	2.5	26
Slim-Fast Bars: Fudge Bar, 2.8 oz	114	1.5	22
Breakfast and Lunch Bars, avg.	150	6	19
Chewy; Meal On-the-Go, avg.	220	5	36
Snack Bar, avg. all flavors	120	4	21
Snackwell's: Cereal Bars	120	0	29
Other varieties	130	3	26
Solid Protein Meal, 2.75 oz	270	6	28
Special K Cereal Bars, 0.8 oz	85	1.5	18
Spiru-tein Energy Bar, 1.4 oz	150	4	20
Steel Bar (ABB), 65g	330	6	52
Steel Pro, 85g	330	6	18
Strive (Biochem), avg., 2.1 oz	190	8	25
Sweet Rewards: Choc. Chip	110	2	23
Brownie; Fat Free	120	2	30
Think Protein Bar, 2.3 oz	280	9	18
Think Thin! Low Carb Diet,			
average all bars, 2.1 oz	250	10	22
Thunder Bar, all flavors	220	2	44
Tiger's Milk: 35g Bar	130	2.5	24
Peanut Butter varieties	150	6	19
Protein Rich	145	5	18
Tiger Sport, 65g	230	2	43
Ultimate Lo Carb, 2.1 oz	240	6	25
Ultimate Protein Bar, 78g	290	4.5	18
Universal Muscle, 56.7g	280	5	35
Usana: Nutribar, 41g	150	4	20
Fibergy Bar	100	1.5	23
Verve (Wholefoods Mkt), 2.4 oz	240	5	41
Viactive (Mead Johnson), 1.6 oz	180	4.5	29
Vyo-Pro (AST) Chocolate, 2.2 oz	210	7	17
Weider Body Shaper: Diet Protein	200	4.5	18
Protein Layered, avg., 60g	220	7	27
Whole Foods: Everyday Bars, avg.	190	4.5	18
Choc Fudge/Raspberry	172	4	17
Honey Peanut Yogurt	200	4.5	18
Worldwide Sport Nutrition:			
Pure Protein Bars, 2.75 oz			
Peanut Butter	310	10	24
Honey Nut; Maple Pecan	310	9	26
Other varieties, average	290	7	27
Xetalean (Nature's Bounty), 40g	140	4.5	21
You Are What You Eat, 56g	220	5	39
Zone Perfect, average, 1.76 oz	210	7	24

Nuts	C	F	Cb
Per 1 oz Unless Indicated			
Acorns, raw 1 oz	105	7	12
Almonds, Dried/Dry Roasted:			
Whole, 24-28 med., 1 oz	170	15	7
1/2 cup, 21/2 oz	420	37	17
Chopped, 1/2 cup, 21/4 oz	380	34	16
Sliced, 1/2 cup, 12/3 oz	280	25	12
Choc. coated (5-6), 1 oz	160	11	14
Oil Rstd *(Blue Diamond)*, 1 oz	175	17	3.5
Almond Meal (partially defatted)			
1 cup (not packed), 21/4 oz	260	11	11
Honey Roasted, 1 oz	170	13	8
Brazil Nuts, 8 medium, 1 oz	185	19	3.5
Cashews, Dry or Oil Roasted:			
14 large/18 med./26 small, 1 oz	165	14	10
1/2 cup, 2.4 oz	400	33	23
Honey Roasted, 1 oz	160	12	11
Chestnuts, avg. all: Dried, 1 oz	105	1	22
Raw/Fresh, 5-6 nuts, 1 oz	60	0	13
Canned, water chestnuts			
sliced/whole/drained, 1 oz	23	0	5
Coconut: Flesh (no shell), 1 oz	100	10	4
Raw: 1 pce. (2"x2"x1/2"), 1.6 oz	160	15	7
1/2 medium (41/2" diam.)	650	62	30
Dried (Desiccated):			
Unsweetened, 1 oz	187	18	17
Sweetened, shredded, 1 oz	140	9	13
Grated, 1/2 cup, 1.3 oz	185	12	18
Cream (canned), 1/2 cup, 5.2 oz	285	26	12
Milk (canned), 1/2 cup, 4 oz	225	24	3
Water (center liq.), 1/2 c., 41/4 oz	23	0	4.5
Filberts or Hazelnuts:			
Shelled, 18-20 nuts	180	18	4.5
Chopped, 1/4 cup	180	18	4.5
Ground, 1/4 cup	120	12	3
Ginko Nuts, can., 14 med., 1 oz	32	0	6
Hickory, 30 small nuts	190	18	5
Macadamia Nuts, shelled:			
Raw, 7 med./14 small, 1 oz	200	21	4
1/2 cup, 2.3 oz	460	48	10
Oil roasted, 1 oz	205	22	3.5
1/2 cup, 2.4 oz	490	52	8
Choc. coated, 2-3 pces, 1 oz	180	13	15
Mixed Nuts: 18-22 nuts, 1 oz	175	13	7
Planters: Dry Roasted/Honey	170	15	7
Oil Roasted, all types	180	16	7
Sweet Roasts, 26 pces, 1 oz	160	12	10
Kettle: Choc Lover's Mix, 1 oz	130	17	16

Per 1 oz Unless Indicated	C	F	Cb
Nut Toppings:			
Chopped, 1 Tbsp, 1/4 oz	40	4	1.5
Peanuts:			
Raw/Dried: In shell, 1 oz	117	10	3
Shelled, 1 oz	160	14	4.5
Boiled: 1/2 cup, 1.1 oz	102	7	7
Roasted, 30 lge./60 sml., 1 oz	165	14	6
1 cup, 5.1 oz	840	71	31
Chopped, 3 Tbsp, 1 oz	165	14	6
Planters: Oil Roasted, 1 oz	170	15	5
Beer Nuts, 1 oz pkg	170	14	7
Choc-coated, 1/2 cup, 21/2 oz	380	25	36
Cocktail, oil roasted, 1 oz	170	14	5
Dry Roasted, 1 oz	160	14	6
Honey Roasted, 1 oz	150	11	10
Honey/Dry Roasted, 1 oz	160	13	7
Spanish Oil Roasted, 1 oz	170	14	5
Sweet 'n Crunchy, 1 oz	140	8	16
Pecans: Kernel halves, 1 oz	190	19	5
(20 Jumbo or 31 large halves)			
1 cup halves, 3.8 oz	720	73	20
Chopped, 1/2 cup, 2 oz	380	30	10
Oil Roasted, 1 oz	195	20	4.5
Honey Roasted, 1 oz	200	18	5
Pilinuts, dried, 1/4 cup, 1 oz	205	23	1
Pinenuts, dried, 1 Tbsp, 10g	50	5	1.5
Pistachios:			
Unshelled, 1/2 cup, 2 oz	165	14	7
Shelled, 1/4 cup, 45 nuts, 1 oz	170	14	8
Lance, 11/8 oz package	180	14	8
Planters: Dry Roasted, 1oz	170	15	6
Fruit 'n Nut Mix, 1 oz	150	9	13
Nut Topping, 1 oz	180	16	6
Tavern Nuts, 1 oz	170	15	6
Trail Mix, 3 Tbsp, 1 oz	140	9	15
Sesame Nut Mix: *Planters,* 1 oz	160	12	8
Soy Nuts: Dry Roasted, 1 oz	130	6	9
1/2 cup, 3 oz	390	18	28
Dr Soy: Choc coated, 1 oz pkg	130	4.5	18
Honey Roasted, 1 oz pkg	140	6	21
Flavors, average, 1 oz	150	7	9
Walnuts:			
Black, 15-20 halves, 1 oz	175	16	3.5
Chopped, 1/4 cup	190	18	4
Ground, 1/4 cup	120	12	2.5
English/Persian:			
14 halves, 1 oz	185	18	5
Chopped, 1/4 cup	195	19	5

Seeds ◆ Supplements

Seeds | C | F | Cb |

Seeds	C	F	Cb
Alfalfa Seeds, sprouted, 1/2 c., 1/2 oz	5	0	1
Caraway, Fennel, 1 tsp	10	0.5	1
Cottonseed Kernels, rst., 1 Tbsp	50	4	2
Flax Seeds, 3 Tbsp, 1 oz	150	10	11
Lotus Seeds, dried, 1/2 c., 1/2 oz	50	0.5	10
Poppy Seeds, 1 tsp	15	1	1
Pumpkin & Squash Seeds, whole:			
Roasted/Tamari, 1 oz	125	5.5	3
1/2 cup (32g)	140	6	3.5
Dried, 1 oz	155	13	4
Safflower Kernels, dried, 1 oz	150	11	10
Sesame Seeds: Dried, 1 Tbsp, 9g	50	4.5	2
Roasted/Toasted, 1 oz	160	14	7
Sunflower Kernels/Seed:			
Dry Roasted, 1 Tbsp, 8g	45	4	1.5
1/4 cup, 1 oz	160	14	6
Oil Roasted, 1/4 cup, 1 oz	180	17	6
Watermelon, dried, 1/4 cup, 1 oz	160	14	4.5

Quick Guide

Peanut Butter

Average All Brands:

1 tsp, 6g	35	3	1.5
1 Tbsp, 0.6 oz, (17g)	105	8.5	3.5
2 Tbsp, 1.2 oz, (34g)	210	17	7
1 oz Quantity (28g)	170	14	6
1/2 cup, 5 oz	850	70	30
Jif "Sensations" Berry Blend, 1 T.	100	8.5	5
Chocolate Silk, 1 Tbsp, 0.6 oz	95	7.5	7
Peanut Wonder, 1 Tbsp	50	2	5.5
Smucker's Honey Swtnd., 1 Tbsp	100	8	4
Goober Grape/Strawb., 1 Tbsp	90	5	4
Skippy, honeynut, 1 Tbsp, 16g	95	8	4

Other Nut & Seed Butters

Almond Butter, 1 Tbsp, 1/2 oz	105	9	2.5
Almond Butter Honey Roasted	90	7	5.5
Beanut Butter, 1 Tbsp, 1/2 oz	88	5.5	7
Cashew Butter, 1 Tbsp	92	7	4.5
Cashew Peanut Date Butter	95	7	4
Hazelnut Butter, 1 Tbsp	100	10	2.5
Pecan Butter, 1 Tbsp	110	11	3.5
Pistachio Butter, 1 Tbsp	100	8.5	5
Sesame Butter/Tahini, 1 Tbsp	30	3	1
1 Tbsp, 1/2 oz	90	8.5	2
Sunflower Seed Butter, 1 Tbsp	95	8	4

Supplements | C | F | Cb |

Supplements	C	F	Cb
Aloe Vera Juice, undiluted, 2 fl.oz	5	0	1
Barlean's Flax Oil, 3 capsules	27	3	0
Cod Liver Oil, 1 Tbsp	120	13	0
Evening Primrose Oil, capsules, 1	5	0.5	0
Fiber Supplements: Tabs, 1	1	0	0
Bios Life 2, 1 packet	10	0	2
Metamucil, 1 packet	5	0	0
Regular, 1 rounded Tbsp	34	0	8
Sugar-Free, 1 Tbsp	6	0	1
Fish Oil Capsules, average, 1	10	1	0
Flax Oil Capsules, 2	10	1	0
Garlic Tablets/Capsules, each	3	0	0
Lecithin Granules, 1 Tbsp, 10g	50	5	1
Protein; Powders, average, 1 oz	100	0.5	0
Tablets, 20 tabs, 1/2 oz	70	0	0
Seaweed: Dried, 1 oz	85	0.5	22
Soaked, drained, 1 oz	15	0.5	3
Spirulina, 1 tablet	2	0	0.5
Vitamins/Minerals: Tabs/Caps, 1	2	0	0
Vitamin E Capsules, each	5	0.5	0
Yeast: Tablets, 2 tabs	4	0	0.5
Flakes, 1 heaping Tbsp, 1/3 oz	30	0.5	4
Powder, 1 heaping Tbsp, 1/2 oz	50	0.5	6

Cough & Pharmaceutical

	C	F	Cb
Cough/Cold Syrups: *Per Tablespoon*			
Regular: w. sugar, 1 Tbsp	35	0	9
w. alcohol, 1 Tbsp	46	0	9
Sugar-Free *(Diabetic Tussin),* 1 T.	0	0	0
Cough Drops/Lozenges: See Page 135			
Antacids: Average, 1 tablet	4	0	1
Liquid, 1 Tbsp	6	0	1
***Sudafed* Syrup,** 1 tsp	14	0	3
***Tylenol* Liquid:** Child, 1 tsp	17	0	4
Extra Strength, 1 tsp	11	0	3

𝒩ut eaters are healthier and live longer say medical researchers.

Nuts are a nutritious source of protein, vitamins, minerals and fiber. Their fat and fiber content can help to lower blood cholesterol, but watch the quantity if overweight.

Fresh Fruit

Weights As Purchased	C	F	Cb
Acerola, 1 cup, 20 pcs, 3 1/2 oz	30	0	7.5
Apples: whole, average all varieties:			
1 small (4 per lb), 4 oz	70	0	17
1 medium (3 per lb), 5 1/2 oz	90	0	23
1 large (2 per lb), 8 oz	135	0	34
I extra large, 11 oz	185	0	46
without skin, 1/2 medium	35	0	9
Caramel Apple, 1 medium	170	0	42
Nut Coated, 1 medium	230	5	46
Apricots: 1 small (12 per lb)	17	0	4
1 medium (8 per lb), 2 oz	25	0	6
1 large (5-6 per lb), 3 oz	35	0	8
Avocado (w/out seed/skin):			
Average, 1/2 medium, 3 1/2 oz	160	15	6
1 salad slice, 1/2 oz	25	2	1
Mashed/Puree, 2 Tbsp, 1 oz	50	4.5	2
1/4 cup, 2 oz	90	9	4
Californian, 1/2 medium, 3 oz	160	14	8
Mashed/Puree, 1/2 c., 4 oz	210	18	12
Florida, 1/2 medium, 5 1/2 oz	170	13	14
Mashed/Puree, 1/2 c., 4 oz	125	10	9
1/2 cup cubed, 3 oz	105	8	8

Note: Avocados are nutritious and contain no cholesterol. Fat is mainly monounsaturated and benefits blood cholesterol. Excellent substitute for butter or margarine on bread or crackers.

	C	F	Cb
Banana: 1 small (4 lb), 4 oz	55	0	13
1 medium (3 per lb), 5 oz	80	0	20
1 large (2 1/2 per lb), 7 oz	105	0	25
w/out skin, 1 medium, 3 1/4 oz	80	0	20
1/2 cup, mashed, 4 oz	105	0	25
Berries: (Blueberries/Black/Boysenberries)			
1/2 cup, 2.5 oz	40	0	10
1 pint, 14 oz	220	1	56
Breadfruit, 1/2 cup, 4 oz	115	0	28
Cantaloupe: Flesh/no skin, 1 oz	8	0	2
1/2 small, 20oz (w.skin/seeds)	125	1	30
1/2 medium, 28oz (w.skin/seeds)	175	1.5	42
1 slice, 2.5 oz (w/out skin)	20	0	5
1 cup pieces/balls, 5.5 oz	55	0	13
Carambola (Star Fruit), 1 med	50	0	4
Cassava, 1/3 cup	120	0	27
Cherimoya (Custard Apple), 4 oz	110	1	27
Cherries: Sweet, 8 fruit, 2 oz	40	0	10
1/2 lb (30 cherries)	145	0	37
Sour, 8 fruit, 2 oz	25	0	6
1/2 lb (30 cherries)	100	0	23
Clementine, 1 med., 3 oz	50	0	15

Weights As Purchased	C	F	Cb
Coconut: Fresh, 1 piece, 1 oz	100	10	3
Shredded, fresh, 1/2 cup	150	14	6
Sweetened, dried, 1/2 cup	235	16	22
Crabapples, 1/2 cup slices, 2 oz	40	0	9
Cranberries, 1/2 cup, 2 oz	20	0	5
Currants ~ Per 1/2 Cup			
European Black, raw, 2 oz	35	0	8
Red & White, raw, 2 oz	30	0	7
Custard Apple, raw, 4 oz	110	1	27
Dates ~ See Dried Fruits			
Dragon Pearl Fruit, med., 11.6 oz	100	0.5	23
Durian, flesh, 4 oz	165	6	28
Elderberries, 1/2 cup, 2 1/2 oz	55	0	13
Feijoas, 1 medium, 2 1/2 oz	35	0	7
Figs, green/black: 1 med., 2 oz	40	0	10
1 large, 3 oz	60	0	15
Fruit Salad, fresh, average,			
1/2 cup, 3 1/2 oz	60	0	15
1 cup, 7 oz	120	0	30
Gooseberries, raw, 1/2 c., 2 1/2 oz	30	0	7
Grapefruit: Average all types,			
1/2 fruit, 10 oz (6 oz flesh)	55	0	13
1 cup sections w. juice, 8 oz	75	0	17
Grapes: Average, 1 cup, 5 1/2 oz	100	0	24
1 small bunch, 4 oz	70	0	17
1 medium bunch, 7 oz	125	0	31
1 large bunch, 16 oz	285	0	71
Granadilla, flesh, 3 1/2 oz	95	0	23
Groundcherries, 1/2 cup, 2 1/2 oz	35	0	8
Guava: 1 fruit, 4 oz	80	0	15
1/2 cup, 3 oz	40	0	9
Honeydew, 1 wedge (7" x 2" wide),			
8 oz (with skin)	50	0	12
1 cup cubes/balls, 6 oz	60	0	14
Honey Murcots, 1 only, 5 oz	45	0	11
Jaboticaba, flesh, 4 oz	75	2	15
Jackfruit, flesh, 1/8 average, 4 oz	105	0	25
Jambos (Brazil Cherry), flesh 4 oz	35	0	8
Java-Plum, 4 plums, 1/2 oz	25	0	6
Jujube, 3 oz	65	0	16
Kiwifruit, 1 medium, 3 oz	45	0	11
1 large, 4 oz	60	0	15
Kumquats, 5 medium, 3 1/2 oz	60	0	15
Kiwano, 1/2 medium, 5 oz	35	0	8
Langsat, Duku, 1 medium, 2 oz	25	0	5
Lemon: 1 medium, 4 oz	20	0	5
1 wedge, 1 oz	5	0	1.5
Peel, 1 Tbsp	4	0	1
Limes, 1 only, 2 oz	20	0	5
Loganberries, froz., 1/2 c., 2 1/2 oz	40	0	9

145

Fresh Fruit (Cont)

Weights As Purchased	C	F	Cb
Longans, 5 fruit, $^1/_2$ oz	10	0	2.5
Loquats, 4 fruit, $2^1/_4$ oz	25	0	6
Lychees, 4 fruit, $2^1/_4$ oz	25	0	6
Mamey Apple, 1 whole, 3 lb	430	4	100
$^1/_4$ fruit (1 cup flesh), 7 oz	100	1	23
Mandarin: 1 small, 3 oz	25	0	6
1 medium, 4 oz	35	0	8
1 large, 6 oz	55	0	13
Mango: flesh, $^1/_2$ cup sl., 3 oz	48	0	11
1 whole, medium, 11 oz	140	0	34
Melon, avg, 1 cup, cubes/balls, 6 oz	60	0	14
Monstera Deliciosa (Taxonia),			
Edible part, 4 oz	50	0	11
Mulberries, 20 fruit, 1 oz	15	0	3
Nashi Fruit (Asian Pear), 1 med., 7 oz	85	0	21
Nectarines, 1 medium, 4 oz	50	0	12
1 large, $5^1/_2$ oz	70	0	17
Oheloberries, $^1/_2$ cup, $2^1/_2$ oz	20	0	5
Olives (Pickled): Green, 10 lrg, $1^1/_2$ oz	45	5	0.5
Ripe, Grk. Style, 10 med., 1 oz	70	7	2
Ripe (Black), Californian:			
1 small/medium	5	0.5	0.5
1 large/extra large	6	0.5	0.5
1 jumbo	7	0.5	0.5
1 colossal	11	1	0.5
1 super colossal	13	1	1
Oranges: Average all varieties,			
1 small, 5 oz (with skin)	50	0	12
1 medium (3" diam.), 7 oz	70	0	17
1 large, 10 oz	100	0	24
Flesh only, 1 cup, 6 oz	80	0	19
Californian Valencia,			
1 medium ($2^3/_4$" diam.), 6 oz	60	0	15
Californ. Navels (3" diam.), 7 oz	60	0	15
Sunkist Navel, 14 oz	130	0	32
Florida Orange, 1 medium, 7 oz	70	0	17
Peel, 1 Tbsp	0	0	0
Papaya: $^1/_2$ cup, cubed, $2^1/_2$ oz	30	0	7
1 medium, 16 oz	120	0	28
Green (unripe), $^1/_2$ cup, $3^1/_2$ oz	20	0	5
Passionfruit, 1 medium, $1^1/_4$ oz	20	0	4.5
PawPaw (see Papaya)			
Peaches: 1 med. (4 per lb), 4 oz	35	0	8
1 large, 6 oz	55	0	13
1 extra large, 10 oz	90	0	22

Weights As Purchased	C	F	Cb
Pears: Bartlett, 1 small, 4 oz	60	0	15
1 medium, 6 oz	90	0	22
1 large, 8 oz	120	0	30
1 cup slices, 5.8oz	100	0.5	25
Asian, 1 medium, 7 oz	85	0	21
Bosc, 6 oz	90	0	22
D'Anjou, 1 medium, 8 oz	120	0	30
Forelle, 1 medium, 7 oz	85	0	21
Red Pear, 5 oz	80	0	20
Seckel (Wash'ton), $2^1/_4$ oz	35	0	9
Pepino, $^1/_2$ medium, 4 oz	20	0	4
Persimmons: Native, 1 oz	30	0	7
Japan. ($2^1/_2$"d. x $2^1/_2$"h), 7 oz	120	0	30
Seedless (Maui), 1 med., 5 oz	100	0	25
Pineapple (no skin):			
1 thin slice, ($^1/_2$"), 2 oz	28	0	7
1 thick slice, ($^3/_4$"), 3 oz	40	0	10
1 cup, diced, $5^1/_2$ oz	75	0	19
1 medium, $1^1/_2$ lb (peeled)	525	0	130
Canned: See Page 148			
Pitanga, 3 fruit, 1 oz	6	0	1
Plaintains, $^1/_2$ cup slices, $2^1/_2$ oz	90	0	22
Plums: Average all types,			
Mini/Damson, (1" diam.), $^1/_2$ oz	8	0	2
Small ($1^3/_4$" diam.), 2 oz	30	0	7
Medium ($2^1/_4$" diam.), 3 oz	45	0	10
Large ($2^1/_2$" diam.), 4 oz	65	0	15
Pluot (plum-apricot), 1 med., 5 oz	80	0	19
Pomegranates, $^1/_2$ fruit, 5 oz	55	0	13
Pummelo, flesh, $^1/_2$ cup, 4 oz	35	0	8
Prickly Pears, 1 fruit, 5 oz	50	0	11
Quince, 1 medium, $3^1/_2$ oz	55	0	14
Rambutan (Rambotang),			
Red/Yellow, 1 medium, 2 oz	15	0	4
Raspberries, $^1/_2$ cup, 2 oz	30	0	7
Rhubarb, raw, $^1/_2$ cup, 2 oz	15	0	3
Sapodilla (Chico), 1 md., $7^1/_2$ oz	140	2	33
Sapotes, $^1/_2$ medium, 5.5 oz	150	0	37
Satsuma Tangerine, 1 med., 3 oz	50	0	15
Soursop, 1 cup pulp, 8 oz	150	0	38
Strawberries: 1 cup, $5^1/_2$ oz	45	0	10
6 medium/3 large, 2 oz	15	0	3
1 pint, 12 oz	95	0	22
Chocolate Dipped, 2 medium	45	2.5	6
Sugar Apples, $^1/_2$ cup pulp, 4 oz	120	0	30
Tamarillo, 1 medium, 3 oz	20	0	3
Tamarind: 1 fruit, $^1/_4$ oz	5	0	0

Weights As Purchased	C	F	Cb
Tangelo: 1 small, 4 oz	30	0	7
1 medium, 5 oz	40	0	9
Tangelo: 1 large, 7 oz	55	0	12
Tangerine, 1 medium, 4 oz	50	0	12
Tangor, 1 medium, 4 oz	35	0	7
Tomatillos, (3) 3 oz	20	0	4
Tomato: Grape, 3 medium	8	0	2
Yellow Tear Drop, 4 med., 1 oz	8	0	2
Cherry, 1 medium, 3/4 oz	5	0	1
1 small, 3 oz	25	0	6
1 medium, 5 oz	35	0	8
1 medium slice	5	0	1
1 large, 7 oz	50	0.5	11
1 giant salad, 10 oz	70	1	16
Canned Tomatoes/Products: See Page 91			
Tree Tomato (Tamarillo), 3 oz	20	0	5
Ugli Fruit, Tangelo type, 5 oz	40	0	9
Watermelon: Flesh only/no skin, 1 oz	9	0	2
1 cup cubes or balls, 4 1/2 oz	50	0	12
1 thick (1") slice (1/4 circle, 4 1/2"radius)			
9 oz w. skin / 5 1/2 oz no skin	50	0	12
1 thin (1/2") slice (1/4 circle)	25	0	6
1 thick (1") slice (1/2 circle)			
18 oz w.skin	100	1	24
1 whole melon (15" long, 7 1/2"diam.)			
20 lb w.skin/10lb no skin	1450	19	324
Wax Jambu (Rose Apple), 2 oz	10	0	2

Dried Fruit

	C	F	Cb
Apples, 5 rings, 1 oz	75	0	18
Apricots, 8 halves, 1 oz	65	0	15
Banana Chips, 1/2 cup, 1 1/2 oz	160	5	18
Banana Flakes, 4 Tbsp, 1 oz	80	0	20
Cranberries, swtn, dr.,1/3 c., 1.4 oz	130	0	33
Currants, 1/4 cup, 1 1/4 oz	100	0	24
Dates: 5 medium dates, 1 1/2 oz	120	0	28
Large Calif., 3 dates, 2 oz	160	0	37
1/2 cup, chopped, 3 oz	240	0	57
Figs, 3 medium figs, 2 oz	145	0	34
Longans; Lychees, 1 oz	80	0	19
Mango Slices, 4 strips, 1 oz	70	0	15
Mixed Fruit, 1 oz	70	0	16
Papaya Spears, 1 oz	75	0	17
Peaches, 2 halves, 1 oz	60	0	14
Pears, 3 halves, 2 oz	75	0	17
Pineapple, 1 oz	80	0	18
Prunes (dried Plums): w. pits, 1 oz	60	0	14
1 Medium (60/lb)	16	0	4
1 Large (50/lb)	22	0	5
1 Extra Large (40/lb)	27	0	6
Without pits, 4 med., 1 oz	70	0	17
Cooked: w. sugar, 1/2 c, 5 oz	200	0	47
w/out sugar, 1/2 c, 4 1/2 oz	125	0	30
Raisins: 2 Tbsp, 1 oz package	90	0	22
1/2 cup, 2.8 oz	260	0	62
Sunsweet: Fruitlings, 1/3 c., 1.5 oz	130	0	31
Plums (5) 1.4 oz	100	0	24

Candied Glacé Fruit

	C	F	Cb
Apricot, 1 medium, 1 oz	100	0	25
Cherry, 3 large, 1/2 oz	50	0	12
Citron/Fruit Peel, 1 oz	90	0	21
Fig, 1 piece, 1 oz	90	0	21
Ginger, 1 oz	95	0	23
Pineapple, 1 slice, 1 1/4 oz	120	0	30

Fruit Leather/Rolls

	C	F	Cb
Average All Brands, 1 oz	100	0	24
Fruit By The Foot, 1 roll, 3/4 oz	80	0	17
Fruit Gushers, 1 pouch, 1 oz	90	1	20
Fruit Roll-Ups, 1 roll, 1/2 oz	50	0	12
Stretch Island Leathers, 2 pces, 1 oz	90	0	21
Sunkist Fruit Roll, 1 roll	75	0	18
Other Fruit Confectionery/Snacks/Bars			
~ See Snacks/Granola Bars Page 140-142			

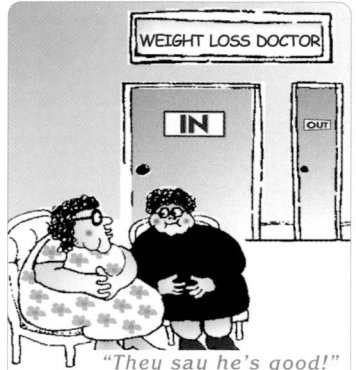

WEIGHT LOSS DOCTOR

IN

OUT

"They say he's good!"

Canned/Bottled Fruit ◆ Fruit Snacks

Canned/Bottled Fruit

Solids & Liquids: Per 1/2 Cup (Approx. 4 1/2 oz)	C	F	Cb
Apples: sweetened	70	0	17
Apricots: In water/diet	35	0	9
In juice/lite	60	0	15
In syrup	105	0	27
Black/Blueberries: Heavy syrup	115	0	30
In light syrup	110	0	26
Cherries, pitted, in water	55	0	14
In light syrup	85	0	21
In heavy syrup	110	0	28
In extra heavy syrup	130	0	33
Maraschino, 5, 1 oz	50	0	12
Pie, 2/3 cup, 5 oz	60	0	14
Fruit Salad: In water/diet	35	0	9
In juice/Light	60	0	16
In heavy syrup	95	0	25
Gooseberries: Light syrup	90	0	23
Grapefruit: Juice pack	45	0	15
In light syrup	75	0	20
Lychees: Canned, 1/2 cup, 4.5 oz	105	0	26
Mixed Fruit: In water/diet	40	0	10
In fruit juices/light syrup	60	0	15
In heavy syrup	100	0	25
Peaches (halves/slices): In water/diet	30	0	8
In juice/light	50	0	14
In light syrup	70	0	20
drained, 1/2 peach	40	0	11
In heavy syrup	100	0	26
Pears: In water/diet	35	0	10
In juice/light	60	0	16
In heavy syrup	100	0	26
Pineapple: All types			
In own juice	70	0	17
In heavy syrup	90	0	22
Slices, drained, 2 slices			
In own juice, drained	30	0	7
In heavy syrup, drained	45	0	11
Plums: In water	50	0	14
In juice	75	0	20
In light syrup, 3 plums	85	0	21
In heavy syrup, 1/2 cup	160	0	41
Prunes: In heavy syrup	120	0	32
In Liqueur, 1/2 cup, 125g	280	0	70
In Water, 1/2 cup	135	0	32
Raspberries, in heavy syrup	120	0	30
Strawberries: In water	25	0	7
In heavy syrup	120	0	31
Tropical Fruit Salad: In light syrup	80	0	18
In heavy syrup	95	0	21

Fruit Snack Cups C F Cb

	C	F	Cb
Mott's: Healthy Harvest, 4 oz cup	50	0	13
Blues Clues; Fruitsations, 4 oz c.	90	0	22
Del Monte Fruit Cups: Per 4 oz Cup			
Fruit Cocktail: In water/diet	40	0	11
In juice/light	55	0	15
In light syrup	80	0	21
In heavy syrup	95	0	25
Mandarin Orange cup	70	0	17
Mandarin Oranges: In water	40	0	10
In light syrup	80	0	20
Peach/Pear/Lite	50	0	13
Fruit Rageous cup	90	0	22
Fruit to Go, 4 oz cup	70	0	18
Pop Top Snack Cans:			
Fruit Cocktail, 8 1/2 oz can	190	0	47
Lite Sliced Peaches, 8 1/4 oz can	115	0	28
Dole Fruit Bowls			
4 oz Bowls: Peaches/Mandarin Or.	70	0	17
Mixed Fruit	80	0	19
Pineapple/Tropical Fruit	65	0	15
7 oz Bowls: Pineapple Chunks	90	0	23
Sliced Peaches	120	0	29
Tropical Fruit	100	0	25
Fruit 'n Gel Bowls 4.3 oz: Reg.	90	0	22
Reduced Sugar	50	0	13
Tree Top: Fruit Rocketz, 1 tube	45	0	11
Natural Apple, 1 Pkg., 4 oz	50	0	12
Vons: Mixed Fruit,			
In heavy syrup, 1 cup, 4.5 oz	90	0	22
In lite syrup, 1 cup, 4.5 oz	60	0	13

Apple & Fruit Sauces

	C	F	Cb
Apple Sauce:			
Regular/sweetened, 2 Tbsp, 1.1 oz	23	0	5
4 oz package cup	80	0	20
1/2 cup, 4.5 oz	90	0	22
Mott's Cinnamon, 1/2 cup, 4.5 oz	110	0	27
Cranberry Sce: Whole Berry, 1 T.	14	0	3
1/4 cup, 2 1/2 oz	110	0	27
Jellied Cranberry, 1/4 cup	110	0	27

Vegetables

Vegetables

Edible Portion ~ Raw Weight | **C** | **F** | **Cb**

Item	C	F	Cb
Alfalfa Sprouts, 1/2 cup, 1/2 oz	5	0	1
Artichokes, Globe/French:			
1 medium, 4 1/2 oz	65	0	15
1 large, 8 oz	105	0	23
Artichoke Heart, 1/2 cup, 3 oz	40	0	10
Asparagus, raw/froz.: 4 med. spears	15	0	3
Cuts & tips, 1/2 cup, 3 oz	25	0	5
Bamboo Shoots, ckd, 1/2 c, 4 oz	15	0	3
Beans: Green/Snap, 1/2 c, 2 oz	20	0	4
Dried Beans, average all types:			
(Kidney, Brown, Haricot, Lima,			
Mung, Navy, Pinto, Red, White)			
Raw, 2 Tbsp, 1 oz	95	0.5	18
1 cup, 7 oz	665	3	126
Cooked, 1 oz	35	0	7
1/2 cup, 3 oz	105	0	21
Bean Sprouts, avg, 1/2 cup, 3 oz	25	0	3
Beets: Cooked, 1/2 c, slices, 3 oz	25	0	6
1 beet, 2" diam., 2 oz	17	0	4
Beet Greens, ckd, 1/2 c., 2 1/2 oz	20	0	4
Bell Pepper: See Peppers			
Bitter Melon/Gourd, 1 c. pieces, 4 oz	22	0	5
Black Eyed Peas, ckd, 1/2 c., 2 oz	160	0	32
Bok Choy (Chinese Chard), 3 oz	13	0	3
Breadfruit, 1/4 small fruit	100	0	25
Broadbeans (Fava Beans):			
Green (in pod), raw: 4 pods			
(3 1/2 oz w. shell; 1.2 oz beans)	30	0	6
1 cup beans (no shell), 4 1/2 oz	110	1	22
Mature Seeds: Raw, 1 c., 5.3 oz	510	2	87
Cooked, 1/2 cup, 3 oz	95	0	17
Broccoli: Raw, 1/2 cup, 1 1/2 oz	12	0	2
1 spear (5 oz edible)	40	0	8
Cooked, 1/2 cup, 3 oz	25	0	5
BroccoSprouts, 1/2 cup, 1 oz	16	0	2
Brussel Sprouts, ckd, 1/2 c, 3 oz	35	0	8
Butterbeans, ckd, 1/2 c, 3 oz	90	0	20
Cabbage: Avg, ckd, 1/2 c., 2 1/2 oz	15	0	2
Raw, shred., 1/2 cup, 1 1/4 oz	8	0	1
Cactus (Nopal), chopped, 1 cup	60	0	14
Carrot: Ckd, 1/2 cup slices, 3 oz	35	0	8
Raw, 1 medium (7 1/2"), 3 oz	33	0	8
Raw, 1 lb, (5-6 med)	175	0	44
4 sticks (4"), 1 1/2 oz	15	0	3
Shredded, 1/2 cup, 2 oz	25	0	6
Cauliflower: 3 florets, 1/2 c., 3 oz	15	0	3
1/2 medium, 15 oz raw	100	0	20

Vegetables (Cont)

Edible Portion ~ Raw Weight | **C** | **F** | **Cb**

Item	C	F	Cb
Celeriac, 1/2 cup, raw, 2 3/4 oz	30	0	7
Celery: 1 stalk, 7 1/2", 1 1/2 oz	5	0	1
Diced, 1/2 cup, 2 1/4 oz	10	0	3
Chard (Swiss), 1/2 cup, 3 oz	20	0	4
Chayote Squash, 4 1/2 oz	30	0	7
Chick Peas (Garbanzo Beans):			
Dry, 1 cup, 6 oz	550	10	92
Cooked, 1 cup, 6 oz	270	4	45
Chicory, Greens, 1/2 cup, 3 oz	20	0	4
Chicory/Witloof: See Endive			
Chili Peppers: See Peppers			
Chinese Long Bean, sliced, 1 c., 3.2 oz	45	0	8
Chives, chopped, 1 Tbsp	1	0	0
Choy Sum, 3 oz	13	0	3
Cilantro (Coriander), 1 Tbsp	1	0	0
Collards, 1/2 cup, 3 oz	15	0	4
Corn, yellow/white:			
Raw, kernels, 1/2 c., 2 3/4 oz	65	1	14
Ear (5"x 1 3/4"), 5 1/2 oz	80	1	17
Trimmed to 3 1/2" long	65	1	14
Cooked, kernels, 1/4 c., 1 1/2 oz	35	0.5	7
(Also see Frozen & Canned Corn Page 151-152)			
Courgette: See Zucchini			
Cress, Garden, 1/2 cup, 1 oz	10	0	2
Cucumber, 1 whole, 11 oz	40	0	12
1/2 cup slices, 2 oz	5	0	1
Daikon Radish, 3 oz	18	0	4
Dandelion Greens, 1/2 cup, 1 oz	15	0	3
Edamame: Shelled, 2/3 cup, 3 oz	120	5	9
in pods, 4 oz	60	3	5
Eggplant: 1/4 medium, 4 oz	35	0	8
1/2 cup, 1" pieces, 1 1/2 oz	10	0	2
1 slice, fried, 1 oz	75	4	10
Endive, Belgian/French:			
1 med. head (6"), 2 1/2 oz	12	0	3
Fava Beans: See Broadbeans			
Fennel, 2 oz	10	0	2
Gai Choy Cabbage, ckd, 1 cup	20	0	5
Gai Lan (Chinese Kale), 3 oz	35	0	7
Garlic, 1 clove	4	0	1
Ginger, 1/4 cup slices, 1 oz	20	0	4
Crystallized (sugared), 1 oz	95	0	20
Horseradish, 1 pod, 3/4 oz	4	0	1
Jerusalem Artichoke, 1/2 cup	60	0	14
Jicama, raw, 1/2 cup, 3 oz	25	0	5
Kale, 1/2 cup, 3 oz	20	0	4
Kohlrabi, 1/2 cup, cooked, 3 oz	25	0	6

Edible Portion ~ Raw Weight	C	F	Cb
Leek, cooked, 1 whole, 4 oz	40	0	9
Lentils, green/brown: Dry, 1 oz	95	0.5	16
Dry, 1 cup, 6 3/4 oz	650	2	109
Cooked, 1/2 cup, 3 1/2 oz	115	0.5	20
Lettuce: 1 c., chop./shred., 2 1/2 oz	10	0	2
Butterhead, 2 leaves, 1/2 oz	2	0	0.5
Cos/Romaine, 1/2., shred., 2 1/2 oz	4	0	1
Iceberg: 1 leaf, 3/4 oz	3	0	1
1 medium head, 15-16 oz	60	0	15
Lima Beans, baby, ckd, 1/2 c., 3 oz	90	0	17
Lotus Root, 10 slices, ckd, 3 oz	60	0	15
Mung Bean Sprouts, 1/2 cup	15	0	3
Mushroom: Raw, 1/2 cup, 1 oz	10	0	2
Cooked, 1/2 cup, 2 1/2 oz	20	0	3
Mustard Greens, 1/2 cup, 1 oz	7	0	1
Nopal (Cactus), chopped, 1 cup	60	0	14
Okra, ckd, 1/2 cup, slices, 2 3/4 oz	25	0	6
Onions: Raw, 1 small, 2 oz	20	0	5
1 medium, 4 oz	40	0	9
1 large, 8 oz	80	0	19
1 jumbo, 16 oz	160	0	38
1/2 cup, chopped, 3 oz	30	0	7
Blossom/Blooming ~ *See Fast-Foods (Chili's/Outback)*			
Dehydrated flakes, 1/4 c, 1/2 oz	45	0	11
Rings, breaded/fried, 2 rings	80	5	9
Ore-Ida, 4 pces	220	11	27
Scallions, 1/2 cup, 2 oz	15	0	4
Spring, 1/4 cup, chopped, 1 oz	6	0	1
Parsley, chopped, 1/2 cup, 1 oz	10	0	2
Parsnips, 1 medium, 4 oz	80	0	20
Cooked, 1/2 cup slices, 2 3/4 oz	65	0	16
Peas: Green, 1/4 cup, 1 1/2 oz	35	0	6
Raw, with pods, 1/2 lb	70	0	13
Snow Peas (8-9 pods), 1 oz	10	0	2
Split, dry, hulled, 1 oz	50	0	10
cooked, 1 cup, 7 oz	230	1	41
Peppers: Sweet, 1 medium, 5 oz	35	0	9
Bell: 1 medium, 5 oz	25	0	6
1/2 cup, chopped, raw, 1 3/4 oz	12	0	3
1 ring (3" diam. x 1/4" thick)	2	0	0
Chile: Green/Red, 1 1/2 oz	18	0	4
Habanero, 1 only, 8g	11	0	2
Pigeon Peas, cooked, 1/2 cup	85	1	16
Pimientos, 3 medium, 3 1/2 oz	25	0	5
Poi, 1/2 cup, 4.2 oz	135	0	33
Pumpkin, mashed, 1/2 cup, 4 oz	25	0	6
Purslane, cooked, 1/2 c., 2 oz	10	0	2

Edible Portion ~ Raw Weight	C	F	Cb
Potatoes: Raw (with skin)			
1 Baby, Gourmet, 2 oz	45	0	11
1 Small, 3 oz	65	0	15
1 Medium, 5 oz	110	0	26
1 Peeled, 4 oz	90	0	22
1 Large, 8 oz	180	0	44
1 Extra large (Russet), 12 oz	270	0	65
1 Jumbo (Russet), 16 oz	360	0	88
Baked (no fat); large, 10 oz raw:			
Plain, with skin, 7 oz	220	0	51
without skin, 5 1/2 oz	145	0	34
With Toppings: + 2 tsp fat	290	8	51
+ Sour Cr./Chives, 2 Tbsp	270	6	53
+ Plain Yogurt, 2 Tbsp	240	1	55
+ Grated Cheese, 1 oz	330	9	56
+ Cottage Cheese, 2 oz	280	2	56
Mashed w. milk and fat, 1/2 c.	110	4	14
Roasted (w. fat), 1 small	155	8	21
Garlic Potatoes, 4 oz	120	2	22
Hash Browns: w. Butt. Sce, 2 1/2 oz	125	6	10
Homemade, 1/2 cup, 2 1/2 oz	165	10	10
Potato Skins: (w. Cheese topping), 1/2 whole (8 oz baking), 4 oz	240	13	22
French Fries: Small serve, 2 1/2 oz	220	12	14
Medium serve, 4 oz	350	20	22
Froz., uncooked, 18 fries, 4 oz	185	7	22
Oven-heated, 18 fries, 4 oz	185	7	22
Take-Out, 1 cup, 5 oz	440	25	28
McDonald's: Small, 2.4 oz	210	10	26
Medium, 5 oz	450	22	57
Supersize, 7 oz	610	29	77
Fried, 18 fries, 3 oz	275	15	16
Au Gratin, 1/2 cup, 4.3 oz	160	9	22
Pancakes, 1 only, 5 oz	90	5	9
Kugel, 5 oz	300	20	26
Puffs, fried, 4 puffs, 1 oz	65	3	37
Scalloped, 1/2 cup, 4 1/4 oz	105	4	13
Ore-Ida Frozen Potatoes: See Page 152			
Potato Salad, 1/2 cup, 4 1/2 oz	180	10	14
Radish: avg., 10 only, 1 1/2 oz	10	0	2
Oriental, 1/2 c. slices, 1 1/2 oz	10	0	2
Rutabagas, ckd., 1/2 c. cubes, 3 oz	30	0	7
Salsify, ckd, 1/2 c. slices, 2 1/2 oz	45	0	11
Sauerkraut, 1/2 cup, 4 oz	25	0	5
Seaweed: Average, dried, 1 oz	50	0	13
Soaked, drained, 1 oz	15	0	4
Nori/Laver, dried, 6 sheets, 1/2 oz	35	0	5

Vegetables - Fresh or Frozen

Edible Portion ~ Raw Weight	C	F	Cb
Shallots, chopped, 1 Tbsp	7	0	1
Sorrel, raw, 1/2 cup, 4 oz	23	0.5	4
Soybeans: Mature, dry, 1 oz	110	5	7
Dry, 1/2 cup, 31/2 oz	385	18	22
Cooked, 1/2 cup, 3 oz	105	5	6
(Soy Products/Tofu/Tempeh: See Page 83)			
Spinach, cooked, 1/2 cup, 3 oz	20	0	4
Creamed, 1/2 cup, 41/2 oz	140	12	8
Raw 1 cup, 1 oz	20	0	4
Squash: Summer, raw, 1/2 c., 21/4 oz	13	0	3
cooked, 1/2 cup slices, 3 oz	18	0	4
Winter, cooked,			
Acorn, 1/2 cup cubes, 31/2 oz	55	0	14
1/2 medium (10 oz raw wt.)	85	0	22
Butternut, 1/2 c. cubes, 31/2 oz	40	0	10
1/4 medium (9 oz raw wt.)	95	0	23
Spaghetti, 1/2 cup, 23/4 oz	23	0	5
Succotash, ckd, 1/2 cup, 31/3 oz	110	1	23
Sweetcorn: See Corn			
Sweet Potatoes: Cooked with Skin (no fat)			
1 medium, 4 oz	120	0	28
No skin, mashed, 1/2 c., 51/2 oz	170	0	40
Swedes, 1/2 cup, 3 oz	45	0	10
Swiss Chard, ckd, chopped, 1 c., 6 oz	35	0	7
Taro, cooked, 1/2 cup, 2 oz	95	0	23
Tomatoes *(See Pg. 147):*			
1 small, 3 oz	20	0	5
1 medium, 5 oz	35	0	8
1 large, 7 oz	45	0	10
Cooked, 1/2 cup, 41/4 oz	30	0	7
Fried, 1 small, 3 oz	60	4	5
Tomatillo, 1 oz	7	0	1
Turnips: White, ckd, 1/2 cup, 3 oz	15	0	4
Greens, ckd, 1/2 cup, 21/2 oz	15	0	3
Water Chestnuts: 4 nuts	40	0	10
1/2 cup slices, 21/4 oz	65	0	15
Watercress: 10 sprigs, 1 oz	4	0	1
Yam: Cooked, 1/2 cup, 21/2 oz	80	0	20
Baked, 1 medium (6") 8 oz	260	0	62
1 large (9") 12 oz	390	0	93
Yardlong Bean, 1 pod, 1/2 oz	7	0	1
Yucca Root, 1/2 cup, 2.5 oz	60	0	14
Zucchini: 1 medium, 10 oz	45	0	10
1/2 cup slices, cooked, 3 oz	13	0	3

Frozen Vegetables

Birds Eye	C	F	Cb
Brocc./Carrots/W. Chestnuts, 1 cup	35	0	6
Broccoli/Corn/Red Peppers, 3/4 cup	50	0.5	11
Broccoli/Cauli./Carrots, 1 cup	30	0	4
Brussels Sprouts/Cauli./Carrots	35	0	5
Carrots/Corn/Green Beans, 2/3 cup	60	0.5	11
Cauliflower/Carrots/Pea Pods, 1 cup	30	0	5
Chopped Spinach, 1/3 cup	20	0	2
Baby: Bean & Carrot Blend, 1 cup	30	0	5
Broccoli Florets, 1 cup	25	0	4
Corn & Bean Blend, 3/4 cup	60	0.5	12
Pea Blend, 3/4 cup	40	0	7
Sweet Peas, 2/3 cup	70	0.5	12
White Corn, 2/3 cup	110	1	22
Simply Grillin':			
Garden Herb, 1 cup, 4.3 oz	140	6	19
Potatoes & Onions, 1 c., 4.4 oz	180	7	25
Rstd Corn & Pot., 3/4 cup, 3.5 oz	140	5	19
Roasted Garlic, 1 c., 31/2 oz	120	4.5	17
Pasta Secrets: Ranch, 1 c., 6.6 oz	300	15	29
Italian Pesto, 1 cup, 6.4 oz	240	9	32
Primavera, 1 c. 6.7 oz	230	10	26
Three Cheese, 1 cup, 6 oz	230	8	31
Zesty Garlic, 1 cup, ckd, 6 oz	240	10	31
Stir Fry: *Prepared (Includes Pasta)*			
Asparagus, 2 cups	90	0.5	16
Green Bean, 13/4 cup	100	0.5	19
Voila! Meals: See Page 62			

Green Giant	C	F	Cb
Vegetables: Asparagus Cuts, 2/3 c.	25	0	4
Corn: Nibblers, 1 ear	70	0.5	14
Extra Sweet Niblets, 2/3 cup	70	1	13
S/Western & Rst Peppers, 3/4 c.	90	1	18
Green Bean Casserole, 2/3 cup	100	5	11
Honey Glazed Carrots, 1 cup	90	3.5	13
Le Sueur Baby Sweet Peas, 2/3 cup	60	0.5	11
Spinach, 1/2 cup	25	0	3
Veges In Cheese & Cream Sauce: *Prepared*			
Alfredo Vegetables, 3/4 cup	80	3	9
Broccoli & Cheese, 2/3 cup	70	2.5	9
Brocc., Cauliflower, Carrots, 2/3 c.	70	2.5	10
Cauliflower & Cheese Sce, 1/2 cup	60	2.5	8
Creamed Spinach, 1/2 cup	80	3	9
Cream Style Corn, 1/2 cup	110	1	23
Green Bean Casserole, 2/3 cup	90	5	9

Vegetables - Frozen, Canned, Bottled

Frozen (Cont)   **C F Cb**

Green Giant (Cont)

Rice & Vegetables: *Prepared*

	C	F	Cb
Cheesy Rice & Brocc., 1 pkt, 10 oz	300	5	56
Oriental Rice, 1 pkt, 10 oz	340	12	52
Rice Medley, 1 pkt, 10 oz	280	4	52
Rice Pilaf, 1 pkt, 10 oz	230	3.5	44
White & Wild Rice, 1 pkt, 10 oz	280	6	51
French Fries: Country, 18 fries, 3 oz	120	4	19
Crispers 1 pkt, 3 oz	210	12	23
Crispy Crunchies, 13 fries, 3 oz	160	8	20
Fast Food Fries, 35 fries, 3 oz	160	7	22

Ore-Ida (As Purchased):

Pasta Accents: *Per Cup (Cooked)*

	C	F	Cb
Alfredo Broccoli	105	4	14
Crmy Cheddar w. Broc./Carrots	125	4	18
Garden Herb	115	3.5	16
Garlic Seas. w. Broc/Corn/Carrots	130	5	18
Primavera	140	4.5	19
Three Cheese	150	4.5	21
White Cheddar	135	4	18
Funky Fries: Cinna-Stiks (17) 3 oz	300	17	37
Cocoa Crispers, 17 pces, 3 oz	300	16	31
Crunchy Rings, 11 pces, 3 oz	230	11	26
Kool Blue, 17 pces, 3 oz	250	15	21
Golden Crinkles, 13 pces, 3 oz	120	3.5	19
Golden Fries, 17 pces, 3 oz	120	4	20
Golden Twirls, 17 pces, 3 oz	160	7	22
Oven Chips, 7 pces, 3 oz	160	7	22
Shoestrings, 40 pces, 3 oz	150	6	22
Steak Fries, 9 fries, 3 oz	110	3.3	19
Texas Crispers, 8 pces, 3 oz	140	6	20
Waffle Fries, 9 fries, 3 oz	150	7	21
Zesties, 12 pces, 3 oz	150	7	20
Hash Browns: Toaster, 2 patties	220	12	25
Potatoes O'Brien, ³/₄ c., 2 oz	60	0	14
Onion Rings: Gourmet, 4 pces, 3 oz	210	10	28
Onion Ringers, 6 pces, 3.2 oz	220	12	25
Sweet Potatoes: 4 oz	80	0	18
Tater Tots: 9 pces, 3 oz	170	8	21
Mini, 19 pces, 3 oz	180	10	18
Onion 9 pces, 3 oz	150	7	21
Twiced Baked: Potatoes, 1, 5 oz	190	7	26

TGI Friday's

	C	F	Cb
Potato Skins, 3 pces, 3¹/₂ oz	210	11	19

Wild Oats: Oven Fries, (18) 3 oz | 130 | 4 | 24

Potato Poppers (Bites), (10) 3 oz | 130 | 8 | 14

Canned/Bottled   **C F Cb**

Solids & Liquid

	C	F	Cb
Artichoke Hearts: Plain, 1 oz (1)	30	0	8
Marinated, 1 oz	60	5	2
Asparagus, ¹/₂ cup, 4¹/₂ oz	20	0	3
Bamboo Shoots, 1 cup, 4¹/₂ oz	25	0	4
Bean Salad, ¹/₂ cup, 3 oz	90	0	23
Bean Sprouts, ²/₃ cup	10	0	2
Beans: Green, ¹/₂ cup, 4¹/₄ oz	20	0	4
Baked Beans, ¹/₂ cup, 4¹/₂ oz	120	<1	18
Butter Beans, ¹/₂ cup, 4¹/₂ oz	90	0	20
Italian, cut, ¹/₂ cup, 4¹/₂ oz	30	0	7
Kidney Beans, ¹/₂ cup, 4¹/₂ oz	105	<1	20
Lima Beans, ¹/₂ cup, 4¹/₂ oz	80	0	15
Pinto Beans, ¹/₂ cup, 4¹/₂ oz	100	<1	20
Beets: Sliced/Whole, ¹/₂ c., 4¹/₂ oz	35	0	7
Crinkle/Pickled (Del Monte) ¹/₂ c.	80	0	20
Carrots: Sliced, ¹/₂ cup	35	0	8
Honey Glazed (Green Giant) ¹/₂ c.	45	3.5	13
Corn: Kernels, ¹/₂ cup	90	1	14
Drained Solids, ¹/₂ cup, 3oz	65	0.5	15
Creamed style, ¹/₂ cup, 4¹/₂ oz	100	0.5	24
Garbanzo/Chick Peas, 3 oz	100	2	20
Green Chilies: diced, 2 Tbsp,	5	0	1
Hearts of Palm, (1), 1.2 oz	9	0	2
Mushrooms: ¹/₂ cup, 2¹/₂ oz	20	0	4
in Butter Sauce, 2 oz	30	1	3
Onions: Pickled, 1 med., ³/₄ oz	10	0	2
Cocktail, 1 onion	2	0	0.5
Peas, ¹/₂ cup, 3 oz	60	0	10
Peppers: Hot Chilli, 1 only, 1 oz	8	0	2
Sweet, undrained, 2¹/₂ oz	15	0	3
Jalapeno, w. liq., ¹/₂ c. chopped	17	0	3
Fried, drain, 2 Tbsp	60	5	3
Salsa, average all types, 2 Tbsp	15	0	3.5
Sauerkraut, undrained, ¹/₂ c., 4 oz	25	0	6
Spinach, ¹/₂ cup, 3¹/₂ oz	25	0	3.5
Succotash: w. Cr. Style Corn,¹/₂ c.	100	1	23
w. whole kernels, undrained	80	1	17
Sweetcorn: See Corn			
Sweet Potato: ¹/₂ cup, 3¹/₂ oz	105	0	24
Candied (Green Giant) ³/₄ cup	240	7	41
Tomatoes, Sundr.: Natural, 5-6 pce	22	0	5
In Oil, drained, 6 pces, ¹/₂ oz	60	4	6
Tomato Products: See Page 91			
Vegetables, mixed, ¹/₂ cup, 4 oz	45	0	8
Yams in Light Syrup, ¹/₂ cup, 4 oz	105	0	25
Candied, ¹/₂ cup, 5 oz	170	0	46
Zucchini in Tom. Sce., ¹/₂ c., 4 oz	30	0	8

Vegetables, Canned or Bottled • Salads

Take-Out Salads & Vegetables

Avg. All Outlets: Per Serving	C	F	Cb
Antipasto Salad, 1 cup	140	10	2
Bean Salad, 1/2 cup	110	4	17
Bulgur Salad, 1/2 cup	70	2	12
Caesar Salad, Classic, 1 cup	200	14	15
Side Salad, no Dressing	25	0	6
Carrot Raisin: No Dressing, 1/2 cup	20	0	5
with Dressing, 1/2 cup	65	5	5
Chef Salad: Regular, no Dressing	620	37	8
w. 2 oz 1000 Island	860	61	8
Chicken Salad Platter, 6 oz	200	8	12
Coleslaw: Traditional, 1/2 cup	150	8	18
w. Low Cal Dressing	60	1	12
Corn, Mexican, 1/2 cup	240	12	33
Cucumber, Non-Oil Dressing, 1/2 c.	60	0	14
w. Oil Dressing, 1/2 cup	140	12	8
Eggplant Salad, 1/2 cup	75	5	7
Fettucini w. veges, 1/2 cup	110	5	15
Garden Salad, no Dressing	35	0	8
Greek Salad, 1 cup	120	10	7
Greek Vegetables, 1/2 cup	140	12	7
Lettuce, hearts, 1/4 head	20	0	4
Lobster Salad Platter, 6 oz	200	8	12
Macaroni Salad, 1/2 cup, 4 oz	180	13	13
Nicoise, 1 cup	450	32	18
Pasta Salad, 1/2 cup	160	8	16
Pineapple Coconut Slaw, 1/2 cup	150	10	14
Potato Salad: Dijon	140	7	17
w. Mayonnaise, 1/2 cup	170	10	17
Lowfat, 1/2 cup	110	1.5	21
Rice Salad, 1/2 cup	150	10	13
Saffron Rice, 1/2 cup	130	3	24
Spinach Salad	180	13	13
Tomato & Mozzarella, 1/2 cup	180	14	10
Tabouli, 1/2 cup	150	6	22
Three Bean Salad, 1/2 cup	80	5	9
Tortelini w. Basil Pesto, 1/2 cup	170	10	19
Waldorf w. Mayo, 1/2 cup	160	12	12

Signature Salads: Per Serving (6 oz) (Supplied to Deli's and Institutions)			
Antipasto Salad, 6 oz	510	50	4
Artichoke Salad, marinated	400	41	8
California Medley	120	7	15
Cheese Agnolotti	250	8	23
Chicken Salad	420	33	11
Crabmeat Flavored	450	38	20

Take-Out Salads (Cont)

Signature Salads (Cont)	C	F	Cb
Egg Salad	300	23	14
Fresh Button Mushroom	190	16	6
Garden Olive	630	67	3
Ham Salad	400	32	14
Prima Pasta Salad	360	30	18
Seafood Pasta Del Mar	170	10	21
Seafood with Crab & Shrimp	420	34	20
Shrimp Salad	360	32	8
Tuna Salad	450	36	14

Fast-Food Restaurants: See Page 183

Fresh Salad Packs

Pre-Packaged (Supermarkets)			
Dole: Complete Caesar, 3 1/2 oz	170	13	8
Complete Oriental, 3 1/2 oz	120	6	13
Complete Romano, 3 1/2 oz	150	12	9
Complete Spinach Bacon, 3 1/2 oz	170	10	18
Complete Sunflower Ranch, 3 1/2 oz	160	16	5
Special Blends (no added dressing), avg. all varieties, 2 cups, 3 oz	15	0	3
Regular Salad Packs (no added dressing):			
Classic Coleslaw, 3 oz	25	0	5
Classic Iceberg, 3 oz	15	0	4
Zesty Italian, 7 oz	110	0	4
Fresh Express: Per Package			
Chicken Caesar, 1 pkg, 183g	240	16	13
Chick. Crmy. Ranch, 1pkg. 194g	230	14	15
Chicken Teriyaki 1pkg, 193g	250	15	17
Salad Kits: Per Serving (Prepared)			
Caesar, 2 cups	160	14	7
Caesar w. Light Dress., 2 cups	100	7	8
Caesar Supreme, 2 cups	150	12	7
Oriental, 1 1/2 cups	140	9	13
European, 2 1/2 cups	15	0	3
Ready Pac: Average all types	15	0	2

Salad Toppings

Bacon Bits, average, 1 Tbsp	30	1.5	2
Chow Mein Noodles, dry, 1/2 cup	120	5	13
Croutons, 2 Tbsp, 10g	35	1	6
Olives, 5 medium	25	2	0
Potato Chips, 1 oz	150	10	15
Sunflower Seeds, 1 Tbsp, 8 g	45	4	1.5
Tortilla Chips, 1 oz	150	8	16

Fruit & Vegetable Juices/Smoothies

Quick Guide

Orange Juice 🅒 🅕 🅒ᵇ

Average ~ Fresh or Sweetened:

	C	F	Cb
1/2 Cup, 4 fl.oz	55	0	13
Small Glass, 6 fl.oz	82	0	20
Regular Glass, 8 fl.oz	110	0	26
8 3/4 fl.oz Box	120	0	28
10 fl.oz Bottle	140	0	32
11 1/2 fl.oz Can	160	0	36
16 fl.oz Bottle	220	0	52
20 fl.oz Bottle	280	0	72
64 fl.oz/1/2 Gallon	880	0	208

Juices ~ Generic

Average All Brands: Per 8 fl.oz Unless Indicated

	C	F	Cb
Aloe Vera Juice, unsweet., 2 oz	5	0	1
Apple Juice: 8 fl.oz	115	0	30
10 fl.oz Bottle	145	0	36
16 fl.oz	230	0	60
Carrot Juice: Fresh, 6 fl.oz	60	0	14
Sweetened, 6 fl.oz	75	0	17
Cranberry Juice, Cocktail/Blend	120	0	34
Fruit Blends, average, 8 fl.oz	120	0	31
Fruit Nectars, average, 8 fl.oz	140	0	35
Grape Juice, 8 fl.oz	160	0	40
Grapefruit Juice, 8 fl.oz	100	0	23
Lemon/Lime Juice: 1 Tbsp	4	0	1.5
1 cup, 8 fl.oz	60	0	21
Concentrate, 1 tsp	0	0	0
Noni Juice: *Tahitian*, 2 Tbsp, 1 fl.oz	10	0	2
Southern Cross Botanicals, 1 fl.oz	6	0	2
Tahiti Traders, 1 fl.oz	20	0	5
Orange Juice, 8 fl.oz	110	0	26
Passion Fruit Juice (Fresh):			
Purple, 1 cup, 8 fl.oz	125	0	34
Yellow, 1 cup, 8 fl.oz	150	0	36
Papaya/Peach Nectar, 8 fl.oz	140	0	35
Pear Nectar, 8 fl.oz	150	0	40
Pineapple Juice, 8 fl.oz	110	0	27
Prune Juice, 8 fl.oz	180	0	43
Strawb./Raspberry Juice, 8 fl.oz	100	0	23
Tangerine Juice, 8 fl.oz	100	0	25
Tomato Juice, 8 fl.oz	50	0	12
Vegetable Juice, 8 fl.oz	50	0	12
Wheat Grass Juice: 1 fl.oz 'Shot'	5	0	1
2 fl.oz 'Shot'	10	0	2

Quick Guide

Fruit Smoothies 🅒 🅕 🅒ᵇ

Average All Brands

	C	F	Cb
Fruit Only: 8 fl.oz	105	0	25
12 fl.oz	160	0	38
16 fl.oz	210	0	50
24 fl.oz	320	0.5	76
Fruit + Nonfat Milk/Soy:			
12 fl.oz	190	0.5	40
16 fl.oz	250	0.5	53
24 fl.oz	380	1	80
Fruit + Nonfat Frozen Yogurt/Sherbet:			
12 fl.oz	210	0.5	47
16 fl.oz	280	0.5	62
24 fl.oz	420	1	94

Juice Brands

Per 8 fl.oz Unless Indicated 🅒 🅕 🅒ᵇ

	C	F	Cb
Ame			
Sparkling Fruit Juice: *Per 8 fl.oz*			
Ame Dry	60	0	15
Ame Red/Rose	80	0	20
Ame White	90	0	23
Apple & Eve			
Naturally Cranberry	120	0	30
Cranberry/Raspberry Apple	120	0	30
Cranberry Grape	140	0	34
Bright & Early			
Orange Juice (Chilled/Frozen)	120	0	30
Grape Juice (Frozen)	140	0	33
Campbell's			
Tomato Juice: 5.5 fl.oz can	35	0	7
10.5 fl.oz	60	0	12
Capri Sun			
Sport, all flavors, 8 fl.oz	120	0	31
Big Pouch: *Per 8 fl.oz*			
Dragonfruit	170	0	44
Rasberry Lemonade	200	0	52
Wild Cherry	190	0	49
Average other flavors	160	0	40

Success is 1% Inspiration and 99% Perspiration.

Fruit & Vegetable Drinks & Juices (Cont)

Per 8 fl.oz Unless Indicated	C	F	Cb
Clamato			
Tomato Cocktails, avg, 8 fl.oz	60	0	13
Crystal Geyser			
Juice Squeeze: *Per Bottle (12 fl.oz)*			
Blackberry Pomegranate	170	0	43
Orange Lime	160	0	40
Ruby Grapefruit	150	0	36
Average other flavors	140	0	32
Dole			
100% Fruit Juice Blends, 8 fl.oz	120	0	29
Donald Duck			
100% Orange Jce (+Calcium), 8 fl.oz	120	0	29
Eden: Organic Apple, 8 fl.oz	80	0	23
Five Alive: Frozen Concentrate,			
made up, 8 fl.oz	120	0	30
Florida's Natural			
Cranberry Apple, 8 fl.oz	120	0	30
Grapefruit Juice, 8 fl.oz	100	0	24
Orange Juice, 8 fl.oz	110	0	26
Fresh Samantha: *Per 8 fl.oz*			
Apple	120	0	30
Banana Strawberry Smoothie	150	1	36
Carrot/Orange; The Big Bang	100	0	25
Crazy Cranberry	130	0	32
Desperately Seeking C	130	0	31
Grapefruit	90	0	24
Mango Mama; Get Smart	130	0	33
Raspberry Dream	120	1	29
Soy Shake, 16 fl.oz	320	8	33
Super Juice w. Echinacea	140	1	33
Fruit Whips: *Per 8 fl.oz Bottle*			
Smoothies, 236ml (8 oz)	125	0	29
Fruitopia			
All flavors, average, 8 fl.oz	115	0	29
20 fl.oz Bottle	290	0	72
Frulatte Smoothies: *Per Bottle (10.5 fl.oz)*			
Orange Mango	230	0	47
Strawberry Kiwi	220	0	45
Avg. other flavors	240	0	50
Fuze: *Per 8 fl.oz*			
Focus (11% Juice), Mojo Mango	100	0	25
Lemonaid	70	0	18
Vitamin Tea	60	0	16
Average other varieties	90	0	22

Per 8 fl.oz Unless Indicated	C	F	Cb
Good Day: Fruit Juice, 8 fl.oz	110	0	28
Goya Nectar			
Apricot Nectar, 12 fl.oz	130	0	31
Pear Nectar, 12 fl.oz can	240	0	59
Hansen's: Natural Juice Cocktail			
Regular, all flavors, 8 fl.oz	110	0	28
Low Calorie Peach Mango	10	0	4
Apple Varieties, 8 fl.oz	120	0	28
Junior Juice, 4.32 fl.oz box	60	0	15
Juice Slam: *Per Box (8.45 fl.oz)*			
Apple; Paradise Punch	120	0	28
Strawb. Banana; Wildberry	110	0	28
Smoothies: *Per Can (10.8 fl.oz)*			
Fruit Flavors, regular	170	0	43
Lite Cranberry Raspberry	50	0	13
Energy Smoothies: *See Page 160*			
100% Fruit Juice Boxes: *Per Box (4.2 fl.oz)*			
White Grape	90	0	22
Average other flavors	60	0	15
Hawaiian Punch			
Fruit Juicy, Red, 6 fl.oz	90	0	22
Box, 8.45 fl.oz	120	0	30
Hawaii's Own			
Frozen Concentrate: *Per 8 fl.oz (Prep'd)*			
Average all varieties	105	0	28
Hi-C Juice Drinks:			
Average, 8 fl.oz	130	0	32
6.75 fl.oz box, average	100	0	27
11.5 fl.oz can	180	0	45
Jamba Juice (California): *See Page 213*			
Jera's Juice (Boston): *Per 24 fl.oz*			
Berry Blitz	440	2	105
Cape Codder	335	0.5	80
Citrus Burst	320	1.5	75
Mango Passion	290	0	68
Orange Bite; Flu Fighter, avg.	280	1.5	65
Razzle Dazzle	380	1	94
Soy Smoothie (7g protein)	320	3.5	68
Strawberry Smile	345	0.5	84
Triathlete (15g protein)	300	1.5	71
Whey-Out Protein (27g protein)	325	1.5	56
Juicy Juice (Libby's): *Per Box (6.75 fl.oz)*			
Grape	110	0	26
Avg. other flavors	100	0	25
4.23 fl.oz box, average	60	0	15

Fruit & Vegetable Drinks & Juices (Cont)

Per 8 fl.oz Unless Indicated	C	F	Cb
Kerns All Nectars			
Canned Juice: *Per Can (11.5 fl.oz)*			
Pear	220	0	54
Pineapple Coconut	280	8	53
Other flavors, average	210	0	52
Kool Aid			
Jammers: Lemonade, 1 pouch	110	0	29
Other varieties, 6.75 fl.oz pouch	90	0	24
Knudsen: *Per 8 fl.oz*			
Fruit Juices: Apple	110	0	28
Cranberry Raspberry	140	0	36
Creamed Papaya	40	0	10
Grapefruit; Just Blueberry	100	0	23
Guava Strawberry	110	0	27
Hibiscus Cooler; Just Boysenberry	90	0	23
Just Concord	160	0	40
Prune	180	0	43
Tomato	60	0	14
Other varieties, average	125	0	32
Sparkling Juice, 8 fl.oz	105	0	29
Nectars: Coconut	140	5	26
Peach	120	0	30
Boysenberry, average	130	0	36
Floats: Orange	140	0	33
Very Veggie, 8 fl.oz	50	0	10
Simply Nutritious:			
Blackberry Hibiscus Mist	100	0	24
Mega C	130	0	31
Average other varieties	120	0	30

Per 8 fl.oz Unless Indicated	C	F	Cb
Krasdale: Cranberry Apple	170	0	42
Cranberry Juice Cocktail	130	0	32
Cranberry Raspberry	150	0	37
L & A *Per 8 fl.oz:* Black Cherry	180	0	45
Grape Juice	160	0	40
Mixed Berry	120	0	30
Prime Juice	180	0	41
Average other varieties	140	0	32
Lakewood Organic			
Carrot Beverage, 6 fl.oz	85	0	19
Coconut, 6 fl.oz	90	1.5	20
Cranberry/Lemonade, 8 fl.oz	85	0	21
Mango, 6 fl.oz	90	0	22
Papaya; Pure Carrot, 6 fl.oz	75	0	18
Pure Cranberry, 6 fl.oz	50	0	12
Pure Pineapple, 6 fl.oz	95	0	23
Pure Pine, 6 fl.oz	165	0	40
Pure Pink Grapefruit, 8 fl.oz	90	0	22
Red Tart Cherry, 6 fl.oz	110	0	19
Super Veggie, 6 fl.oz	40	0	9
Average other varieties	105	0	26
Langers: *Per 8 fl.oz*			
Apple Juice; White Cranberry avg.	120	0	28
Cranberry/100 Varieties, avg .	140	0	35
Cranberry Berry	135	0	34
Cranberry Grape; White Grape	165	0	41
Cranberry Raspberry	150	0	36
Diet Apple Juice	60	0	40
Diet Cranberry	30	0	8
Diet Cranberry Grape	120	0	28
Frozen Concentrate: *Per 8 fl.oz (Prepared)*			
Cranberry	140	0	29
Avg. other flavors	120	0	29
Luzianne: *Per 8 fl.oz (Prepared)*			
Smoothies: Mixed Berry	90	0.5	19
Peach Mango	90	0	19
Strawberry Banana	80	0.5	18
Martinellis			
Sparkling Juice: *Per 8 fl.oz*			
Apple-Cranberry	110	0	27
Apple-Grape	120	0	31
Cider	140	0	35
Mauna La'i Hawaiian: 8 fl.oz	140	0	32
Mistic (Mega 24 fl.oz)			
Average All flavors, 8 fl.oz	120	0	30
24 fl.oz	360	0	90

"I've worked on vitamins for years and I've discovered that the three most important elements necessary to life are breakfast, lunch and dinner."

Per 8 fl.oz Unless Indicated	**C**	**F**	**Cb**

Minute Maid

	C	F	Cb
Orange Juice, Premium, 8 fl.oz	110	0	27
Blends, Avg. all flavors, 8 fl.oz	120	0	30
Pink Lemonade, 8 fl.oz	110	0	28
Chilled Singles: *Per Bottle (16 fl.oz)*			
Berry/Tropical Punch	240	0	60
Lemonade/ Orange Juice	220	0	55
Juices to Go: Avg. all flav., 10 fl.oz	160	0	40
Boxed Juices: *Per 6.75 fl.oz*			
Apple; Lemonade, avg.	90	0	24
Orange Tropical	110	0	32
Other varieties, average	100	0	25
Calcium Juices, 8 fl.oz	120	0	29
Coolers: *Per Pouch (6.75 fl.oz)*			
Clear Cherry	110	0	29
Other varieties, average	100	0	26
Disney, 6.75 fl.oz box	100	0	25
Frozen Concentrates: *Per 8 fl.oz (Prep'd)*			
Average all varieties	105	0	28

Mott's

	C	F	Cb
Apple Juice, 8 fl.oz	120	0	29
Apple Raspb., Fruit Punch, 10 fl.oz	145	0	36
Apple Cranb., Grape Apple, 10 fl.oz	180	0	42
Fruitsations, all flavors, 4 oz	85	0	22
Juice Paks: All flavors, 8.45 fl.oz	120	0	30
Mini Motts, 4.23 oz	60	0	14

Naked Juice: *Per $^1/_2$ Bottle (8 fl.oz)*

	C	F	Cb
Blue Nanas	140	2	34
Grapefruit Juice; Mighty Mango	110	0	23
Carrot-O-Copia	80	0	13
Green Machine	140	0.5	35
Lemons Juiced	130	0	32
Power-C	120	5	29
Protein Zone (17g protein)	220	4	32
Raspberry Ade; Well-Being	140	0	35
Tangerine Scream	110	0	25
Zenergy	160	0	37
Avg. other varieties	120	0	30
Soy Shakes: Choc (9g protein)	210	2	38
Vanilla (8g protein)	170	1	33

Nantucket Nectars

	C	F	Cb
Juice Cocktails: Cranberry/Apple	140	0	34
Guava; Grapeade	130	0	33
Fruit Punch; Orange Mango	130	0	32
Kiwi Berry	120	0	30
Average other varieties	120	0	30

Per 8 fl.oz Unless Indicated	**C**	**F**	**Cb**

Nantucket Nectars (Cont)

	C	F	Cb
100% Juices: Grape Juice	160	0	39
Apple Cider; Nectar Fizz	90	0	23
Peach Orange	130	0	31
Pineapple Orange Banana	140	0	35
Premium Orange Juice	120	0	29
The Original Peach	120	0	30
Average other varieties	100	0	25
Lemonades: Authentic/Pink	120	0	30

Newman's Own

	C	F	Cb
Lemonade (Reg./Pink), 8 fl.oz	110	0	27

Northland

	C	F	Cb
100% Juice: *Per 8 fl.oz*			
Cranberry; Cranberry Peach	140	0	35
Cranberry Blackberry	140	0	35
Cranberry Grape/Raspberry	150	0	38

Ocean Spray: *Per 8 fl.oz*

	C	F	Cb
Cranberry Cherry	150	0	39
Cranapple	160	0	41
Fruit Punch; Tangerine	130	0	32
Lite Cranberry varieties, avg.	40	0	30
Grapefruit: 100% Juice	100	0	24
Kiwi Strawb.; Summer Cooler	120	0	31
Lemonade flavors, average	130	0	32
Pink Grapefruit	110	0	28
Ruby Red & Strawberry	140	0	34
Ruby Red & Mango/Tangerine	130	0	33
Ruby Red; White Cranberry varieties	120	0	29
White Grapefruit	100	0	24
Cranberry: Cranberry Grape	170	0	41
Cranberry Juice Cocktail	140	0	34
Light Style (Low Calorie)	40	0	10
Other Cranberry flavors, avg	150	0	35
Cravin' Less Sugar: Kiwi Strawb.	70	0	17
Tropical; Cranberry Wildberry	60	0	15

Odwalla: *Per 8 fl.oz*

	C	F	Cb
Carrot	70	0	15
Carrot, Orange, Apple	100	0	23
C Monster	150	0	34
Femme Vitale	130	0	29
Fruitshake Blackberry	160	0	40
Glorious Morning; Blueb. C	140	0	33
Grapefruit Juice	90	0	34
Lemonade; Lime	90	0	24
Mango Tango; Serious Energy	150	0	37
Mo Beta	140	0	35

Fruit & Vegetable Drinks & Juices (Cont)

Per 8 fl.oz Unless Indicated   **C** **F** **Cb**

Odwalla (Cont)

	C	F	Cb
Orange Juice	120	0	34
Strawberry Banana/Go Man Go	100	0	25
Strawberry C Monster	150	0	34
Strawberry Lemonade	110	0	28
Super Protein	190	1	35
Superfood	140	1	32
Wellness (Echinacea)	150	1	33

Old Orchard

	C	F	Cb
Apple Juice, all varieties, 8 fl.oz	120	0	29

Frozen Concentrate: *Per 8 fl.oz (Prep'd)*

	C	F	Cb
Apple	120	0	29
Other flavors	130	0	31

Orange Julius: Original (Orange, Strawberry),

	C	F	Cb
16 fl.oz	225	0	55
20 fl.oz	280	0	68
32 fl.oz	450	0	109

Other Drinks: *See Fast-Foods, Page 226*

PS - Private Selection (Ralphs)

	C	F	Cb
Lemonade (Premium Juice), 8 fl.oz	110	0	29
Orange Juice, 8 fl.oz	110	0	27
Mango Nectar, 8 fl.oz	140	0	35

Realemon - Realime (Borden)

Lemon/Lime Juice (from concentrate)

	C	F	Cb
1 teaspoon	0	0	0
2 Tbsp, 1 fl.oz	6	0	2

Pom Wonderful

100% Juice: *Per 8 fl.oz*

	C	F	Cb
Pomegranate	145	0	35
Blueberry; Mango	140	0	34
Cherry	135	0	33
Tangerine	150	0	37

S&W

	C	F	Cb
Apple Juice, 8 fl.oz	120	0	30
Orange Juice, 6 fl.oz can	90	0	22
Grapefruit Juice, unswt'd, 8 fl.oz	105	0	25
Tomato Juice, 8 fl.oz	30	0	7

Santa Cruz

	C	F	Cb
Apple Juice; Cider & Spice	120	0	30
Concord Grape; White Grape	160	0	40
Orange Mango	130	0	31
Tropical Blend	140	0	33
Average other varieties	100	0	24

Nectars: Apricot; Cranberry

	C	F	Cb
	110	0	27
Berry	110	0	30
Average other varieties	120	0	30

Snapple

	C	F	Cb
Fruit Drink Blends, 8 fl.oz	120	0	30
Grapeade; Orangeade 8 fl.oz	120	0	30
Vitamin Supreme	150	0	44
Diet: Snapple Apple	15	0	4
Kiwi Strawberry	15	0	4
Avg. other flavors	10	0	2

Snap.E Tom

	C	F	Cb
Tom. & Chile Cocktail, 11.5 oz can	70	0	15

Squeezit

	C	F	Cb
Average all flavors, 6.75 oz	90	0	23

Stonyfield Farm: Per Bottle (10 fl.oz)

	C	F	Cb
Peach Smoothie	250	3	49
Wildberry; Strawberry Smoothie	250	3	45

Sunny Delight

	C	F	Cb
Florida Citrus, 6 fl.oz	90	0	22
Calcium Rich, 6 fl.oz	150	0	37
Mango Citrus	130	0	31
Smooth (California Style)	130	0	32
Sunny Delight Lite, 6 fl.oz	20	0	5
Tangy Original (Florida Style)	120	0	29
Tropical Fruit Punch, 6 fl.oz	90	0	22

Sunsweet

	C	F	Cb
Prune Juice/w. Pulp, 8 fl.oz	170	0	42
Superfood: Juice, 8 fl.oz	140	1	32
Tampico: Citrus Punch, 1 cup	100	0	25
Mango/Trop. Frt. Punch, 1 cup	110	0	28

Tang

	C	F	Cb
Pouches, average all flavors (1)	100	0	26
Mix: Made Up, 6 fl.oz			
Regular (2 Tbsp dry)	90	0	22

Trader Joes: Per 8 fl.oz

	C	F	Cb
Carrot Juice	80	0	13
Ginger Lemonade	150	0	37
Organic Carrots & Greens	80	0	19
Strawberry Lemonade	160	0	41
Strawberry Smoothie	140	2	30
Avg. other varieties	110	0	25

Trader Darwin's (100%):

	C	F	Cb
Dairy Free Protein w. Pzazz	170	0	32
Very Green Juice Blend	110	0	32
Avg. other varieties	130	0	31

100% Juice: *Per 8 fl.oz*

	C	F	Cb
Apple Cranberry Blend	130	0	30
Original Lemonade	110	0	27
Other Apple varieties	140	0	33

Fruit & Vegetable Drinks & Juices (Cont)

Per 8 fl.oz Unless Indicated	C	F	Cb
Trader Joes: (Cont)			
All Natural Pasteurized: Per 8 fl.oz			
Combat; Lemon Ginger	110	0	26
Cranberry Harvest	135	0	35
Cranberry; White Grape	140	0	36
Garden Patch; Vege -10	50	0	12
Hawaiian Pineapple	110	0	29
Just Pomegranate; Concord Grape	160	0	40
Mango Lemonade	135	0	35
Mango Passion Fruit Blend	130	0	33
Rio Red Grapefruit	140	0	35
Tropical Papaya Nectar	130	0	34
Average other varieties	125	0	30
Tree of Life			
Black Cherry	180	0	43
Concord Grape	160	0	40
Cranberry Nectar	150	0	38
Other varieties, average	130	0	33
Tree Top: Per 6 fl.oz			
Apple Cranberry/Grape	130	0	32
Avg. other varieties	120	0	30
Frozen Concentrates: Per 8 fl.oz (Prep'd)			
Apple Juice	120	0	29
Tropicana: Per 8 fl.oz			
Blends: Berry; P'apple, 8 fl.oz	130	0	32
Pure Premium: Orange-Strawb.	130	0	30
Avg. other varieties	120	0	26
Twister: Average, 8 fl.oz	120	0	32
10 fl.oz bottle	150	0	40
11.5 fl.oz can	160	0	40
Light: Average, 8 fl.oz	35	0	10
10 fl.oz bottle	50	0	11
100% Juice Blends: Per 8 fl.oz			
Pineapple Orange	120	0	30
Average other flavors	140	0	33
V8® Juices & Drinks			
V8 100% Vegetable Juice, 8 fl.oz	50	0	10
1 Can, 12 fl.oz	70	0	15
V-8 Splash, all flavors, 8 fl.oz	110	0	28
V-8 Splash Smoothies, 8 fl.oz	125	0	27
Diet V-8 Splash, all flavors, 8 fl.oz	10	0	3
Veryfine			
Grape Juice (100%)	150	0	37
Grapefruit Juice (100%)	90	0	20
Pink	120	0	30
Papaya Punch (100%)	120	0	30

Per 8 fl.oz Unless Indicated	C	F	Cb
Walnut Acres: Per 8 fl.oz			
Black Cherry; Plain Apple	120	0	30
Lemonade; Cranberry	110	0	27
Limeade	100	0	24
Other flavors	130	0	32
Welch's: Per 8 fl.oz			
100% Grape Juice	170	0	42
100% Red Grape Juice	170	0	44
100% White Grape Juice	160	0	39
Mountain Berry	140	0	34
Tomato Juice, 8 fl.oz	50	0	10
Concentrate: Per 8 fl.oz Made Up			
Apple	120	0	29
Grape	170	0	41
Fruit Fantastic	130	0	32
Wild Berry	140	0	36
Fruit Juice Cocktails: Per 8 fl.oz			
Grape; Strawberry Breeze	130	0	33
Country Pear; Wild Raspberry	145	0	35
Frozen Concentrates: Per 8 fl.oz (Prep'd)			
Grape	150	0	38
100% Grape	165	0	41
Strawberry Breeze	130	0	33
Orange Pineapple Apple	140	0	36
Sparkling Juice	160	0	40
Wild Oats			
Down to Earth, average, 8 fl.oz	140	0	34
Beautiful Juices, average, 8 fl.oz	120	0	27

"And how long has celery been your basic diet."

Nutritional/Sports Shakes & Drinks

Nutritional Shakes/Drinks

Per 8 fl.oz Unless Indicated   **C F Cb**

	C	F	Cb
ABB			
Performance: Mass Recovery	380	0	60
Avg., other varieties, 18 fl.oz	100	0	23
Power Drinks, 22 fl.oz	310	0	43
Weight Gain: Pure Pro, 22 fl.oz	180	0	2
Extreme XXL, 24 fl.oz	1025	0.5	215
Pure Pro Shake: Choc., 12 fl.oz	175	1	6
Vanilla, 12 fl.oz	160	0.5	4
AllSport, all flavors, 8 fl.oz	70	0	18
AMP Energy Drink, 8.4 fl.oz can	120	0	30
Amway Positrim Drink Mix, 1 pkt	160	4	27
Fat Free Mix, 1 pkt, 65g	230	0	50
Appeal, avg. all flavors, 1 pkt	210	2	33
Arbonne Meal Shakes, 1 pkt, 46g	190	4.5	25
Arizona: Rx Energy, 16 fl.oz	240	0	60
Rx Health/Stress, avg.	75	0	19
Rx Power, 16 fl.oz	210	0	52
Rx Total Trim, 8 fl.oz	5	0	1
Atkins: Shake Mix, avg., 2 scoops	170	8	1.5
Shake Pwdr., avg. all flav., 1 scp	85	4	4
Ready-to-Drink Shakes, 1 can	170	9	4
Balanced: Diet, avg., 11 fl.oz	180	2	35
Choc., Strawb.; Van., 11 fl.oz	230	3	36
Kids Chocolate, 8 fl.oz can	160	3	30
Bariatrix Shakes, 1 serving	100	2	6
Proti-Max Meal, 67g	250	3	20
Bawls Guarana, 12 fl.oz	130	0	32
Blue Sky, Blue Energy, 8.3 fl.oz	110	0	27
Blue Thunder, 22 fl.oz	300	0	43
Body Design Shakes			
Average., 2 scoops	250	3.5	36
Lite, average, 2 scoops	170	4	16
Body Fuel (w. NutraSweet), 8 fl.oz	4	0	1
Boost: Ready-To-Drink, 8 oz	240	4	41
Boost High Protein, 8 fl.oz	240	6	33
Boost Plus, 8 fl.oz can	360	14	45
Breeze Juice Drink, 8 fl.oz can	160	0	31
Carboplex (Unipro),			
mix, 1/2 cup, 2 oz	210	0	52
Carnation Instant Breakfast			
Powder: 1 reg. envelope, 37g	130	1	28
No Sugar Added, 1 envel., 21g	70	1	12
Ready-To-Drink, avg., 10 oz	220	3	37
CeraSport, 27 Liquid, 11 fl.oz	70	0	17
34g packet (makes 16 fl.oz)	110	0	32

Per 8 fl.oz Unless Indicated   **C F Cb**

	C	F	Cb
Champion Nutrition:			
Heavywt Gainer 900, 4 sc., 5.4 oz	630	10	101
Lean Gainer, 3 scoops, 2.7 oz	280	4	11
Super H. Wt Gainer, 4 scoops	900	29	108
Choice dm (Mead Johnson), 8 fl.oz	250	12	25
Cytomax: 8 fl.oz	65	0	13
Powdered Mix, 1 scoop	95	0	20
Designer Whey, Prot. Blast, 16 fl.oz	170	1	1
Elements: Avg., all varieties	125	0	31
Diet Air/Ice, 8 fl.oz	10	0	2
Endura (Unipro), 2 scoops, 1.3 oz	120	0	29
Perfect Protein Shake, 8.3 fl.oz	110	0	28
Ensure: High Calcium, 8 oz can	225	6	31
Enlive! 8.1 fl.oz	300	0	65
Ensure Fiber, 8 fl.oz can	250	6	42
Ensure Light, 8 fl.oz can	200	3	33
Ensure Plus, 8 fl.oz can	360	11	50
Ensure Regular, 8 fl.oz can	250	6	40
Glucerna, 8 fl.oz can	220	11	22
Powder, made up, 1/2 cup	250	9	34
Enterex Diabetic (w/fiber), 8 fl.oz			
(Carbohydrates as Maltodextrin)	237	9	27
4Kick Energy, 8.3 fl.oz	120	0	29
Fruit2O (Veryfine), 8/16/20 fl.oz	0	0	0
G-Up, 8.4 fl.oz	220	0.5	55
Gatorade: Energy Drink, 12 fl.oz	310	0	78
ThirstQuencher, 8 fl.oz	50	0	14
Nutrition Shake, 325ml can	370	6	62
Genisoy: Shake, 1 scoop, 35g	120	0	17
Protein Powder, 1 scoop, 29g	100	0	0
Glaceau: Vitamin Water, 20 fl.oz	110	0	28
Smart Water	0	0	0
HMR: 70 Plus, 1 pkt	110	0.5	13
120	120	1.5	16
500	100	0	17
800	170	2	21
Hansen's: Per Can (8.3 fl.oz)			
Energy Original	130	0	32
Power	120	0	30
Slim Down	0	0	0
D-Stress; B-Well; Stamina	125	0	31
Diet Red Energy	10	0	3
Energade, 8 fl.oz	65	0	16
Smoothies: See Page 155			
Health Source Soy, 2 scps, 1 oz	100	1	4
Hydra Fuel (Tury Labs)	65	0	16
Isopure Perfect, 1 pkt (88g)	100	0	25

Nutritional/Sports Shakes & Drinks (Cont)

Per 8 fl.oz Unless Indicated	C	F	Cb
Jarrow: Whey Protein, 1 scoop	90	1	1
Muscle Optimal, 1½ scoops	155	2.5	10
Jones, avg., 1 can/8 fl.oz	120	0	30
Kashi GoLEAN Shakes: Vanilla	220	2.5	36
Chocolate, 325ml can	230	3	32
Powdered, avg., 2 scoops	220	1	32
Keto: Nutritional Shake, 8 fl.oz	160	8	2
Knudsen: ReCharge, all flavors	80	0	18
Simply Nutritious, ½ bot., 16 fl.oz	60	0	14
Kombucha: Vit. Enriched, 8 fl.oz	30	0	11
Wonder Drink, 8.5 fl.oz	65	0	16
Lipovitan: EB[3], 8.2 fl.oz	110	0	29
Met-Rx: Original, 1 pkt	250	2.5	19
Lite, 1 pkt	175	1.5	21
Ultra, 1 pkt	265	2.5	20
Ultra Pure Protein, 11 fl.oz can	170	1	2
RTD 40, 15 fl.oz can	200	3	15
Metabolol: Endurance, 2 scp, 52g	200	5	24
Metabolol II, 2 scoops, 66g	260	3	40
Met Max, mix, 2 scoops	230	2	11
MRM: Low Carb Protein, 1 scoop	120	2.5	4
Whey Protein Isolate, 1 scoop	115	1.5	1
Whey Pumped, 1 scoop	100	1	5
Myoplex: Original Shake, 17 fl.oz	300	0.5	20
Carb Sense Shake, 11 fl.oz	150	3.5	5
Low Carb Sense Shake, 11 fl.oz	120	3.5	2
Light Nutritional Shake, 11 fl.oz	190	2.5	20
Powder, 1 pkt, 2.7 oz	280	2	24
Lite Powder, 1 pkt, 2 oz	190	1.5	20
Nature's Best: Isopure			
Zero Carb, 2 scoops, 2.1 oz	200	0	0
Low Carb, 2 scoops, 2.3 oz	210	0	3
Perfect Whey, 1 scoop, 0.7 oz	90	1.5	1
Nitro Speed, all flavors, 18 fl.oz	110	0	7
Noni: Tahiti/Pacific, 2 Tbsp	5	0	1
Noni Juice, 1 fl.oz	20	0	5
Liquid Hawaiian/Tahitian, 1 Tbsp	30	0	8
Nutrament (Mead Johnson), 12 fl.oz	360	10	52
Ny-Tro Pro 40, average	260	1	23
Optifast 800: Powder, 1 serving	160	3	20
Ready-To-Drink, Chocolate	160	3	20
Pedialyte (Abbott)	25	0	6
Pitbull Energy Drink, 1 can	110	0	28
Power Dream (Imagine Foods):			
Java Jolt, 11 fl.oz	240	4.5	42
Mango Passion, 11 fl.oz	320	4.5	65
X-Treme Choc, 11 fl.oz	280	5	48
Vanilla Blast, 11 fl.oz	240	5	39

Per 8 fl.oz Unless Indicated	C	F	Cb
Powerade: Regular, 8 fl.oz	70	0	19
20 fl.oz bottle	175	0	48
Light, 8 fl.oz	25	0	7
20 fl.oz bottle	65	0	17
Rev-up, all flavors, 20 fl.oz	70	0	18
PowerBar Power Gel: Choc.	120	1.5	28
Other flavors, 41g pack	110	0	28
ProBalance, 8.45 fl.oz	300	10	39
Pro-Cal 100 (R-Kane), 1 pkt	105	2	7
Red Bull Energy Drink, 8.3 fl.oz	113	0	28
Sugar-Free, 1 can	10	0	3
Red Devil: Energy Drink, 12 fl.oz	120	0	31
Red Tiger Energy Drink, 8.2 fl.oz	115	0	28
Resource (Novartis): Plus, 8 fl.oz	360	11	52
Agrinard Extra, 1 bikpak	250	0	52
Health Shake, 4 fl.oz	200	4	35
Shake, 8 fl.oz	270	6	45
Standard 8 fl.oz pak	250	6	40
Diabetic, 8 fl.oz pak	250	11	23
Revenge Pro (Champ. Nutr.), 1 oz	100	0	20
Pro-Score 100, 2 scoops	160	2	1.5
Revival Soy Mix: Plain Soy, 1 pkg	110	1.5	1
Chocolate Day Dream, 1 pkg	240	2.5	36
Other varieties, avg., 1 pkg	225	2	33
Rite Aid: Nutritional Suppl., 8 oz	250	6	40
Rite Aid Plus, 8 oz	360	11	50
Rockstar: Energy Drink, 8 fl.oz	130	0	32
Diet Energy Drink, 8 fl.oz	10	0	2
Sav-on Nut'l: 8 fl.oz can	360	13	47
Light, 8 fl.oz can	200	3	33
Scan Diet (Soy-base), 1 scoop	160	3	21
Shark Energy Drink, 1 can	140	0	35
Slim-Fast: Ready-To-Drink Cans,			
Shakes, all flavors, 325ml	220	3	40
Juices, all flavors, 340ml	220	1	46
Powder Mix: 1 scoop, 1 oz	100	1	20
w. 8 oz fat-free milk	190	1	32
Slim-Fast Soy Protein:			
Café Mocha, 2 scoop, ⅓ cup	170	1.5	26
Ultra Slim-Fast Mixes: Reg.flavors, avg.,			
1 scoop, ⅓ cup, 33g	120	1	25
w. 8 oz fat free milk	200	1.5	36
Choc Delite w. Soy Protein,			
2 scoops, ½ cup, 48g	170	2	25
w. Fruit Juice Mix,			
1 scoop, ¼ cup, 31g	100	1	17
w. 8 oz fruit juice	220	1	42

Nutritional/Sports Shakes & Drinks (Cont)

Per 8 fl.oz Unless Indicated

	C	F	Cb
Snapple Sport, all flavors	80	0	20
SoBe: Power, avg., 8 fl.oz	140	0	35
Juice Elixers, 8 fl.oz	90	0	24
Lean, all flavors, 8 fl.oz	5	0	1
Lizard, avg. all types, 8 fl.oz	130	0	33
Love Bus Brew, 8 fl.oz	140	1	28
No Fear, 8 fl.oz	145	0	36
Sports System, 591 mL	190	0	45
Solaray Soytein *(Protein Energy Meal)*,			
Natural, 1 heaping scoop, 24g	70	0.5	5
Flav., avg., 1 heaping scoop, 32g	115	1	13
Sport Pharma Piomax, 2 scoops	250	3.5	6
Spiru-Tein: 8 fl.oz can	220	5	23
Powder, 1 scoop, 34 g	100	1	11
Sweet Success *(Nestlé):*			
Healthy Shake, 10 fl.oz can	200	3	32
Fruit Flavors, 10 fl.oz	200	0.5	39
Powder, 2 scoops, 32g (1.1 oz)	100	1	25
Synergy: Mystic Mango, 16 fl.oz	100	0	24
Other flavors, 16 fl.oz	70	0	16
ToppFast, 2 scoops (32g)	140	1	13
Total Balance, 9.5 oz can	230	7	25
Drink Mix, avg., 2 scoops	190	6	20
Twin Lab: Ultra Fuel, 16 fl.oz	400	0	100
RxFuel, 1 pkt	250	0	62
Energy Fuel, 250ml can	0	0	0
Ultima Replenisher, 12g pkt	40	0	10

	C	F	Cb
Usana: Nutrimeal, 2 scoops, 43g	150	4	20
Fiergy Drink, 2 scoops	120	1.5	31
SoyaMax, 2 scoops	110	1	1
Venom Energy *(Elements)*, 8.2 fl.oz	130	0	29
VP2 *(AST):* Vanilla, 1 scoop, 1 oz	105	0.5	1
Chocolate, 1 scoop, 1 oz	110	0.5	2
Walgreens Nutritional Supplements:			
Advanced Formula, 8 oz can	250	6	40
Plus, 8 oz can	355	13	47
Light, 8 oz can	200	3	33
Weider (Powders):			
Body Shaper Powder, 1 pkt	140	1	8
Body Shaper Shake, 1 can	160	1	5
Celt Recovery Stack, 1 scoops	200	0	25
Creatine ATP, $^1/_2$ cup, 1.7 oz	210	0	37
Mass 1000, $1^1/_3$ cups	740	4	146
Ultra Whey Pro, $^1/_3$ cup, 1 oz	110	1	4
Dynamic:			
Muscle Builder, 2 scoops, 45g	190	0	27
Weight Gainer, 4 scoops, 85g	330	0.5	62
Worldwide: Carbo Rush, 20 fl.oz	280	0	60
Fat Shredder, 20 fl.oz bottle	0	0	0
Pure Protein, 22 fl.oz bottle	170	0	0
Rapid Recovery, 20 fl.oz	280	0	25
Thermo 525, 20 fl.oz bottle	5	0	1
XS Energy Citrus/Energy, 8.4 fl.oz	8	0	0
Zone Perfect: Shake Mix, 2 scps	225	7	23
Protein Powder, 1 scoop	30	0	0
Nutritional Drinks, avg., 8 fl.oz	270	8	30

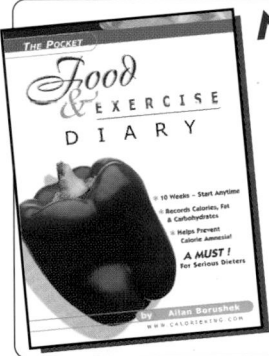

Soft Drinks • Soda

Quick Guide

Cola Soda Drinks

Average All Brands
Coca-Cola and Pepsi

	C	F	Cb
8 fl.oz Cup	100	0	25
12 fl.oz Can	150	0	37
16 fl.oz Bottle	200	0	50
20 fl.oz Bottle	250	0	63
24 fl.oz *(Pepsi)*	300	0	75
1 Liter Bottle	400	0	100
2 Liter Bottle	800	0	200

Other Soda Drinks

	C	F	Cb
Club Soda, 12 fl.oz	0	0	0
Club Soda Cream, 12 fl.oz	170	0	42
Diet Soft Drinks, avg., 12 fl.oz	0	0	0
Ginger Ale, 12 fl.oz	120	0	30
Lemon Lime, 12 fl.oz	220	0	55
Orange, 12 fl.oz	180	0	45
Root Beer, 12 fl.oz	165	0	41
Tonic Water, 12 fl.oz	135	0	34
Mineral Water: Plain, 12 fl.oz	0	0	0
Sweetened/flavored, 12 fl.oz	150	0	37
w. Fruit Juice, 12 fl.oz	120	0	30
Seltzers: Plain/Diet, 12 fl.oz	0	0	0
Sweetened/flavored, 12 fl.oz	150	0	37
w. Fruit Juice, 12 fl.oz	120	0	30

Movie Theater & Take-Out

Average All Flavors (Figures allow for 1/3rd Ice)

	C	F	Cb
Small, 12 fl.oz	110	0	27
Regular, 16 fl.oz	150	0	37
Medium, 22 fl.oz	210	0	52
Large, 32 fl.oz	300	0	75
Cinnabon: Icescapes, 16 fl.oz			
Orange Cream	360	16	50
Root Beer	470	22	63
Mochalatta	390	12	62

Soda Brands

Per 12 fl.oz Unless Indicated

	C	F	Cb
A&W: Cream Soda	165	0	41
Diet Cream Soda/Root Beer	1	0	0
Root Beer	180	0	45
Albertson's: Cola	160	0	43
Lemon Lime	140	0	38
Other flavors, average	170	0	47

Soda Brands (Cont)

Per 12 fl.oz Unless Indicated

	C	F	Cb
Arizona: Lemonade, 8 fl.oz	110	0	28
Barq's Root Beer	165	0	41
Barrelhead, Rootbeer	165	0	41
Big Red, 12 fl.oz	150	0	38
Big Red, 12 fl.oz	150	0	38
Blue Sky: Cola; Orange Cream	160	0	44
Cherry; Raspberry; Root Beer	180	0	45
Grape; Lemon Lime; Dr Becker	140	0	36
Organic, all flavors	170	0	43
Other varieties, average	150	0	39
Cactus Cooler	150	0	40
Canada Dry: Club Soda	0	0	0
Ginger Ale, all flavors	135	0	37
Tonic Water/Twist Lime	150	0	37
Diet	0	0	0
Clearly Canadian, 11 fl.oz, avg.	90	0	33
Coca-Cola: Classic/Caffeine Free	140	0	35
Diet Coke, all flavors	0	0	0
Cherry Coke/Vanilla Coke	150	0	40
Cragmont: Cola	165	0	41
Cherry	180	0	45
Diet, all flavors	0	0	0
Crush, all flavors	210	0	52
Crystal Light, all flavors	8	0	2
Diet Rite, all flavors	1	0	0
Dr Diablo, Cola	140	0	35
Dr Nehi	150	0	41
Dr Pepper: Reg./Red Fusion	150	0	40
Diet (Reg.; Caffeine Free)	3	0	0.5
Fanta: Orange; Grape	180	0	45
Strawberry; Pineapple	180	0	48
Fresca	4	0	1
Frutopia: See Page 155			
GuS, avg. all flavors	100	0	25
Hansen's: Diet Soda, average	0	0	0
Natural Soda, all flavors, 8 fl.oz	110	0	30
Natural Lemonade(s), 16 fl.oz	200	0	52
Signature Soda, avg.	150	0	42
Hawaiian Punch, all flavors	180	0	45
Health Valley			
Ginger Ale; Sarsp. Root Beer	150	0	41
Rootbeer Old Fashioned	120	0	30
Hires: Cream; Root Beer	180	0	45
IBC: Root Beer	110	0	29
Cream Soda; Black Cherry	180	0	48
Diet Root Beer	0	0	0

Soft Drinks (Cont)

Per 12 fl.oz Unless Indicated	C	F	Cb
Jolt Cola	150	0	41
Knudsen: Spritzers, average	170	0	43
Lucozade, 7 fl.oz	136	0	34
Mello Yello: Regular	180	0	45
Diet	5	0	0
Minute Maid: Lemonade	160	0	40
Berry; Black Cherry; Orange	165	0	41
Fruit Punch; Grape; Strawberry	180	0	45
Lemonade	160	0	40
Peach; P'apple; Raspb.; Grapefr.	165	0	41
Valencia Orange; Mixed Berry	180	0	50
Light Valencia Orange	10	0	2
Mistic: Punch, 16 fl.oz	230	0	57
'N Juice, average	155	0	38
Sparkling, average, 11.1 fl.oz	115	0	28
Mountain Dew, 24 fl.oz bottle	170	0	46
Live Wire; Code Red	170	0	45
Diet flavors	0	0	0
Mr Pibb Regular	150	0	37
Mug Root Beer	160	0	43
Natural Brew: Vanilla, Cream	170	0	43
Ginseng Cola, Ginger Ale	170	0	43
Orange; Grapefruit, avg.	155	0	39
Nehi (Royal Crown): Cream	180	0	45
Ginger Ale, Quinine Water	135	0	45
Other flavors, average	195	0	45
Orangina: 10 fl.oz bottle	120	0	45
Rouge, 8 fl.oz	90	0	22
Pepsi: Regular/Blue/Caffeine Free	150	0	41
Diet Pepsi/Twist/Vanilla	0	0	0
One	1	0	0
Twist	150	0	40
Wild Cherry; Vanilla	160	0	43
Perrier Regular or flavors	0	0	0
Ramblin' Root Beer	180	0	45
RC Cola: Regular; Cherry	160	0	40
Diet Cola	1	0	0
Reed's: Spiced Apple Brew	160	0	41
Ginger Brew, avg. all varieties	145	0	38
Santa Cruz: Sparkling, all types	150	0	37
Schweppes: Bitter Lemon/Sour	165	0	41
Ginger Ale, Regular; Raspberry	120	0	30
Seltzer	0	0	0
Tonic Water	120	0	30
7UP: Regular	140	0	38
Cherry, Gold	155	0	38
Caffeinated	170	0	46
Diet varieties	0	0	0

Per 12 fl.oz Unless Indicated	C	F	Cb
Shasta: Black Cherry	170	0	46
Cherry Cola; Doc Shasta	160	0	40
Club Soda; Diet, all flavors	0	0	0
Cola, regular	170	0	46
Caffeine Free	160	0	40
Cream Soda	190	0	47
Fruit Punch, Pineapple	200	0	50
French Vanilla Cola	180	0	45
Ginger Ale	130	0	33
Orange	200	0	49
Root Beer	170	0	42
Sierra Mist Lemon Lime	150	0	39
Slice: Lemon Lime	150	0	38
Diet Lemon Lime	0	0	0
Orange	190	0	50
Diet Orange	0	0	0
Sprite: Regular	150	0	37
Diet	4	0	1
Tropical Remix	140	0	38
Squirt: Citrus Burst	150	0	40
Diet Citrus Burst	0	0	0
Ruby Red Soda	170	0	46
Star Ruby: Dry Valencia Orange	100	0	26
Other flavors	95	0	24
Sunkist: Average all flavors	210	0	52
Diet Citrus	0	0	0
Diet Orange	7	0	1.5
Surge Citrus	170	0	46
TAB	0	0	0
Think!: Root Beer, 8.4 fl.oz	118	0	27
Sparkling Citrus, 8.4 fl.oz	130	0	31
Cola, 8.4 fl.oz	112	0	29
Upper 10 (RC): Regular	150	0	37
Diet	4	0	1
Vernor's: Ginger Ale	150	0	37
Diet, 10 fl.oz	0	0	0
Welch's: Sparkling, average	180	0	45
Wild Oats: Down to Earth	150	0	37
Wink	195	0	48

Powdered Soft Drink Mix

Per 8 fl.oz (Prep'd)	C	F	Cb
Country Time: Lemonade	60	0	16
Other flavors, avg.	85	0	22
Crystal Light, 8 fl.oz	5	0	1
Flavoraid, 1/8 pkg	2	0	0.5
Sugar-Free, 6 fl.oz	5	0	1
Kool-Aid: All flavors	70	0	17
Unsweetened, 6 fl.oz	2	0	0.5
Tang, 8 fl.oz	100	0	24

Coffee • Hot Chocolate

Instant Coffee

	C	F	Cb
Powder/Granules: Regular or Decaffeinated,			
1 level tsp	2	0	0.5
1 rounded tsp	4	0	1
Ground, 1 Tbsp	5	0	1
Brewed/Percolated, 1 cup, 8 fl.oz	5	0	1
Coffee With Milk/Cream/Creamers:			
1 Cup Coffee (8 fl.oz):			
w. Whole Milk: Dash, 1 Tbsp	10	0.5	1
2 Tbsp, 1 fl.oz	20	1	1.5
w. 2% Milk, 2 Tbsp	15	0.5	1.5
w. 1% Milk, 2 Tbsp	12	0.3	1.5
w. Fat Free Milk, 2 Tbsp	10	0	1.5
w. Half & Half: 2 Tbsp	45	4	1
w. Cream (light coffee): 2 Tbsp	65	6	1
w. *Coffee Mate:* Liquid, reg., 1T.	40	2	5
Liquid Fat Free, 1 Tbsp	15	0	2
Powder, 1 heaping tsp	20	1	2
Sugar ~ Add Extra: 1 heaping tsp	25	0	6
Single portion, 1 pkt	25	0	6

Flavored Coffee Mixes

	C	F	Cb
Caffé D'Vita: 1 tsp	20	1	4
Coffee Essence, 1 tsp	16	0	4
General Foods, Cafe Intl: Regular	60	3	10
Sugar-free, average	30	2	3
Maxwell House: Mocha, 1 envelope	100	2.5	17
Mocha, sugar-free, 1 envelope	60	3	7
Van., Irish Cream, 1 envelope	90	1	20
Nescafé: Frothé, all flavors, average	90	1.5	19
Chicory: Instant Coffee, 1 tsp	6	0	1
Coffee Essence, 1 tsp	16	0	4

Coffee Substitute Mixes

Roasted Cereal Beverages: (No Caffeine)

	C	F	Cb
Cafix Instant Beverage, 1 tsp	6	0	1
Kaffree Roma (Natural Touch) , 1 tsp	6	0	1
Postum, Instant Hot Beverage, 1 tsp	12	0	3
Revival Soy "Coffee", 1 Tbsp	5	0	1
Teeccino Caffe, 1 tsp	10	0	2

Vending Machine

	C	F	Cb
Cappuccino, 1 cup, 8 fl.oz	70	4	6

Coffee Shops/Restaurants

Per 8 fl.oz Cup (Unless Indicated)	C	F	Cb
Coffee (Regular/Percolated/Filtered)	5	0	1
Americano Drip Coffee, 1 cup	5	0	1
Cafe Au Lait: 1 cup, 8 fl.oz	65	2.5	6
Nonfat Milk, 1 cup	45	0	7
Caffe Latté:			
8 fl.oz cup: w. Whole Milk	100	5	8
w. 2% Milk	80	2.5	8
w. Nonfat Milk	60	0	8
12 fl.oz: w. Whole Milk	180	10	14
w. Nonfat Milk	110	0.5	15
16 fl.oz: w. Whole Milk	200	10	16
w. Nonfat Milk	120	0	16
Cafe Mocha (Mochaccino): 1 c.	120	3	15
12 fl.oz	180	4.5	15
16 fl.oz	240	6	15
Cappuccino:			
8 fl.oz cup: w. Whole Milk	70	4	6
w. 2% Milk	60	2	6
w. Nonfat Milk	40	0	6
12 fl.oz: w. Whole Milk	110	6	9
w. 2% Milk	80	3	9
w. Nonfat Milk	60	0	9
16 fl.oz: w. Whole Milk	140	7	12
w. Nonfat Milk	80	0	12
Mocha, with Cream			
8 fl.oz: w. Whole Milk	180	12	16
w. Nonfat Milk	150	8	16
Tall, 12 fl.oz: Whole Milk	290	18	25
w. Nonfat Milk	230	11	26
Iced Mocha (no cream)			
Tall, 12 fl.oz: w. Whole Milk	190	9	24
w. Nonfat Milk	140	2	24
Espresso: Regular	4	0	1
Doppio (Double)	8	0	2
Espresso Con Panna			
(w. dollop whipped cream)	30	3	1
Espresso Macchiato	15	0.5	2
Frappuccino: Tall, 12 fl.oz	200	3	39
Grande, 16 fl.oz	270	4	52
Frappuccino Mocha:			
Large/Tall, 12 fl.oz	230	3	44
Grande, 16 fl.oz	310	4.5	59
Iced Latte: Similar to Caffe Latte			
Intellicino: 12 fl.oz	150	7	15
Lowfat (2% Milk)	120	3.5	5
Starbucks: *See Page 249*			

Starbucks: *See Page 249*

Hot Chocolate ✦ Caffeine Counter

Irish & Liqueur Coffees

	C	F	Cb
Irish Coffee (no sugar)	175	10	0
Liqueur Coffee, avg. all types	200	10	16

Cocoa & Hot Chocolate

	C	F	Cb
Cocoa: 8 fl.oz cup: w. Whole Milk	210	14	19
w. Nonfat Milk	80	8	2
Tall (12 fl.oz): w. Whole Milk	300	20	26
w. Nonfat Milk	120	11	5
Hot Chocolate:			
8 fl.oz cup: w. Whole Milk	200	10	25
w. Nonfat Milk	140	2	25
Tall (12 fl.oz): w. Whole Milk	300	15	38
w. Nonfat Milk	210	3	38
Cinnabon: Mocholatta Chill, 16 oz	410	18	54

Coffee Extras

	C	F	Cb
Chocolate (Cocoa) Topping, 1/2 tsp	10	0	2
Flavored Syrups, 2 Tbsp	80	0	20
Sugar-free, 2 Tbsp	0	0	0
Hershey's Chocolate Syrup, 2 Tbsp	100	0	24
Half & Half Cream, 2 Tbsp	40	3	3
Light Whipped Cream, 2 Tbsp	30	2	2
Marshmallows, miniature, 2	20	0	5

Bottled Coffee (Chilled)

Ready-To-Drink: Per Bottle

	C	F	Cb
Arizona Mocha Latte 10 1/2 fl.oz	130	2	24
Blue Luna: Cafe Latte 12 1/2 fl.oz	195	3	36
Lite Cafe Mocha, 12 1/2 fl.oz	114	3	15
Jakada (Folgers) Coffee Latte:			
French Roast, 10 1/2 fl.oz	170	3.5	31
Mocha, 10 1/2 fl.oz	180	3.5	33
Jaradelic (Planet Java), 9 1/2 fl.oz	180	3	34
Kahlúa Cappuccino Shake 15 1/2 fl.oz	195	3	36
Main St Cafe:			
French Van. Ice Latte, 12 fl.oz	190	3	31
Meadow Gold Mocha Latte	450	16	61
Nescafe: Caffe Latte	140	3.5	23
Mocha	140	3	26
Royal Mills: Per Can			
Hawaiian Kona; Iced, 10.8 oz	125	2	27
Iced Cappuccino, 10.8 oz	165	3	32
Island Mocha, 10.8 oz	220	3.5	42
Kona Blend, 11.5 oz	90	1.5	18
Starbucks: Per 9.5 fl.oz Bottle			
Frappuccino: Caramel	200	3	37
Coffee	190	3.5	35
Hazelnut; Mocha	200	3.5	37
DoubleShot, 6.5 fl.oz can	140	6	18

Caffeine Counter

Moderate caffeine intake is not harmful to healthy adults. However, regular large amounts (over 350mg/day) may cause dependency ('caffeinism') and adversely affect health. To be safe, limit caffeine to 200mg/day. Avoid if pregnant; breast feeding; a child under 8; or have heart arrhythmias.

Caffeine	(mg)
Coffee: Instant, Weak, 1 level teaspoon	45
Medium, 1 rounded teaspoon	70
Strong, 1 heaping teaspoon	100
Decaffeinated, 1 round teaspoon	2
Bags*(Folgers),* 1 bag (6-8 fl.oz)	115
Ground, 1 Tbsp, 6g	60
Bottled (Ready-to-Drink), 9.5 fl.oz	70
Coffee Shop: Brewed, 8 fl.oz	110-150
Cappuccino: 1 cup, 8 fl.oz	80
Tall, 12 fl.oz	120
Large, 16 fl.oz	160
Decappuccino (decaffeinated)	5
Espresso: Regular/Solo	80
Double (Doppio) Espresso	160
Iced Coffee, 12 fl.oz	80
Latte, 1 cup, 8 fl.oz	80
Mocha, 8 fl.oz	90
Hot Chocolate, 8 fl.oz	10
Tea (Black/Green): Weak, 1 cup	20
Medium Strength, 1 cup	40
Strong, 1 cup	70
Herbal Tea	0
Iced Tea, Tall Glass/Can, 12 fl.oz	25
Soda Drinks: *Per 12 fl.oz Can*	
Coca-Cola (Classic/Van./Cherry); *Pepsi* (Reg./Diet)	35
Diet Coke; TAB; RC Cola (Regular)	45
Dr. Pepper (Reg./Diet); *Diet Dr. Pepper*	40
Sunkist Orange Soda; Mr PiBB	40
Jolt Cola; SunDrop	65-70
Pepsi One; Mtn Dew; Mellow Yellow; Surge	55
Chocolate Bars: Milk Chocolate, 2 oz	12
Dark Chocolate, 2 oz	30
Cocoa/Hot Choc. Mix, 1 oz pkt	5
Chocolate Milk, 1 cup, 8 fl.oz	3
Choc Chip Cookies, 1 medium, 1 oz	3
Chocolate Cake, 3 oz	5
Chocolate Icecream, 1/2 cup	2
Chocolate Syrup, 2 Tbsp, 1.4 oz	7

Extensive Caffeine Counter ~ www.CalorieKing.com

Teas

	C	**F**	**Cb**
Regular: Bag, Loose or Instant			
Brewed, 1 cup, 8 fl.oz	1	0	0
(Add extra for sugar/milk)			
Herbal: Average all varieties, 1 cup	1	0	0
Bigelow: Apple Orchard, 1 cup	5	0	1
Other Varieties	2	0	0.5
Celestial Seasonings:			
Bengal Spice; Spearmint	5	0	0.5
Lemon Zinger	4	0	1
Roastaroma	10	0	2
Other varieties	2	0	0.5
Chai Tea Latté (Starbucks): See Page 249			
Bubble Tea, 12 fl.oz	240	0	55

Quick Guide

Iced Tea

	C	**F**	**Cb**
Average All Brands			
Pre-Sweetened: 8 fl.oz	100	0	25
12 fl.oz	150	0	38
16 fl.oz	200	0	50
Unsweetened: 8 fl.oz	2	0	0

Iced Tea Mixes

Per Serving (1 Cup, Made-Up)

4C Instant	90	0	22
Bigelow, Nice Over Ice	1	0	0.5
Celestial Seasonings, Iced Delight	4	0	1
Crystal Light, Sugar Free	3	0	0
Kool-Aid Fruit T's	70	0	17
Lipton: Instant	0	0	0
Instant Lemon/Raspberry	3	0	1
Lemon	55	0	14
Peach/Raspb, Sugar Free	5	0	1
Nestea: 100% Instant	2	0	0
Decaffeinated	6	0	1
Ice Teasers, all flavors	6	0	1
Peach, Raspberry	90	0	22

> *A woman is like a teabag. You never know her strength until she's in hot water.*
>
> ~ Nancy Reagan

Bottled & Canned Teas

Per 8 fl.oz Unless Indicated

	C	**F**	**Cb**
Arizona:			
Original Iced Tea	100	0	25
Green Tea(s)/Asian Plum	70	0	18
Diet Green/Lemon	0	0	0
Iced Tea w. Ginseng Extract	60	0	15
Herb Tea w. Honey	70	0	17
Peach/Raspberry	90	0	22
Brisk: 1 liter Bottle, avg, 1 cup	90	0	24
12 fl.oz Can: Lemon, 1 can	120	0	33
Raspberry, 1 can	130	0	35
24 fl.oz Bottle: Lemon, 1 cup	80	0	22
Hansen's: Natural Iced Tea, 8 fl.oz	70	0	21
Low Calorie Blueberry/Raspberry	10	0	3
Knudsen: Coolers, all flavors	90	0	23
Lipton (16 fl.oz Bottle): *Per 8 fl.oz*			
No Lemon	70	0	18
Lemon	90	0	21
Peach; Raspberry	110	0	26
Mistic: Tropical Cooler, 8 fl.oz	45	0	12
Nantucket: Blueberry Tea, 8 fl.oz	80	0	20
Original Lemon Tea; Half & Half	90	0	23
Diet Lemon Tea	10	0	2
Nestea Iced Tea: Diet Lemon	3	0	0.5
Cool from Nestea, 1 cup, 8 fl.oz	80	0	20
Diet Cool from Nestea	2	0	0.5
Lemon/Peach/Raspberry	90	0	22
Sweetened Ice Tea	65	0	17
Oregon Chai: Herbal Bliss, 1/2 cup	70	0	18
Nirvana/Kashmir Green, 1/2 cup	80	0	20
Royal Mistic: Regular, 12 fl.oz	145	0	36
Diet, 12 fl.oz	8	0	2
Schweppes, 8 fl.oz	90	0	22
Shasta, 8 fl.oz	80	0	20
Snapple: Regular, sweetened	70	0	17
Diet/Unsweetened	0	0	0
Lemon; Peach, Raspberry	100	0	25
SoBe: Green/Lemon Tea, 8 fl.oz	90	0	23
20 fl.oz bottle	225	0	57
Ssips (Johanna Farms), 8.45 fl.oz	100	0	25
Tropicana: Lemonfruit	100	0	25
Diet Lemon Fruit	15	0	4
Peach/Rasp./Tangerine, 8 fl.oz	120	0	28
11.5 fl.oz can	160	0	40
Twister: Apple Berry, 8 fl.oz	100	0	28
Turkey Hill: Regular	90	0	22
Raspberry Cooler	110	0	28

Alcohol Guide

♦ **Health Hazards: Excess alcohol** contributes to obesity, high blood pressure, stroke, heart and liver disease, some cancers, and even impotence. **Concentration and short-term memory** are reduced as well as sporting performance.

Other alcohol hazards include stomach upsets, menstrual problems, anxiety, headaches, insomnia, work absenteeism, risky behaviors, and family arguments.

♦ **Alcohol contributes to obesity** through its high calories and by lessening the body's ability to burn fat. Fat storage is promoted, particularly in the belly - a health danger zone. Alcohol can also stimulate appetite.

♦ **Alcohol is potentially more harmful while dieting.** Blood sugar levels may drop with resultant tiredness and further impairment of concentration, reflexes and driving skills - and maybe even the dieter's resolve!

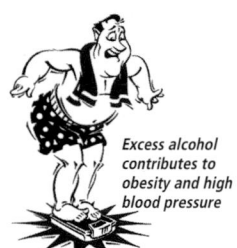

Excess alcohol contributes to obesity and high blood pressure

SAFE ALCOHOL LIMITS

Women: No more than **1 drink** per day.
Men: No more than **2 drinks** per day.
(At least 2 days a week should be alcohol-free.)

1 Drink = 12 fl.oz regular beer, or 5 fl.oz wine,
or 1½ fl.oz spirits (80 proof).
Each drink contains approximately 14g alcohol.

For some people, **safe drinking** will mean no alcohol drinks at all. (Even one drink may impair driving skills, particularly if tired; and 3-4 drinks daily has been linked to brain shrinkage in some social drinkers).

♦ **It is advisable not to drink at all if you are:**
- pregnant or trying to conceive
- taking drug medication (unless approved by your doctor or pharmacist)
- have a condition such as liver or heart disease
- planning to drive, use machinery or play sport
- studying or needing to concentrate
- a child or adolescent

♦ **Women and adolescents are more prone** to alcohol's ill-effects due to their lower body weight, smaller livers and lesser capacity to metabolize alcohol.

Note: You cannot save daily drinks for one occasion.
Binge drinking is particularly harmful ~ 4 drinks 'in a row' for males or 3 drinks for females.

Extra Information: www.CalorieKing.com

HOW TO CALCULATE ALCOHOL CONTENT

Percent alcohol on label refers to alcohol volume (ml alcohol/100ml).

100ml = 3½ fl. oz

To convert to grams (weight) of alcohol, multiply the percent volume by 0.8 - since 1 ml of alcohol weighs only 0.8 grams (actually 0.789g).

EXAMPLE

12 fl.oz Can Beer (5% alcohol)

5% alc.volume = 5% of 12 fl.oz
= 0.6 fl.oz
= 18ml alcohol
(1 fl.oz = 30ml)

Weight (18ml x 0.8) = 14.4g alc.

GOVERNMENT WARNING

(1) According to the Surgeon General, women should not drink alcoholic beverages during pregnancy because of the risk of birth defects.

(2) Consumption of alcoholic beverages impairs your ability to drive a car or operate machinery, and may cause health problems.

Beers • Ales (with Alcohol Counts)

Quick Guide Alc ~ Alcohol (Grams)

Beer Cb ~ Carbohydrate

Beer Contains Zero Fat

Regular Beer (5% Alc. Vol.)

	C	Alc	Cb
7 fl.oz Glass	80	8.5	4
12 fl.oz Bottle/Can/Glass	140	14	10
16 fl.oz Bottle/Can	185	19	13
22 fl.oz Bottle	260	25	20
24 fl.oz Can	280	28	20
32 fl.oz Bottle	370	35	28
40 fl.oz Bottle	470	46	35
50 fl.oz Football	590	57	50

Light Beer (4.2% Alc. Vol.)

	C	Alc	Cb
7 fl.oz Glass	65	7	4
12 fl.oz Bottle/Can/Glass	110	12	7
16 fl.oz Bottle/Can	145	16	9
22 fl.oz Bottle	200	22	13
24 fl.oz Can	220	24	14

Non-Alcoholic/Near Beer

(Less than 0.5% alcohol by volume)

	C	Alc	Cb
Average All Brands, 12 fl.oz	70	1	16

Beer Brands

Per 12 fl.oz Serving Alc ~ Alcohol (Grams)
*Percentage alcohol listed below
is by volume - not by weight.*

	C	Alc	Cb
Amber Ice (5.3% alcohol)	130	15	6
Amstel Light (3.5%)	100	10	5
Anchor Steam (4.6%)	155	13	16
Arrogant Bastard Ale (7.2%)	190	20	12
Artic Ice (5.3%)	150	15	8
Artic Ice Light (3.9%)	100	11	6
Asahi Super Dry (5.2%)	150	15	11
Augsburger Bock (4.9%)	170	14	17
Bass (5.51%)	140	16	13
Beck's (5%)	150	14	12
Big Sky (4.8%)	150	14	12
Big Sky Light (4.5%)	105	13	5
Black Label (5.6%)	155	15	11
Blackhook Porter (4.9%)	160	14	14
Blatz (4.6%)	145	13	13
Blatz LA (2.3%)	75	7	6
Blatz Light (3.9%)	110	11	8
Blonde (4.3%)	140	12	10
Bud Dry (4.9%)	130	14	8
Bud Light (4.2%)	110	12	7
Bud Ice (5.5%)	150	16	9
Bud Ice Light (4.1%)	110	12	7

Brands (Cont)

Beer Contains Zero Fat

	C	Alc	Cb
Budweiser (4.9%)	145	14	11
Natural Light (4.2%)	110	12	7
Natural Ice (5.8%)	160	16	10
Busch (4.6%)	135	13	10
Busch Ice (5.9%)	175	16	13
Busch Light (4.2%)	110	12	7
Carling (4.4%)	140	13	10
Carlsberg (5%)	135	13	10
Carta Blanca (4.0%)	125	11	11
Castlemaine XXXX (4.7%)	140	13	9
Colt 45 Malt (5.6%)	160	15	11
Coors (5%)	150	14	12
Coors Extra Gold (5%)	150	14	11
Coors Light (4.2%)	105	12	5
Corona Extra (4.6%)	150	13	13
Corona Light (4.1%)	105	12	5
Dos Equis Lager (5%)	130	14	9
Drop Top Amber Ale (4.8%)	165	13	15
Fosters Lager (4.9%)	135	14	9
George Killian's: Irish Brown (5.2%)	185	15	15
Irish Red (5%)	160	14	13
Goebel (4.1%)	130	11	12
Goebel Light (3.9%)	110	11	8
Grolsch Premium (5%)	140	14	10
Guinness Draught (4.2%)	125	12	10
Guinness Extra Stout (5.8%)	175	17	14
Hamm's (4.7%)	145	13	12
Special Light (4.1%)	110	12	7
Harp (4.5%)	150	12	13
Heineken (5%)	150	14	12
Heineken Special Dark (5.2%)	175	15	16
Hop Jack Pale Ale (5%)	185	14	14
Hurricane (5.8%)	160	16	10
Icehouse (5.0%)	135	14	8
Icehouse (5.5%)	150	15	9
Jacob Best Ice (5.8%)	160	16	11
Keystone: Premium (4.4%)	125	12	6
Ice (5.9%)	130	17	5
Light, (4.2%)	100	12	5
Killarney's Red Larger (5%)	200	14	23
Killain's (4.9%)	165	14	14
King Cobra (5.9%)	170	16	12
Kirin Lager (4.9%)	145	14	11
Kirin Light (3.2%)	95	9	7
Labatt's Blue (5%)	145	14	9

Beers • Ales (with Alcohol Counts)

Brands (Cont)

Alc ~ Alcohol (Grams)
Cb ~ Carbohydrate

Beer Contains Zero Fat
Per 12 fl.oz Serving

	C	Alc	Cb
Leinenkugel's: Original (4.6%)	150	13	14
Light (4.1%)	105	11	6
Lone Star: Regular (4.7%)	140	13	12
Light (3.9%)	110	11	8
Lowenbrau Dark/Special (4.9%)	160	14	15
Magic Hat #9 (4.8%)	140	14	12
Magnum Malt Liquor (5.6%)	155	16	10
Meister Brau (4.5%)	130	13	12
Memphis Brown (4.6%)	120	13	6
Michelob: Regular (5%)	155	14	14
Light (4.3%)	135	12	12
Dry (4.9%)	130	14	8
AmberBock (5.2%)	165	15	15
Golden Draft (4.7%)	150	13	13
Golden Draft Light (4.2%)	110	12	7
Hefeweizen (5%)	155	14	12
Honeylarger (4.9%)	175	14	18
ULTRA (4.2%)	95	12	3
Mickey's Malt Liquor (5.6%)	160	16	11
MGD (5%)	145	14	13
MGD Light (4.5%)	110	13	7
Miller High Life (5%)	145	14	13
Miller High Life Light (4.5%)	110	13	6
Miller Lite (4.5%)	100	13	4
Milwaukee's Best (4.5%)	130	13	12
Milwaukee's Best Ice (5.9%)	145	16	6
Milwaukee's Best Light (4.5%)	100	13	4
Minnesota's Best (4.9%)	140	14	10
Molson Canadian (5%)	150	14	14
Molson Ice (5.6%)	160	16	12
Molson Special Dry (5%)	145	14	10
Moosehead (5%)	125	14	14
Negra Modela (5%)	155	14	14
Newcastle Brown Ale (4.5%)	140	12	13
Northstone Amber Ale (4.9%)	150	14	8
Olde English "800" (5.9%)	160	16	11
Old Milwaukee (4.6%)	145	13	13
Light (3.9%)	110	11	8
Ice (5.9%)	180	16	15
Old Style (4.7%)	140	13	12
Old Style Light (4.2%)	115	12	7
Old Style LA (2.2%)	75	6	6
Pabst (4.3%)	145	13	12
Pabst Blue Ribbon (4.7%)	145	14	12
Pabst Light (3.9%)	110	11	8
Pabst Extra Light (2.2%)	70	6	6
Pete's Wicked Ale (5%)	180	14	20
Piels (4.3%)	125	12	9
Red Dog (5%)	150	14	14
Red Hook ESB (5.7%)	180	17	16
Red Hook India Pale Ale (4.7%)	180	13	19
Red Stripe Jamaican Ale (5.0%)	155	14	14
Red Wolf (5.4%)	150	15	10
Rolling Rock (4.5%)	120	12	7
Sam Adams Light (4%)	130	11	10
Samuel Adams (4.6%)	170	13	17
Samuel Adams Lager (4.7%)	180	13	19
Sapporo Draft (3.9%)	135	11	14
Schaefer (4.6%)	145	13	12
Schaefer Light (3.9%)	110	11	8
Schlitz (4.6%)	145	13	12
Schlitz Light (3.9%)	110	11	8
Schmidt's (4.6%)	145	13	13
Schmidt's Light (3.9%)	110	11	8
Sheaf Stout, 5.7%	180	16	17
Sierra Nevada: Pale Ale (5.6%)	200	16	12
Big Foot (9.6%)	295	28	25
Porter (5.6%)	200	16	16
Wheat Beer (4.4%)	150	12	12
Silver Thunder (5.9%)	165	17	11
Sol Cerveza Especial (4%)	125	11	11
Southpaw Light (5%)	125	14	7
St Pauli Girl (5%)	135	14	9
Stella Artois, 5%, 330ml	135	14	9
Stroh's (4.6%)	145	13	12
Stroh's Light (4.0%)	130	12	10
Tecate (4.7%)	155	13	16
Tequiza (4.5%)	125	12	9
Warsteiner: Verum/Dunkel (5%)	155	14	13
Weinhard's: Pale Ale (4/6%)	150	13	13
Hefeweízen (4.9%)	155	14	12
Wheat Hook (4.8%)	150	14	12
Widmer: Hefeweizen (4.7%)	155	13	16
Zeigenbock Amber (4.4%)	145	12	13

Home-Brewed Beer: Similar to regular beers, according to alcohol content.

Cider • Wine (with Alcohol Counts)

Non-Alcoholic Brews

Less Than 0.5% Alcohol **C** **Alc** **Cb**
Average All Brands (Busch NA, Coors NA, Kaliber, Kingsbury, O'Douls NA, Old Milwaukee NA, Pabst NA, Stroh's NA, Sharp's, Haakebeck, Texas Select)

	C	Alc	Cb
12 fl.oz Can/Bottle	65	1	14

Cider **Alc** ~ Alcohol (Grams) **Cb** ~ Carbohydrate

	C	Alc	Cb
Alcoholic Cider: Average, 6% alcohol,			
Dry, 12 fl.oz	130	17	12
Sweet, 12 fl.oz	170	17	15
Hardcore Crisp Hard Cider (6%)	190	17	19
Hornsby's: Draft Cider (6%)	170	17	16
Hard Apple Cider (5.5%)	200	16	27
Woodchuck (5%) Amber, 12 fl.oz	200	15	21
Dark & Dry, 12 fl.oz	180	15	21
Granny Smith, 12 fl.oz	165	15	11
Wyder's: Raspb. (4%), 11.5 fl.oz	140	11	15
Peach (5%) 11.5 fl.oz	150	13	16
Pear (5%), 11.5 fl.oz	130	13	14
22 fl.oz bottle	250	25	28

Quick Guide

Table Wine **C** **Alc** **Cb**
Average All Varieties (11.5% Alcohol)

	C	Alc	Cb
4 fl.oz 1 small wine glass OR 1/2 large wine glass	85	11	2
6 fl.oz (3/4 large wine glass)	125	16	3
8 fl.oz (1 large wine glass)	170	22	4
1/2 Carafe/Bottle, 375ml	265	34	6
1 Bottle, 750ml	530	68	13

Table Wines **C** **Alc** **Cb**

	C	Alc	Cb
Red: Claret/Burgundy/Chianti, 4 fl.oz	80	11	2
Sparkling Reds, 4 fl.oz	90	11	3
Rose: Medium, 4 fl.oz	80	11	1.5
White: *Per 4 fl.oz*			
Dry (Chablis/Hock/Riesling)	75	11	1
Zinfandel Sweet (Moselle/Sauterne), 4 fl.oz	85	11	2
Sparkling, 4 fl.oz	95	11	4

Table Wines (Cont)

	C	Alc	Cb
Champagne: *Per 4 fl.oz Serving*			
Average 1 glass, 4 fl.oz	85	11	2
w. Orange Jce (3:1 orange)	75	8	4
w. Orange Jce (1:1 orange)	65	5	7
Cold Duck, 4. fl.oz	108	11	8
Mulled Wine: (Gluhwein), 4 fl.oz	180	14	20
Non-Alcoholic Wine, avg., 4 fl.oz	50	0	12
Reduced Alcohol Wine (6%):			
Average all types, 4 fl.oz	50	0	12
Sake: Rice Wine (16% alc.), 4 oz	125	15	5

Flavored Wine

Average All Brands (6% alcohol)
(Examples: Arbor Mist, Wild Vines, Boones)

	C	Alc	Cb
1 small wine glass, 4 fl.oz	80	6	11
1 large wine glass, 8 fl.oz	160	11	21
1 bottle, 750 ml (25.4 fl.oz)	510	36	67

Dessert Wines

	C	Alc	Cb
Madeira (18% alc), 2 oz	85	9	5
Marsala (18%), 2 oz	110	9	11
Port, Muscatel, (18%), 2 oz	85	9	5
Sherry (18%), 2 oz			
Dry, 1 Sherry glass	65	9	0.5
Sweet/Cream, average	85	9	5
Vermouth: Dry (18%), 2 oz	65	9	0.5
Sweet (15%), 2 oz	85	7	8

Cooking Wine

Average All Brands

	C	Alc	Cb
Red/White: 2 Tbsp, 1 oz	20	3	1
1 cup, 8 fl.oz	160	22	12
Marsala, 2 Tbsp, 1 oz	35	4	2
Sherry, 2 Tbsp, 1 oz	40	4	2

Cooking with Wine:
For alcohol to evaporate, sufficient heat and cooking time (at least 30 minutes) is required.
Red and white table wines would then contain negligible residual calories.
Sweetened wines (marsala/sherry) would contain 10 calories per 1 fl.oz used.
Flambé Desserts: Only surface alcohol is burnt off, so negligible reduction in alcohol or calories.

Liquors ◆ Coolers ◆ Cocktails

Spirits/Liquors

Includes Bourbon, Brandy, Gin, Rum, Scotch, Tequila, Vodka, Whiskey.
Note: All spirits with same proof (alcohol) have similar calories and zero fat.

Average All Brands

	C	**Alc**	**Cb**
80 Proof (40% Alcohol by Volume):			
1 fl.oz (1 shot)	**65**	9.5	0
2 fl.oz (Double shot)	**130**	19	0
1/2 Bottle, 375 ml	**810**	120	0
1 Bottle, 750 ml	**1620**	240	0
86 Proof (43% Alcohol):			
1 fl.oz (1 shot)	**70**	10	0
2 fl.oz (Double shot)	**140**	20	0
1/2 Bottle, 375 ml	**870**	125	0
1 Bottle, 750 ml	**1750**	250	0
100 Proof (50% Alcohol):			
1 fl.oz (1 shot)	**82**	12	0
1/2 Bottle, 375 ml	**1025**	150	0
1 Bottle, 750ml	**2050**	300	0

Flavored Spirits ~ Average All Brands

	C	**Alc**	**Cb**
70 Proof (35% Alcohol)			
1 fl.oz (1 shot)	**70**	8.5	2
2 fl.oz (Double shot)	**140**	17	0.5

Hard Lemonade

	C	**Alc**	**Cb**
Average All Brands (5%), 12 fl.oz	**250**	14	39
Doc Otis Lemon (4.8%), 12 fl.oz	**250**	14	39
Henry's Hard Lem'ade (5%), 12 fl.oz	**285**	14	46
Hooch Hard (5.2%), 330ml	**215**	14	32
Hooch Ice (5.7%), 330ml	**230**	15	32
Mike's (5.2%), 11.2 fl.oz	**250**	14	38
24 fl.oz bottle	**530**	29	80
Rick's Spiked (5.2%), 12 fl.oz	**250**	14	39

Enjoy a beer but watch the portion size. Those footballs hold 50 fl.oz !

Coolers & Premix Cocktails

Ready-To-Drink
Zero Fat Unless Indicated

	C	**Alc**	**Cb**
Arbor Mist: Blenders,			
all flavors (12.5%), 4 fl.oz	**100**	11	14
Bacardi: Silver (5%), 12 fl.oz	**220**	14	35
Silver O³ (5%), 12 fl.oz	**225**	14	33
Silver Raz (5%), 12 fl.oz	**225**	14	33
Ready to Pour (1.75 liter bottle)			
Bahama Mama (10%), 4 fl.oz	**130**	13	16
Hurricane (12.5%), 4 fl.oz	**144**	12	16
Rum Island Ice Tea (12.5%), 4 fl.oz	**150**	12	16
Bartles & Jaymes			
Malt Based Coolers (3.9% alc): Per 12 fl.oz			
Black Cherry; Classic Original	**200**	11	30
Exotic Berry, Juicy Peach	**210**	11	33
Fuzzy Navel; Hard Lemonade	**230**	11	38
Margarita, Pina Colada	**270**	11	48
Raspberry Daiquiri	**220**	11	38
Strawb. Cosmopolitan/Daiquiri	**230**	11	35
Raspb. Lemonade, Lusc. Blackb.	**230**	11	38
Cruzan Island Cocktails (5% alc): Per 12 fl.oz			
Jumbie Brew	**230**	14	32
Mojito	**300**	14	50
Wazi Koki	**285**	14	46
Jack Daniels Country Cocktails (5.9%)			
average all flavors, 6.8 fl.oz	**170**	10	25
Jack Daniels Hard Cola (5%) 12 oz	**234**	14	34
Jose Cuervo Authentic Margarita (5.9% alc)			
Margarita/ Lime.Strawb. 200ml	**180**	12	27
Sauza Diablo (5%), 12 fl.oz	**260**	14	40
Seagram's Coolers (5%)			
Smooth Red/Citrus 12 fl.oz	**240**	14	35
Skyy Blue (5%), 12 fl.oz	**280**	14	45
Stolichnayar Citr. (5%), 12 fl.oz	**240**	14	36
Smirnoff Ice (5%), 330ml	**225**	13	35
Triple Black, 12 fl.oz	**220**	14	29
TGI Friday's: Per 6 fl.oz			
On The Rocks: Margurita (7.5%)	**180**	12	27
Long Island Ice Tea (15%)	**260**	22	27
Mudslide (10%)	**400**	15	36
White Russian (12.5%)	**410**	17	38
Blenders: Mudslide (12.5%)	**240**	17	31
Orange Dream (12.5%)	**240**	17	31
Strawberry Shortcake (12.5%)	**235**	17	24

Coolers ◆ Cocktails (with Alcohol Counts)

Coolers & Premix Cocktails (Cont)

Ready-to-Drink

	C	**Alc**	**Cb**
The Club Premix Cocktails (8 oz Can): *Per 4 oz Serving (½ can)*			
Long Island Ice Tea; Manhattan	**220**	16	30
Margar.;Screwdriver;Vodka Martini	**210**	7	40
Mudslide (9g fat)	**270**	12	41
Pina Colada; Or. Craze; Whisk. Sour	**260**	10	40
Zima (4.8%), 12 fl.oz	**190**	13	22

Shooters   **Alc** ~ Alcohol (Grams)

	C	**Alc**	**Cb**
Alabama Slammer	**110**	14	2
Amaretto Sours	**120**	6	19
Cranium Meltdown	**75**	7	2
Duck Fart	**85**	7	5
Kamakazie	**150**	20	2
Kool-Aid	**160**	15	14
Liquid Cocaine	**130**	13	10
Mud Slide	**160**	13	17
Fuzzy Navel	**120**	13	7
Pineapple Bomber	**130**	11	13
Turbo	**110**	14	3

Cocktail Mix 'N Drinks

No Alcohol Added

	C	**Alc**	**Cb**
Bacardi: Frozen Concentrate *(Made Up from 2 fl.oz concentrate)*			
Margarita, 8 fl.oz	**90**	0	25
Pina Colada, 8 fl.oz	**170**	0	35
Strawberry, 8 fl.oz	**120**	0	35
Daily's Pina Colada, 3 fl.oz	**160**	0	37
J.Cuervo Margarita, 4 fl.oz	**100**	0	24
Mr & Mrs T: Mai Tai, 4.5 fl.oz	**140**	0	33
Bloody Mary, 8 fl.oz	**40**	0	9
Margarita, 4 fl.oz	**100**	0	26
Pina Colada, 4.5 fl.oz	**180**	0	43
Strawberry Daiquiri, 4 fl.oz	**200**	0	50
Sweet 'n' Sour, 4 fl.oz	**90**	0	23
Sauza Margarita, 3 fl.oz	**70**	0	18
Skyy Cosmo, 4 fl.oz	**140**	0	36
TGI Fridays: Hurricane, 2.3 fl.oz	**60**	0	15
Long Island Ice Tea, 3.3 fl.oz	**55**	0	14
Mudslide, 2.3 fl.oz	**120**	0	24

Cocktails   **Alc** ~ Alcohol (Grams)

Made to Standard Recipes
Main Reference: The New American Bartender's Guide

Zero Fat Unless Indicated	**C**	**Alc**	**Cb**
Bloody Mary	**95**	10	16
Blue Lady	**230**	15	16
Blushin' Russian (9g fat)	**365**	14	47
Bourbon & Soda	**130**	19	0
Brandy Alexander (10g fat)	**300**	20	17
Cerebral Hemorrhage (5g fat)	**290**	17	32
Chupa Naranjas (w. 1½ oz Tequila)	**150**	16	8
Collins (w. 2 oz Gin)	**180**	20	11
Cosmopolitan	**215**	24	12
Daiquiri: Fuzzy Navel	**140**	19	4
Frozen Daiquiri: no fruit	**155**	19	6
w. fruit (and less Rum)	**140**	14	10
Gin & Tonic	**220**	19	22
Grasshopper	**280**	13	30
Green Fantasy	**210**	23	11
Harvey Wallbanger (2 oz Vodka)	**200**	19	17
Highball (1½ oz Whiskey)	**110**	14	3
Irish Coffee (contains 5g fat)	**175**	14	6
Kahlua Mudslide: w.milk (3.5g fat)	**150**	11	10
w. cream (12.5g fat)	**230**	11	0
L.A. Sunrise	**280**	26	21
Lady Killer	**165**	13	20
Leprechaun's Libation	**285**	31	17
London Rock	**165**	18	10
Long Island Iced Tea (w. 8 oz Cola)	**290**	22	31
w. Diet Cola	**190**	22	6
Mai Tai (w. 2 oz Rum)	**220**	21	16
Manhattan	**130**	17	3
Margarita	**150**	18	4
Martini	**135**	20	0
Mind Eraser	**160**	17	10
Mint Julep	**210**	29	4
Mojito (w. 2 oz Rum)	**160**	19	6
Pina Colada (contains 12g fat)	**325**	19	12
Rainbow Room	**265**	30	14
Screwdriver	**160**	14	14
Sex On The Beach	**240**	20	26
Singapore Sling	**210**	25	9
Spritzer (3 oz Wine)	**60**	8	2
Tequila Sunrise	**200**	14	25
Tom Collins	**210**	24	12
Tom & Jerry	**170**	9	8
Whiskey Sour	**150**	19	5
White Russian	**250**	20	16

Liqueurs (with Alcohol Counts)

Liqueurs/Cordials

Per 1 fl.oz	C	Alc	Cb
Advocaat (36 Proof; 2g fat)	85	4	9
Amaretto (56 Proof)	110	6	17
Baileys Irish Cream (34 Proof; 5g fat)	95	4	5
Lite (30 Proof; 2g fat)	75	4	7
Benedictine (80 Proof)	90	10	5
Chartreuse (80 Proof)	100	10	7
Cherry Brandy (48 Proof)	80	6	9
Coffee Liqueur (53 Proof)	90	6.5	11
Cointreau (80 Proof)	100	10	7
Creme de Cacao (54 Proof)	100	6	15
Creme de Menthe (60 Proof)	120	7	14
Curacao (70 Proof)	95	8	6
Drambuie (80 Proof)	105	10	9
Frangelico (48 Proof)	80	6	9
Galliano (80 Proof)	100	10	8
Grand Marnier (80 Proof)	100	10	7
Kahlua (53 Proof)	90	6.5	11
Kirsch (68 Proof)	80	8	6
Midori (42 Proof), average all types	80	5	11
Ouzo (80 Proof)	90	10	5
Pernod (80 Proof)	75	10	2
Sambuca (84 Proof)	100	10	7
Schnapps (80 Proof)	100	10	7
Southern Comfort (78 Proof)	75	9	3
Tia Maria (64 Proof)	90	8	5
Triple Sec (60 Proof)	80	7	4

Liqueur Coffee & Hot Drinks

Liqueur Coffee, avg. all types	200	10	10
Egg Nog	270	10	25
Hot Toddy, w. 2 oz liquor	200	19	17
Irish Coffee, w. 2 Tbsp whip. crm	80	7	4
Mulled Wine (Glühwein), 5 oz	175	14	6

Flavorings/Syrups

Non-Alcoholic, Fat Free

Angostura Bitters, 1/4 tsp	3	0	0
Ginger Ale, 8 fl.oz	80	0	22
Grenadine/Cassis, 2 Tbsp, 1 oz	70	0	17
Lime/Lemon Juice, 2 Tbsp, 1 oz	10	0	2
Maraschino Cherry, 1 small	8	0	2
Sugar Syrup, 2 Tbsp, 1 oz	70	0	17
Sour Mix, 2 Tbsp, 1 oz	10	0	2
Tonic Water, 8 fl.oz	90	0	22

Ten Hints to Avoid Harmful Drinking

1. **Add up the alcohol** you typically drink each day and on social occasions. How does this compare with 'low risk' amounts?

2. **Compare the alcohol content** of different drinks and select the lowest. Request half ounces of alcohol in cocktails and mixed drinks. Dilute them and keep topping off with non-alcoholic drinks.

3. **Try low alcohol** or non-alcohol alternatives such as fruit juices and mineral water. Take your own to parties.

4. **Before drinking alcohol,** quench your thirst with water and non-alcoholic drinks - particularly after vigorous exercise or sport.

5. **Slow the rate of drinking.** Chugging or drinking fast is the major cause of illness and death from alcohol poisoning.

6. **Avoid drinking in 'rounds'.**

7. **Have a non-alcoholic 'spacer'** between drinks (e.g. mineral water, orange juice).

8. **Don't drink on an empty stomach.** Food slows the rate of alcohol absorption.

9. **Keep track of the number of drinks** and know when to stop. Stick to a set limit.

10. **Do not drive, swim, or operate machinery** while under the influence.

Note: Alcohol can be very dangerous when taken with prescription or street drugs or when you are very tired.

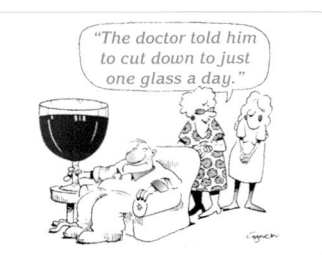

"The doctor told him to cut down to just one glass a day."

Cafeteria-Style Foods

	C	F	Cb
Beef Stroganoff, 5 oz	195	13	7
Beef Stroganoff w. 4 oz noodles	350	13	36
Chicken Lasagna, 1 piece	300	11	32
Chicken Chop Suey w. 4 oz rice	245	4	37
Deep Dish Burrito, 7 oz	265	13	20
Grnd Beef Casserole, 2 scoop, 6 oz	245	13	17
Italian Meat Sce for Spagh., 5 oz	150	9	9
w. 5 oz Spaghetti	350	10	49
Lasagna, 1 piece	275	11	25
Meatloaf, 3 oz	205	13	4
Ranch Beans, 2 scoops, 6 oz	350	11	45
Red Beans & Rice, 7 oz	280	9	37
Scalloped Potato/Ham, 6 scp, 6 oz	160	6	20
Stuffed Shells in Sauce (1)	105	3	17
Swedish Meatballs (3)	205	12	9
Sweet & Sour Pork/Rice, 9 oz	240	3	40
Swiss Steak w/Mushr. Gravy, 6 oz	280	11	4
Tator Tot Casserole, 2 scoops, 6 oz	260	15	20
Tenderloin Tips/Mushr. Gravy, 5 oz	210	13	3
w. 5 oz noodles	395	15	38
Tuna Noodle Casserole, 2 scp, 6 oz	180	6	17
Turkey Tetrazini, 2 scoops, 6 oz	195	7	17
Vegetable Lasagna, 1 piece	250	13	21

Croissants

Unfilled: Medium 1 1/2 oz	180	10	21
Filled: w. Ham (2 oz), Salad	280	14	24
w. Ham (2 oz), Cheese (2 oz)	470	30	20
w. Chick (2 oz) Cheese (2 oz)	470	30	20
w. Turkey/Ham/Chse (2 oz ea.)	580	36	20
Au Bon Pain: Ham & Cheese	290	9	39
Spinach & Cheese	220	9	29
7-Eleven: Page 239			

Bagels

Plain: Large, 3 oz (no filling)	240	2	45
w. 2 Tbsp Cream Cheese	340	12	46
w. 2 oz Lox (Smoked Salmon)	320	4	45
Also see Bagels Section: *Page 108*			
Au Bon Pain: Page 187			
Breugger's: Page 192			
Einstein Bros Bagels: Page 206			
Other Fast-Foods Restaurants: Page 183			

Sandwiches

No Spreads Unless Indicated

	C	F	Cb
(Includes 2 Slices Bread ~ 3 oz)			
BLT (5 strips Bacon, 2 Tbsp Mayo)	600	40	46
Breaded Chicken & Salad	540	28	46
Chicken (5 oz) Salad w. Mayo.	580	30	49
Chopped Liver, Egg, Mayo.	630	25	44
Corned Beef (5 oz) w. Mustard	560	28	44
Cream Cheese w. Olives (5 large)	340	14	46
Egg Salad w. Mayonnaise	570	29	49
Egg Salad Club w. Bacon, Mayo.	780	53	49
Grilled Cheese (3 oz)	540	30	44
Ham (4 oz); Cheese (4 oz), Mayo.	910	56	44
Lobster Salad (4 oz) w. Mayo.	530	25	45
Overstuffed Tuna Salad (7 oz)	870	39	75
Philadelphia Cheese Steak S'wich	550	23	42
Reuben (6 oz Beef/Pastrami, 2 oz Cheese,			
2 Tbsp Dressing)	920	60	28
Roast Beef (4 oz) w. Mustard	460	12	45
Roast Pork (4 oz) w. Apple Sauce	500	16	55
Shrimp Salad Club w. Bacon, Mayo.	800	57	48
Sloppy Joe w. Sauce (7 oz)	600	30	45
Steak Sandwich (5 oz cooked)	680	32	41
Triple Cheese (4 oz) Melt	720	45	46
Tuna (5 oz) Salad w. Mayo.	610	30	49
Turkey Breast (5 oz) w. Mayo.	460	18	44
Turkey Breast (5 oz) w. Mustard	360	7	44
Turkey Club w. Bacon, Mayo.	830	38	31
Vegetarian w. Avocado, Cheese	820	49	72
Subway: Page 251-252			
7-Eleven: Page 239			

Wraps & Roll-Ups

Average All Types

(Meat/Chicken/Fish/Veges)			
Small size, approx. 9 oz	500	25	48
Regular, approx. 15 oz	830	40	80
Large, approx. 22 oz	1400	70	134
Au Bon Pain: See Page 187			
Other Fast-Foods Restaurants: Page 183			

Restaurant & International Foods

Chinese & Asian Dishes

Appetizers — C | F | Cb

	C	F	Cb
Crab Cake, 63g	105	5	0.5
Curried Meat Triangles, 1 pce	150	5	12
Dumplings: Pork, steamed, 1	40	3	4
Pork, fried, 1 dumpling	75	7	4
Vegetable, steamed, 1	25	0.5	4
Egg Rolls, mini, 3 rolls	100	3	11
Fortune Cookies, 1	100	0	23
Spring Roll: Small, 1 1/2 oz	100	7	10
Medium, 3 oz	200	12	20
Large, 5 oz	350	15	33
Wonton, 1 only	55	3	4
Soup: Clear, 1 bowl	30	1	4
with Noodles	100	3	12
Chicken & Corn	150	8	8
Rice: Plain, cooked, 1 cup, 6 1/2 oz	245	0.5	53
Fried: 1 cup, 5 oz	320	13	42
Large dish, 16 oz	1010	40	134
Noodles: Chinese Egg, ckd, 1 cup	200	3	42
Entrees & Mains: *Per Whole Dish*			
Beef Satay, 17 oz	760	50	15
Beef in Black Bean Sce, 17 oz	530	33	17
Beef with Broccoli, 16 oz	650	30	31
Chicken & Almonds, 18 oz	685	50	18
Chicken (sliced) & Broccoli	280	12	13
Chop Suey: Chicken, 20 oz	560	37	7
Pork, 20 oz	680	50	12
Chow Mein: Beef/Chicken, 24 oz	940	60	40
Crab Rangoon, 1 dumpling	70	6	4
Crispy Fried Chicken, 8 oz	485	33	12
Egg Drop Soup: w. Noodles, 1 cup	120	3	15
w/out Noodles, 1 cup	70	3	3
Lemon Chicken, 10 oz	580	32	25
Lo Mein (stir-fried)	620	29	61
Moo Shu Chicken, 2 wrapped crepes	430	16	43
Omelet, Chicken/Shrimp, 16 oz	990	82	10
Steamed Whole Fish, 1/2 Red Snapper	500	11	1
Sweet & Sour: Fish, 20 oz	1160	58	106
Pork, 18 oz	950	50	92
Vegetable Combination, w. oil, 6 oz	250	17	19
Vegetables, Steamed (no oil), 6 oz	120	1	25
Bubble Tea, 12 fl oz	240	0	55
Fortune Cookie: each	25	0.5	5
Extra Listings: *See Frozen Meals*			

Confucious say:

"Man who eat with one chopstick never have problem with obesity"

Cajun & Creole

	C	F	Cb
Alligator, 4 oz cooked	160	2	0
Baked Herb Chicken, 1 serving	850	53	2
Bouillabaisse	400	15	10
Cajun Fried Turkey, 1 serving	630	25	0
Cocktail Sauce, 1 Tbsp	15	0	3
Couche-couche, 1/2 cup	80	0	17
Crawfish Bisque, 1 serving	500	10	10
Crawfish, cooked, 2 oz	45	0.5	0
Creole Jambalaya, 1 serving	550	30	15
Dove, cooked, 1 oz	60	3.5	0
Frog's Legs, steamed (2)	45	0	0
Guinea Fowl, flesh, 1 oz, ckd	40	1	0
Hogshead Cheese, 1/4 cup	80	5.5	0
Jambalaya, Shrimp & Crabmeat	520	14	12
Red Beans & Rice, 1 serving	400	17	52
Roasted Quail, w. Bacon on Toast	550	25	15
Remoulade Sauce, 1 Tbsp	55	5.5	1
Shrimp Creole, 1 serving	450	20	10
Stuffed Smothered Steak, w. 1 cup Rice	890	50	50
Squab, flesh, 1 oz cooked	60	3.5	0
Turtle, cooked, 1 1/2 oz	60	1.5	0

French Foods

	C	F	Cb
Blanquette d'Agneau (Lamb Stew)	800	30	17
Brioche, 1 cake	280	14	34
Bouillabaisse (Fish Stew)	400	15	10
Coq au Vin (Chicken in Wine)	800	30	16
Coquilles St. Jacques, fried, 6 lge.	300	14	2
Crème Brulée, 1 serving	460	40	21
Creme Caramel (Caram. Custard)	260	10	38
Crepe Suzette, 1x 6"crepe/sauce	220	10	13
Duck a l'Orange	780	35	47
Escargots (Snails), in garl. butter, (6)	200	10	4
French Stick Bread, 3 slices, 2.2 oz	150	1	35
Frogs Legs, fried, 4 med. pairs	400	20	10
Lamb Noisettes, fried, 2 chops	500	40	1
Mousse au Chocolat	380	15	33
Potage Creme Crecy (Carrot Soup)	360	18	14
Salade Nicoise (Tuna/Oliv./Veg.)	450	13	14
Veal Cordon Bleu (Veal/Ham/Ch)	650	25	18
Vichyssoise (Pot./Leek Soup), 1 c.	200	9	15
Baguette & French Stick: *Page 107*			
Croissants: *Pages 117, 175*			

Restaurant & International Foods

Cuban

	C	F	Cb
Bl. Beans w. Rice (Moros con Cristianos)	510	22	76
Blk.-eyed Pea Fritters (Bollitos de Carita)	80	5	6
Casserole Corn Tamale (Tammal en Cazuela)	445	20	55
Chkn w. Yellow Rice (Arroz con Pollo)	925	49	87
Cuban Bread (Pan Cubano)	80	1.5	15
Donuts in Syrup (Bunuelos)	170	5	10
with Melado	100	5	10
Grilled Plantains	145	0	40
Gypsy's Arm Cake (Brazo Gitano)	260	18	42
Roast Pork S'wich (Pan con Lechon)	640	30	62
Seasoned Beef w. Olives & Raisins (Picadillo)	435	36	10
Shredded Beef (Ropa Vieja)	550	35	10
Taro Root Mash (Pure de Malanga)	315	3	69
Yuca with Citrus Garlic Dressing (Yuca con Mojo)	190	9	25

German

	C	F	Cb
Bavarian Bread Dumpling, 3 small	330	10	28
Beef Goulash with Veges	520	20	46
Black Forest Cake, 1 slice	380	16	30
Bratwurst, grilled, 1 medium, 6 oz	450	37	2
Chicken: Fried, Viennese-style	530	20	28
Livers w. Apple/On., 6 oz	460	28	10
Herring, Pickled: Rollmops, 4 oz	260	16	3
with Sour Cream, 4 oz	310	20	3
Hot Sausage Curry	300	7	6
Kugelhupf Cake, 1 lge slice, 4 oz	400	23	40
Sauerbraten Pork (Pot Roast)	650	35	15
Torte: Linzer (Alm./Raspb. Jam)	430	18	58
Sacher (Choc./Apricot Jam)	260	12	23
Weiner Schnitzel, 1 medium	750	35	38

Greek

	C	F	Cb
Baklava Pastry, 1 only, 3 3/4 oz	400	21	45
Calamari, deep fried, 1 cup	300	13	17
Galactobureko, 1 only (Filo, Custard, Pastry in Syrup)	360	15	48
Kataifi, (Filo, Nut, Pastry in Syrup)	350	11	56
Moussaka, 1 serve, 8 oz	350	22	22
Souvlakia (Lamb), each, 2 oz	120	6	1
Stuffed Tomatoes, 2 only	250	12	17
Taramosalata, 1 Tbsp, 1/2 oz	40	3	2
Tyropita (Filo/Egg/Cheese Pastry)	350	26	31
Tzatziki (Cucumber/Yog. Dip), 1 T.	20	1	1
Vine Leaves, stuffed, 3 rolls, 6 oz	200	5	13

Hawaiian

	C	F	Cb
Ahi Tuna, grilled (6 oz fillet), no fat	220	2	0
Chicken Long Rice, 1 cup, 7 oz	240	14	12
Gyoza, 1 only	55	2	6
Haupia (Coconut Pudd.), 1 pce (4"x2 1/2")	120	6	17
Hawaiian Sweet Bread, 1/2" slice, 2 oz	180	4.5	29
Kalua Chicken, 4 oz	280	16	0
Pork, 4 oz	350	24	0
Kim Chee (pickled cabbage), 1/2 c., 4 oz	20	0	5
Kulolo (Taro Pudding), 1 slice	125	5	19
Lau Lau: Chicken (1) 7 oz	280	21	3
Pork (1) 7 oz	320	26	5
Loco Moco (rice/burger/egg/gravy)	650	27	63
Lomi Lomi Salmon, 1/2 cup, 4 oz	75	2	6
Lomi Salmon, 1/4 cup, 4 oz	20	1	2
Malasadas (Donut), 2 oz	240	13	26
Manapua (Char Siu Pork Bun), 2.3 oz	180	8	25
Poi (mashed ckd taro), 1 c., 8 1/2 oz	270	0.5	65
Poke, avg all types, 3 oz	90	1	0
Portuguese Sausage, 2 oz	180	15	2
Potato Salad, 1/2 cup, 5 oz	170	10	17
Shave Ice (Matsumoto), all flavors:			
w. Icecream, 1 large	300	4	64
w. Beans, 1 large	290	0	72
Spam Musubi: w. Regular Spam	265	11	34
(4 oz rice+1.3 oz Spam/7-Eleven Hawaii)			
Homemade: w. Lite Spam (50% less fat)	220	5	34
Taro Pancake Mix, 1/3 cup (makes 2)	140	2	26
Plate Lunches:			
Chicken Katsu (9 oz) w. 2 scp Rice	1110	48	108
+ Macaroni Salad, 3/4 cup	1360	68	123
or Tossed Salad + Fr. Dress. (2 T.)	1240	61	111
Hamburger (5 oz) w. 2 scoops Rice	710	24	81
Gravy + Macaroni Salad	1135	49	112
MahiMahi (7 oz) w. 2 scoops Rice	650	12	90
+ Macaroni Salad + Tartar Sce	1150	58	109
or Macaroni Salad, no Tartar Sce	935	34	108
or Tossed Salad + Fr. Dress (3 T.)	815	27	96
or Tossed Salad, no dressing	670	12	93
Teri Beef (5 oz) w. 2 scoops Rice	790	23	94
+ Macaroni Salad, 3/4 cup	1095	47	113
or Tossed Salad, no dressing	800	23	95

Indian & Pakistani

(Meat dishes allow 4 oz meat/serving)

	C	F	Cb
Aloo Samosa, each	155	12	12
Alu Gosht Kari (Meat/Pot. Curry)	600	40	23
Chicken Korma	500	35	6
Chicken Pilaf (Murgh Biriyani)	700	53	50

Restaurant & International Foods

Indian & Pakistani (Cont)

Per Serving

	C	F	Cb
Chicken Tikka	260	16	2
Chicken Vindaloo	400	20	8
Chapati/Roti, 7" diam. piece	60	0.5	11
Dal (Lentil Puree): 1 cup, no oil	230	1	37
1 Tbsp Tadka (oil topping)	120	13	0
Dhakla (Lentil Dish), 1" sq., 1 oz	105	5	13
Dhansak, 1/2 cup	105	3.5	11
Gosht Kari (Meat Curry/Tom./Pot.)	460	25	17
Lamb Pilaf	520	35	40
Lassi (Sweet or Mango), 1 cup, 8 oz	160	4	24
Masala Gosht (Beef/Tom./Gravy)	400	25	18
Mulligatawney Soup, average	300	15	8
Murgh Tikka, 1 cup	300	4	7
Naan Bread, 1/4 (8" x 2"), 1 oz	75	2	11
Pappadum, 1 large/2 small	50	3	5
Pesrattu (Lentil Crepe), 9", 2.6 oz	130	5	15
Pork Vindaloo Curry	620	47	3
Rajmah (Kidney Bean Curry), 1 cup	225	5	35
Rogan Josh (Lamb/Yogurt Sce)	500	30	3
Shahi Korma (Braised Lamb)	430	28	3
Tandoori Chicken: Breast	260	13	5
Leg/Thigh portion	300	17	6

Italian Dishes

	C	F	Cb
Bruschetta, 2 slices	380	17	53
Cannelloni, 1 tube, 6 oz	280	15	18
Chicken Cacciatore	370	22	4
Fettucine Alfredo w. Cream	910	63	60
Gnocchi, Spinach	300	18	17
Lasagne w. Meat, 10 oz	400	17	36
Linguini w. Red Clam Sauce	570	10	95
Manicotti, cheese/tomato	230	14	18
Minestrone Soup, 1 cup	260	6	28
Osso Buco (Veal/Tom./Mushr.)	550	28	5
Ratatouille	76	6	5.5
Ravioli, 8 oz	300	12	30
Risotto (Chicken)	420	12	70
Spaghetti: Plain, 1 cup, 5 oz	185	1	44
Restaurant: 2 cups, plain	370	2	88
+ Bolognese (Meat Sce)	650	16	90
+ Marinara Sauce	540	13	105
Spaghetti & Meatballs	960	42	102
Saltimbocca (Veal/Ham/Cheese)	430	28	5
Shrimp Scampi (w. 8 large shrimp)	830	26	75
Tortellini, 20 pieces	530	20	74
Veal Marsala	400	20	11
Veal Parmigiana	350	20	5

Pizza: *See Fast-Foods Section, Page 183*

Japanese

	C	F	Cb
Sushi Rice: cooked, 1 Tbsp	25	0	5
1 cup, 5 1/4 oz	380	3	82
Sushi (Maki) Rolls: *Per Piece*			
Average all types (California Rolls; Crm Cheese w. Crab; Eel; Salmon; Shrimp; Tuna; Yellowtail; Vegetable)			
Small (1 1/8" diam. x 1 1/8" high), 0.8 oz	22	0.5	0.5
Med. (1 3/4" diam. x 1 3/4" high), 1.6 oz	44	1	1
Large (2 1/4" diam. x 7/8" high), 2 oz	55	1.5	1.5
Sushi Packs: *Per Pack*			
Average all types: 6 large pces	335	7.5	7.5
9 medium pieces	405	9	9
12 small pieces	325	12	6
Futomaki (thick roll), 6 pieces	315	1.5	7
Hand Roll (Cone), 2, 6 oz	225	5	5
Inari (rice filled soybean pocket), 4 pce	260	5	46
Sushi-Nigiri (fish on rice):			
average all types, 1 piece	70	0.5	12
Sushi Plate: Assorted, 6 pieces	420	3	36
Combination (Sushi & Sushi Rolls)			
2 Sushi + 6 sm. & 3 med. rolls	400	7	72
Sashimi (Sliced Raw Seafood/Beef)			
Ika (Squid), 4 oz	105	2	0
Hamachi (Yellowtail), 4 oz	165	6	0
Naguro (Yellowfin Tuna), 4 oz	120	1	0
Niku (Beef), 5 oz	200	10	0
Saba (Mackerel), 4 oz	160	7	0
Suzuki (Sea Bass), 4 oz	110	0.5	0
Tako (Octopus), 4 oz	95	1	0
Dipping Sauces: Average, 2 Tbsp	30	0	7
Ginger Vinegar Dressing, 2 Tbsp	20	0	5
Edamame (young green soybeans)			
Steamed/Salad (in pods), 4 oz	60	3	5
Boiled beans (no pods), 4 oz	160	7	12
Katsu-don Pork w. Rice	1100	39	141
Miso Soup w. Tofu pces, 1 cup	85	3	11
Seaweed Salad, 1.5 oz	20	2	0
Sukiyaki (Beef/Tofu/Veg.), 8 oz	400	24	32
Tempura (Batter-fried Shrimp & Veges)			
3 large shrimp & veges	320	18	25
1 shrimp only	60	4	3
Teppan Yaki (Steak, Seafood & Veges)			
10 oz serving	470	30	15
Teriyaki: Beef, 4 oz serving	350	25	4
Chicken, 4 oz serving	260	9	7
Salmon, medium, 6 oz serving	270	8	3
Sake Wine (16% alc.), 3 fl.oz	115	0	7
Yakatori, 1 skewer, 2 1/2 oz	140	5	1

Restaurant & International Foods

Kosher/Deli Foods · C · F · Cb

	C	F	Cb
Bagel/Bialy, 1 small, 2 oz	160	2	32
Beiglach (Cheese Knish)	350	17	35
Blintzes: Average, 1 only	120	1	26
w. Sour Crm. & Preserves	370	10	30
Borscht: (no cream), 1 cup	85	3	14
Diet/Reduced Cal., 1 cup	30	1	7
Cabbage Roll (meat/rice), 5 oz	170	6	21
Chicken Broth: 1 cup	80	8	0
with vegetables	100	8	5
with noodles	150	9	16
Lowfat, plain, 1 cup	25	1	0
Cholent, 1 med serve, 1 cup	350	16	48
Chopped Liver: 1 serve, 3 oz	110	6	5
with Egg Salad, 1/4 cup	100	7	3
Farfel, dry, 1/2 cup	90	0.5	21
Hallah (Yeast Bread), 1 sl., 1 oz	85	2	14
Gefilte Fish Balls:			
Regular, medium, 2 oz	55	2	4
with jelled broth	80	2	6
Cocktail size, 1 oz	30	1	2
Sweet, medium, 2 oz	65	2	4
with jelled broth	95	2	9
Herring: Smoked, 2 oz	120	8	0
in Sour Cream, 2 oz	150	10	0
Kasha, cooked, 1/2 cup	100	0.5	20
Kipfel (Vanilla/Almd. Cookie), 1 pce	60	2	7
Knaidlach, 1 ball	40	2	5
Knish: Kasha/Potato, 1 only	130	4	22
Cheese, 1 only	350	17	35
Knishette (Gabila's) Potato,			
4 piece, 4 oz	140	1	29
Spinach, 4 piece, 4 oz	110	1	20
Kreplach, beef, 1 piece	40	1	6
Kugel, potato/noodle, 1 serve	150	7	20
Latkes (Potato Pancake), 2 oz	200	11	22
3 Latkes w. Sour Cr./Apple Sce	750	25	95
Lochshen: Plain, 1 cup	130	2	26
Pudding, 1 cup	380	13	48
Lox (Smoked Salmon), 2 oz	65	2	0
Mandelbrot (Almond Bread),			
1 slice, 1/4" thick	45	2	5
Matzo (See Page 109), 1 oz board	110	0.5	21
Matzo Balls, 2 small, 1 large	90	3	12
Matzo Soup, with 1 large ball	180	7	24
New York Cheesecake, 4 oz	350	24	26
Pierogi, potato/cheese, 1 pce	90	4	11
Reuben Sandwich	920	60	28
Schmaltz (Rend'd chick. fat), 1 T.	90	10	0

Lebanese/Middle East

	C	F	Cb
Baba Ghannouj, 2 Tbsp, 1 oz	70	6	2
(Eggplant/Sesame Dip)			
Baklava, 1 pastry, 1 3/4 oz	245	18	18
(Pastry, Nuts, Syrup)			
Cabbage Rolls, 1 roll, 3 oz	100	3	12
(Cabbage Leaf, Meat, Rice)			
Cous Cous, 1 serve	400	21	43
(Semolina, Milk, Fruit, Nuts)			
Felafel (Chick Pea Fritter):			
Fried, 1 medium, 1 oz	60	4	4
Hummus, 1/4 cup, 2.2 oz	105	3	5
Fried Kibbi, 1 piece, 3 oz	180	8	15
(Wheat, Meat, Pinenuts)			
Kafta, 1 skewer, 1 1/2 oz	85	5	2
(Ground Lamb Saus. on Skewer)			
Kibbeh Naye, 1 cup, 9 oz	450	18	28
(Raw Lamb, Bulgur & Spices)			
Lebanese Omelet, 1 serving, 4 oz	200	12	13
(Egg, Spinach, Pinenuts, Onion)			
Pilaf, 1 cup	400	11	60
(Rice, Onion, Rais., Apr. Spice)			
Shawourma, 1 serve, 4 oz	280	15	2
(Spit Roast Beef)			
Shish Kabob, 1 stick, 2 1/2 oz	130	7	2
Spinach Pie, 1 piece, 3 1/2 oz	290	21	20
Sweet Almond Sanbusak, 1 pce	200	15	11
(Pastry, Almonds, Spices)			
Tabouli, 1 serve, 4 oz	170	14	7
Tahini Sauce, avg., 1 Tbsp	90	8	2

Sal Monella Restaurant

"I wonder why business is so bad these days?"

Restaurant & International Foods

Mexican

	C	F	Cb
Black Bean Soup, 1 bowl	200	3	34
Bueso Fresco, 1/4 cup	80	4.5	8
Burritos *(Taco Bell)*: Bean	370	10	55
Supreme® Beef	440	18	50
Chili, plain, 1 cup	90	6	8
Chili con Carne: w. Beans, 1 cup	310	17	15
w/out Beans, 1 cup	370	28	10
Chimichangas, Beef, 5 oz	400	19	43
Chorizo Sausage, 2 oz	265	23	0
Churros, 1 1/2 oz	150	8	18
Corn Chips, 1/2 cup, 1 oz	160	10	17
Empanadas, average, 1 small	230	10	28
Enchilada, average	330	10	49
Fajitas, Chicken (Soft)	200	7	20
Guacamole, 2 Tbsp, 1 oz	120	12	2
Horchata: *Don Jose,* 1 cup, 8 fl. oz	140	4	25
Cacique, 1 pint bottle, 16 fl. oz	320	7	62
Margarita (w. 1 1/2 oz Tequila)	160	0	6
Menudo, 1/2 cup	55	1.5	10
Nachos: *Del Taco,* Regular	395	24	40
Macho Nachos	1145	63	113
Taco Bell: BellGrande®	760	43	80
Supreme®	470	26	42
Piloncillo (Brown Sugar): 1 Tbsp, 4g	15	0	4
Cone, small, 3", 3 oz	325	0	81
Quesadilla, Cheese *(Taco Bell)*	490	28	39
Refried Beans, 3/4 cup, 6 oz	160	3	26
Rice Pudding (Arroz Con Leche), 4 oz	140	3	24
Sopaipillas (flaky pastry puffs), 1 pce	100	7	10
w. Honey & Cream	200	14	18
Sopes (Gorditas), 2 oz	120	0	27
Taco *(Taco Bell)*: Regular	170	10	13
Chicken	190	6	19
Taco Supreme®	220	14	14
Double Decker® Taco	340	14	39
Taco Salad w. Salsa	840	52	85
Taco Sauce, average, 1/4 cup	15	0	3
Taco Shell, regular	50	2	8
Tamales, Beef/Chicken, avg, 4.5 oz	250	11	27
Taquitos, Beef & Cheese, 4.5 oz	330	15	36
Tostada *(Taco Bell)*	250	10	29
Tortilla, Corn, 6" diam.	70	1	14
Tortilla Chips, 1 oz	150	8	18

Extra Listings of Mexican Dishes:
• Frozen Entrees/Meals: *See Page 61-73*
• Fast Foods Section *(Taco Bell, Del Taco)*
• Canned Bean/Chili Products: *See Page 77-83*

Polish

	C	F	Cb
Cabbage Rolls w. Sour Cr., 2 sm.	220	10	30
Chicken Casserole w. Mush., 1 c.	520	27	5
Kielbasa (Sausages, Onions, fried, 2 large.)	350	28	2
Meatballs in Sour Cream, 3 x 1 1/2" balls	300	16	11
Pierogi, Fruit/Veg, 3" ball	80	2	15
Pork Goulash (Pork/Veg. Stew)	550	21	38
Pot Roast with Vegetables	630	21	28

Soul Foods

	C	F	Cb
Breakfast Sausage, fried, 2 patties	250	17	0
Brunswick Stew, 1 cup, 8.5 oz	320	14	19
Cornbread, home-made, 3 oz	200	7.5	28
Fatback, raw, 1/4 oz	60	6.5	0
Ham Hock	90	6.5	0
Hog Maw	45	2.5	0
Hominy, 3/4 cup	85	1	17
Hush Puppies, 5 pieces	260	12	35
Kale, cooked, 1/2 cup	20	0.5	4
Opossum	65	3	0
Oxtail	70	3.5	0
Pig Ear, 1/4 ear	50	3	0
Pig Foot, 1/2 foot	70	4.5	0
Pig Tail, 1/3 tail	115	10	0
Poke Salad, cooked, 1/2 cup	16	0.5	3
Pork Brains	40	2.5	0
Pork Chitterlings, simmered, 3 oz	260	25	0
Pork Cracklings, 1/2 oz	80	6	0
Pork Neck Bones	65	4	0
Pork Skin, 1 oz	70	4.5	0
Pork Tongue, 1/3 tongue	75	5.5	0
Sousemeat	60	4.5	0
Succotash, 1/2 cup	80	1	17
Sweet Potato Pie, 1/8 of 9" pie	250	12	34
Tripe, 2 oz	55	2	0
Vienna Sausage, 2 small	90	8	1
small	45	4	0.5

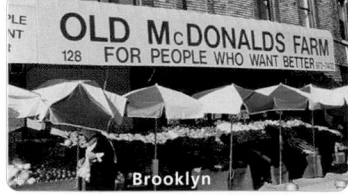

OLD McDONALDS FARM
128 FOR PEOPLE WHO WANT BETTER

Brooklyn

Restaurant & International Foods

Thai Foods

	C	F	Cb
Appetizers: Satay Pork, 1 oz	100	4	2
Spring Roll, 1¼ oz	110	6	13
Soups: Tom Yam (Hot & Sour):			
Spicy Shrimp/Seafood, 1 cup	100	4	6
1 bowl	160	7	10
Vegetarian, 1 cup	50	0	11
Curries: Chicken w. Ginger, 1 cup	390	34	4
Thick Red Curry w. Beef, 1 cup	600	50	7
Thai Chicken Curry, 1 cup	340	23	4
Massaman Curry, 1 cup	680	57	8
Green Curry w. Pork, 1 cup	480	44	5
Pad Thai, Large serving, 18 oz	990	38	125
Fish: Steamed w. Spicy Thai Sce	450	8	46
Crispy Fried, 5 oz	290	15	9
Spicy Chicken (w. veges), stir-fry	450	22	14
Spicy Garlic Tofu w. veges, stir-fry	340	18	18
Sticky Thai Rice, plain 1 cup, 6oz	170	0.5	36
w. Coconut & Sesame Seeds, 1 cup	880	28	120
Stir-fried Rice Noodles, 1 c., 5½ oz	270	9	40
Stir-fried Vegetables, 1 cup	100	3	18
Salads: Green Papaya Salad	160	0	44
Spicy Prawn, 9 shrimp	170	3	15
Thai Chicken, 1 serving	330	9	17
Thai Beef Salad, 1 serving	260	9	15
Thai Noodle, 1 serving	410	13	45
Satay Chicken & Peanut Sauce:			
1 satay stick	390	24	20
Sauces: Peanut Satay, ½ cup, 4 oz	160	10	13

Spanish

	C	F	Cb
Arroz Abanda (Fish with Rice)	340	8	31
Arroz Con Pollo (Rice/Chick. Sal)	500	23	50
Clams Marinera, 8 clams	330	16	22
Cochifrito (Lamb w. Lemon/Garlic)	650	25	5
Cochinillo Asado, 2 sl. (Rst Suckling Pig)	300	15	3
Cocido Madrileno			
(Madrid-Style Boiled Dinner)	450	27	18
Flan de Leche (Caramel Custard)	325	9	52
Fritadera de Ternera (Sauteed Veal)	450	27	2
Gazpacho, 1 bowl	60	0	15
Paella a la Valenciana			
(Chicken & Shellfish Rice)	900	42	70
Pollo a la Espanola (Chicken)	475	30	4
Ternera al Jerez (Veal w. Sherry)	660	29	6
Zarzuela (Fish & Shellfish Medley)	530	27	40

Vietnamese

	C	F	Cb
Bo Xao Dau Phong: *Per Whole Dish*			
(Ginger Beef w.Onion, Fish Sce.)	750	30	10
Bo Nuong (Beef Satay), 2 sticks	265	9	4
Ca Chien Gung (Whole Snapper/Ging.)	600	16	6
Canh Chay (Veg./Tofu Soup)	80	3	13
Chicken & Rice Noodle Soup	400	3	55
Cuu Xao Lan (Curried Lamb,			
Veges in Coconut)	900	40	80
Ga Chien (Crisp Chick + Plum Sce)	900	40	105
Ga Nuong (Chicken Satay + Sce)	240	10	4
Ga Xao Rau (Marinated Chicken			
Braised w. Veg.)	800	26	100
Rau Cai Xao Chay			
(Stir Fried Vege., Soy Sauce)	400	15	65
Thit Heo Goi Baup Cai, each			
(Spicy Cabbage Rolls w. Pork)	200	7	11

Gourmet & Miscellaneous

	C	F	Cb
Ants Eggs/Larvae, 1 Tbsp	20	0	0
Ants, Choc. coated, 3 Tbsp	140	7	2
Bee Maggots, canned, 3 Tbsp	65	2	0
Caviar, black/red, 1 Tbsp	40	3	0
Caterpillars, canned, 2 oz	60	2	0
Frogs Legs, fried, 1 pair (large)	125	7	0
Haggis, boiled, 4 oz	350	24	22
Locusts, raw, 1 oz	35	1	0
Silkworms, raw, 1 oz	60	2	0
Snails in garlic butter, 6 large	200	10	4
Snake, roasted, 4 oz	160	6	0

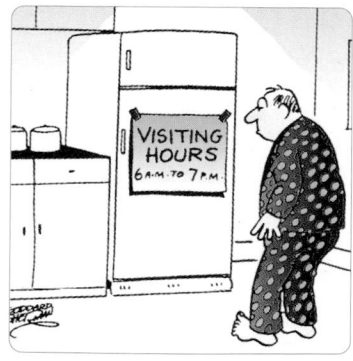

VISITING HOURS 6 A.M. TO 7 P.M.

181

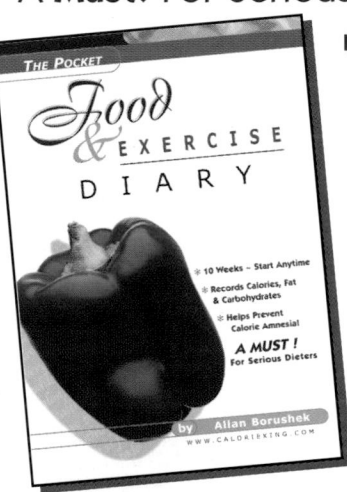
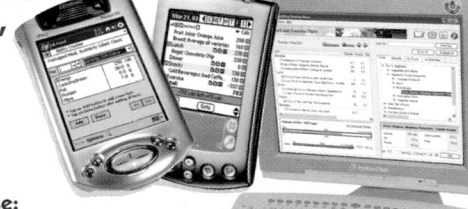

Fast-Food Chains & *Restaurants*

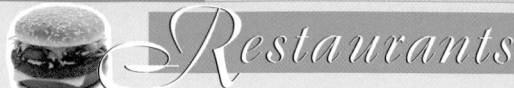

©2004
Allan Borushek

A&W®

Sandwiches

	C	F	Cb
Baby Burger	265	10	28
Cheeseburger	475	22	42
Cheeseburger Deluxe	525	27	43
Cheeseburger Deluxe Bacon	620	32	43
Chseburger Deluxe Bacon Double	880	51	50
Cheeseburger Deluxe Double	795	44	50
Cheeseburger Jr.	500	24	42
Crispy Chicken Sandwich	485	25	57
Grilled Chicken Sandwich	275	11	37
Hamburger	440	21	39
Hamburger Deluxe	475	25	39
Hamburger Jr	435	21	38
Mama Burger	480	28	36
Papa Burger	700	40	36
Grandpa Burger	910	55	36
Teen Burger	565	33	36
Double Teen Burger	790	48	36
Mozza Burger	630	36	38
Double Mozza Burger	830	53	38

Chicken: Chicken Grill

	C	F	Cb
Chicken: Chicken Grill	350	11	40
Chubby Chicken Burger	490	23	48
Chubby Chicken Pces: Breast	330	19	10
Drumstick	140	8	5
Thigh	410	31	9
Wing	205	14	6
Chubby Chicken Strips, 1	120	5	10

Dipping Sauces: Barbeque

	C	F	Cb
Dipping Sauces: Barbeque	35	0	7
Dijon Honey Mustard	105	6	11
Sweet and Sour	45	0	11

Hot Dog: Plain, 3.2 oz

	C	F	Cb
Hot Dog: Plain, 3.2 oz	285	17	22
Regular, 4 oz	375	22	31
Cheese Dog, 4.4 oz	325	20	25
Chili Coney, 4.4 oz	310	18	24
Whistle Dog, 5.4 oz	490	30	39

Fries & Sides: Per Serving

	C	F	Cb
A&W Fries, regular, 4.75 oz	375	16	54
Poutine, small	420	24	38
Fresh Onion Rings	395	25	37
Gravy, small	80	5	6

Salads

	C	F	Cb
Coleslaw, Individual	90	6	7
Potato Salad, Individual	160	8	22
Macaroni Salad, Individual	175	9	22

Breakfast

	C	F	Cb
Bacon 'n Egger	510	35	32
Bacon & Eggs	575	40	28
Hash Brown	175	11	18
Sausages & Egger	595	42	34
Sausages & Eggs	515	40	28
French Toast, 2 pces	800	34	98
Cinnamon Bun	390	11	65

Desserts

	C	F	Cb
Cookies, average all types, 2	250	11	36
Apple Turnover	195	8	29
Soft Icecream Cone, regular	220	11	30

Drinks: Per 18 fl.oz

	C	F	Cb
A&W Root Beer	300	5	36
Diet A&W Root Beer; Diet Coke	3	0	0
Coco-Cola	190	0	53
Sprite	195	0	50
Minute Orange Maid Soda	240	0	60
Hestea Iced Tea	195	0	50

Milkshakes & Floats: Per Regular Size

	C	F	Cb
Chocolate Milkshake	460	13	75
Strawberry Milkshake	455	11	76
Vanilla Milkshake	450	13	74
A&W Root Beer Milkshake	455	11	78
A&W Root Beer Float	300	5	60

For Complete Nutritional Data ~ see CalorieKing.com

Applebee's®

Low Fat Menu: Per Serving

	C	F	Cb
Asian Chicken Salad	715	9	121
Blackened Chicken Salad	425	8.5	39
Chicken Fajita Quesadilla	520	11	63
Chicken Quesadilla	740	14	89
Chicken Rancho Rollup	590	12	80
Chicken Roma Rollup	640	10	83
Chicken Pasta	530	10	76
Garlic/Lemon Chicken Pasta	530	11	78
Veggie Quesadilla	595	12	86
Whitefish w. Mango Salsa	435	10	54

Desserts, Sundaes

	C	F	Cb
Low Fat Brownie Sundae	325	3	49
Marble Cheesecake	260	2	50
Bikini Banana Strawb. Shortcake	230	3	49

Restaurants & Fast-Foods

Arby's®

Breakfast Items	C	F	Cb
Biscuit: w. Butter	280	17	27
w. Bacon	320	21	27
w. Ham	330	20	28
w. Sausage	460	33	28
Croissant: Plain	220	12	25
w. Bacon	325	20	28
w. Ham	310	20	28
w. Sausage	420	32	28
Sourdough: w. Bacon	235	7	29
w. Ham	190	7	30
w. Sausage	330	19	29
French-Toastix, no syrup	370	17	48
French Toast Syrup	130	0	32
Swiss Cheese, 1 slice	45	3	0

Roast Beef Sandwich: Arby-Q®	C	F	Cb
Arby-Q®	360	14	40
Arby's Melt w. Cheddar	340	15	36
Big Montana®	630	32	41
Giant Roast Beef	480	23	41
Junior Roast Beef	310	13	34
Regular Roast Beef	350	16	34
Super Roast Beef	470	23	47

Sub Sandwiches: French Dip	C	F	Cb
French Dip	440	16	42
Hot Ham 'N Swiss	530	27	45
Italian	780	53	49
Philly Beef 'N Swiss	700	42	46
Roast Beef	760	48	47
Turkey	630	37	51

Other Sandwiches	C	F	Cb
Chicken Bacon 'N Swiss	610	33	49
Chicken Breast Fillet	540	30	47
Chicken Cordon Bleu	630	35	47
Grilled Chicken Deluxe	450	22	37
Hot Ham 'N Swiss	340	13	35
Roast Chicken Club	520	28	38

Market Fresh™ Sandwiches	C	F	Cb
Roast Beef & Swiss	810	42	73
Roast Chicken Caesar	820	38	75
Roast Ham & Swiss	730	34	74
Roast Turkey Ranch & Bacon	880	44	74
Roast Turkey & Swiss	760	33	75
Ultimate BLT	820	49	72

Market Fresh™ Salads (no Dressing)	C	F	Cb
Caesar Salad	90	4	8
Caesar Side Salad	45	2	4
Chicken Finger Salad	570	34	39
Grilled Chicken Caesar Salad	230	8	8
Turkey Club Salad	350	21	9

Light Menu	C	F	Cb
Garden Salad	70	1	14
Grilled Chicken	280	5	30
Grilled Chicken Salad	210	4.5	14
Roast Chicken Deluxe	260	5	33
Roast Chicken Salad	160	2.5	15
Roast Turkey Deluxe	260	5	33
Side Salad	25	0	5

Sides	C	F	Cb
Cheddar Curly Fries w. Sce	460	24	54
Chicken Finger 4-Pack	640	38	42
Chicken Finger Snack w. Fries	580	32	55
Curly Fries, small	310	15	39
Homestyle Fries, small	300	13	42
Jalapeno Bites™	330	21	30
Mozzarella Sticks (4)	470	29	34
Onion Petals	410	24	43
Potato Cakes (2)	250	16	26
Baked Potato: Plain	355	0	82
w. Butter & Sour Cream	500	24	65
w. Broccoli 'N Cheddar	540	24	71
Deluxe Baked Potato	650	34	67

Desserts/Shakes	C	F	Cb
Apple Turnover (Iced)	420	16	65
Cherry Turnover (Iced)	410	16	63
Shakes: Chocolate, 14 oz	480	16	84
Jamocha/Vanilla, 14 oz	470	15	82
Strawberry, 14 oz	500	13	87

Condiments	C	F	Cb
Arby's Sauce	15	0	4
Au Jus Sauce	5	0	1
BBQ Vinaigrette	140	11	9
Bronco Berry Sauce™	90	0	23
Buttermilk Ranch Dressing	360	30	3
Light	100	6	12
Caesar Dressing	310	34	1
Croutons: Cheese & Garlic	100	6	10
Seasoned	30	1	5
German Mustard	5	0	1
Honey French Dressing	290	24	18
Horsey Sauce®, packet	60	5	3
Italian Dressing, Reduced Calorie	25	1	3
Marinara Sauce	35	1	4
Mayonnaise	90	10	0
Light Cholesterol Free	20	1.5	1
Tangy Southwest Sauce™	250	26	3

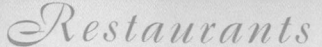

Arthur Treachers

C F Cb

Meals			
Fish N Chips	1540	101	132
Seafood Sampler	3380	270	227
1/4 Sampler	845	67	56
Shrimp N Chips	2050	124	225

Sides: Per Serving			
Coleslaw	210	8.5	34
Hush Puppy	275	10	42

Atlanta Bread Company®

Bagel: Per Bagel			
Asiago; Banana	350	3	67
Blueberry; Plain; Cinnamon Raisin	340	1.5	68
Chocolate Chip	330	3	62
Everything; Poppy Seed; Sesame	310	1.5	61
Honey Wheat; Jalapeno	330	1.5	66
Onion; Pumpernickel	300	1.5	60

Bread: Per Thick Slice (2 oz)			
Asiago	150	2.5	29
Cinnamon Raisin	170	2.5	31
Cracked Wheat	160	2	30
French	140	0.5	29
Honey Wheat; Nine Grain: Pesto	150	1.5	29
Pumpernickel; Rye	150	1	28
Sourdough	140	0	29
Sundried Tomato	150	0	30

Bread Rolls: French	180	0.5	37
Sourdough	190	0	38

Muffins: Apple Cinnamon	400	19	52
Banana Walnut	440	22	53
Blueberry	430	20	55
Chocolate Chip/Mocha avg.	470	23	61
Cranberry Apple	390	18	51
Cranberry Orange Walnut	440	23	51
Honey Raisin Bran	460	21	65
Lemon Poppy Seed	460	23	57
Low Fat varieties, average	320	5	60
Peaches/Creme	530	25	68
Pumpkin	370	13	58
Zucchini	480	24	60

Muffin Tops: Blueberry	320	15	41
Banana Walnut	330	16	40
Chocolate Chip	340	16	45
Chocolate Mocha	350	17	45
Pumpkin	280	10	43

Atlanta Bread (Cont)

C F Cb

Salads:			
Caesar, no dressing	35	0	8
Chicken	305	21	0.5
Chicken Caesar, no dressing	115	2.5	8
Chicken Curry	340	24	10
Chicken House, no dressing	115	2.5	8
Chopstix Chicken, no dressing	470	24	38
Fruit Salad	140	1	32
Greek Chicken, no dressing	210	10	12
Greek, no dressing	120	8	12
House Salad	35	0	8
Tuna Salad	240	16	0

Sandwiches (Sourdough)			
ABC Special, no dressing	450	6	67
Avocado, no dressing	630	32	75
Bella Basil Chicken	795	37	76
Chicken Curry, no dressing	630	25	70
Chicken Salad, no dressing	600	23	61
Honey Maple Ham, no dressing	310	4.5	60
Pastrami, no dressing	440	7	62
Roast Beef, no dressing	450	5	62
Tuna, no dressing	530	18	61
Turkey Breast, no dressing	420	4.5	60
Veggie, no dressing	290	1	60

Panini: Cordon Bleu	590	15	76
Chargrilled Chicken Pesto	740	30	78
Cuban Pork Loin	740	30	82
Italian Vegetable	620	21	81
Turkey Club	780	32	76

Soup: Per Cup			
Black Bean & Rice; Chkn Gumbo	110	3	14
Black Bean w/Ham	200	7	32
Chicken 'n Dumpling	240	13	21
Chicken Chili	220	6	27
Chicken Noodle	110	4	12
Chili w. Beans	280	11	24
Clam Chowder	270	16	22
French Onion	60	2	9
Garden Veg.; Mushr., Barley & Sage	80	1	15
Lentil & Roasted Garlic	200	2.5	33
Seven Bean w. Ham	240	12	27
Szechuan Hot & Sour	80	2	12
Tomato Florentine	120	3	17
Vegetable Chili	180	3.5	31
Wisconsin Cheese	210	11	20

For Complete Nutritional Data ~ see CalorieKing.com

Au Bon Pain®

Bagels: Per Bagel	C	F	Cb
Asiago Cheese	380	6	66
Cinnamon Raisin	360	1.5	77
Dutch Apple w. Walnut Streussel	350	5	77
Plain	350	1.5	72
Wild Blueberry	380	1.5	80
Spreads: Plain Cream Cheese, 2 oz	130	11	1
Honey Walnut, 2 oz	150	10	10
Sundried Tomato; Veggie, 2 oz	140	12	3

Breakfast Sandwiches: Per Sandwich			
Bagel & Egg	500	5	83
Bagel & Egg w. Bacon or Cheese	580	12	83
Bagel & Egg w. Bacon & Cheese	660	19	83

Sandwiches: Per 1/2 Sandwich			
Arizona Chicken	300	7	28
Chicken & Mozzarella Foccacia	400	7	36
Chicken Tarragon w. Field Onions	435	23	32
Croque Madame	285	11	26
Croque Monsieur	295	12	26
Fresh Mozzarella, Tomato & Pesto	395	21	30
Garden Vege Goat Chse w. Artichoke	285	10	37
Hickory Smoked Ham & Brie	310	13	36
Honey Dijon Chicken	375	12	32
Smoked Turkey & Swiss	405	21	34
Smoked Turkey Club	315	14	26
Wraps: Chicken Caesar	320	13	30
Fields & Feta	310	9	50
Honey Smoked Turkey	260	3	42
Southwestern Tuna	355	15	34

Brownies: Blonde	570	36	57
Average other varieties	490	28	55

Soups: Per Serving (8 oz)			
Black Bean	180	0	33
Chicken Noodle	100	2	12
Corn Chowder	270	15	28
Garden Vegetable	50	1	8
Split Pea	160	1	27
Vegetarian Chili	170	1	31

Breads: Average, 1.75 oz slice	130	1	27
Bread Bowl (1)	600	2	118
Foccacia (1)	430	16	34
Four Grain Bread, 1 slice	400	4	74
French Sandwich Roll (1)	260	1	53
Rosemary Garlic Breadstick	200	2	37
Bread Rolls: Hearth (1)	210	2	38
Petit Pain (1)	180	0	37

Yogurt & Fruit Cups: Per Serving	C	F	Cb
Yogurt, average all types	220	3	43
Fruit Cup: Small, 1 cup	60	0	16
Large, 1 cup	130	1	32

Salads: Per Serving (Container)			
Caesar Salad	240	12	19
Charbr. Salmon Filet, Yellow Peppers	220	11	9
Chef's Salad	290	15	11
Chicken Caesar	380	18	19
Garden Salad, large	160	4	26
Garden Salad, small	90	2	14
Mediterranean Chicken	290	16	11
Pear, Field Greens, Gorgonzola	350	26	23
Tomato, Mozzarella w. Basil Pesto	280	19	11
Tuna Garden	440	24	28
Watercress, Chicken & Gorgonzola	250	15	3

Cookies: Per Cookie			
Chocolate Chip; English Toffee	230	7	39
Choc Macadamia; Walnut Raisin	250	13	31
Oatmeal Raisin	210	6	38
Shortbread	240	7	44

Cakes & Bars			
Apple Strudel	400	26	48
Cinnamon Scone, 4.4 oz	440	17	82
Cherry Strudel	360	23	37
Pecan Roll	620	24	94

Croissants: Ham & Cheese	290	9	39
Spinach & Cheese	220	9	29
Filled: Plain	220	6	38
Almond	480	25	58
Apple	200	3	40
Chocolate	330	10	53
Raspberry	290	9	47
Sweet Cheese	320	12	46

Muffins: Blueberry	470	15	79
Carrot Walnut Spice	520	25	67
Chocolate Chip; Double Choc	530	23	77
Pumpkin	510	18	74
Raisin Bran	400	12	77
Lowfat: Chocolate Cake	280	2	64
Triple Berry	270	2	58

Drinks			
Mocha Blast, large, 24 oz	480	4	96
Iced Cappuccino, medium, 12 fl.oz	150	6	15
Iced Tea, medium, 12 fl.oz	130	0	33
Frozen Mocha Blast, 16 oz	320	3	64

Fast–Foods & *Restaurants*

Auntie Anne's®

	C	F	Cb
Pretzels: With Butter			
Almond	400	8	72
Cinnamon Sugar	450	9	83
Garlic	350	4.5	68
Glazin' Raisin®	510	4	107
Jalapeno	310	4.5	59
Kidstix, 4 sticks	250	3	48
Original	370	4	72
Parmesan Herb	440	13	72
Sesame	410	12	64
Sour Cream & Onion	340	5	66
Whole Wheat	370	4.5	72
Pretzels: Without Butter			
Almond Pretzel; Whole Wheat	350	1.5	72
Cinnamon Sugar	350	2	74
Garlic Pretzel; Sour Crm & Onion	320	1	66
Glazin' Raisin®	470	0.5	104
Jalapeno Pretzel	270	1	58
Kidstix, 4 sticks	230	1	48
Original Pretzel	340	1	72
Parmesan Herb	390	5	74
Sesame Pretzel	350	6	63
Dipping Sauces			
Caramel Dip	135	3	27
Cheese Sce; Hot Salsa Chse, avg.	100	8	4
Chocolate Flavored Dip	130	4	24
Light Cream Cheese	70	6	1
Marinara Sauce	10	0	4
Strawberry Cream Cheese	110	10	4
Sweet Mustard	60	1.5	8
Beverages: Per Serving			
Auntie Anne's Lemonade, 22 fl.oz	180	0	43
Dutch Ice (20 fl.oz): Kiwi-Banana	270	0	63
Blue Raspberry	230	0	55
Lemonade	450	0	110
Mocha	570	15	105
Orange Crème	400	0	92
Pina Colada	535	0	125
Strawberry	315	0	72
Wild Cherry	300	0	69
Dutch Ice (14 fl.oz): Kiwi-Banana	190	0	44
Blue Raspberry	165	0	38
Lemonade	315	0	77
Mocha	400	10	74
Orange Crème	280	0	64
Pina Colada; Strawberry	220	0	53
Wild Cherry	210	0	48

Back Yard Burgers®

	C	F	Cb
Burgers			
Back Yard Burger 1/3 lb., 9 oz	525	29	38
w. Cheese	580	34	38
Bacon Cheddar, 9 oz	675	42	38
Barbecue Bacon, 9.5 oz	680	39	47
Black Jack	580	39	36
Chili Cheese, 9.8 oz	620	36	41
Gardenburger®, 7 oz	320	6	54
Great Little Burger®, 6 oz	345	15	38
Hawaiian, 9.5 oz	600	33	44
Miz Grazi's, 9 oz	585	34	39
Mushroom Swiss, 9.4 oz	605	36	37
Worcestershire, 10 oz	550	34	41
Chicken Sandwiches			
Barbecue, 7 oz	344	8	44
Blackened, 7 oz	350	11	39
Hawaiian, 7.8 oz	350	8	45
Honey Mustard, 7 oz	385	11	46
Lemon Butter, 6.5 oz	325	9	37
Savory, 6.3 oz	295	6	36
Bacon Swiss	455	20	37
Buffalo Ranch	545	30	51
Specialties: BLT, 5 oz	270	16	36
Chicken Tenderloins, 3 piece	415	28	22
Chili Dog, 5 oz	340	20	29
Chili Cheese Dog, 5.4 oz	400	25	29
Hot Dog, 4 oz	310	18	27
Baked Potatoes			
Chili & Cheddar, 9 oz	330	11	48
Ranch, 7.7 oz	415	22	45
Salsa, 7.7 oz	260	5	47
Traditional/Plain, 6 oz	190	0	43
Fries: Chili Cheese Fries, 6.7 oz	340	22	28
Seasoned Fries, regular, 3 oz	260	16	28
Waffle Fries, regular, 3 oz	245	22	28
Salads (No Dressing)			
Blackened Chicken, 10 oz	165	4	11
Charbroiled Chicken, 10 oz	155	3	11
Garden Fresh, 3.6 oz	25	0	5
Cobblers: Apple, 6 oz	430	20	60
Blackberry; Peach, 6 oz	435	20	60
Cherry, 6 oz	470	20	68
Shakes			
Chocolate/Vanilla, 12 oz	560	26	72
Strawberry, 12 oz	580	26	79

Baja Fresh® **C** **F** **Cb**

Burritos: Includes Cheese

	C	F	Cb
"Dos Manos": Steak, 1/2 meal	785	24	101
Chicken, 1/2 meal	735	20	101
Mexicano: Chicken	815	13	124
Steak	900	20	124
Ultimo Burrito: Steak, no sour crm	930	37	90
Chicken, no sour cream	850	30	90
Baja Burrito: Chicken	670	35	75
Steak	915	42	75
Bare Burrito	640	7	99
Bare Burrito Vegetarian	560	8	102
Bean & Cheese Burrito: Chicken	990	33	104
Steak	1080	41	104
Vegetarian	860	31	104

Enchiladas: Verano

	C	F	Cb
Verano	580	9	87
Cheese Enchilada	855	37	92
Chicken Enchilada	780	25	91
Steak Enchilada	875	33	94

Ensalada: Mahi Mahi, no dressing

	C	F	Cb
Mahi Mahi, no dressing	295	9	20
Shrimp, no dressing	190	4	17
Baja Ensalada: Chicken, no dress.	320	7	17
Fish, no dressing	385	15	27
Steak, no dressing	450	18	17

Fajitas: Chicken w. Corn Tortillas

	C	F	Cb
Chicken w. Corn Tortillas	1225	29	164
Steak w. Corn Tortillas	1380	42	164

Mini Tosta-Dita: Chicken

	C	F	Cb
Chicken	550	17	67
Steak	605	22	67

Mini-Quesa-Dita: Steak

	C	F	Cb
Steak	685	23	81
Cheese; Chicken, avg.	630	21	81

Nachos: Cheese; Chicken, avg.

	C	F	Cb
Cheese; Chicken, avg.	1900	104	166
Steak	2075	113	166

Picado: Chicken

	C	F	Cb
Chicken	670	31	31
Steak	835	45	31

Quesadilla: Chicken

	C	F	Cb
Chicken	1265	71	80
Steak	1355	79	80
Vegetarian; Cheese, avg.	1155	70	92

Tacos: Chilito Chicken

	C	F	Cb
Chilito Chicken	320	10	38
Chillito Steak	345	12	38
Baja Style Tacos: Chicken	200	5	26
Steak	225	7	26
Wild Gulf Shrimp	195	5	26
Fish Taco Baja	275	13	31
Fish Taco Charbroiled	270	10	32
Grilled Veggie Taco	440	10	72

Taquitos: Includes Sour Cream

	C	F	Cb
Chicken w. Beans/Rice, avg.	720	36	66
Steak w. Beans, Crema Salsa	815	42	69
Steak w. Rice, Crema Salsa	775	42	67

Tostada: Steak w. chse & sr crm

	C	F	Cb
Steak w. chse & sr crm	1210	60	102
Chicken w. chse & sour crm	1120	52	102
Vegetarian w. cheese & sour crm	990	50	102

Banana's® **C** **F** **Cb**

Frosty: Per 8 oz Serving

	C	F	Cb
Banana Berry Cream	180	0.5	40
Citrus Blend	110	0	26
Mango Magic	150	0	38
Melon Banana	140	0.5	36
Orange Swirl Creamy	170	0.5	37
P-nut Butter Cup Creamy	380	20	35
Raspberry Creamy	170	2	31
Strawberry	50	0.5	12
Strawberry Creamy	150	0	32

Smoothie: Per 8 oz Serving

	C	F	Cb
Banana Berry	130	1	32
Chococino	350	19	39
Cookies N Cream	300	4	57
Mocha ala Orange	160	1	37
Pina Colada	170	0	44
Raspberry Flavored Lemony Batch	290	0	73
Strawberry Flavored Lemony Batch	250	0	66

Ben & Jerry's®

Icecream & Frozen Yogurt ~ See Page 32
Novelty Bars ~ See Page 36

Big Apple Bagels®

Bagels: All types, 5 oz

	C	F	Cb
All types, 5 oz	380	2	77
1/2 bagel, 2.5 oz	190	1	38

My Favorite Muffin® Bagels: Per Bagel (4 oz)

	C	F	Cb
Honey Grain	310	3	61
Avg. other varieties	310	1	66

My Favorite Muffin® Muffins: Each (6 oz)

	C	F	Cb
Plain	600	30	75
Plain, Fat Free	390	0	90
Chocolate	510	24	69
Chocolate, Fat Free	375	0	87

Cream Cheese: Per 2 Tbsp (1 oz)

	C	F	Cb
Plain	100	10	1
Honey Cinnamon; Very Berry, avg.	130	12	3
Lite varieties, average	70	5	2

Soups: Per Cup (8 fl.oz)

	C	F	Cb
Boston Clam/Potato Chowder	210	13	20
Chicken Gumbo; Beef Pot Roast	110	4	12
Garden Vege; Hearty Vegetable	110	1	18
Minestrone	150	3	26
Split Pea w. Ham	90	2	15

Baskin Robbins® C F Cb

Hard Scooped Icecream
Per Regular Scoop

	C	F	Cb
Cherries Jubilee	240	13	29
Chocolate: Regular Scoop	270	16	31
Small Scoop	180	10	20
Chocolate Chip	270	17	26
Chocolate Chip Cookie Dough	300	15	36
Chocolate Fudge	290	15	34
Cookies 'N Cream	300	17	30
French Vanilla	280	18	25
German Choc Cake	310	15	39
Gold Medal Ribbon	270	13	35
Jamoca	250	15	25
Jamoca Almond Fudge	280	16	30
Mint Choc Chip	270	15	28
Old Fashion Butter Pecan	290	18	24
Peanut Butter 'N Chocolate	330	20	30
Pink Bubblegum	270	14	34
Pistachio Almond	290	19	25
Pralines 'N Cream	280	15	33
Quarterback Crunch	290	17	32
Reeses Peanut Butter	310	19	30
Rocky Road	300	14	35
Vanilla: Regular Scoop	250	16	24
Small Scoop	160	10	15
Very Berry Strawberry	230	10	30
World Class Chocolate	280	14	33
Lowfat Icecream: Espresso 'N Crm	180	2.5	31
No Sugar Added Icecream, avg.	160	4	27

Ices, Sherbets, Sorbets: Regular Scoop

	C	F	Cb
Ices: Daiquiri	130	0	33
Sherbets: Rainbow	160	2	34
Sorbets: Average all flavors	115	0	29

Lowfat Yogurt (Hard): Regular Scoop

	C	F	Cb
Maui Brownie Madness	250	9	38

Nonfat Yogurt (Soft Serve): Small Scoop

	C	F	Cb
Nonfat Frozen Yogurt, 5 oz	190	0.5	39
Truly Free Yogurt, Cafe Mocha	140	0.5	27

Shakes, Smoothies, Blasts: Regular (16 fl.oz)

	C	F	Cb
Shakes: Chocolate Icecream	750	43	80
Vanilla Icecream	630	35	69
Smoothies: Average all flavors	320	1	70
Blasts: Cappuccino w/whipped crm	340	16	44
Cones: Sugar Cone	60	3	7
Cake Cone	25	0.5	4
Waffle Cone: Large	120	1.5	14
Fresh Baked	145	2	30

Big Boy® C F Cb

Sandwiches

	C	F	Cb
Big Boy	600	26	35
Brawny Lad™	420	21	30
Buddie Boy	760	34	80
Fish Sandwich	690	48	41
Small Hamburger	445	30	30
Super Big Boy™	830	66	34
Swiss Miss	635	44	28
Tuna Salad Sandwich	545	40	30

Sides & Salad

	C	F	Cb
French Fries	360	19	45
Chili	315	18	19
Onion Rings	580	41	45
Tartare Sauce, 2 oz	370	40	1
Trio Salad	620	46	18

Blimpie®

Cold Subs: Per 6" Sub on White

	C	F	Cb
Blimpie Best	475	16	52
Club Sub	440	12	50
Ham & Cheese	435	12	52
Roast Beef	470	13	50
Seafood	355	7.5	58
Tuna	495	23	50
Turkey Sub	425	11	49

Hot Subs: Per 6" Sub on White

	C	F	Cb
BLT	590	32	49
Grilled Chicken	380	9	50
ChickMax	510	13	71
Meatball	570	27	55
MexiMax	425	9	65
Steak & Onion	440	16	49
VegiMax	395	7	60
Grilled Subs: Reuben, 6"	630	33	55
Pastrami, 6"	460	14	52
Wraps: Zesty Italian	640	33	74
Chicken Caesar, regular	645	35	56
Salads: Chef, regular	210	9	9
Coleslaw, 5 oz	180	13	13
Potato Salad, 5 oz	270	19	19
Turkey, regular	370	19	31
Dressings: Fat Free Italian, 1 fl.oz	20	0	5
Blimpie Dressing, 1 fl.oz	120	8	16
Blimpie Special Sub, 3/4 fl.oz	70	7	2
Soup: Chicken Noodle, 1 cup	120	2.5	18
Desserts: Oatmeal Raisin Cookie	190	8	27
Sugar Cookie	330	17	24
Average other varieties	2100	10	26

For Complete Nutritional Data ~ see CalorieKing.com

Boston Market®

C F Cb

Entrees

	C	F	Cb
1/4 Chicken:			
White meat w. skin & wing	280	12	2
No skin or wing	170	4	2
1/4 Chicken: Dark meat w. skin	320	21	2
No skin	190	10	1
1/2 Chicken w. skin	590	33	4
Chicken Pot Pie, 1 pie	750	46	57
Chunky Chicken Salad, 6.4 oz	480	39	4
Grilled Chicken BBQ	400	19	16
Grilled Chicken Teriyaki	290	10	14
Honey Glazed Ham (lean), 5 oz	210	8	10
Marinated Grilled Chkn, 1 breast	230	10	1
Meatloaf, 5 oz	325	19	16
Meatloaf & Brown Gravy	360	23	19
Meatloaf & Chunky Tom. Sauce	350	19	25
Rotisserie Turkey Breast: no skin	170	1	3
w. Stuffing & Gravy	600	18	67
Turkey Pot Pie	710	41	58
Soup: Chicken Noodle, 3/4 cup	100	4.5	8
Chicken Tortilla w. toppings, 6 oz	170	8	18
Turkey Tortilla w. toppings, 6 oz	160	7	18
Salads: Caesar Side Salad, 4 oz	300	26	13
Caesar Salad Entree, 9.5 oz	470	40	17
no Dressing, 8 oz	260	18	24
Chunky Chicken Salad, 3/4 cup	480	39	4
Grilled Chicken Caesar, 13.5 oz	710	50	18
Old Fashioned Potato Salad	200	12	22
Oriental Gr. Ckn, no dress./noodles	320	10	20
Sandwiches: BBQ Chicken	830	45	59
BBQ Chicken, no cheese/mayo	550	15	58
Chicken w. Cheese & Sauce	640	29	61
no Cheese or Sauce	400	6	60
Ham w. Cheese & Sauce	660	32	67
no Cheese or Sauce	420	9	65
Meatloaf w. Cheese	730	29	85
Open-Faced, w. sides	730	36	74
Turkey: Bacon Club	770	37	64
Open-Faced	720	20	93
Turkey w. Cheese & Sauce	630	26	64
no Cheese or Sauce	400	4.5	61
Side Dishes: Rice Pilaf, 1 cup	140	4	24
Whole Corn, 3/4 cup	180	4	30
Hot Cinnamon Apples, 3/4 cup	250	4.5	56
Macaroni & Cheese, 3/4 cup	280	11	33
Mash Potatoes (3/4 c.) & Gravy	230	9	32
Creamed Spinach, 3/4 cup	260	20	11

Bojangles®

C F Cb

Cajun & Southern Style Chicken	C	F	Cb
Breast, average	280	17	12
Leg, average	265	16	11
Thigh, average	310	23	11
Wing, average	355	25	11
Sandwiches			
Cajun Filet: w/out Mayo	335	11	41
w. Mayonnaise	435	22	41
Grilled Filet: w/out mayo	235	5	25
w. Mayonnaise	335	16	25
Snacks: Buffalo Bites	180	5	5
Chicken Supremes	335	16	26
Biscuit Sandwiches: Bacon	290	17	26
Bacon, Egg & Cheese	550	42	27
Biscuit (plain)	245	12	29
Cajun Filet	455	21	46
Country Ham	270	15	26
Egg	400	30	26
Sausage	350	23	26
Smoked Sausage	380	26	27
Steak	650	49	37
Fixins': Botato Rounds	235	11	31
Cajun Pintos	110	0	18
Corn on the Cob	140	2	34
Dirty Rice	165	6	24
Green Beans	25	0	5
Macaroni & Cheese	200	14	12
Marinated Cole Slaw	135	3	26
Potatoes, no Gravy	80	1	16
Seasoned Fries	345	19	39
Sweet Biscuits: Bo Berry™	220	10	29
Cinnamon	320	18	37

Braum's

C F Cb

	C	F	Cb
Cinnamon Rolls, with Icing	340	11	56
Frozen Custard: Avg. all flavors	185	8	25
Frozen Yogurt: Per 1/2 Cup			
Banana Pecan	170	7	23
Bordeaux Cherry Amaretto	155	5	24
Capp. Chunky Choc.; Toffee Bark	170	6	26
Chocolate varieties, avg.	150	4.5	23
Coconut Chocolate Walnut	175	7	24
Peach; Strawberry/Banana	145	3.5	25
Pineapple Almond	155	5	24
Toffee Bark	170	6	25
Vanilla	115	0.5	24
Diet Yogurt: Avg. all flav., 2 1/2 oz	140	5	20

Braum's cont..

Frozen Yogurt (Cont)	C	F	Cb
Fat Free, No Sugar Added Yogurt:			
Brownie Fudge Sundae	100	0	21
Strawberry; Vanilla Bean	90	0	18
Icecream: Per $^{1}/_{2}$ Cup			
Light: Average all varieties	165	5	26
Premium: Black Walnut	200	11	21
Dream Cooler	315	9	55
Homestyle Vanilla	200	9	26
Peanut Butter Cups	235	14	23
Strawberry	165	7	22
Average other flavors	190	9	25
Sherbet: Avg. all varieties	170	3	36
Muffins: Banana Nut; Blueberry	415	21	50
Carrot Walnut	500	27	56
Cherry Pecan	435	21	56
English	145	2	27
Strawberry	470	21	64
Pie: Cappuccino; Chunky Choc	235	9	34
Ice Cream, Choc Pecan	235	13	27
Mint Choc. Chip; Pumpkin	220	10	30
Strawberry Cheesecake	210	8	31
Icecream Bars: Icecream Cups	160	7.5	20
Chocolate Covered Vanilla	215	14	19
Icecream Sandwiches: Brownie	370	17	49
Vanilla	295	11	44
Cones: Nutty Cones	320	18	34
Pecan Caramel Fudge Sundaes	330	20	35
Twin Pops, 2.5 oz	60	0	15
Yogurt Bars No Sugar Added:			
Chocolate Choc. w. Almonds	160	10	15
Chocolate Coated Vanilla	155	9	15
Choc. Covered Vanilla/Almonds	320	18	34
Fudge Bars	95	0.5	21

Breugger's Bagels®

	C	F	Cb
Bagels: Plain	300	2	61
Classic Blueberry/Cranberry Orange	330	2	68
Classic Cinnamon Raisin	320	2	68
Classic Everything	310	2	62
Cream Cheese: Average, 1 oz	100	9	3
Light varieties, average	70	4	4
Breakfast Sandwiches: Per Sandwich			
Egg & Cheese	480	15	66
Egg & Cheese & Bacon	560	22	66
Egg & Cheese & Ham	520	17	66
Egg & Cheese & Sausage	680	33	66

Breugger's cont..

Sandwiches	C	F	Cb
Atlantic Smoked Salmon	475	12	66
Chicken Breast	440	6	62
Chicken Fajita	520	12	74
Chicken Salad w. Mayo; Leonardo	460	12	67
Deli-Style Ham w. Honey Mustard	440	4.5	77
Garden Veggie	390	2.5	80
Herby Turkey	530	14	73
Santa Fe Turkey	480	10	71
Turkey w. Mayonnaise	480	14	65

Briazz®

	C	F	Cb
Paninis: Chicken Mozzarella	605	27	58
Chicken Pesto	680	12	104
Pepperjack Smoked Turkey	625	17	72
Philly Cheesesteak	700	32	75
Sunflower Chicken	790	44	52
Tuscan Turkey	590	29	50
Rustic Slice Sandwich: Per Sandwich			
Low Fat Salami, 8.3 oz	295	3.5	38
Smoked Turkey & Havarti	455	25	36
Turkey Breast & Provolone	355	11	35
Subzz: Per Sandwich w. Dressing			
Beef & Cheddar	490	19	51
Briazz Tuna 'n Cheese	625	30	53
Demi Tuna 'n Cheese	390	24	26
Ham & Swiss	475	13	57
Italian Ham, Salami & Provolone	605	27	59
Turkey Provolone	500	17	54
Cafe Salads: Greek Orzo	260	10	33
Chicken Breast w. Dressing	200	12	11
Classic w. Dressing; Parisian	160	11	11
Greek Island w. Dressing	290	24	10
Orzo Almondine w. Dressing	430	21	50
Tuna w. Dressing	240	16	8
Togas: Per Package			
Chicken Club	680	42	46
Chop Chop Veggie	545	24	63
Classy Tuna	640	33	46
Italian w. Italian Dressing	760	47	49
Smokin' Turkey Club w. Ranch Dr.	740	43	55
Southwest Turkey	600	27	46
Cakes, Muffins, Desserts: Per Serving			
Banana Muffin	520	26	64
Chocolate Marble Pound Cake	410	21	49
Classic Brownie	375	16	55
Iced Lemon Pound Cake	505	23	69
Mixed Fruit Cup	110	0	25
Sour Cream Coffee Cake Muffin	710	40	78
Yogurt & Lowfat Granola Parfait	510	6	100

Restaurants & Fast−Foods

Burger King®

Burgers & Sandwiches	C	F	Cb
¼lb Burger	490	21	50
Fish Fillet	520	30	44
Bacon Double Cheeseburger	580	34	32
Cheeseburger	360	17	31
Chicken Whopper	580	26	48
without Mayonnaise	420	9	47
Chicken Whopper JR	350	14	30
without Mayonnaise	270	6	30
Double Cheeseburger	540	31	32
Double Hamburger	450	24	31
Hamburger	310	13	31
Homestyle Griller	480	27	35
King Supreme	550	34	32
Original Double Whopper	980	62	52
without Mayonnaise	820	45	52
Original Whopper	720	43	52
without Mayonnaise	550	25	52
Jr Whopper w. Cheese	440	21	33
without Mayonnaise	360	17	33
Smokehouse Cheddar Griller	720	48	32
Chicken Specialty	560	28	52
without Mayonnaise	460	17	52
Veggie w. Red Fat Mayonnaise	340	10	47
Baguettes, all types w. Sauce	350	5	47
Breakfast			
Bacon, 3 half slices	40	3	0
Breakfast Syrup	80	0	21
Biscuit, Plain	300	15	35
Cini-Minis, without Vanilla Icing			
serving, 4 rolls	440	23	51
Vanilla Icing	110	3	20
Croissant	170	7	22
Croissan'wich w. Egg, Cheese	320	19	24
w. Sausage, Cheese	420	31	23
w. Sausage, Egg, Cheese	520	39	24
Egg'wich: w. Canadian Bac. & Egg	380	19	35
w. Canadian Bacon, Egg, Chse	420	23	36
French Toast Sticks, 5 sticks	390	20	46
Grape or Strawberry Jam	30	0	7
Ham, 2 slices	35	1	0
Hash Brown Rounds: Large	390	25	38
Small	230	15	23
Puffed Scrambled Egg Portion	100	8	2
Sausage Patty, 2 oz	260	25	0
Sourdough: w. Bacon, Egg & Chse	380	22	30
w. Ham, Egg & Cheese	380	20	30
w. Sausage, Egg & Cheese	540	39	30

Chicken Tenders: *Per Serving*	C	F	Cb
4 pieces	170	9	10
5 pieces	210	12	13
6 pieces	250	14	15
8 pieces	340	19	20
Dipping Sauces (1 oz): Barbecue	35	0	9
Honey Flavored	90	0	23
Honey Mustard	90	6	9
Ranch	140	15	1
Sweet & Sour	40	0	10
Zesty Onion Ring	150	15	3
French Fries: *Per Serving*			
Small, 2.6 oz	230	11	29
Medium, 4 oz	360	18	46
Large, 5.6 oz	600	30	76
Value, 3.8 oz	340	17	43
Onion Rings: Small, 1.8 oz	180	9	22
Medium, 3.2 oz	320	16	40
Large, 4.8 oz	480	23	60
King Size, 5.6 oz	550	27	70
Salads: *No Dressing*			
Chicken Caesar, croutons	160	6	5
Garden Salad	25	0	5
Sides			
Baked Potato w. Chives, 8.5 oz	260	0	61
Chili, 7.6 oz	190	8	17
Jalapeno Poppers , 4 pieces	230	13	22
Mozzarella Sticks , 4 pieces	290	16	25
Desserts: Dutch Apple Pie	340	14	52
Hershey's Sundae Pie	300	18	31
Nestle Toll House Cookies (2)	440	16	68
Vanilla Bean Cheesecake	190	9	26
Drinks			
Coca-Cola Classic, medium	230	0	56
Coffee, medium	5	0	1
Diet Coke, medium	0	0	0
Dr. Pepper, medium	220	0	54
Chocolate, Strawb., Vanilla Shake (syrup added),			
Small, 11 fl.oz	620	32	72
Medium, 14 fl.oz	790	42	89

For Complete Nutritional Data ~ see CalorieKing.com

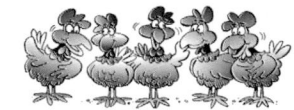

Captain D's Seafood®

	C	F	Cb
Platters: Per Platter			
Broiled Shrimp	720	8	131
Broiled Chicken	800	10	131
Broiled Fish	735	7	131
Broiled Fish & Chicken	775	10	131
Lunches Per Lunch Platter			
Broiled Shrimp	420	7	64
Broiled Chicken	505	9	65
Broiled Fish	435	7	65
Broiled Fish & Chicken	480	8	68
Stuffed Crab	95	7	1
Sandwiches: Per Sandwich			
Broiled Chicken	450	19	29
Desserts: Per Slice			
Carrot Cake	435	23	49
Cheesecake	420	31	30
Chocolate Cake	305	10	49
Pecan Pie	460	20	64

Caribou Coffee

	C	F	Cb
Drinks: Per Serving			
Cappuccino: 2% Capp, 12 fl.oz	120	4	13
Skim Capp, 12 fl.oz	80	0.5	11
Latte: 2% Latte, 12 fl.oz	125	4.5	13
Skim Latte, 12 fl.oz	90	0.5	12
Chai Latte: 2% Chai Latte, 12 fl.oz	210	4	38
Skim Chai, 12 fl.oz	150	0	32
Mocha: 2% Mocha, 12 fl.oz	260	12	30
Skim Mocha, 12 fl.oz	225	9	26
Turtle Mocha, 16 fl.oz	370	9	63
Coolers: Caramel Cooler, 12 fl.oz	345	9	64
Chocolate Cooler, 12 fl.oz	190	2	40
Coffee Cooler, 12 fl.oz	175	2	36
Espresso Cooler, 12 fl.oz	140	2	28
Mint Oreo Cooler, 12 fl.oz	520	17	83
Vanilla Cooler, 12 fl.oz	195	3	39
Hot Apple Blast: Small	195	8	31
Medium	235	8	41
Large	270	8	50
Smoothies: Raspberry, 12 fl.oz	220	0	53
Strawberry Banana, 12 fl.oz	190	0	46
Wild Berry, 12 fl.oz	175	0	42
Caramel Hirise, 16 fl.oz	260	10	35
Lite White Berry, 16 fl.oz	310	5	57
Mint Condition, 16 fl.oz	370	9	61

Carl's Jr.®

	C	F	Cb
Burgers/Sandwiches			
Bacon Swiss Crispy Chicken	760	38	72
Carl's Catch Fish Sandwich™	530	28	55
Carl's Famous Star® Hamburger	590	32	50
Charbroiled: BBQ Chicken S'wich™	290	3.5	41
Chicken Club Sandwich™	470	23	37
Santa Fe Chicken Sandwich™	540	31	37
Sirloin Steak	550	24	52
Dble Sourdough Bacon Chseburger	880	59	37
Dble Western Bacon Chseburger®	920	50	65
Famous Bacon Cheeseburger™	700	41	51
Hamburger	280	9	36
Ranch Crispy Chicken Sandwich	660	31	71
Sourdough Bacon Cheeseburger	640	41	37
Sourdough Ranch Bacon Chseburger	720	46	43
Spicy Chicken Sandwich	480	26	47
Southwest Spicy Chicken S'wich	620	41	48
Super Star® Hamburger	790	47	51
The Six Dollar Burger™	960	62	62
Bacon Cheese Burger	1010	69	52
Chili Cheese Burger	930	57	58
Guacamole Bacon Burger	1120	81	54
Western Bacon Cheeseburger®	660	30	64
Western Bacon Crispy Chkn S'wich	750	28	91
Potatoes: Plain	290	0	68
Bacon & Cheese	640	29	75
Broccoli & Cheese	530	21	76
Sour Cream & Chives	430	14	70
Breakfast: Breakfast Burrito	550	32	36
Breakfast Quesadilla	370	17	38
English Muffin w. Margarine	210	9	28
French Toast Dips, no Syrup	370	20	42
Sourdough Breakfast	410	20	33
Scrambled Eggs	180	14	1
Sunrise Sandwich, no Bacon/Saus.	360	21	28
Bakery/Desserts: Cheese Danish	400	23	49
Blueberry Muffin	340	14	49
Bran Raisin Muffin	370	14	61
Chocolate Chip Cookie, 2.5 oz	350	18	46
Strawberry Swirl Cheesecake, 3.5 oz	290	17	30
Side Orders: Chicken Stars, 6 pces	260	16	14
CrissCut Fries®, 5 oz	410	24	43
French Fries, small, 3 oz	290	14	37
Hash Brown Nuggets, 4 oz	330	21	32
Onion Rings, 4.5 oz	430	22	53
Salads: w. Fat Free Italian Dressing			
Charbroiled Chicken Salad-to-Go™	200	7	12
Garden Salad-to-Go™	50	2.5	4

Restaurants & Fast−Foods

Carvel Icecream®

	C	F	Cb
***Soft Serve Icecream:** Per Serving (4 fl.oz)*			
Chocolate	195	10	22
Vanilla	195	10	21
No Fat Chocolate	120	0	28
No Fat Vanilla	115	0	25
No Sugar Added Vanilla	130	3	25
Sherbet, assorted flavors	140	1	31
***Flying Saucer:** Per Sandwich*			
Chocolate; Vanilla, avg.	240	10	33
98% Fat Free: Choc., Raspberry	190	1.5	40
***Fountain Beverages:** Per 16 fl.oz*			
Thick Shakes: Chocolate	735	31	96
Vanilla	655	30	79
Reduced Fat: Chocolate	540	8	100
Vanilla	465	7	84
Fizzlers®, regular	350	4.5	75
Carvelanche™ w. Topping (8 oz)	600	30	71
***Icecream Cakes:** Per Serving (4 fl.oz)*			
Butterscotch Dream	260	10	37
Celebration; Lil' Love, Holiday Ice	200	10	24
Cookies n'Cream	240	12	29
Fudge Drizzle	245	11	32
Gameball	335	17	41
Sinfully Chocolate	245	10	34
Strawberries n'Cream	270	10	40
***Italian Ices:** Per Serving (4 fl.oz)*			
Cherry	100	0	25
Chocolate Cream	90	1	20
Vanilla Cream	100	2	20
Average other flavors	75	0	19

For Complete Nutritional Data ~ see CalorieKing.com

Checkers

*~ Same Menu & Data as
Rally's Hamburgers® See Page 234 ~*

Cheesecake Factory®

Per Slice			
Adam's P. B. Cup Fudge Ripple	940	59	95
Banana Cream Cheesecake	860	61	70
Brownie Sundae Cheesecake	960	62	96
Choc Chip Cookie Dough	1080	71	100
Dulce de Leche Caramel Ch/cake	1000	70	83
Kahlua Cocoa Coffee	840	55	80
Keylime Cheesecake	700	48	63
Original Cheesecake	640	45	55
Vanilla Bean Cheesecake	870	62	69
White Choc. Raspberry Truffle	900	60	80

Chick-Fil-A®

	C	F	Cb
Chick-Fil-A Sandwiches			
Chicken Sandwich	410	16	38
Chargrilled Chicken Sandwich	290	7	30
Chargrilled Chicken Club 370	13	31	
Chicken Salad Sandwich	350	15	32
Cool Wraps®: Spicy Chicken	380	6	52
Chargrilled Chicken	380	6	54
Chicken Caesar	460	10	52
***Breakfast:** Per Serving*			
Plain Biscuit	260	6	38
Hot Buttered Biscuit	165	4	28
Biscuit and Gravy	340	21	30
Biscuit: w. Bacon	340	21	30
w. Bacon, Egg & Cheese	370	21	39
w. Egg & Cheese	230	6	38
Biscuit: w. Sausage	160	4	28
w. Sausage & Egg	320	10	51
w. Sausage, Egg & Cheese	320	15	45
Danish	370	21	39
Hashbrowns	360	21	38
***Salads:** Chick-n-Strips® Salad*	390	18	22
Chargrilled Chicken Garden	180	6	9
Southwest Chargrilled	240	8	17
***Salad Dressing:** Per Packet (1.25 oz)*			
Caesar	200	21	1
Raspberry Vinaigrette	80	2	14
Bleu Cheese; Buttermilk Ranch	190	20	2
Fat Free Dijon Honey Mustard	60	0	14
Light Italian	20	0.5	3
Spicy	170	17	2
Thousand Island	170	16	6
***Strips, Nuggets:** Per Serving*			
Chick-n-Strips® (4-count)	290	13	14
Nuggets (8-pack)	260	12	12
***Dipping Sauces:** Polynesian, 1 oz*	110	6	13
Dijon Honey Mustard, ¹/₂ oz	50	5	2
Barbecue; Honey Mustard, 1 oz	45	0	10
***Sides:** Carrot & Raisin Salad, small*	130	5	22
Coleslaw, small	210	17	14
Garlic and Butter Croutons, ¹/₂ oz	50	2.5	6
Rstd Unsalted Sunflower Kernel,, ¹/₂ oz	80	7	3
Side Salad	60	3	4
Tortilla Strips, 1 pkt	60	3.5	9
Waffle Potato Fries™,small	280	14	37

Chick-Fil-A® cont...

	C	F	Cb
Soup: Hearty Breast of Chicken	140	3.5	18
Desserts: Cheesecake, 3.3 oz slice	340	21	30
with Fruit Topping, avg.	370	21	39
Icedream® Cup, small	230	6	38
Icedream® Cone, small	160	4	28
Lemon Pie, 4 oz slice	320	10	51
Fudge Nut Brownie (1), 2.6 oz	330	15	45

Chili's®

Starters:

Awesome Blossom w. sauce	2880	222	191
1/4 Whole w. Blossom Sauce	720	55	48
Boneless Buffalo Wings + sauce	1140	74	64
Boneless Shanghai Wings	1340	84	90
Fajita Nachos: Chicken	995	36	94
Beef	1130	50	100
Wings over Buffalo w. Dressing	760	58	6
Guiltless Grill®: Chicken Platter	565	9	83
Chicken Grill Pita	545	9	77
Chicken Sandwich	525	8	70
Tomato Basil Pasta	670	15	106
Burgers (No Fries): Ranch Burger	1070	66	64
Old Timer Burger	790	45	52
Chipotle Bleu Chse Bacon Burger	1120	75	54
Mushroom Swiss Burger	910	48	62
Ground Peppercorn Burger			
w. Strings & Dressing	1200	79	78
Meals: Chili's Filet	1215	78	69
Bottomless Tostada Chips w. Salsa	910	46	109
Cajun Chicken Pasta	1190	56	103
Cajun Chicken Sandwich	850	41	77
Cheese Steak Sandwich (no Fries)	740	29	67
Chicken Caesar Pita (no Fries)	520	19	33
Chick. Crispers w. fries, corn, dress.	1630	95	105
Citrus Fire Chicken & Shrimp	660	12	73
Country Fried Steak	1335	70	126
Flame Grilled Rib Eye	1080	66	70
Ginger Citrus Glazed Salmon	710	22	70
Grilled Baby Back Ribs	1130	54	109
Grilled Margarita Chicken	725	25	72
Grilled Margarita Tuna	880	25	97
Grilled Shrimp Alfredo	1290	53	142
Hawaiian Steak	685	13	88
South Western Egg Rolls	830	40	86
Veggie & Smoked Chse Quesadilla	1160	67	95

Chili's® cont...

	C	F	Cb
Fajitas: Includes 3 Tortillas & Garnishes			
Mushroom Jack	1270	60	103
Chicken	1020	41	97
Steak	1070	51	93
Salads: Includes Dressing			
Chicken Fajita Salad	795	55	47
Crispy Chicken Salad	930	59	60
Grilled Caribbean Salad	650	34	74
Grilled Chicken Caesar Salad	660	32	53
Lettuce Wraps w. Dipping Sauce	730	37	60
Southwestern Chicken Salad	1185	86	44
Desserts: Choc Chip Paradise Pie	1250	47	188
Molten Choc Cake	1505	67	207

For Complete Nutritional Data ~ see CalorieKing.com

Chuck E. Cheese®

	C	F	Cb
Appetizers: Per Serving			
Blended Pizza Sauce, 1/4 cup	35	0	7
Buffalo Wings, 4 pieces	220	15	1
Lamb Wesson Fr. Fries, ckd, 4 oz	285	10	43
Sargento Mozzarella Sticks, 2	380	24	26
Sandwiches: Fries Not Included			
Grilled Chicken Sub	740	39	57
Ham & Cheese	770	41	60
Hot Dog	430	29	27
Italian Sub	770	47	52
Pizza (Medium): Per 2 Slices			
BBQ Chicken	410	13	51
Beef	410	17	43
Cheese	330	10	43
Pepperoni	370	14	43
Sausage	385	15	44
Birthday Items: Per Slice (1/12 Cake)			
8" Chocolate Cake w. Whip Cream	210	11	25
8" White Cake w. Whip Cream	210	11	26
Breakfast: Per Serving			
Kellogg's Snack Um's: Cinn. Blast	140	5	24
Froot Loops; Rice Krispy, avg.	125	1	26
PCB Banana Loaf Cake (1)	350	11	50
PCB Cinn. Crumb Pound Cake (1)	385	17	55
Desserts: Per Serving			
PCB Brownie (1)	380	18	46
PCB Choc Chunk Cookie (1)	410	19	56
PCB Original Krispy Treat (1)	340	9	50

Church's Chicken®

	C	**F**	**Cb**
Fried Chicken (Edible Portion Only)			
Breast, 1 piece	200	12	4
Leg, 1 piece	140	9	2
Thigh, 1 piece	230	16	5
Wing, 1 piece	250	16	5
Krispy Tender Strips™, 1 piece	140	5	11
Tender Crunchers™, 6-8 pces	410	15	32
Side Items: Per Serving			
Apple Pie, 1 piece	280	12	41
Honey Butter Biscuits (1)	250	16	26
Cajun Rice, regular	130	7	16
Chicken Fried Steak w. White Gravy	470	28	36
Cole Slaw, regular	90	6	8
Corn on the Cob, 1 ear	140	3	24
French Fries, regular	210	11	29
Okra, regular	210	16	19
Mashed Potatoes & Gravy, reg.	90	3	14

For Complete Nutritional Data ~ see CalorieKing.com

CinnaMonster®

	C	**F**	**Cb**
Cinnamon Roll: Per 1/4 Roll (2 oz)			
Caramel Pecan	210	8	30
Original	220	6	25

For Complete Nutritional Data ~ see CalorieKing.com

Coco's

Menu Items	**C**	**F**	**Cb**
3 Egg Omelettes: Per Serving			
California Omelette, 10 oz	720	60	5
Denver Cheese Omelette, 10 oz	645	51	6
Haystack Burger w. Chse & Sauce	985	54	82
Southern Style Chkn Strips, 11 oz	940	58	59
Cinn. Roll/French Toast, Combo	1205	76	96
Pot Roast Entree, 23 oz	670	28	65
Salads: Per Serving			
Cobb Salad, 14 oz	510	32	17
Oriental Chicken, 18 oz	955	57	86
Thai Chicken, 25 oz	890	53	65

Cosi®

	C	**F**	**Cb**
Melts: Bacon Turkey Cheddar, 12 oz	890	39	79
Grilled Chicken Parmesan, 10 oz	615	19	60
Pesto Chicken, 11 oz	745	29	67
Tomato Bazil Mozzarella, 9 oz	620	28	63
Tuna Melt, 12 oz	930	52	57
Pasta: Penne Marinara, 14 oz	935	4	190
Penne Pesto w. Chicken, 19 oz	1510	48	195
Penne a la Cosi, 17 oz	1255	34	194
Thai Chicken & Peanut Noodle	1535	45	208
Pizzas: Four Cheese, 16 oz	950	35	124
Meatlovers, 21 oz	1280	60	124
Spinach & Fresh Tomato, 16 oz	905	30	129
Sandwiches: Buffalo Blue	700	30	58
Cosi Club	755	38	62
Country Ham & Brie	725	35	71
Grilled Chicken TBM	670	29	58
Hummus & Fresh Vegetables	435	8	75
Sesame Ginger Chicken	515	7	71
Smoked Turkey & Brie	780	35	73
Tandoori Chicken	810	34	78
Tuna & Cheddar	940	54	56
Turkey Light	495	8	75
Tuscan Pesto Chicken	600	18	62
Salads: (No Dressing): Cobb, 11 oz	460	28	8
Bombay; Chicken Caesar	310	8	27
Caesar, 7 oz	200	6	25
Greek, 12 oz	235	17	10
Mixed Greens, 8 oz	55	1	9
Shanghai Chicken, 9 oz	220	5	16
Signature, 10 oz	405	21	39
Dressings (Per 2 oz Pkg.):			
Balsamic Vinaigrette, Fat Free	45	0	11
Average other varieties	330	35	5
Lowfat varieties, average	85	3	13
Desserts: Apple Pie, 14 oz	990	40	147
Caramel Coated Brd Pudding, 9 oz	645	31	84
Cheesecake, 8 oz	740	46	73
Dble Trouble Brownie Sundae, 18 oz	1155	77	198
Extra Chocolate Bar, 2 oz	225	13	24
Ice Cream, Double Scoop, 6 oz	230	14	22
Mud Pie, 9 oz	915	49	109
S'mmm...oreos, for two, 7 oz	850	24	147
S'mores, for two, 7 oz	760	21	133
Sundae, medium, 8 oz	410	24	43

For Complete Listings ~ see CalorieKing.com

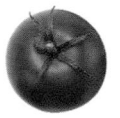
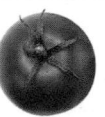

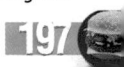

Fast-Foods & 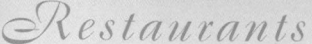*Restaurants*

Cousins Subs®

	C	F	Cb
Italian 7¹/₂" Subs: Per Sandwich			
Cappocolla & Cheese/Genoa	630	40	48
Special	800	53	48
Genoa & Cheese	730	49	48
Regular	685	44	48
Cold 7¹/₂" Subs: BLT	615	44	45
Club Sub	745	43	48
Club Sub, no mayo/cheese	370	6	48
Cold Veggie	365	11	49
Cold Veggie, no mayo/cheese	245	2	49
Chicken Salad	570	26	61
Ham	310	5	47
Ham & Cheese	640	40	47
Provolone (Cheese) Sub	685	45	46
Roast Beef	620	34	46
Roast Beef, no mayo/cheese	365	6	46
Seafood with Crab	555	32	53
Tuna	830	60	46
Turkey Breast	560	32	48
Turkey Breast, no mayo/cheese	305	3	48
Hot 7¹/₂" Subs: Cheese Steak	540	24	46
Double Cheese Steak	850	46	46
Chicken Breast	620	34	46
Chicken Breast, no mayo/cheese	365	6	46
Gyro	680	40	55
Hot Veggie; Italian Sausage	490	23	49
Meatball & Cheese	585	27	50
Pepperoni Melt	785	52	47
Philly Cheese Steak	680	36	50
Extras: Hot Dog	300	16	29
Italian/Wheat Bread, half loaf	210	3	42
French Fries: Medium	400	19	55
Soups: Per Regular Serving			
Cheese Broccoli	190	12	15
Cheese	240	16	18
Chicken w. Wild Rice	230	12	21
Chicken Dumpling; Clam	170	5	19
Chili	250	9	26
Cream of Potato	190	9	24
Salads: Chef Salad	190	10	7
Garden	135	8	7
Italian	295	20	7
Seafood	175	8	12
Side Salad	70	4	4
Tuna Salad	310	23	7

Coldstone Creamery®

Icecream & Sorbet (Small)	C	F	Cb
Sweet Cream Icecream, 4 oz	260	16	24
Yogurt, 4 oz	140	0	24
Chocolate Icecream, 4 oz	240	16	20
Italian Sorbet, 4 oz	110	0	32
Waffle Cone, cone only	100	1	22

Culver's®

	C	F	Cb
Butterburgers: Cheese	385	31	32
Bacon Deluxe Double	710	51	35
Deluxe, Single	415	22	30
Double	460	23	32
Double Cheese	590	32	32
Mushroom & Swiss Double	570	32	33
Mushroom & Swiss Single	320	16	32
Sourdough Melt Double	655	26	37
Wisconsin Swiss Melt Double	635	27	36
Favorite Sandwiches: Chkn Filet	515	13	61
Beef Pot Roast	405	10	34
Chicken Tenders	465	25	28
Grilled Chicken Breast	310	9	35
Grilled Ham & Swiss	405	20	35
Norwegian Cod Filet	605	10	52
Philly Ribeye Steak	345	21	43
Pork Tenderloin	530	27	72
Smoked Turkey	315	21	44
Turkey Sourdough BLT	525	24	38
Garden Fresh Salads: Chef	405	20	17
Chicken Caesar	410	11	18
Chicken Cashew	525	29	21
Taco Salad	700	45	52
Tossed Salad, small	105	6	7
Fish & Chicken: Shrimp Basket	1250	63	119
Chicken Dinner, 2 pieces	1660	89	129
Chicken Tenders, 4 pieces	420	18	32
Norwegian Cod, 2 pces	1155	58	120

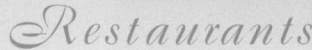

Restaurants & Fast−Foods

Culver's® cont...

Sides	C	F	Cb
Cheese Curds	600	43	54
Chili Cheddar Fries, regular	620	32	52
French Fries, regular	355	16	44
Mashed Potatoes & Gravy, small	100	5	32
Onion Rings	395	29	73
Desserts: Lemon Ice, 9 oz	210	0	46
Lemon Smoothie	670	28	94
Root Beer Float	650	18	116
Frozen Van. Custard: Dish, Single	310	18	32
Cake Cone, Single	340	18	38
Waffle Cone, Single	410	21	51
Sundaes: Turtle, 15.4 oz	1245	68	141
Caramel Cashew, small	1185	55	152
Hot Fudge Sundae, small	1015	65	91

D'Angelo's®

Sandwiches	C	F	Cb
Number 9 Steak Sandwich: Pokket	440	18	36
Large	880	36	72
Chicken Stir Fry: D'Lite Pokket	430	6	57
Sub, small	490	11	57
Sub, large	980	22	114
Classic Vegetable D'Lite Pokket	380	7	64
Grilled Chkn Stir Fry D'Lite Pokket	395	7	52
Italian: Sub, small	645	35	54
Sub, large	1290	70	108
Roast Beef: D'Lite Pokket	360	5	51
Sub, small	355	5	50
Sub, large	710	10	100
Steak Pokket, small	410	13	30
Turkey: D'Lite Pokket	370	4	51
Sub, small	305	3	39
Sub, large	610	6	78

Salads: No Dressing Unless Indicated			
Asian Chicken Salad	235	4	23
Caesar Salad w. Dressing	485	39	20
Chef Salad	275	12	17
Chicken Stir Fry	165	3	10
Roast Beef	155	3	9
Lobster	390	27	11
Turkey	160	2	9

For Complete Nutritional Data ~ see CalorieKing.com

Dairy Queen®

Burgers/Sandwiches	C	F	Cb
Chicken Breast Fillet Sandwich	500	26	48
Chili 'n' Cheese Dog	330	21	22
DQ® Homestyle: Hamburger	290	12	29
Bacon Double Cheeseburger	610	36	31
Cheeseburger	340	17	29
Double Cheeseburger	540	31	30
Ultimate Burger	670	43	29
Grilled Chicken Sandwich	310	10	30
Hot Dog, regular	240	14	19
Sides: Chkn Strip Basket w. Gravy	1000	50	102
Onion Rings	320	16	39
French Fries, medium	440	23	53
Icecream Cones/Soft Serve			
DQ® Vanilla Soft Serve, 1/2 cup	140	4.5	22
DQ® Choc. Soft Serve, 1/2 cup	150	5	22
Chocolate Cone, medium	340	11	53
Dipped Cone, medium	490	24	59
Vanilla Cone, medium	330	9	53
Salads: With Dressing			
Crispy Chicken w. Fat Free Italian	460	26	27
Grilled Chicken w. Fat Free Italian	230	9	13
Novelties: Buster Bar®	450	28	41
Chocolate Dilly® Bar	210	13	21
DQ® Fudge Bar, No Sugar Added	50	0	13
DQ® Sandwich	200	6	31
DQ® Vanilla Orange Bar, NAS	60	0	17
Lemon DQ Freez'r®;Starkiss®	80	0	21
Blizzards® & Sundaes			
Choc. Chip Cookie Dough, medium	950	36	143
Choc. Sandwich Cookie, medium	640	23	97
Chocolate Sundae, medium	400	10	71
DQ® Treatzza Cake® 1/8 cake	370	13	56
DQ® Treatzza Pizza™, 1/8 pizza	180	7	28
Royal Treats®: Banana Split	510	12	96
Peanut Buster® Parfait	730	31	99
Strawberry Shortcake	430	14	70
Frozen Yogurt: Cup, medium	230	0.5	48
DQ® Nonfat Frozen Yogurt, 1/2 cup	100	0	21
Heath® Breeze®, medium	710	18	123
Strawberry Breeze®, medium	460	1	99
Yogurt Cone, medium	260	1	56
Yogurt Strawberry Sundae, medium	280	0.5	61
Misty® Slushes, medium	290	0	74

For Complete Nutritional Data ~ see CalorieKing.com

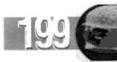

Fast-Foods & *Restaurants*

Davanni's®

	C	F	Cb
Hoagies: Per Half Hoagie (6"): Includes Mayonnaise:			
Assorted	405	31	21
Chicken Breast	495	33	23
Chicken Parmigana	385	19	22
Club	400	27	22
Ham	380	25	22
Italian Sausage	520	37	28
Meatball	465	31	31
Mediterranean	510	38	22
Pastrami	460	27	22
Pizza	315	18	23
Cheese	400	29	21
Roast Beef	385	25	21
Salami	485	38	21
Tuna	565	44	22
Turkey	370	24	22
Vegie	445	29	29
Without Butter ~ Deduct	35	5	0
Without Cheese ~ Deduct	40	3	0
Without Mayo ~ Deduct	100	11	1
Pizzas: **Canadian Bacon & Vegie Works:**			
Thin, 1 slice	225	9	18
Traditional, 1 slice	275	10	28
Solo	675	23	71
Mediterranean: Thin, 1 slice	210	8	20
Traditional, 1 slice	260	8.5	30
Solo	670	22	76
Pepperoni & Vegie Works:			
Thin, 1 slice	245	12	18
Traditional, 1 slice	295	12	28
Solo	775	35	70
The Works: Thin, 1 slice	250	13	18
Traditional, 1 slice	300	14	28
Solo	735	32	70
Vegie Works: Thin, 1 slice	210	9	18
Traditional, 1 slice	260	9	28
Solo	635	22	70
Deep Dish ~ Add 10 Calories			
If no extra cheese ('light')			
deduct per slice on Vegie Works	50	4	0
Sauce Type: Above figures are for red sauce			
White Sauce: Add Per Slice	45	5	0
Calzones: Chicken Tomato	660	28	66
Pepperoni Sausage	730	38	66
Average other varieties	700	35	66
Desserts: Chocolate Cookie	240	10	36
Fabulous Brownie	270	8	45
Rice Crispy Treat	460	11	88
Barq's Root Beer: 16 fl.oz	165	0	45
20 fl.oz	220	0	60

Del Taco®

	C	F	Cb
Breakfast			
Breakfast Burrito	235	11	24
Bacon & Egg Quesadilla	450	23	40
Egg & Cheese Burrito	465	24	39
Macho Bacon & Egg Burrito™	1030	60	82
Steak & Egg Burrito	600	34	41
Tacos: Big Fat Chicken Taco™	340	13	38
Big Fat Crispy Chicken Taco™	620	38	52
Big Fat Steak Taco™	395	19	38
Big Fat Taco™	320	11	39
Chicken Soft Taco	210	12	16
Taco; Soft Taco, average	160	10	11
Ultimate Taco	260	17	13
Burritos: Combo Burrito™	555	22	61
Bean & Chse Red/Green Burrito	270	8	38
Chicken Works Burrito	540	23	57
Del Beef Burrito™	560	30	42
Del Classic Chicken Burrito™	585	36	41
Deluxe Combo Burrito™	600	25	64
Deluxe Del Beef Burrito™	605	33	45
Half Pound Red/Green Burrito	450	12	65
Macho Beef Burrito™	1155	62	89
Macho Combo Burrito™	1045	44	113
Spicy Chicken/Veggie Works, avg.	490	18	69
Steak Works Burrito	620	31	58
Quesadillas: Chicken	575	31	41
Cheddar	490	27	39
Spicy Jack Chicken	560	30	40
Spicy Jack	480	26	38
Salads: Deluxe Chicken Salad	745	34	77
Deluxe Taco Salad™	795	40	76
Taco Salad	350	30	10
Burgers: Cheeseburger	330	13	37
Double Del Cheeseburger™	560	35	35
Del Cheeseburger™	430	25	35
Nachos: Regular	395	24	40
Macho Nachos®	1145	63	113
Sides: Beans 'n Chse Cup, 7.7 oz	265	3	44
Rice Cup, 4 oz	140	2	27
Fries: Chili Cheese, 10.5 oz	685	46	51
Deluxe Chili Cheese™, 12 oz	720	49	53
Large, 7 oz	495	32	47
Regular, 5 oz	355	23	34
Shakes: Choc., small, 11 fl.oz	510	12	89
Vanilla; Strawb., sm., 11 fl.oz	420	7	77
Chocolate, large, 15 fl.oz	765	16	117
Vanilla; Strawb., large, 15 fl.oz	550	10	97

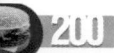
200

Restaurants & Fast-Foods

Denny's®

Breakfast	C	F	Cb
All American Slam®, no bread	800	67	3
Dagwood Breakfast, no bread	1460	90	81
Farmer's Slam, no syrup	1250	80	81
French Slam®, no syrup	1160	77	71
Grand Slam Slugger, no brd/pot.	925	55	74
Lumberjack Slam, no syrup	1020	58	51
Moons Over My Hammy	845	51	42
Original Grand Slam®, no bread	675	49	33
w. Syrup & Margarine	1030	60	101
Scram Slam, no bread	825	68	8
Slim Slam (no topping/sides)	440	6	56

Breakfast Skillets (No Bread)	C	F	Cb
Chicken Fajita	855	49	30
Meat Lover's Skillet	1030	74	27

Breakfast Sides	C	F	Cb
Applesauce, Musselman's	60	0	15
Bacon, 4 strips	160	18	0
Bagel, 1 only	235	1	46
Biscuit: Buttered	270	11	40
w. Sausage Gravy	400	21	45
Country Fried Potatoes, 5 oz	285	20	23
Cream Cheese, 1 oz	100	10	1
Egg: 1 only	120	10	1
Two Egg w. Hashbrowns	825	67	24
Egg Beaters® (Substitute), 2 oz	70	5	1
English Muffins, each	125	1	24
Flour Tortillas and Salsa	290	8	50
Grits, 4 oz	80	0	18
Ham, grilled slice, 3 oz	95	3	2
Hashed Browns, 4 oz	200	12	20
Covered, 6 oz	285	19	21
Covered & Smothered, 8 oz	500	25	54
Kellogg's® Dry Cereal, avg., 1 oz	100	0	23
Oatmeal Deluxe	485	6	95
Quaker® Oatmeal, 4 oz	100	2	18
Sausage, 4 links	355	32	0
Sausage Gravy, 4 oz	125	10	6
Syrup: Blueberry/Strawberry, avg.	100	0	23
Maple-flavored, 3 Tbsp	145	0	36
Sugar-free, 3 Tbsp	25	0	9
Toast, 1 slice dry	90	1	17
Toppings, average, 3 oz	105	0	26
Whipped Cream, dollop, 2 oz	25	2	2
Whipped Margarine, 1/2 oz	90	10	0

French Toast: Plain	C	F	Cb
	770	71	104

Omelette (No Extras)	C	F	Cb
Ham'n Cheddar	605	47	5
Ultimate	630	50	11
Veggie-Cheese	515	39	11

Waffles (No Extras):	C	F	Cb
Plain Belgian	605	45	28
w. Syrup & Butter	835	55	37

Buttermilk Hot Cakes: Plain (3)	675	23	47
w. Syrup & Butter	905	33	83

Steak & Eggs (No Extras)	C	F	Cb
Country Fried Steak	475	34	13
Sirloin Steak	655	45	1
T-Bone Steak	990	77	1

Soup: Per Cup	C	F	Cb
Chicken Noodle	60	2	8
Chili w. Cheese topping	400	19	21
Clam Chowder	625	42	55
Cream of Broccoli	575	43	41
Cream of Potato	220	12	21
Split Pea	145	5	18
Vegetable Beef	80	1	11

Sandwiches (No Fries/Sides)	C	F	Cb
Albacore Tuna Melt	640	39	42
BBQ Burger	965	52	72
BBQ Chicken	1095	62	86
BLT	600	38	50
Bacon Cheddar Burger	910	52	58
Boca Burger®	625	27	64
Buffalo Chicken Sandwich	720	28	80
Chicken Ranch Melt	760	45	44
Classic Burger	700	35	56
w. Cheese	855	48	57
Club Sandwich	720	38	62
Grilled Chicken	480	14	53
Ham & Swiss on Rye	430	16	39
Hoagie Chicken Melt	750	44	43
Hoagie Philly Melt	870	50	58
Mushroom Swiss Burger	900	49	63
Patty Melt	790	50	37
The Super Bird® Sandwich	620	32	48
Turkey Breast w. Multigrain	290	4	41

Denny's® cont...

Appetizers	C	F	Cb
Buffalo Chicken Strips (5)	740	42	43
Buffalo Wings (12)	855	54	1
Chicken Strips (5)	710	33	56
Mozzarella Sticks (8)	710	41	4
Onion Rings, 4 oz	380	23	38
Sampler, no condiments	1405	80	124

Entrees (No Sides)			
Chicken Strips, 10 oz	635	25	55
Country Fried Steak	645	17	14
Pot Roast Dinner w. Gravy	290	11	5
Fish & Chips	955	57	77
Fried Shrimp Dinner	230	10	18
Fried Shrimp & Scampi	350	20	15
Grilled Chicken Breast Dinner	130	4	0
Pot Roast Dinner w. Gravy	290	11	5
Roast Turkey & Stuffing w. Gravy	365	3	38
Shrimp Scampi Skillet Dinner	285	19	3
Sirloin Steak Dinner	330	28	1
Steak & Shrimp Dinner	645	42	31
T-Bone Steak Dinner	845	65	0

Sides: Bread Stuffing, plain	100	1	19
Carrots in Honey Glaze	80	3	12
Corn in Butter Sauce	125	4	19
Fries: Unsalted, 6 oz	430	20	57
Seasoned, 6 oz	270	12	35
Smothered Cheese, 9 oz	815	48	69
Gravy, all types, average	15	0.5	2
Green Beans w. Bacon	65	4	6
Potato: Baked, plain w. skin	225	0	51
Mashed	165	7	23

Salads (No Dressing/Bread Unless Indicated)			
Garden Deluxe Salad: w. Chkn Brst	230	11	10
w. Fried Chicken Strips	470	26	26
w. Albacore Tuna	450	29	12
Grilled Chkn Caesar w. Dressing	600	41	20
Side Caesar w. Dressing	360	26	20
Side Garden Salad, no Dressing	115	4	16

Dressings & Sauces: BBQ Sauce	55	1	11
Blue Cheese, 1 oz	170	18	1
Caesar; Ranch, 1 oz	135	14	1
French, regular, 1 oz	105	10	3
Honey Mustard, 1 oz	215	15	20
Italian Dressing, Low Calorie; Salsa	15	0.5	3
Marinara Sauce, 1.5 oz	50	2	7
Sour Cream, 1.5 oz	95	9	2
Tartar Sauce, 1.5 oz	220	23	3
Thousand Island, 1 oz	120	11	5

Denny's® cont...

Desserts:	C	F	Cb
Choc. Layer Cake, 3 oz	275	12	42
Hot Fudge Brownie, 7 oz	1015	42	147
Pies: Per 1/6 Whole			
Apple, 7 oz	485	24	64
Cheesecake, no topping, 4 oz	630	38	51
Chocolate Peanut Butter, 6 oz	665	39	64
Sundaes: Banana Split	930	43	121
Single Scoop, no topping	195	14	14
Double Scoop, no topping	385	27	29
Dessert Toppings: Choc., 2 oz	340	25	27
Blueberry, 2 oz	70	0	17
Fudge, 2 oz	215	10	31
Strawberry, 2 oz	80	1	17
Drinks: Cappuccino, avg., 8 oz	100	2	28
Floats, Rootbeer/Cola	290	10	47
Milkshake, Van./Choc.	580	26	76
Ruby Red Grapefruit Juice, 10 oz	165	0	41
Raspberry Iced Tea, 16 fl.oz	85	0	21
Oreo Blender Blaster, 15 oz	925	46	112

Dippin' Dots

Icecream: Average all types, 5 oz	190	9	22
Red. Fat/No Sugar Vanilla, 5 oz	120	6	17
Fat-Free/No Sugar Fudge, 5 oz	60	0	14
Nonfat Yogurt, 5 oz	110	0	23
Flavored Ice, 5 oz	50	0	13
Flavored Sherbet, 5 oz	100	1	21
Vanilla; Strawb., large, 15 fl.oz	550	10	97

Donato's® Pizza

Original Crust Pizza: Per Slice (1/8 Large)			
Chicken Vegy Medley	255	9	28
Founders Fav.; The Works, avg.	370	21	35
Hawaiian; Serious Cheese, avg.	310	15	29
Mariachi Beef/Marlachi Chkn, avg.	305	16	26
Original	330	17	29
Serious Meat	410	23	34
Vegy	280	12	30
Vegy (without Cheese)	185	6	27

Salads: Grilled Chicken, no dress.	315	18	12
Side Salad, no dressing	105	7	6

Subs: Big Don, w. Dressing	705	33	68
Big Don w. Lite Italian w. Dressing	630	25	69
Grilled Chicken Club	785	43	68
Ham & Cheese w. Dressing	610	22	70
Ham & Cheese w. Lite Dressing	535	14	70
Vegy w. Lite Dressing	660	28	78

Domino's®Pizza

	C	F	Cb
Buffalo Chicken Kickers™:			
1 average piece, 24g	47	2	3
1 order, 10 pieces, 240g	470	21	32
Hot Sauce, 1.5 oz Cup	15	0	4
Blue Cheese; Ranch, 1.5 oz	220	23	2

Classic Hand Tossed Pizza

Medium (12") Pizza: *Per 2 Slices (¹/₄ Pizza)*

	C	F	Cb
Cheese Pizza (base only)	375	11	55
America's Favorite Feast	510	22	57
Bacon Cheeseburger Feast	550	26	55
Barbeque Feast	505	20	62
Deluxe Feast	465	18	57
Hawaiian Feast	450	15	58
MeatZZa Feast	560	26	57
Pepperoni Feast	535	25	56
Vegi Feast	440	16	57

Large (14") Pizza: *Per 2 Slices (¹/₄ Pizza)*

	C	F	Cb
Cheese Pizza (base only)	520	15	75
America's Favorite Feast	710	30	78
Bacon Cheeseburger Feast	770	36	75
Barbeque Feast	700	27	85
Deluxe Feast	640	24	78
ExtravaganZZa Feast	780	36	80
Hawaiian Feast	630	22	80
MeatZZa Feast	760	34	78
Pepperoni Feast	740	34	76
Vegi Feast	620	22	78

Thin Crust Pizza

Medium (12") Pizza: *Per 2 Slices (¹/₄ Pizza)*

	C	F	Cb
Cheese Pizza (base only)	275	12	31
With Topping: Bacon	375	20	31
Beef	350	19	31
Cheddar Cheese	330	17	31
Pepperoni	350	19	31
X-tra Cheese & Pepperoni	400	23	32
Ham	300	13	31
Italian Sausage & Mushroom	360	18	34
Vegi (olive/mushr./onion/peppers)	340	17	34

	C	F	Cb
Large (14") Pizza: *Per 2 Slices (¹/₄ Pizza)*			
Cheese Pizza (base only)	380	17	43
With Topping: Bacon	530	30	43
Beef	490	27	44
Cheddar Cheese	450	23	44
Pepperoni	480	25	44
X-tra Cheese & Pepperoni	550	30	45
Ham	415	18	44
Italian Sausage & Mushroom	500	25	48
Vegi (olive/mushr./onion/peppers)	470	23	47

Ultimate Deep Dish Pizza

Medium (12') Pizza: *Per 2 Slices (¹/₄ Pizza)*

	C	F	Cb
Cheese Pizza (base only)	480	22	56
With Topping: Bacon	580	30	56
Beef	560	29	56
Cheddar Cheese	540	27	56
Pepperoni	555	29	56
Ham	505	23	56
Italian Sausage & Mushroom	565	28	59
Vegi	550	27	58

Large (14") Pizza: *Per 2 Slices (¹/₄ Pizza)*

	C	F	Cb
Cheese Pizza (base only)	675	30	80
With Topping: Bacon	830	43	80
Beef	785	40	80
Cheddar Cheese	745	36	80
Pepperoni	775	39	80
X-tra Cheese & Pepperoni	845	44	82
Ham	705	31	80
Italian Sausage & Mushroom	795	39	85
Vegi	765	36	83

Sides: Dots™, 1 oz	100	4	15
Breadstick, 1 stick, 37g	120	4	18
Cheesy Bread, 1 stick, 43g	145	6	18
Barbeque Wings, 1 piece	50	2.5	2
Hot Wings, 1 piece	45	2	0.5
CinnaStix®, 1 stick	110	5	15
Sweet Icing, 2¹/₂ oz cup	280	5	60

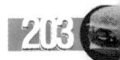

Fast-Foods & *Restaurants*

Don Pablos®

Appetizers: Per Serving	C	F	Cb
Beef Taquito (1), no garnish	125	6	10
Buffalo Chicken Wings	1035	77	43
Chicken Flauta (1), no garnish	130	8	11
Nachos: Acapulco	1625	113	85
Beef Fajita	1465	99	71
Chicken Fajita	1405	87	83
Pizza, avg. all types, 1 slice	160	9	10

Quesadillas: Incl. Sour Cream & Guacamole			
Mesquite Grilled Chicken	1320	65	110
Mesquite Grilled Steak	1550	91	122
Portabello Mushroom & Vege	1525	83	136
Combo Gr. Chicken & Steak	1435	78	116
Combo Cheese & Vegetable	1440	81	120

Dips: Per Cup (No Chips)			
Queso Blanco	345	27	13
Prairie Fire Bean w. Cheese	385	25	23
Spinach & Artichoke	340	29	14

Burritos (No Sides): Chkn w. Rice	875	35	133
Beef & Bean w. Rice	1415	73	123

Chimichangas: Includes Rice & Refritos			
Spicy Beef	1205	63	109
Pollo Chimi	1085	49	117

Combinaciones: Includes Everything on Plate			
El Matador	1890	87	179
Conquistador (no rice)	1110	51	100
Primo Combo Chicken	1035	54	93
Primo Combo Steak & Chicken	1085	62	90

Salads (No Dress.): Steak Fajita	1290	88	80
Chicken Fajita	1055	62	68
Traditional Taco Salad	1430	85	104

Salad Dressing: Per 3 oz			
Blue Cheese	455	48	2.5
House Vinaigrette	360	31	14
Honey Mustard	300	26	17
Low Fat French	290	3.5	30
Ranch	330	34	3.5

Sides: Chips & Salsa	345	17	43
Guacamole, 1.2 oz	60	5	2.5
Mexican Rice, 3 oz	100	1.5	20
Refritos, 5 oz	160	4	23
Salsa, 1 oz	5	0	1
Side Salad	110	6.5	8
Sour Cream, 1.25 oz	80	7.5	1.5
Sour Crema, 1 oz	60	5.5	1
Tortilla Shell	475	27	50

Dunkin Donuts®

Donuts: Each	C	F	Cb
Apple/Blueberry Crumb Donut	230	10	34
Apple N' Spice Donut	200	8	29
Black Raspberry/Strawberry Donut	210	8	32
Blueberry Cake Donut	290	16	35
Boston Kreme Donut	240	9	36
Butternut Cake Donut	300	16	36
Chocolate Coconut Cake Donut	300	19	31
Chocolate Frosted Cake Donut	360	20	40
Chocolate Frosted Donut	200	9	29
Chocolate Glazed Cake Donut	290	16	33
Cinnamon Cake Donut	330	20	34
Coconut Cake Donut	290	17	33
Double Chocolate Cake Donut	310	17	37
Dunkin' Donut	240	15	25
Glazed Donut	350	19	41
Jelly Filled Donut	210	8	32
Jelly Stick Donut	290	12	44
Kreme Filled (Choc./Vanilla)Donut	270	13	35
Lemon Donut	240	14	28
Maple/Marble Frosted Donut	210	9	29
Old Fashioned Cake Donut	300	19	28
Powdered Cake Donut	330	19	36
Strawb./Van. Frosted; Bavarian	210	9	32
Sugared Donut	250	15	27
Toasted Coconut Cake Donut	300	17	35
Whole Wheat Glazed Cake Donut	310	19	32

Muffins			
Apple Danish, 3 oz	250	10	36
Banana Nut	540	23	73
Blueberry: Regular	490	17	76
Reduced Fat	450	13	74
Cheese Danish, 3 oz	270	14	32
Chocolate Chip	585	23	85
Coffee Cake Muffin, 6.5 oz	710	29	102
Corn	515	17	81
Cranberry Orange	460	16	71
Honey Raisin Bran	490	14	81
Raspberry White Chocolate, 4 oz	450	22	59
Strawberry Cheese Danish, 3 oz	250	12	33

Crullers: Glazed Cruller	290	15	37
Glazed Chocolate Cruller	280	15	35
Plain Cruller	240	15	25
Powdered Sugar Cruller	270	15	30
French Cruller	150	8	17

204

Restaurants & Fast−Foods

Dunkin Donuts® cont...

C F Cb

Sandwiches: Per Sandwich

Biscuit Sandwiches:

	C	F	Cb
Egg/Cheese Sandwich	360	20	31
Sausage/Egg/Cheese Sandwich	560	13	31
Croissant: Plain, USA, each	330	18	37
Pizza; Spanish Cheese	520	35	33
Eng. Muffin S'wich:Ham/Egg/Chse	310	10	35

Bagels: Biscuit Bagel

Everything	430	7	75
Onion	375	4	71
Sesame	455	11	71
Salt; Plain	360	3	69
Cream Cheese (Per Packet): Lite	130	11	3
Average of other flavors	180	17	3

Cake Munchkins

Plain (4)	270	16	27
Cinnamon; Powdered, (4)	250	14	29
Coconut; Coconut Toasted (3)	200	12	23
Sugared (4)	240	14	28

Yeast Munchkins: Per Serving

Glazed; Jelly Filled (5)	210	9	28
Lemon Filled (4)	170	8	23
Sugar Raised (7)	220	12	26

Cake Sticks: Per Stick

Cinnamon	455	30	42
Glazed/Chocolate	475	29	50
Jelly	260	29	61
Plain	420	29	35
Powdered	450	29	42

Scones: Blueberry, 3 oz

Scones: Blueberry, 3 oz	410	19	55
Cinnamon Apple	460	19	67
Maple Walnut	470	22	62
Strawberry Cheese Danish	250	12	33

Cookies

Chocolate varieties, average (1)	220	11	27
Oatmeal Raisin Pecan	220	10	29

Drinks: Dunkacinno, 10 fl.oz

Drinks: Dunkacinno, 10 fl.oz	240	10	35
Hot Chocolate, 10 fl.oz	230	8	38
Iced Coffee, 16 fl.oz	5	0	1
w. Cream, 16 fl.oz	50	6	1
w. Milk, 16 fl.oz	15	0	3
Vanilla Chai, 10 fl.oz	235	8	40

Coolatta®: Per 16 fl.oz

Coffee Coolatta®: w. Cream	370	22	40
w. Milk	220	4	42
w. 2% Milk	200	2	41
Orange Mango Fruit Coolatta®	270	0	66
Strawberry Fruit Coolatta®	290	0	72
Vanilla Bean Coolatta®	440	17	70

Eat 'N Park®

C F Cb

Breakfast

	C	F	Cb
Cornbeef Hash, 7.5 oz	340	23	17
Egg Beaters® Breakfast	75	0	5
Eggs Benedict	600	31	35
Fruit Cup	60	0.5	15
Hash Browns, 6 oz	235	12	28
Homefries, 6 oz	210	12	24
Omelette: Bacon & Cheese	500	39	2
Cheese	390	30	2
Ham & Cheese	465	33	3
Supreme	420	30	9
Western	345	21	7
Pancake, Plain (1)	225	3	43
Apple Waffles	960	45	125

Burgers: American Grill

Burgers: American Grill	785	51	37
Amer./Swiss/Provolone Gourmet	775	47	36
Bacon & Cheese	615	36	33
Cheeseburger	540	30	33
Gardenburger	355	6.5	60
Hamburger	495	26	32
Southwest	680	37	57
Super	705	49	38
Swiss	580	32	34
Turkey	500	22	38

Sandwiches: BLT

Sandwiches: BLT	290	15	27
Bacon Turkey Swiss	525	38	16
Chicken Bacon Deluxe	565	23	50
Chicken (Breaded)	515	20	50
Chicken Chargrill/Spicy, 4 oz	330	6	35
Chicken Fiesta, 4 oz	325	12	21
Cod (Breaded)	670	25	67
Croissants: Chicken Salad; Tuna	595	39	36
Dutch Ham & Swiss	570	31	36
Grilled Cheese	505	36	26
Hot Roast Beef	280	5.5	25
Turkey	390	19	31
Pita: Chicken Fajita	620	19	69
Tuna	640	26	72
Turkey	445	5	68
Reuben	720	49	31
Shredded Pot Roast	530	31	28
Steak'n Cheese	765	51	43
Tuna Melt	610	41	35
Turkey Club	775	47	50
Turkey Pastrami	715	46	40
Whitefish (Breaded)	790	36	69

205

Fast-Foods & *Restaurants*

Eat 'N Park® cont...

	C	F	Cb
Appetizers: Cheese Fries	880	50	93
Cheese Sticks	410	25	17
Onion Rings	210	13	20
Wings	400	28	0.5
Dinners: Chicken Breast, stuffed	370	17	28
Chicken Fillets, 5 oz	530	26	28
Chicken Milano	215	10	4
Chicken Naturelle, 4 oz	140	3.5	0
Chicken Parmigiana: Marinara	840	33	90
Meat	900	38	86
Chicken Stir-Fry	555	25	48
Chicken'n Biscuits	495	20	30
Chicken, 3 piece	1195	70	57
Cod (Breaded)	925	46	57
Floridian Scrod	120	1.5	4
Spaghetti Marinara	620	8	20
Veal Parmigiana w. Meat Sauce	820	27	108
Whitefish (Breaded)	790	36	69
Ziti w. Meat Balls & Meat Sauce	960	42	102
Salads & Dressings: Chef Salad	460	28	10
Chicken Salad	440	19	30
Chicken Caesar Salad	270	9	16
Chicken Portabella Salad	345	12	23
Fruit w. Sherbet	310	3	74
Garden Salad	100	3	17
Steak Salad	615	39	30
Taco Salad	385	20	36
Dressings: Bleu Cheese	90	7	7
French Fat Free	70	0	17
Fruit Salad	150	14	6
Italian Fat Free	10	0	3
Light Burgundy Vinaigrette	35	1.5	6
Thousand Island	95	9	3
Desserts: Cheesecake	505	36	40
Banana Fudge Sensation	975	44	48
Grilled Sticky Loaf	485	28	53
Icecream, 2 scoops	285	16	36
Pies: Apple Reduced Fat	340	11	62
Peach Lite	300	10	50
Pudding (Sugar Free)	90	2.5	13
Strawberry Shortcake	685	26	113

For Complete Nutritional Data ~ see CalorieKing.com

Einstein Bros®

	C	F	Cb
Bagels			
Average all types, 4 oz	330	1	70
Chocolate Chip Bagel, 4 oz	370	3	76
Egg Bagel, 3$\frac{1}{2}$ oz	340	3	69
Sesame Dip	380	5	75
Cream Cheese: Plain, 2 Tbsp	70	7	1
Plain Lite, 2 Tbsp	60	5	2
Smoked Salmon, 2 Tbsp	60	5	2
Flavors, average, 2 Tbsp	70	5	5
Spreads: Fruit, 2 Tbsp	75	0	19
Honey Butter, 1 Tbsp	90	8	4
Peanut Butter, 2 Tbsp	190	15	8
Sandwiches: BBQ Chicken	550	11	83
Baguette, Our Big Hero	920	39	98
Chicago Bagel Dog Asiago	740	34	78
Classic NY Lox & Bagel	660	27	79
Egg Santa Fe	650	24	78
Ham Deli	450	6	74
Holey Cow	900	50	77
Mediterranean Hummus	540	13	89
Roast Beef Deli	460	4	76
Roast Chicken & Smoked Gouda	520	11	68
Smoked Turkey Deli	420	1.5	75
The Veg-Out	490	13	77
Tuna Salad Deli	500	7	77
Turkey Pastrami Deli	440	2	76
Turkey Pastrami Reuben Deli	660	19	83
Bagel Shtick: Asiago	450	9	72
Cinnamon Sugar	570	24	79
Everything; Potato	380	4.5	73
Sesame Bagel Shtick	420	8	75
Bagel Chips: Plain, 1 oz serving	90	3	15
Flavors, average, 1 oz	90	3	15
Roll-Ups: Albuquerque Turkey	790	39	81
Baja Shaved Beef	720	36	67
Pacific Smoked Salmon	590	31	55
Cookies: Big Brownie	500	21	76
Chocolate Chunk, 4 oz	600	28	78
Oatmeal Raisin, 4 oz	550	21	82
Muffins: Banana Nut	520	29	59
Blueberry	460	24	57
Chocolate Chip	240	13	67
Lowfat Lemon Poppyseed	370	7	69
Mocha Chocolate Chip	550	29	66
97% Fat Free Apple Cinnamon	560	2	77
Scones: All types, 5 oz	490	17	75
Coffee: Cafe Latte, regular	140	5	13
Cappuccino	90	3.5	9

Restaurants & Fast—Foods

El Pollo Loco®

Flame-Broiled Chicken	**C**	**F**	**Cb**
Breast	160	6	0
Leg	90	5	0
Thigh	180	12	0
Wing	110	6	0
Tortillas: 6" Corn	70	1	14
6.5" Flour	110	4	13
Burritos: Bean, Rice & Cheese	505	16	73
Chicken Lover's	475	19	47
Classic	580	22	66
Mexican Chicken Caesar	735	35	65
Spicy	635	21	80
Tacos: Chicken Soft Taco	235	12	15
Taco Al Carbon	180	8	20
Bowls: Flame Broiled Chkn Salad	355	13	39
Mexican Chicken Caesar Salad	495	30	32
Nacho Pollo Bowl	765	33	64
Pollo Bowl	470	11	66
Smokey Black Bean Pollo Bowl	605	23	75
Specialties: Chicken Nachos	1420	91	105
Chicken Quesadilla	595	29	48
Chicken Sticks (Kids), 4 oz	225	12	15
Chicken Tamale	180	8	21
Chicken Tostada Salad	990	52	91
Side Dishes: Cole Slaw	205	16	12
Corn Cobbette (3")	80	1	18
French Fries	445	19	61
Garden Salad	105	7	7
Pinto Beans	185	4	29
Spanish Rice	130	3	24
Pollo Salads: Chicken Fiesta	755	58	28
Chicken Fiesta, no Dressing	450	26	25
Chicken Caesar: w. Dressing	565	45	18
no Dressing	250	11	16
Condiments: Guacamole	30	2	3
House/Spicy Chipotle Salsa	6	0	2
Jalapeno Hot Sauce, 1 pkt	5	0	1
Sour Cream	60	5	1
Pico de Gallo Salsa	10	0.5	1.5
Desserts: Banana Split	715	28	107
Churros	180	11	18
Foster's Freeze without cone	180	5	30
Smoothies, all types	365	7	68

For Complete Nutritional Data ~ see CalorieKing.com

Fatburger®

Burgers: Baby Fat	**C**	**F**	**Cb**
Burgers: Baby Fat	295	13	25
Bacon & Egg Sandwich	440	27	31
Chicken Sandwich	400	15	32
Chili Dog	510	26	45
Fatburger	600	34	39
Fatburger w. Cheese	625	36	38
Kingburger	825	46	56
Kingburger w. Cheese	1020	58	65
Turkey Burger	590	33	41
Shakes (21 fl.oz):			
Chocolate Shake	920	43	115
Strawberry Shake	850	41	103
Vanilla Shake	810	44	85
Fries & Sides: Chili Cup, 7 oz	345	23	14
Fat Fries, 7.6 oz	540	26	70
Skinny Fries, 5 oz	515	26	65
Onion Rings, 6.1 oz	235	23	0.5

For Complete Nutritional Data ~ see CalorieKing.com

Fazoli's® Italian Food

Soup & Bread Stick	**C**	**F**	**Cb**
Minestrone Soup	120	1	23
Breadstick (1)	90	1	17
Salads (No Dressing Unless Indicated)			
Chicken & Pasta Caesar Salad	370	13	33
Chicken Finger Salad	190	9	8
w. Bacon Honey Mustard Dress.	400	28	17
Chicken Caesar Salad	420	29	17
Garden Salad	30	0	6
Italian Chef Salad	260	21	13
Pasta Salad	590	25	70
Side Pasta Salad	240	10	29
Dressings: Honey French, 1 oz	150	12	9
House Italian, 1 oz	110	9	5
Reduced Calorie Italian, 1 oz	50	5	3
Ranch, 1 oz	150	17	1
Thousand Island, 1 oz	130	13	4
Submarinos: Per 1/2 Sandwich			
Club	1100	44	121
Ham & Swiss	1000	37	120
Meatball	1260	59	128
Original	1160	55	124
Pepperoni Pizza	1060	40	133
Turkey	990	34	121

Fast–Foods & *Restaurants*

Fazoli's® cont...

	C	**F**	**Cb**
Paninis: Chicken Caesar Club	660	35	51
Chicken Pesto	510	20	51
Four Cheese & Tomato	720	43	55
Ham & Swiss	600	30	53
Italian Deli	660	35	61
Italian Club	670	37	54
Smoked Turkey	710	38	57
Pasta: Per Serving			
Fettucine Alfredo: Small	530	15	80
Regular	800	22	119
Peppery Chicken Alfredo	610	16	80
Small Spaghetti: w. Marinara	420	6	74
w. Meat Sauce	450	8	74
w. Meatballs	720	31	80
Regular Spaghetti: w. Marinara	620	8	111
w. Meat Sauce	670	11	111
w. Meatballs	1020	42	119
Pizza (Per Double Slice):			
Cheese	460	15	58
Combination	570	25	63
Pepperoni	530	22	61
Italian Specialties: Per Serving			
Baked Chicken Alfredo	790	29	82
Baked Chicken Parmesan	740	20	99
Baked Spaghetti Parmesan	700	25	76
Baked Ziti: Small	490	17	56
Regular	750	26	87
Broccoli Fettucine Alfredo: Small	560	15	85
Regular	830	23	125
Cheese Ravioli: w. Marinara	480	15	65
w. Meat Sauce	510	17	65
Classic Sampler	830	22	90
Lasagna: Homestyle	680	23	27
Broccoli	750	27	34
Pizza Baked Spaghetti	750	31	78
Shrimp & Scallop Fettucine	610	16	81
Desserts: Lemon Ice	190	0	45
Cheesecake: Plain	290	22	17
Turtle	420	34	24
Chocolate Chip	300	22	22
Lemon Ice	190	0	45
Milk Chocolate Chunk Cookie	360	15	54
Strawberry Topping, 1 oz	35	0	8

Frisch's Big Boy®
~ Same Menu & Data as Big Boy

Freshens®

	C	**F**	**Cb**
Yogurt Smoothies: Per 21 oz			
Blueberry Sunset	385	0.5	84
Jamaican Jammer	475	1	110
Peachy Pineapple	405	1	91
Pina Collider	560	4	126
Raspberry Rapture	515	1	121
Raspberry Rocker	490	1	113
Strawberry Squeeze	390	0.5	88
Tropical Fruit Juice Smoothies: Per 21 oz			
Blueberry Wave; Caribbean Craze	330	0.5	84
Peach Sunset; Raspberry Rumba	365	0.5	93
Pineapple Passion	420	4	100
Raspberry Rhapsody	345	0.5	88
Strawberry Shooter	245	0	63
Orange Smoothies: Per 21 oz			
Aruba Orange; Orange Wave	420	3.5	97
Orange Shooter	370	3	81
Orange Sunrise	415	3	90
Coffee Smoothies: Per 21 oz			
Original Coffee	340	3.5	70
Caramel Coffee	425	4	89
Mocha Coffee	375	3.5	79
Oreo® Coffee	520	11	96
Decadent Smoothies: Per 21 oz			
Fudge Oreo® Supreme	640	11	126
Peanut Butter Cup	930	34	141
Pretzel Logic Pretzels (1/2), 3 oz	255	3	49
Freshen® Farms Icecream, 1/2 c.	150	6	21
MET-Rx® Performance Supplements			
Protein Booster, 1 scoop, 10g	35	0	0
Soy Booster, 1 scoop, 16g	60	0.5	5
Avg. other varieties, 1 sachet	5	0	1

Golden Corral®

Chicken: Grilled	170	5	0
Fried	370	19	14
Shrimp, fried	250	12	24
Steak: Ribeye, 6 oz	450	35	0
Sirloin, 5 oz	230	14	0
Chopped, 4 oz	320	23	0
Tips w. Onions	290	13	8
Sides: Baked Potato	225	2	46
Texas Toast	170	6	26

208

Godfather's™ Pizza

Original Crust: *Per Slice* | **C** | **F** | **Cb**

	C	F	Cb
Cheese Pizza: Mini, 1/4 pizza	130	3	19
Medium, 1/8 pizza	230	5	34
Large, 1/10 pizza	260	6	36
Jumbo, 1/10 pizza	380	9	53
Combo Pizza: Mini, 1/4 pizza	175	7	21
Medium, 1/8 pizza	305	11	36
Large, 1/10 pizza	340	12	38
Jumbo, 1/10 pizza	505	18	56

Golden Crust:

	C	F	Cb
Cheese Pizza: Medium, 1/8 pizza	210	10	26
Large, 1/10 pizza	240	9	28
Combo Pizza: Medium, 1/8 pizza	270	12	28
Large, 1/10 pizza	305	14	31

(The) Great American Bagel Co®

Bagels: 4-Grain Honey; Cinn. Rais.

	C	F	Cb
4-Grain Honey; Cinn. Rais.	420	1.5	88
Apple/Blueberry Crumb, average	570	8	106
Banana Nut; Cheddar Herb, aver.	410	5	82
Blueberry; Onion; Strawberry	380	1	83
Cheddar Salsa	430	11	63
Cheese Twist	740	20	107
Chocolate Chip	390	4	75
Cinnamon Sugar; Egg	390	2	83
Cranb. Nut; P'nut Butter Choc Chip	400	6	72
Hot Tomazzo; Tomazzo	360	7	57
Jalapeno Cheddar	330	4.5	58
Plain	390	1.5	85
Pumpernickel; Pumpkin, average	330	1.5	72
Pumpkin Chocolate Chip	350	3.5	67
Spinach Herb	300	1	60
Stuffed Pepperoni	500	12	74
Stuffed Spinach	720	22	98
Sun-Dried Tomato Basil	390	1.5	77
Veggie; Whole Wheat; Salt	340	1	70
Other varieties, average	370	2	75

Gretel's Pretzels®

Pretzels

	C	F	Cb
Cinnamon/Sugar	195	3	38
Original	170	3	31
Poppy Seed	175	3.5	31
Raisin Danish/Icing	350	2	79
Sesame Seed	175	3.5	31
Sweet Dough	115	0.5	23

Haagen-Dazs®

Icecream: *Per 1/2 Cup*

	C	F	Cb
Baileys Irish Crm; Cookies & Crm	270	17	23
Bananas Foster	260	15	28
Belgian Chocolate; Pecan Pie	330	21	29
Butter Pecan	310	23	21
Cafe Mocha Frappe	310	19	30
Cherry Vanilla; Strawberry	240	15	23
Chocolate; Coffee	270	18	22
Chocolate Brownie w. Walnuts	290	19	25
Chocolate Chsecake; Rocky Road	300	18	29
Chocolate Chocolate Chip	300	20	26
Chocolate Cookies & Cream	270	17	24
Chocolate/Fr. Vanilla Mousse	310	19	30
Chocolate Peanut Butter	360	24	27
Chocolate Raspberry Torte	270	15	29
Coffee Almond Swirl	320	21	27
Cookie Dough Chip; Van. Cherry	310	20	29
Creme Brulee	280	19	23
Cr. Caramel Pecan; Choc. Caramel	320	20	29
Dulce De Leche; German Choc.	290	17	28
Macadamia Brittle; Mint Chip	300	20	25
Mango	250	14	28
Mocha Almond Fudge	340	23	28
Peanut Butter Fudge Chunk	340	23	25
Pineapple Coconut	230	13	25
Pistachio	290	20	22
Rum Raisin; Vanilla	270	17	22
Strawberry Cheesecake	270	16	28
Tres Leche; Vanilla Fudge	290	19	25
Vanilla Caramel Brownie	300	18	30
Vanilla Chocolate Chip	310	20	26
Vanilla Fudge/Brownie; Pralines	300	18	28
Vanilla Swiss Almond	300	20	24
Sorbet: Orchard Peach	130	0	33
Average other flavors	120	0	30
Gelato: Cappuccino; Raspberry	240	7	40
Chocolate	240	8	37
Hazelnut	260	12	33
Frozen Yogurt: *Per 1/2 Cup*			
Apple Pie; Strawberry Chsecake	220	6	35
Banana Cream Pie	220	6	34
Choc. Fudge Brownie	190	2.5	34
Coffee; Vanilla	200	4.5	31
Dulce De Leche	190	2.5	35
Lemon Pie	260	7	41
Peach Melba	210	3.5	37
Pumpkin Cheesecake	240	8	35
Strawberry Non Fat	140	0	31
Vanilla Raspberry Swirl	170	2.5	31

Icecream Bars ~ See Page 37

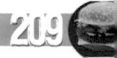

Hardees®

Breakfast Items	C	F	Cb
Hash Rounds™, regular	230	14	24
Biscuits: Bacon, Egg & Cheese	520	30	45
Apple Cinnamon 'N' Raisin™	250	8	42
Biscuit 'N' Gravy™	530	30	56
Chicken Biscuit	590	27	62
Cinnamon 'N' Raisin™	370	18	48
Country Ham	440	22	44
Frisco™ Breakfast S'wich (Ham)	450	22	42
Ham	410	20	45
Jelly Biscuit	440	21	57
Made From Scratch® Biscuit	390	21	44
Omelet™	550	32	45
Pork Chop	530	22	56
Sausage	550	36	44
Sausage & Egg	620	40	45
Steak	580	32	56
Sunrise Croissant: Bacon	410	25	28
Ham	410	23	31
Sausage	560	40	28
Hamburgers: All Star	660	43	42
Bacon Swiss Crispy Chicken	670	44	45
Cheeseburger	320	15	30
Double Cheeseburger	480	28	31
Famous Star	570	35	42
Frisco™ Burger	740	51	38
Hamburger	270	10	29
Monster Burger®	990	72	37
Monster Roast Beef	610	39	26
Mushroom 'N' Swiss™	500	26	39
Six Dollar Burger	950	62	58
Super Star	790	53	42
1/3 lb Bacon Cheeseburger	615	34	41
Sandwiches: Big Roast Beef™	410	24	26
Chicken Fillet Sandwich	430	18	42
Fisherman's Fillet™	520	28	47
Grilled Chicken Sandwich	350	16	28
Ham 'N' Cheese Supreme	490	27	45
Hot Dog w. Condiments	450	32	25
Hot Ham 'N' Cheese	300	12	34
Roast Beef Sandwich	310	16	26
Roast Beef Supreme	500	31	38
Turkey Supreme	480	25	40
Fried Chicken: Breast, each	370	15	30
Wing, each	200	8	23
Thigh, each	330	15	30
Leg, each	170	7	15

Hardees® cont...

French Fries: Regular	C	F	Cb
Large	440	21	60
Monster	510	24	67
Sides: Coleslaw, small	240	20	13
Chicken Strips: 3 pieces	120	5	8
5 pieces	200	8	13
Crispy Curls: Regular	340	18	41
Large	520	28	62
Monster	590	31	70
Gravy, 1.5 oz	20	0.5	3
Honey Mustard, 1 oz	50	0	12
Mashed Potatoes & Gravy, small	90	0.5	17
Desserts: Apple Turnover	270	12	38
Chocolate Chip Cookie	370	19	61
Peach Cobbler, small	310	7	60
Orange Juice, 10 oz	140	0	34

Harvey's®

Main Menu	C	F	Cb
Original Hamburger	355	18	32
Original Cheeseburger	405	21	32
Ultra Burger	410	19	33
w. Cheese	455	22	34
Ultra Patty by itself	240	17	0
Value Burger	300	13	30
w. Cheese	350	16	31
Hot Dog	315	12	39
Fish Sandwich	350	10	49
Harvey's Grilled Chicken	300	5	35
Harvey's Crispy Chicken	380	10	48
Chicken Fajita	450	16	54
Chicken Nuggets	170	9	11
Veggie Burger, 3.2 oz	330	9	41
Crispy Fries: Junior, 3.2 oz	290	15	34
Regular, 4.2 oz	380	20	46
Large, 5.3 oz	475	25	57
Onion Rings: Regular, 2.8 oz	285	20	23
Large	430	30	34
Side Orders			
Poutine, 10 oz	700	40	67
Gravy, 3 oz	45	0.5	9
Garden Salad	120	6	11
Caesar Salad	55	1.5	5
Chicken Caesar Salad	145	4.5	6
Chicken Garden Salad	210	8	12
Soup: Harvest Vegetable, 1 cup	120	1.5	25
Cream of Broccoli/Mushr., 1 cup	170	7	25
Chicken Noodle, 1 cup	100	1.5	17

Harvey's® cont...

	C	F	Cb
Breakfast: Bagel	295	2	55
Breakfast Club Sandwich	310	15	26
Eggs (2): Fried	175	13	1
Scrambled Eggs	165	11	2
Hashbrowns	130	7	15
Home Fries	270	11	38
Muffins: Blueberry	375	19	62
Bran Muffin	435	17	57
Pancakes (2)	225	3	42
Pancake Syrup	165	0	42
Sausage	135	11	3
Toasted Western Sandwich	370	15	52
Dressings: Light Caesar/Italian	35	2.5	3
Average, other flavors	70	7	1
Desserts			
Apple Turnover, 3 oz	245	15	25
Shakes: Choc.; Vanilla, 14.5 fl.oz	370	10	59
Strawberry, 14.5 fl.oz	355	9	56

Hot Dog on a Stick®

Menu Items			
Hot Dog on a Bun	470	26	41
Hot Dog on a Stick	250	14	23
Veggie Dog	180	3	24
American Cheese on a Stick	240	13	22
Pepper Jack Cheese on a Stick	240	13	21
French Fries, 7 oz	550	7	113
Lemonade (12 fl.oz): Original	140	0	24
Cherry/Lime	170	0	42
Sugar Free Lemonade	10	0	2

I Can't Believe It's Yogurt®

Original Frozen Yogurt: Regular Serving (9 fl.oz)			
Awesome Amaretto	280	6	51
Cookies 'N Cream	260	3	54
French Vanilla	260	6	47
Peanut Butter Bliss	310	12	46
White Chocolate Mousse	280	7	49
Nonfat Frozen Yogurt: Regular	220	0.5	48
Small, 6.2 fl.oz	160	0.5	32
Nonfat (with NutraSweet): Reg.	190	0.5	40
Small, 6.2 fl.oz	140	0.5	29

In-N-Out Burger®

Burgers	C	F	Cb
Hamburger w. Onion	390	19	39
w. Mustard/Ketchup, no Spread	310	10	41
Protein Style, no Bun	240	17	11
Cheeseburger w. Onion	480	27	39
w. Mustard/Ketchup, no Spread	400	18	41
Protein Style, no Bun	330	25	11
Double Double® (2 patty/2 sl. chse)	670	41	40
w. Mustard/Ketchup, no Spread	590	32	42
Protein Style, no Bun	520	39	11
French Fries, 125g	400	18	54
Drinks: Milk, 10 fl.oz	180	6	18
Coca-Cola®; Dr. Pepper, 16 fl.oz	200	0	54
Diet Coca-Cola®, 16 fl.oz	0	0	0
Lemonade, 16 fl.oz	180	0	40
Root Beer, 16 fl.oz	220	0	60
Seven-Up®, 16 fl.oz	220	0	54
Shakes: Chocolate, 15 fl.oz	690	36	83
Strawberry, 15 fl.oz	690	33	91
Vanilla, 15 fl.oz	680	37	78

For Complete Nutritional Data ~ see CalorieKing.com

International House of Pancakes®

Pancakes: (Syrup/Butter extra)	C	F	Cb
Buttermilk, 1 (1.7 oz)	110	3	17
Short Stack, 3	330	9	51
Full Stack, 5	550	15	85
Buckwheat, 1 (1.7 oz)	110	4	15
Country Griddle, 1 (2 oz)	120	3.5	19
Harvest Grain 'N Nut, 1 (2¹/4 oz)	180	9	20
Crepes (Egg Pancakes), 1 (2 oz)	120	6	14
Syrup: 1 Tbsp	50	0	12
Whipped Butter, 1 Tbsp	80	9	0
Waffles (Plain)			
Regular, 1 (3 oz)	310	15	37
Belgian: Regular, 1 (4 oz)	390	19	48

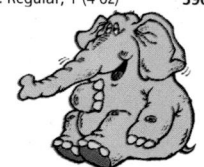

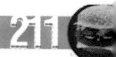

Fast–Foods & *Restaurants*

Jack in the Box®

Breakfast	C	F	Cb
Biscuit	190	9	24
Breakfast Jack®	310	14	33
Extreme Sausage Sandwich	720	53	35
French Toast Sticks, 4 pces	430	18	57
Hash Brown	150	10	13
Sausage Biscuit	380	27	25
Sausage Croissant	680	50	41
Sausage, Egg & Cheese Biscuit	760	60	33
Sourdough Breakfast Sandwich	450	26	36
Supreme Croissant	570	37	41
Ultimate Breakfast Sandwich	730	40	66
Country Crock Spread	25	3	0
Grape Jelly, 1 packet	35	0	10
Syrup	130	0	32

Burgers			
Hamburger	310	14	30
Hamburger w. Cheese	360	18	31
Bacon Bacon Cheeseburger	910	59	58
Bacon Ultimate Cheeseburger	1120	75	59
Big Cheeseburger	700	40	59
Big Texas Cheeseburger	610	32	55
Ultimate Cheeseburger	990	66	59
Jumbo Jack®: Regular	600	31	58
w. Cheese	690	38	61
Philly Cheesesteak	580	22	55
Sourdough Jack®	700	49	36
Turkey Jack	700	32	69
Teriyaki Bowls: Chicken	550	3	103
Mexican Food: Monster Taco	260	15	21
Taco	170	9	15
Snacks: Onion Rings	500	30	51
Bacon Cheddar Potato Wedges	770	53	52
Cheese Sticks, 3 piece	240	12	21
Chicken Breast Pieces, 5 piece	360	17	24
Curly Fries: Chili Cheese, 8.3 oz	630	40	54
Seasoned, 4.4 oz	400	23	45
French Fries: Small	330	16	44
Medium	410	20	55
Large	580	28	77
Egg Rolls, 1 piece, 2 oz	130	6	15
Fish & Chips	610	31	66
Stuffed Jalapenos, 3 piece	230	13	22
Taquitos: 3 piece	320	17	28
5 piece	480	24	47

Sandwiches	C	F	Cb
Chicken Chipotle	380	18	29
Chicken Fajita Pita	330	11	35
Chicken Sandwich	410	21	39
Chicken Supreme	710	39	62
Grilled Chicken Fillet	430	22	34
Jack's Spicy Chicken®	730	31	69
Sourdough Grilled Chicken Club	520	28	33

Salads: No Dressing			
Asian Chicken Salad, 16 oz	145	1.5	18
Chicken Club, 17 oz	305	16	12
Side Salad	50	3	5
Southwest Chicken, 19 oz	340	13	28

Salad Dressing: Asian Sesame	230	17	20
Bacon Ranch	320	33	5
Creamy Southwest	270	26	7
Low Fat Balsamic Viniagrette	40	2	6
Ranch	390	41	4
Lite Ranch	190	18	3
Croutons, 1/2 oz	60	2	10
housand Island, 2 oz	160	12	12

Condiments			
Cheese: American, 1 slice	45	3.5	1
Swiss-style, 1 slice	40	3	1
Dipping Sauce: Buttermilk, 1 oz	130	13	3
Frank's Red Hot Buffalo®, 1 oz	10	0	2
Marinara, 1 oz	15	0	3
Barbeque; Sweet & Sour, 1 oz	45	0	11
Tartar	210	22	2
Packet Sauce: Ketchup; Salsa	10	0	2
Mayonnaise	150	17	0
Mustard; Soy Sauce	5	0	0
Taco	0	0	0
Sour Cream	60	6	1

Desserts: Apple Turnover	320	16	41
Cheesecake	310	16	34
Double Fudge Cake	310	11	49

Icecream Shakes: Per 16 fl.oz			
Strawberry Banana	700	28	100
Chocolate	660	29	89
Oreo Cookie Classic	670	33	81
Strawberry	640	28	84
Vanilla	570	29	65

Drinks: Barq's Root Beer®, 20 fl.oz	180	0	50
Coca-Cola Classic®, 20 fl.oz	170	0	46
Dr Pepper®; Minute Maid, 20 fl.oz	190	0	49
Orange Juice, 10 fl.oz	140	0	32
Sprite®, 20 fl.oz	160	0	41

For Complete Nutritional Data ~ see CalorieKing.com

Jamba Juice®

Smoothies: Per 24 fl.oz	**C**	**F**	**Cb**
Aloha Pineapple™	400	1.5	89
Banana Berry™	480	1.5	112
Berry Lime Sublime®	445	2	104
Bounce Back Blast™	485	2	109
Caribbean Passion™, Orange-A-Peel	440	2	102
Chocolate Moo'd™	705	8	142
Citrus Squeeze™	405	2	93
Coldbuster®	440	2.5	100
Cranberry Craze®	430	2	97
Jamba Powerboost®	450	1.5	103
Kiwi Berry Burner™	465	0	112
Mango-A-Go-Go™	500	2	117
Orange Berry Blitz™	420	2.5	94
Orange Dream Machine®	540	2.5	112
Peach Pleasure®	465	2	108
Peanut Butter Moo'd™	860	21	145
Peenya Kowlada®	550	5	118
Pineappalooza™	450	2.5	103
Protein Berry Pizzazz™	460	1.5	92
Razzmatazz®	480	2	112
Strawberries Wild®	445	0	105

For Complete Nutritional Data ~ see CalorieKing.com

KarmelKorn®Popcorn

Popcorn: Per 24 fl.oz	**C**	**F**	**Cb**
Buttery flavored, 3 cups, 1 oz	135	8	15
Butter Rum, 1¼ cups, 1 oz	120	1.5	25
Carmel Coated, 1 cup, 1 oz	130	3	24
w. Peanuts, 1 cup, 1 oz	150	6	23
Cheese-coated, 2¼ cups, 1 oz	170	13	11
White Cheddar Chse, 2 cups, 1 oz	170	13	12

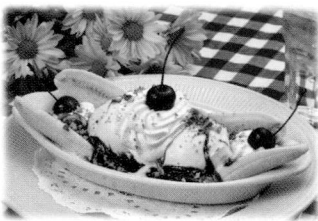

Jimmy John's®

Club Sandwiches	**C**	**F**	**Cb**
Figures based on 7 Grain Wheat, Mayo, Cheese, Sce			
Beach	915	51	74
Billy	855	46	69
Bootlegger's	710	33	66
Club Lulu	765	40	67
Country	830	43	69
Hunter's	835	44	69
Italian Night Club	970	58	70
Smoked Ham	850	47	68
Tuna	820	41	75
Veggie	1040	63	74
Club Sandwiches			
Figures based on 8" French Bread, Mayo, Chse, Sce			
Beach	900	47	79
Billy	845	42	75
Bootlegger's	695	29	71
Club Lulu	750	35	72
Country	815	39	74
Hunter's	820	39	74
Italian Night Club	950	54	75
Smoked Ham	830	42	73
Tuna	790	35	80
Veggie	1020	59	79
Gargantuan™ Sandwich	1070	57	75
Slim Jim's: *Figures based on 8" French Bread without Mayo/Sauce*			
Baked Turkey Breast	385	0.5	69
Double Provolone	545	16	71
Ham & Cheese	515	13	71
Rare Roast Beef	400	2.5	69
Salami & Capicola	595	20	71
Tuna Salad	570	20	74
Subs: *Figures based on 7 Grain Wheat*			
Big John	660	33	66
JJBLT	735	41	67
Sorry Charlie	610	25	73
The Pepe	770	43	68
Turkey Tom	645	31	67
Vegetarian	830	47	72
Vito	665	29	70
Subs: *Figures based on 8" French Bread*			
Big John	550	28	52
JJBLT	630	37	53
Sorry Charlie	500	20	59
The Pepe	665	38	54
Turkey Tom	540	26	53
Vegetarian	720	43	58
Vito	555	24	56

For Complete Nutritional Data ~ see CalorieKing.com

 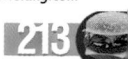

Kenny Rogers Roasters®

Chicken	C	F	Cb
1/2 Chicken: No Skin or Wing	315	10	1
w. Skin	515	28	1
1/4 Dark Meat: No Skin	170	7	1
w. Skin	270	17	1
1/4 White Meat: No Skin or Wing	145	2	1
w. Skin	245	11	1
Pies: Chicken Pot Pie	710	33	78
Pitas: BBQ Chicken	400	7	51
Chicken Caesar	605	35	34
Roasted Chicken	685	35	42
Turkey: Sliced Breast	160	2	0
Sandwiches: Chicken Tender Pita	610	38	45
Chicken Tender Sandwich	725	47	55
Grilled Chicken	525	30	42
Meals: Chicken Breast Platter	945	54	88
Chicken Tender Platter	1300	83	109
Salads (No Dressing): Per Serving			
Chicken Caesar	285	9	18
Pasta	230	12	28
Roasted Chicken	290	10	19
Side	25	0	6
Sour Cream & Dill Pasta	230	16	20
Tomato Cucumber	125	2	10
Sandwiches: Turkey	385	12	30
Side Dishes: Chicken Tenders (3)	510	37	24
Cinnamon Apples	200	5	41
Cole Slaw	225	16	18
Corn Muffin	160	6	25
Corn: on the Cob	70	0.5	14
Cornbread Stuffing	325	19	34
Muffin	175	8	24
Sweet Corn Niblets	115	0.5	28
Creamy Parmesan Spinach	120	6	10
Honey Baked Beans	150	1	32
Italian Green Beans	115	8	10
Macaroni & Cheese	200	6	24
Potatoes: Baked Sweet	265	0	62
Garlic Parsley	260	12	37
Potato Salad	390	27	34
Real Mashed	295	14	39
Rice Pilaf	175	5	43
Steamed Vegetables	50	0	8
Zucchini & Squash Santa Fe	70	5	8
Soup: Chicken Noodle, 1 bowl	90	2	12
Chicken Noodle, 1 cup	55	1	7

KFC®

	C	F	Cb
Extra Crispy™: Breast, 5.7 oz	470	28	19
Drumstick, 2.1 oz	160	10	5
Thigh, 4 oz	370	26	12
Whole Wing, 1.8 oz	190	12	10
Hot & Spicy: Breast, 6.3 oz	450	27	20
Drumstick, 2.1 oz	140	9	4
Thigh, 4.5 oz	390	28	14
Whole Wing, 1.9 oz	180	11	9
Original Recipe®: Breast, 5.7 oz	370	19	11
Drumstick, 2 oz	140	8	4
Thigh, 4.4 oz	360	25	12
Whole Wing, 1.6 oz	145	9	5
Tender Roast: Per Serving			
Breast w. Skin	250	10	1
Breast without Skin	170	4.5	1
Leg w. Skin	100	4.5	1
Leg without Skin	70	2.5	1
Thigh w. Skin	210	12	1.5
Thigh without Skin	105	6	1
Wing w. Skin	120	8	1
Crispy Strips: Per 3 Pieces			
Blazin Strips, 4.5 oz	315	16	21
Colonel's Crispy Strips, 5.3 oz	340	16	20
Honey BBQ Strips, 6.3 oz	375	15	33
Spicy Crispy Strips, 4 oz	335	15	23
Desserts: Per Serving			
Colonel's Pies: Apple Pie Slice, 4 oz	310	14	44
Pecan Pie Slice, 4 oz	490	23	66
Strawberry Creme Pie Slice	280	15	32
Double Choc. Chip Cake, 2.7 oz	320	16	41
Little Bucket™ Parfaits:			
Chocolate Cream, 4 oz	290	15	37
Fudge Brownie, 3.5 oz	280	10	44
Lemon Creme, 4.5 oz	410	14	62
Strawberry Shortcake, 3.5 oz	200	7	33
Entrees			
Chunky Chicken Pot Pie, 13 oz	770	42	69
Honey BBQ Wings, 6 pces, 6.7 oz	605	38	33
Hot Wings, 6 pieces, 4.8 oz	470	33	18
Kentucky Nuggets, 6 pieces	285	18	15
Popcorn Chicken: Large, 6 oz	620	40	36
Small, 3.5 oz	360	23	21

KFC® cont...

Sandwiches

	C	F	Cb
Blazin Twister, 8.7 oz	720	43	56
Chicken Twister Wrap, 8.5 oz	600	34	52
Crispy Caesar Twister, 9.5 oz	745	41	66
Honey BBQ Crunch Melt, 8.1 oz	555	26	48
Honey BBQ Flav. Chicken w. Sce	310	6	37
Original Recipe Chicken: w. Sauce	450	22	33
without Sauce, 6.6 oz	360	13	21
Tender Roast Chicken: w. Sauce	350	15	26
without Sauce, 6.2 oz	270	5	23
Triple Crunch Chicken: w. Sauce	490	29	39
without Sauce, 6.2 oz	390	15	39
Triple Crunch Zinger™: w. Sauce	550	32	39
without Sauce, 6.2 oz	390	15	36

Side Dishes: Per Serving

	C	F	Cb
BBQ Baked Beans, 5.5 oz	190	3	33
Biscuit, 2 oz	180	10	20
Coleslaw, 5 oz	230	13	26
Corn on the Cob, 5.7 oz	150	1.5	35
Cornbread	230	13	25
Green Beans, 4.6 oz	45	1.5	7
Macaroni & Cheese, 5.4 oz	180	8	21
Mashed Potatoes w. Gravy, 4.8 oz	120	6	17
Mean Greens, 5.4 oz	70	3	11
Potato Salad, 5.6 oz	230	14	23
Potato Wedges, 4.8 oz	375	15	53

For Complete Nutritional Data ~ see CalorieKing.com

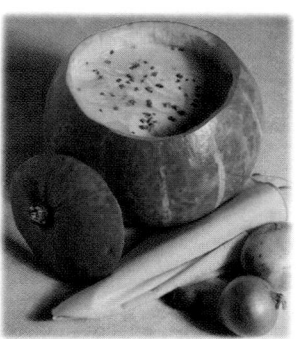

Kilwin's®

Icecream: Per 1/2 Cup

	C	F	Cb
Black Cherry; Caramel Revel	90	0	23
Butter Pecan	190	13	16
Butter Pecan Yogurt	130	6	17
Chocolate	170	10	17
Chocolate Chip Cookie Dough	190	10	22
Chocolate Ripple	100	0	23
French Silk; Mud	190	11	20
Lemon/Raspberry Sorbetto	100	0	25
Old Fashioned Vanilla	180	9	20
Toppings: Caramel, 40g	160	4.5	31
Fudge, 40g	110	6	28

Fudge: Per Piece (40g)

	C	F	Cb
Butter/Vanilla Pecan	160	5	29
Chocolate	150	4.5	30
Chocolate Peanut Butter	160	5	29
Chocolate Pecan/Walnut; P. Butter	160	6	28
German Chocolate	160	7	27
Heavenly Hash	200	11	24
Walnut Maple	160	5	29

Chocolate Bars: Per 1 oz Bar

	C	F	Cb
Chocolate Sea Foam, Dark/Milk	190	9	28
Happy Birthday; Teacher; Thank You	160	9	17
Kilwin's Molded	270	13	24

Clusters: Per Serving

	C	F	Cb
Almond Cluster: Dark (4)	250	19	20
Milk (3)	210	19	17
Cashew Cluster: Dark (4)	190	13	16
Milk (3)	250	16	20
Coconut Cluster: Dark (4)	230	15	24
Milk (4)	210	13	21
Peanut Cluster (3)	220	16	16
Dark/Milk (4)	230	16	19
Pecan Cluster: Dark (4)	240	11	20
Milk (4)	250	18	21
Raisin Cluster: Dark (3)	190	9	28
Milk (4)	170	1	25

Chocolate-Coated Candy: Per Serving

	C	F	Cb
Coated Almonds: Dark (5); Milk (6)	220	15	20
Coated Brazils: Dark (6)	230	19	14
Milk (7)	250	20	15
Coated Cashews: Dark (6)	220	16	16
Milk (7)	240	17	17
Coated Pecans: Dark (7)	230	20	14
Milk (8)	270	23	17

For Complete Nutritional Data ~ see CalorieKing.com

Fast-Foods & *Restaurants*

Koo•Koo•Roo®

Rotisserie Chicken	C	F	Cb
Leg & Thigh, 4.8 oz	300	18	1
Breast & Wing, 6.5 oz	355	16	1
Half Rotisserie Chicken, 11.3 oz	655	34	2
Original Skinless Flame Broiled Chicken™			
3 Piece Original Dark, 5 oz	320	16	5
Original Breast, 4.1 oz	190	5.5	0
Fresh Roasted Turkey			
Hand-Carved Turkey Sandwich	600	32	31
Traditional Turkey Dinner			
w. pot., veges, stuffing, gravy, sce	690	29	67
Turkey Pot Pie (1)	885	44	83
Sliced Turkey Breast (1)	180	8	0
Salads: Per Regular (no dressing)			
BBQ Chicken Salad	365	14	22
Chicken Caesar Salad	285	11	13
Chinese Chicken Salad	550	29	39
Koo Koo Roo House Salad	115	4	16
Chicken Bowls (No Sce): Chargrill	570	18	57
Southwest	570	19	66
Spicy Ginger Garlic	485	6	62
Tostade (no shell)	530	22	45
Soup: Chicken Noodle, 5 oz	70	3	4
Chicken Tortilla, 5 oz	110	6	7
Ten Vegetable, 5 oz	95	2	16
Sandwiches: BBQ Chicken w. Sce	560	11	71
Original Chkn Breast w. Dressing	660	28	62
Chicken Caesar w. Dressing	780	36	62
Wraps: Caesar Chicken	755	39	59
Chipotle Chicken	925	43	88
Sides: Baked French Fries, 5 oz	250	7.5	42
Baked Yams, 6 oz	200	0	47
Black Beans, 6 oz	125	2.5	22
Buffalo Wings (no sauce), 6 wings	605	27	42
Creamed Spinach, 5 oz	100	7	10
Mashed Potatoes, 6.5 oz	185	5	32
Macaroni & Cheese, 6 oz	340	17	32
Roasted Garlic Potatoes, 5 oz	135	4.5	21
Dressings/Extras:			
BBQ Sauce, 2 Tbsp	45	2	7
Caesar Dressing, 1½ oz	235	26	1
Chinese Salad Dressing, 3 oz	325	26	26
Chipotle Sauce, 1 oz	130	14	0
Cranberry Sauce, 1 oz	45	0	11
Lahvash (flatbread), each	60	0	12

For Complete Nutritional Data ~ see CalorieKing.com

Krispy Kreme®

Doughnuts	C	F	Cb
Apple Fritter	380	21	46
Caramel Kreme Crunch	350	19	43
Chocolate Iced Cake	270	14	36
w. Sprinkles	290	14	40
Chocolate Iced Creme Filled	350	21	39
Chocolate Iced Cruller	290	15	37
Chocolate Iced Custard Filled	300	17	35
Chocolate Iced Glazed	250	12	33
w. Sprinkles	260	12	38
Chocolate Malted Kreme	390	21	49
Cinnamon Apple Filled	290	16	32
Cinnamon Bun	260	16	28
Cinnamon Sugar Cake	280	14	37
Cinnamon Twist	230	9	33
Coffee & Kreme	360	20	43
Dulce De Leche	290	18	30
Glazed Cinnamon	210	12	24
Glazed Creme Filled	340	20	39
Glazed Cruller	240	14	26
Glazed Custard Strawberry Filled	290	16	34
Glazed Devil's Food; Blueberry	340	18	42
Glazed Lemon Filled	290	16	34
Glazed Raspberry Filled	300	16	39
Glazed Sour Cream	340	18	42
Glazed Twist	210	9	28
Honey and Oat	340	18	42
Key Lime Pie	330	18	40
Maple Iced	240	12	32
Maple Iced Cake	270	13	35
New York Cheesecake	330	19	36
Original Glazed	205	12	22
Powdered Cake	280	14	37
Powdered Creme Filled	340	21	36
Powdered/Glazed Blueberry Filled	290	16	32
Powdered Raspberry	300	16	36
Powdered Strawberry Filled	260	16	32
Pumpkin Spice Cake	340	18	42
Sugar Coated	200	12	21
Traditional Cake Doughnut	230	13	25
Vanilla Iced Cake w. Sprinkles	270	13	35
Vanilla Iced Creme Filled	340	20	38
Vanilla Iced Custard Filled	290	16	33
Vanilla Iced Glazed	240	12	32
Vanilla Iced Raspb. Filled/Glazed	350	16	50

For Complete Nutritional Data ~ see CalorieKing.com

Krystal®

Breakfast	C	F	Cb
Biscuit: Plain	260	15	27
Bacon, Egg & Cheese	390	25	28
Chik	340	17	34
Sausage	440	32	27
Country Breakfast	660	42	46
Hash Browns	190	13	17
Sunriser™	240	14	14

Sandwiches			
Krystal: Regular	160	7	17
Double	260	13	24
Bacon Cheese	190	10	16
Cheese	180	9	16
Double Cheese	310	16	26
Krystal Chik	240	11	24
Krystal Chili	200	7	22
Chili Cheese Pup	210	12	17
Corn Pup	260	19	19
Plain Pup	170	9	15

Fries: Per Serving			
Regular, 3.8 oz	370	18	49
Chili Cheese, 7.3 oz	540	28	59

Desserts/Drinks			
Chocolate Shake	380	11	58
Krystal Chill	200	7	22
Apple Turnover	220	10	31
Lemon Meringue Pie	360	10	60

For Complete Nutritional Data ~ see CalorieKing.com

Kohr Bros®

Frozen Custard: Per 1/2 Cup	C	F	Cb
Chocolate	140	6	18
Orange Sherbet	105	2	21
Vanilla	130	6	16

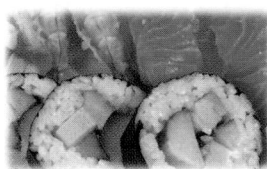

La Rosa's®

Pan Crust Medium Pizza: Per Slice	C	F	Cb
Blanca, medium	350	22	28
Cheese	300	16	30
Deluxe/Pepperoni Topper	370	21	31
Meat Topper	400	23	30
Veggie Topper	320	16	32

Traditional Crust Medium Pizza: Per Slice			
Blanca, medium	260	16	17
Cheese	200	10	19
Deluxe/Pepperoni Topper	280	16	20
Meat Topper	300	18	20
Veggie Topper	220	11	21

Focaccia Style Medium Pizza: Per Slice (1/10 Pizza)			
Cheese, medium	230	12	23
Florentine	240	13	24
Roma	300	18	23

Super Crust Medium Pizza: Per Slice			
Blanca, medium	270	15	23
Cheese	220	8	25
Deluxe/Pepperoni Topper	290	14	26
Meat Topper	310	16	25
Veggie Topper	230	9	27

Calzones: Per Calzone			
3 Meat & 3 Cheese	1080	55	102
3 Veggie & 3 Cheese	860	34	105
Cheese	840	34	101
Cheese & Pepperoni	960	45	101
Cheese Steak	1020	54	93

Hoagy (No Cheese/Dressing/Sauce)			
Baked Buddy	710	40	53
Double Royal Hoagy	920	55	55
Double Steak Hoagy	850	49	54
Filet of Haddock	630	25	62
Meatball Hoagy	590	28	57
Royal Hoagy	610	30	55
Steak Hoagy	560	27	52
Tuna Fish Hoagy	630	32	61
Hoagy Dressing: Chse on Hoagy	220	18	0
Italian Dressing	320	34	3
Mayonnaise	400	11	0
Mushroom Sauce	20	0.5	3
Pizza Sauce	50	2	7
Tartar Sauce	260	24	11

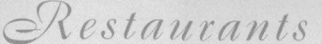

Fast–Foods & *Restaurants*

La Rosa's® cont...

Ciabatta: Includes Chips & Pickle Spear

	C	F	Cb
Garden	680	31	82
Deli	880	44	78
Chicken	780	34	80
Steak	960	55	80
Kitchen Chips & Pickle	235	14	26

Lite & Low Fat Menu

	C	F	Cb
Grilled Chicken Hoagy, low fat	540	10	62
Grilled Chicken Salad, low fat	380	10	40
Lite Deluxe Pizza: Medium, 1 slice	190	6	27
Minestrone Soup, 1 bowl	80	1	15

Pasta Dinner: *Per Entree*

	C	F	Cb
Cheese Ravioli	460	19	53
Lasagna	610	33	48
Meat Ravioli	440	16	54
Spaghetti: w. Meat Sauce	680	18	104
w. Meatballs	890	33	113
w. Sauce	580	10	106

Chicken Wings: BBQ Wings (12)

	C	F	Cb
BBQ Wings (12)	1300	94	48
Special Recipe Wings (12)	1160	94	16
Spicy Hot Wings (12)	1180	94	22

Fresh Baked Bread: *Per Serving*

	C	F	Cb
Garlic Bread, 2 slices	240	9	35
w. Cheese (2)	390	21	35
Garlic Bread Sticks (5)	740	26	109
w. Cheese (5)	1030	49	109

Sauces: Garlic Dipping Sauce

	C	F	Cb
Garlic Dipping Sauce	360	40	0
Pizza Sauce	50	2	7

Rolls: Plain Dinner Roll

	C	F	Cb
Plain Dinner Roll	150	0.5	31
Seasoned Garlic Roll	230	8	32

Salad *(No Dressing)*

	C	F	Cb
Antipasto Meal	260	19	8
Tossed Garden Salad	210	13	14
Tuna Salad Meal	760	48	50

Salad Dressing: *Per Packet*

	C	F	Cb
La Rosa's Creamy Garlic/Italian	250	26	3
Marzetti Blue Cheese	220	24	2
Marzetti Buttermilk Ranch	260	29	1
Marzetti Creamy Caesar	200	22	2
Marzetti Fat Free Honey Dijon	70	0	16
Marzetti Fat Free Italian	20	0	4
Marzetti Fat Free Ranch	40	0	10
Marzetti Honey French	210	18	14
Marzetti Thousand Island	220	21	7

Soup

	C	F	Cb
Minestrone, 12 oz	130	2	22

For Complete Nutritional Data ~ see CalorieKing.com

La Salsa Fresh Mexican Grill®

Figures do not include Corn Chips

	C	F	Cb
If Corn Chips included, add	110	7	10

Appetizers: Salsa & Chips

	C	F	Cb
Salsa & Chips	675	32	87
Guacamole, Salsa & Chips	960	55	103
Nachos: Chicken	1575	83	148

Burritos: Baja Mahi Mahi

	C	F	Cb
Baja Mahi Mahi	855	54	59
3 Pepper: Chicken	830	35	86
Shrimp	765	34	80
Steak	845	37	81
Bean & Cheese	600	19	82
California: Chicken	855	33	95
Steak	875	35	91
Steak Burrito	865	35	89
El Champion Chicken	1495	53	178
Grande Chicken	860	34	97
Los Cabos Shrimp	740	34	77
Original Gourmet: Chicken	640	26	66
Steak	655	28	62
Sonora Mahi Mahi	535	21	56

Meal Platters: Ranch Burrito

	C	F	Cb
Ranch Burrito	1020	35	128
Enchilada: Cheese	930	47	82
Chicken	780	26	90
Fajita Platter	920	32	105
Two Tacos Platter: Chicken	770	19	107
Veggie	805	23	117
Two Taquitos Platter Quesadilla	1625	86	143

Quesadillas: *Per Serving*

	C	F	Cb
Chips w. Quesadillas	200	10	25
Classic: Regular	860	54	56
Chicken or Steak, average	1000	58	60
Grande: Black Bean, Chicken	1185	61	97
Pinto, Chicken	1180	62	95
Black Bean, Steak	1205	63	92
Pinto, Steak	1190	63	90

Salad: Caesar Salad

	C	F	Cb
Caesar Salad	645	44	30
Caesar Salad w. Chips	80	4	10
Chile Lime	780	49	53
Chicken Taco	1010	42	114
Steak Taco	1030	44	110
Salad w. Taco & Chips	205	10	26

Sides: Black Beans

	C	F	Cb
Black Beans	245	1.5	43
Pinto Beans	210	1.5	37
Rice	150	3	28
Rice & Black Beans, (half & half)	275	3.5	49
Rice & Pinto Beans, (half & half)	250	3.5	45

La Salsa Fresh cont...

Tacos: Per Serving	C	F	Cb
Baja: Mahi Mahi	379	23	29
Mahi Mahi Basket	760	46	58
Style Shrimp	325	19	30
Style Shrimp Basket	645	38	60
Chips w. 1 Taco	90	4.5	11
Chips w. Taco Basket	200	10	25
Fajita: Chicken	265	11	24
Steak	275	12	21
La Salsa: Chicken	270	8	32
Steak	275	9	29
Mexico City: Chicken	210	3.5	31
Chicken Basket	410	7	61
Steak	225	5	28
Sonora Mahi Mahi	190	8	17
Taquitos	900	52	73
Vegetarian: Taco	285	10	37
Taco Baskets: Includes Cheese, Sauce, 2 Tacos			
Baja: Mahi Mahi Basket	760	46	58
Style Shrimp Basket	645	38	60
Fajita: Chicken Basket	520	22	46
Steak Basket	545	24	41
La Salsa: Chicken Basket	535	16	64
Steak Basket	560	19	58
Mexico City: Chicken Basket	410	7	61
Steak Basket	440	10	55
Sonora Mahi Mahi Basket	395	17	33
Vegetarian Taco Basket	570	20	74

LaMar's®

Bars: Caramel Iced, Unfilled	430	18	59
Chocolate Iced: Unfilled	540	22	81
Bavarian Cream Filled	600	22	96
Chocolate/White Fluff Filled	800	35	118
Bizmarks: Bavarian Cream	620	22	101
Blueberry/Lemon Filled	530	21	80
Cherry Filled	550	19	88
Donuts: Apple Spice Cake	340	17	44
Bluberry Cake	350	17	47
Chocolate Iced Cake	330	18	37
Old Fashioned Sour Cream	420	18	60
Ray's Chocolate Glazed	290	11	44
Ray's Original Glazed	220	10	31
White Iced Cake	320	17	38
Other Items: Apple Fritter	650	26	91
German Chocolate Knot	480	27	54
Cinnamon Roll	690	25	106
Cinnamon Twist	770	26	120
Raisin Nut Cinnamon Roll	850	27	137

Little Caesar's®

Pizza: Per Slice	C	F	Cb
12" Round: Cheese, 1/8 pizza	185	6	23
Pepperoni, 1/8 pizza	205	7.5	23
12" Deep Dish: Cheese, 1/8 pizza	140	5	19
Pepperoni, 1/8 pizza	160	6	19
12" Thin: Cheese, 1/8 pizza	140	7	13
Pepperoni, 1/8 pizza	170	8.5	13
14" Round: Cheese, 1/10 pizza	200	6.5	25
Meatsa, 1/10 pizza	280	13	26
Pepperoni, 1/10 pizza	230	8	25
Supreme, 1/10 pizza	270	10	31
Veggie, 1/10 pizza	240	7.5	32
14" Deep Dish: Cheese, 1/10	230	9	27
Pepperoni, 1/10 pizza	260	11	27
14" Thin: Cheese, 1/10 pizza	160	7.5	14
Pepperoni, 1/10 pizza	180	9	14
Pizza: Per Slice			
16" Round: Cheese, 1/12 pizza	220	7	27
Pepperoni, 1/12 pizza	240	8.5	27
18" Round: Cheese, 1/12 pizza	230	7	30
Pepperoni, 1/12 pizza	260	9	30
Baby Pan! Pan!, 1 piece	360	16	34
Pizza By The Slice: Cheese, 1/6	330	11	42
Pepperoni, 1/6 medium pizza	390	14	42
Sandwiches:			
Italian	800	45	66
Ham & Cheese	640	29	66
Veggie	600	28	67
Salads: Antipasto, 7 oz	140	7.5	6
Caesar, 4.5 oz	90	3	12
Tossed Salad, 6 oz	100	3	15
Greek, 9.5 oz	120	6.5	11
Dressings: Caesar, 1 oz	230	25	1
Greek, 1.5 oz	270	29	0
Italian, avg., 1.5 oz	220	23	2
Fat Free Italian, 1.5 oz	25	0	5
Ranch, 1.5 oz	230	24	2
Thousand Island, 1 oz	220	21	7
Sides: Chicken Wings, 1 piece	70	5	0
Crazy Bread, 1 stick, 1.2 oz	90	2.5	14
Crazy Sauce, 4 oz	45	0	9
Italian Cheese Bread, 1 piece	130	6	13
Crazy Cinnamon Bread (2)	100	2	19

For Complete Nutritional Data ~ see CalorieKing.com

Fast−Foods & *Restaurants*

Lone Star Steakhouse

	C	F	Cb
Chili: Lone Star, 6 fl.oz	225	15	8
Meals: Grilled Chicken, 6 oz	180	2.5	0
Grilled Pork Chops, 16 oz	1400	100	0
Ribs, 12 oz	960	80	0
Shrimp Dinner, 3½ oz	100	1.5	1
Sweet Bourbon Salmon, 6 oz	230	11	0
Mesquite Grilled Steaks			
Cajun Ribeye, 16 oz	1230	101	0
Chopped Steak, 12 oz	880	71	0
Delmonico, 11 oz	845	70	0
Five Star Filet, 9 oz	725	61	0
New York Strip, 14 oz	1015	80	0
San Antonio Sirloin, 12 oz	755	55	0
T-Bone, 20 oz	1515	124	0
Prime Rib: Whole, ½″ Fat			
Smoked, 16 oz	1230	101	0
Sides: Baked Potato	670	18	114
Baked Sweet Potato	645	8	137
Sauteed Mushrooms	115	9	6
Sauteed Onions	100	7	8
Steamed Vegetables	85	1	14
Texas Rice	75	2	12
Soup: Black Bean, 6 fl.oz	200	4	31
Texas Teasers: Ribs, 6 oz	480	40	0
Dessert: Homemade Cobbler	250	8	43

Long John Silver's®

	C	F	Cb
Sandwiches: Ultimate Fish	480	22	51
Fish Sandwich	440	20	48
Chicken Sandwich	480	22	51
Sides: Fries: Regular	230	10	34
Large, 5 oz	390	17	56
Cheese Sticks (3)	140	8	12
Coleslaw, 4 oz	200	15	15
Corn Cobbette, no butter	90	3	14
Crumblies, 1 oz	170	12	14
Hushpuppies, 1 pup	60	2.5	9
Rice, 4 oz	180	3.5	34
Soup: Clam Chowder, 1 bowl	220	10	23
Chicken: Battered Plank, 1 piece	130	8	9
Seafood: Battered Fish, 1 piece	230	13	16
Battered Shrimp, 1 piece	45	2.5	3
Breaded Clams, 1 order	240	13	22
Desserts: Per Pie			
Chocolate Cream Pie	310	22	24
Pecan Pie	370	15	55
Pineapple Cream Pie	290	13	39

For Complete Nutritional Data ~ see CalorieKing.com

McDonald's®

	C	F	Cb
Burgers/Sandwiches			
Big Mac®	580	33	47
Big N' Tasty®	530	32	37
with Cheese	580	37	37
Cheeseburger	330	14	35
Chicken McGrill®	400	17	37
Plain (no mayo)	300	6	34
Crispy Chicken	500	26	46
Double Cheeseburger	480	27	37
Double Quarter Pounder w. Chse	760	48	38
Filet-O-Fish®	470	26	45
Hamburger	280	10	35
McChicken: Hot & Spicy	450	26	39
Regular	430	23	41
McVeggie Burger®	350	8	47
Quarter Pounder®	420	21	36
with Cheese	530	30	38
Breakfast Menu: Per Serving			
Bacon, Egg & Cheese Biscuit	480	31	31
Bagel, Plain	260	1	54
Big Breakfast	710	48	45
Biscuit, 2.7 oz	240	11	30
Breakfast Burrito, 4 oz	290	16	24
Breakfast Sourdough	560	33	41
Chorizo & Egg Breakfast Burrito	290	16	24
Egg McMuffin®	300	12	29
English Muffin, 2 oz	150	2	27
Ham, Egg & Cheese Bagel	550	23	58
Hash Browns, 2 oz	130	8	14
Hotcakes: Plain, (3)	340	8	58
w. Margarine, 2 pats	420	17	56
w. Margarine, 2 pats & Syrup (1)	600	17	104
McGriddles®:			
Bacon, Egg & Cheese	450	23	43
Sausage	420	23	42
Sausage, Egg & Cheese	550	33	43
Sausage Biscuit	410	28	30
with Egg	490	33	31
Sausage McMuffin®	370	23	28
with Egg	450	28	29
Sausage Patty, 1.5 oz	170	16	0
Scrambled Eggs (2), 3½ oz	160	11	1
Spanish Omelete Bagel	710	40	59
Steak, Egg & Cheese Bagel	640	31	57
French Fries: Small, 2.4 oz	210	10	26
McValue, 3.7 oz	325	16	40
Medium, 5 oz	450	22	57
Large, 6 oz	545	26	68
Super Size, 7 oz	610	29	77

220

McDonald's® cont...

Chicken McNuggets®/Sauces	C	F	Cb
Chicken McNuggets®: 4 pieces	210	13	12
6 pieces	310	20	18
10 pieces	510	33	30
Sauce: Barbecue, 1 oz pkg	45	0	10
Honey, 1/2 oz pkg	45	0	12
Honey Mustard, 1/2 oz pkg	50	4.5	3
Hot Mustard, 1 oz pkg	60	3.5	7
Light Mayonnaise, 1 pkg	45	4.5	1
Sweet 'N' Sour, 1 oz pkg	50	0	11
Muffins/Danishes: Apple Danish	340	15	47
Cheese Danish, 3.7 oz	400	21	45
Cinnamon Roll, 3.5 oz	340	15	52
Lowfat Apple Bran Muffin, 4 oz	300	3	61
Salads: (No Dressing)			
Bacon Ranch Salad, no chicken	140	10	7
Butter Garlic Croutons, 0.5 oz	50	1.5	8
Caesar Salad, no chicken, 6.7 oz	90	4	7
California Cobb Salad, no chicken	160	11	4
Crispy Chicken Bacon Ranch	370	21	20
Crispy Chicken Caesar Salad, 10 oz	310	16	20
Crispy Chicken California Cobb	380	23	20
Grilled Chicken Bacon Ranch	270	13	11
Grilled Chicken Caesar Salad, 9.8 oz	210	7	11
Grilled Chicken California Cobb	280	14	11
Side Salad, 3.1 oz	15	0	3
Salad Dressings: Per 2 fl.oz Pkg.			
Newman's Own: Cobb	120	9	9
Creamy Caesar	190	18	4
Light Balsamic Vinaigrette	90	8	4
Lowfat Balsamic Vinaigrette	40	3	4
Ranch	290	30	4
Desserts/Cookies			
Baked Apple Pie, 2 3/4 oz	260	13	34
Chocolate Chip Cookies (1)	170	9	23
Fruit 'n Yogurt Parfait:			
Regular, with Granola	380	5	76
Regular w/out Granola	280	4	53
Snack Size w. Granola	160	2	30
Snack Size w/out Granola	130	2	25
McDonaldland® Cookies, 2 oz bag	230	8	38

Desserts/Cookies (Cont)	C	F	Cb
McFlurry™: Butterfinger®, small	620	22	90
M&M®, small	630	23	90
Nestlé Crunch®, small	630	24	89
Oreo®, small	570	20	82
Sundaes/Cone			
Sundae: Hot Caramel Sundae	360	10	61
Hot Fudge Sundae, 6.3 oz	340	12	52
Strawberry Sundae, 6.3 oz	290	7	50
Nuts (Sundae/Topping), 1/4 oz	40	3.5	2
Cone: Vanilla Reduced Fat	150	4.5	23
Kiddie Cone	45	1.5	7
Drinks: % Lowfat Milk, 8 fl.oz ctn	100	2.5	13
Orange Juice, 12 fl.oz	180	0	42
Triple Thick Shakes: *Per 16 fl.oz*			
Chocolate	580	17	94
Strawberry; Raspberry	560	16	89
Vanilla	570	16	89
Coca-Cola Classic® (25% Ice):			
Childs, 12 fl.oz	110	0	29
Small, 16 fl.oz	150	0	40
Medium, 21 fl.oz	210	0	58
Large, 32 fl.oz	310	0	86
Super Size, 42 fl.oz	410	0	113
Diet Coke (25% Ice)			
Childs, 12 fl.oz	1	0	0
Small, 16 fl.oz	2	0	0
Medium, 21 fl.oz	3	0	0
Large, 32 fl.oz	4	0	0
Sprite(25% Ice): Childs, 12 fl.oz	110	0	28
Small, 16 fl.oz	150	0	39
Medium, 21 fl.oz	210	0	56
Large, 32 fl. oz	310	0	86
Super Size, 42 fl.oz	410	0	109
Hi-C Orange Drink: Childs, 12 fl.oz	120	0	32
Small, 16 fl.oz	160	0	44
Medium, 21 fl.oz	240	0	64
Large, 32 fl.oz	350	0	94
Super Size, 42 fl.oz	460	0	12

For Complete Nutritional Data ~ see CalorieKing.com

Fast−Foods & *Restaurants*

Manhattan Bagel

Bagel: Per Bagel (4 oz)

	C	F	Cb
Blueberry	255	0.5	54
Cheddar Cheese	270	4	48
Chocolate Chip	285	2.5	56
Cinnamon Raisin	275	0.5	57
Cranberry Orange	270	1	55
Garlic	265	0.5	55
Jalapeno Cheddar; Egg	265	1.5	53
Oat Bran; Sun-Dried Tomato	260	1	53
Oat Bran, Raisin & Walnut	280	2.5	54
Onion	265	0.5	55
Plain; Marble	255	0.5	52
Poppy	295	4	54
Pumpernickel; Rye	255	1	52
Sesame	310	5	55
Spinach	260	0.5	54
Whole Wheat; Salt	255	0.5	52

For Complete Nutritional Data ~ see CalorieKing.com

Mazzio's® Pizza

Pizza: Per Slice (1/8 Medium Pizza)

	C	F	Cb
Cheese: Thin Crust	160	9	18
Original Crust	180	6	29
Deep Pan Crust	310	16	37
Large Pizzeria Crust	320	15	42
Pepperoni: Thin Crust	160	10	18
Original Crust	230	11	29
Deep Pan Crust	320	16	37
Large Pizzeria Crust	330	15	42
Sausage: Thin Crust	190	12	18
Original Crust	250	12	30
Deep Pan Crust	350	19	38
Large Pizzeria Crust	380	20	43
Combo: Thin Crust	200	13	20
Original Crust	250	12	31
Deep Pan Crust	350	19	39
Large Pizzeria Crust	370	19	44
Supremebuster: Thin Crust	190	11	19
Original Crust	240	11	30
Deep Pan Crust	340	18	38
Large Pizzeria Crust	360	18	43

Mazzio's®cont...

	C	F	Cb
Meatbuster: Thin Crust	220	14	19
Original Crust	270	14	30
Deep Pan	370	21	38
Large, Pizzeria Crust	410	22	43
Chicken Club: Thin Crust	180	8	19
Original Crust	250	10	30
Deep Pan Crust	350	17	38
Large Pizzeria Crust	360	15	40
California Alfredo: Thin Crust	210	14	17
Original Crust	260	13	28
Deep Pan Crust	370	20	36
Large Pizzeria Crust	390	20	41
Mexican: Thin Crust	280	14	25
Original Crust	330	13	36
Deep Pan Crust	440	22	44
Large Pizzeria Crust	490	21	52
"Mazzio's Works": Thin Crust	220	14	20
Original Crust	270	14	31
Deep Pan Crust	380	21	39
Large Pizzeria Crust	410	22	44

Appetizers: Per Serving

	C	F	Cb
Cheese Nachos, 1/2 container	440	10	19
Cheese Dippers, 1/4 container	330	16	38
Wings of Fire: Large	370	28	2
Small	360	26	3
Cinnamon Sticks, 3.2 oz	350	16	45
Breadsticks, 2.8 oz	120	2.5	25
Meat Nachos, 5 oz	520	18	20

Pasta: Per Serving

	C	F	Cb
Calzone: Pepperoni, 1/10 whole	240	8	33
Ham-Bacon-Cheddar, 1/10 whole	280	8	32
Fettuccine Alfredo, 14.7 oz	1320	42	195
Italian Sampler, 24 oz	1640	57	218
Lasagne w. Meat Sauce, 16 oz	700	36	60
Spaghetti: w. Meatballs, 21 oz	1560	53	206
w. Meat Sauce, 17 oz	1210	26	200
w. Marinara, 16 oz	940	10	208

Mimi's Cafe®

Menu Items: Per Serving

	C	F	Cb
Broiled 10 oz Halibut Steak	625	16	51
Capellini w. Tomatoes & Basil	680	8	130
EggBeater Fitness Omelette	655	8	110
Half-A-Turkey Sandwich	410	6	55
Maggie's Chicken and Fruit	545	9	59
Roasted Turkey Breast	540	8	52
Two "AA" Large Eggs	395	8	62

Restaurants & Fast−Foods

Miami Subs

Burgers	C	F	Cb
Deluxe	765	59	31
Deluxe Cheeseburger	840	65	32
Deluxe Bacon Cheeseburger	890	70	32

Cheesesteaks: Per 6" Sandwich			
Original	405	11	45
Classic	420	12	47
Works	545	23	51
Chicken Philly	550	27	46

Pitas: Gyros	665	39	46
Chicken	390	13	33

Subs: Per 6" Sandwich			
Ham & Cheese	450	18	49
Italian Deli	510	25	49
Meatball	505	22	49
Tuna	480	18	44
Turkey	485	19	51

Sides: Per Serving			
Mozzarella Sticks	745	57	34
Onion Rings	860	69	55
Spicy Fries, Regular	525	40	39

Platters: Gyros	1410	94	81
Chicken Breast	735	41	57
10 Wings w. Fries, Blue Cheese	995	67	50

Salads			
Caesar w. Dressing	460	34	26
Chicken Caesar w. Dressing	605	39	28
Chicken Club, no Dressing	490	26	23
Garden, no Dressing	315	18	21
Greek, no Dressing	285	15	24
Side Greek w. Dressing	75	6	4

Mr. Goodcents®

Quartermeal: w. Chicken Noodle Soup			
Roast Beef	435	7	60
Turkey	460	9	62

Pasta: w. Breadstick			
Chicken Parmesan (Mostiaccioli)	80	10	110
Mostiaccioli w. Tomato Pasta Sce	540	5	109

Subs: Per 1/2 Sub			
Chkn Parmesan on Wheat, no dress.	480	10	63
Ham & Cheese on Wheat	480	10	70
Oven Roasted Chicken on White, standard dressing, no oil	445	4	74
Penny Club on Wheat	430	7	63
Roast Beef on Wheat	455	6	68
Turkey on Wheat	460	8	70
Veggie on Wheat	385	7	66

Mr. Hero®

Cheesesteaks: Per 7" Serving	C	F	Cb
Grilled Steak Philly	465	14	48
Hot Buttered Cheesesteak Deluxe	595	34	48

Pasta: Per Serving			
Breadsticks w. Sauce, 5 oz	295	9	47
Spaghetti Dinner, 16.8 oz	610	9	112
Spaghetti w. Meatballs, 19.8 oz	850	27	117

Salads			
Garden Salad	40	0.5	7
Grilled Chicken	220	10	7
Seafood Crab	455	37	18
Side Salad	30	0.5	6
Tuna	740	69	8

Dressings: Per Serving			
Buttermilk, 2 oz	285	29	6
Creamy Italian, 2 oz	200	17	11
Croutons, 1/2 oz	60	2	8.5
Fat Free, French	75	0	18
Fat Free, Ranch	65	0	16

Sandwiches: Per 7" Sandwich			
Cold Subs: Classic Italian	610	36	50
Tuna & Cheese	685	47	47
Turkey & Cheese	470	21	46
Ultimate Italian	630	34	52
Hot Subs: Grilled Chicken Philly	455	14	48
Meatball	645	32	53
Romanburger	740	47	50
Round: Bacon Cheeseburger	355	23	23
Chicken	415	23	23
Fish Sandwich	415	23	31
Tuna	435	34	23

Side Orders: Per Serving			
Cheddar Cheese Sauce	65	4.5	5
Onion Rings	575	32	64
Potato Wafers	345	18	42

Desserts: Per Serving			
Cheesecake, plain	365	27	26
Cheesecake w. Cherries	405	27	35

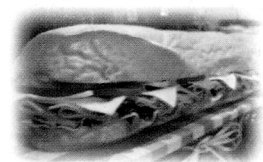

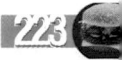

Mr Subb®

Subs (Regular Size)	C	F	Cb
Classic: Assorted	665	20	82
Ham	500	6	87
Meatball	735	26	78
Pizza	590	21	72
Salami	570	18	74
Vegetarian	395	3	73
Premium: Breaded Chicken	755	20	100
Canadian Club	555	11	78
Grilled Chicken	570	7.5	80
Louisiana Chicken	585	14	71
Seafood with Crab	515	5	89
Specialty Subs: BBQ Rib	695	26	73
BLT	540	14	75
Corned Beef	505	10	71
Roast Beef	500	9	70
Tuna	565	9	81
Turkey	470	5	75
Wraps: Louisiana Chicken	360	12	39
Roast Beef	300	8	38
Seafood with Crab	325	5.5	52
Tuna	365	9	46
Turkey	285	5.5	41
Sauces (Per 1/2 oz (1 Tbsp):			
Mayo Lite	60	5	2
MR SUB Secret Sauce	80	9	0
Average, all others	20	0	4
Soups and Chili			
Bean and Spring Vegetable	125	1	23
Caribbean and Black Bean	110	0.5	22
Chicken Noodle	95	2	14
Chili with Beef	185	1.5	31
Clam Chowder	175	8	21
Cream of Mushroom	65	1	10
Cream of Potato and Leek	170	8	20
French Canadian Pea	145	2.5	23
Garden Vegetable	50	0.5	11
Italian Wedding Style	125	3	21
Minestrone	80	0.5	15
Pasta Fagioli	140	1.5	25
Vegetable Beef and Barley	85	1	16
Salad: (No Cheese/Dressing)			
Garden Salad	20	0	4
Mediterranean Greek	60	4	6
Mighty Caesar Salad	100	4	8

For Complete Nutritional Data ~ see CalorieKing.com

Mrs Fields Cookies®

Per Cookie (2.3 oz)	C	F	Cb
Butter Toffee	290	13	40
Chewy Fudge	220	11	30
Cinnamon Sugar	300	12	41
Coconut & Macadamias	280	13	39
Debra's Special	280	12	39
Milk Chocolate	280	13	38
Milk Choc w. Walnuts/Macadamia	320	18	36
Milk Chocolate Chip	280	13	38
Oatmeal Chocolate Chip	280	11	40
Oatmeal Raisins & Walnuts	280	12	39
Peanut Butter	310	16	34
Peanut Butter Milk Chocolate	300	17	35
Pumpkin Harvest	200	10	24
Semi-Sweet Chocolate	280	14	40
w. Pecans/Walnuts	310	16	38
Snickerdoodle Jumbo	640	29	90
Triple Chocolate	220	10	31
White Chunk Macadamia	310	17	37
Bite Size Nibbler™: Per 2 Cookies (1 oz)			
Butter	110	4.5	15
Chewy Chocolate Fudge	110	5	15
Cinnamon Sugar	120	4.5	17
Debra's Special Nibbler	100	4.5	13
M&M Nibbler	110	5	16
Milk Choc w. Walnuts	120	6	14
Milk/Semi-Sweet Chocolate	110	5	15
Peanut Butter; Triple Choc	110	6	13
White Chunk Macadamia	120	7	13
Brownies: Each (2.7 oz)			
Double Fudge	360	19	49
Frosted Fudge	440	21	62
Pecan Fudge;Pie Brownie	340	21	40
Walnut Fudge	380	23	45
Bundt Cakes: Per Piece (3 oz)			
Banana Walnut	350	21	35
Banana Walnut w. Choc Chip	370	22	39
Blueberry	270	12	36
Raspberry	270	12	36
White Cake w. Choc Chips	350	17	45

For Complete Nutritional Data ~ see CalorieKing.com

My Favorite Muffin®

**~ Same Data as
Big Apple Bagel (See Page 238) ~**

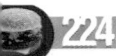

Restaurants & Fast–Foods

Nathan's Famous®

Burgers: 1/4 lb Burger	C	F	Cb
1/4 lb Burger w. Chse	850	61	45
Bacon Cheeseburger	705	44	43
Super Burger	865	62	42
Cheese Steaks: Original	740	43	50
Supreme	785	43	61
Chicken Cheesesteak	565	19	62
Sandwiches: Fish Sandwich	470	20	42
Sides: Nuggets (6)	350	27	20
French Fries: Regular	545	38	46
Large	760	52	65
Supersize	1190	82	100
Onion Rings: Small	560	44	36
Large	750	59	48
Hot Dogs: Nathan's Famous	310	20	22

For Complete Nutritional Data ~ see CalorieKing.com

O'Charley's®

Appetizers: Per Serving			
Buffalo Wings, 3 wings	340	25	0.5
Chicken Quesadilla, 1/2 order	460	26	25
Chicken Tenders (2)	215	11	8
Chips & Salsa, 1/4 order	235	11	29
Fried Cheese Wedges (1)	140	11	5
Loaded Potato Skins (1)	290	17	21
Spinach & Artichoke Dip, 1/2 order	425	25	43
Brunch: Per Order (No Fries or Bread)			
Cajun Chicken Omelette	675	51	5
Spanish Omelette	600	47	5
Ultimate Omelette	700	51	12
Waffles w. Strawberries	1120	44	161
Chicken: Per Order (No Sides or Salads)			
Cajun Chicken	695	35	24
Chicken Parmesan	775	41	31
Chicken Tenders Dinner	730	34	23
Chicken Teriyaki	610	21	33
Grilled Chicken Dinner	595	24	25
Savannah Chicken	1280	86	64
Salad: Per Order			
Black & Blue Caesar	1205	83	18
Caesar Salad	405	32	13
Cajun Chicken w. Ranch Dressing	970	59	33
Chicken Caesar	670	43	13
Salmon Caesar	655	44	13
Southern Fried Chkn w. Dressing	1140	91	38
Sandwiches (No Sides)			
Bacon & Cheese Chicken	630	31	27
Buffalo Chicken	645	35	41
Cajun Chicken	465	18	27

O'Charley's® cont...

Sandwiches (No Sides) (Cont)	C	F	Cb
Chicken Sandwich	430	18	26
Fisherman's Sandwich	650	28	65
French Dip	695	30	47
Half Pound Cheeseburger	895	55	27
The O'Charley's Club, no Dressing	670	34	48
Three Cheese Bacon Burger	1225	87	28
Seafood: Per Order (No Sides or Salad)			
Fisherman's Platter	1110	54	95
Fried Shrimp Platter, 8 shrimp	550	28	26
Sides: Baked Potato, plain	295	0.5	68
Cole Slaw	205	13	20
French Fries	410	21	50
Loaded Baked Potato	560	24	73
Rica Pital	165	6	26
Smashed Potatoes	345	15	43
Vegetable Medley	130	7.5	12
Soup: Loaded Potato Soup, 1 bowl	360	22	31
Vegetable Steamer, 1 order	445	6	84
Steak & Ribs: Per Serving (No Sides or Fries)			
Beef Tips Monterey, 1 order	870	53	36
Choice Sirloin	530	20	0
Filet Mignon	520	25	0
New York Strip Steak	765	56	0
Petite Sirloin	370	14	0.5
Prime Rib: 8 oz	600	42	1
10 oz	760	54	1
16 oz	1270	90	1
Full Rack of Ribs	1075	85	6
1/2 Rack of Ribs	540	42	4
Ribeye Steak	985	72	0
Steak & Fried Shrimp Combo	645	28	13
Steak & Grilled Shrimp Combo	600	20	26
Steak & Rib Combo	910	57	4

For Complete Nutritional Data ~ see CalorieKing.com

Olive Garden®

Garden Fare Selections (Lower Fat)			
Lunch: Capellini Pomodora, 13 oz	350	11	52
Chicken Giardino, 15.5 oz	350	7	40
Linguine alla Marinara, 10.6 oz	280	6	48
Shrimp Primavera, 19 oz	490	15	65
Dinner: Chicken Giardino, 21.5 oz	460	8	59
Capellini Pomodora, 21 oz	560	18	84
Linguine alla Marinara, 17 oz	450	9	79
Shrimp Primavera, 26 oz	730	25	84
Extras: Minestrone Soup, 6 fl.oz	100	1	18
Breadstick, plain, 1 stick	140	1.5	26

Fast-Foods & *Restaurants*

(The) Old Spaghetti Factory®

	C	F	Cb
Garlic Cheese Bread, ½ svg, 6 oz	530	25	60
Entrees: Fettuccine Alfredo	1140	87	61
Spaghetti Pot Pourri	990	40	110
Spaghetti: w. Clam Sauce	720	33	82
w. Meat Sauce	520	11	85
w. Meatballs/Tomato Sauce	720	18	95
w. Mizithra Cheese	910	57	76
w. Mizithra/Mushr./Tomato Sce	680	32	79
w. Mushroom/Tomato Sauce	450	6	83
w. Sausage/Meat Sauce	730	25	86
w. Tomato/Meat Sauce	480	3	84
Favorites: Baked Lasagna, 16 oz	590	32	35
Chicken Marsala, 19 oz	1110	69	61
Chicken Parmigiana, 19 oz	630	16	68
Spinach & Cheese Ravioli, 12 oz	650	19	87
Spinach Tortellini w. Alfredo, 12 oz	1180	68	104
Pies: Mud/Caramel Turtle, avg	580	31	68

Orange Julius®

	C	F	Cb
Original (Orange, Strawberry):			
Small, 16 fl.oz	225	0	55
Medium, 20 fl.oz	280	0.5	68
Large,32 fl.oz	450	1	109
Classic Smoothy® Drinks 16 fl.oz:			
Bananarilla; Tropical	300	7	56
Cool Cappucino	415	10	72
Pina Colada; Raspberry	360	7	72
Strawb. Banana; Tripleberry	380	7	75
20 fl.oz Size ~ Add 25% to above figures			
32 fl.oz Size ~ Double the above figures			
Julius Creations®: Per Serving (20 fl.oz)			
Berry Lively; Blackberry Toner	400	0	93
Blackberry Storm	570	8	114
Blueberrathon	335	1	80
Chai Tea Dragon	515	3	110
Cocoa Latte Swirl	655	9	122
Fruitasia	395	3	90
Muscle Peach	275	0.5	66
Orange Swirl	490	10	96
Pineapple Hardbody	360	0.5	81
Raspberry Slim	395	1	95
Strawb. Treasure; Raspb. Creme	525	8	103
Strawberry Xtreme	385	0.5	87
Tart 'N' Berry	430	3	99
Tropi-Colada	550	8	110
Add Banana, 1 medium	110	0.5	27
Nutrifiers: Avg. all types, ¼ oz	16	0	4

Outback Steakhouse®

	C	F	Cb
Aussie-Tizers:			
Aussie Cheese Fries, 28 oz	2900	182	240
Bloomin Onion, w. dressing	2210	134	241
¼ serving	550	33	60
Gold Coast Coconut Shrimp	690	30	97
Grilled Shrimp on the Barbie	660	42	32
Kookaburra Wings w. Sauce (10)	1160	75	65
Lobster-Crab Cakes w. Sauce (2)	840	72	33
Steaks: Meat Only ~ Add Extra for Sides			
Michael J. "Crocodile" Dundee:			
New York Strip, 14 oz	900	60	0
Outback Special, 12 oz Sirloin	810	50	0
Prime Minister's Prime Ribs:			
8 oz cut	450	38	0
12 oz cut	675	57	0
16 oz cut	905	77	0
Rockhampton Rib-Eye, 14 oz	730	40	0
The Melbourne, P/house, 20 oz	1230	99	0
Lean meat only	590	32	0
Victoria's Filet: Tenderloin, 9 oz	570	44	0
Sides: Aussie Chips w Ketchup	725	32	100
Fresh Veggies	80	1	14
Grilled Onions, 7.5 oz	180	11	19
Jacket Potato, Plain	270	0	63
Jacket Potato, w. Butter/Cheese	400	14	63
Mushrooms, Sauteed	150	11	12
Desserts: Cheesecake Olivia	700	38	79
Choc. Thunder from Down Under	1220	78	134

Panda Express®

	C	F	Cb
Chicken: Black Pepper, 5.5 oz	1800	10	10
Orange Chicken, 5.5 oz	475	21	50
w. Mushrooms, 5.5 oz	135	7	7
w. String Beans, 5.5 oz	165	8	12
Spicy w. Peanuts, 5.5 oz	205	7	17
Beef & Broccoli, 5.5 oz	150	8	9
Sweet & Sour Pork, 4 oz	415	30	17
Mixed Veges, 5 oz	80	3	11
Fried Tofu w. Beans, 5.5 oz	185	11	11
Rice & Noodles: Serving (8 oz)			
Steamed Rice	330	0.5	74
Vegetable Chow Mein	330	11	48
Vegetable Fried Rice	390	12	61
Appetizers: Chkn Egg Roll (1)	190	8	21
Fried Shrimp, 6 pieces	260	12	26
Veggie Spring Roll (1)	85	2.5	14

Restaurants & Fast-Foods

Panera Bread®

	C	F	Cb
Bagels: Asiago Cheese	330	5	57
Blueberry	330	1	70
Chocolate Chip	360	6	67
Cinnamon Crunch	510	9	95
Dutch Apple & Raisin	350	2.5	72
Everything; Sesame Seed	300	1.5	60
Morning Glory	380	7	71
Plain	300	1.5	61
Spreads: Per 2 oz			
Plain Cream Cheese	190	18	2
Reduced Fat, avg.	150	10	5
Roasted Garlic Hummus	90	5	7
Salad: Per Serving			
Asian Sesame Chicken	400	15	43
Caesar Salad	390	26	22
Classic Cafe	400	36	12
Grilled Chicken Caesar	490	27	23
Fandango	400	28	23
Greek	480	45	15
Sandwiches:			
Asiago Roast Beef	960	52	78
Bacon Turkey Bravo	860	34	83
Chicken Salad on Nine Grain	600	26	57
Coronado Carnitas Panini	720	30	72
Frontega Chicken Panini	860	46	82
Italian Combo on Ciabatta	1005	49	80
Peanut Butter & Jelly on French	440	16	64
Sierra Turkey	760	44	68
Smoked Ham & Swiss on Rye	630	31	49
Smoked Turkey on Sourdough	450	15	44
Tuna on Honey Wheat	730	46	52
Turkey Artichoke Panini	850	41	73
Tuscan Chicken	860	52	83
Soup: Per Serving			
Baked Potato	240	15	20
Black Bean	180	0.5	32
Boston Clam Chowder	210	12	19
Broccoli Cheddar	220	17	13
Chicken Chili	180	6	24
Chkn Noodle; Sirloin Steak & Veg	110	2.5	15
Cream of Chicken w. Wild Rice	210	13	18
Fire Roasted Vegetable Bisque	180	11	16
Forest Mushroom	140	8	14
French Onion w. Fetina Cheese	200	9	21
Garden Vege; Mesa Vegetable	110	1.5	23
Gumbo	110	3	18
Moroccan Tomato Lentil	110	1.5	23
Potato Cream Cheese	190	10	21
Savory Vegetable Bean; Vege Lentil	120	2	21

Papa Gino's®

	C	F	Cb
Appetizers: Per Serving			
Buffalo Chick. Tenders, med., 4 oz	225	10	21
Cheese Breadsticks, medium	155	5	21
Cheese Garlic Bread, 11 oz	660	15	110
Chicken Tender, 3 oz	200	10	17
Cinnamon Sticks, 3.5 oz	310	9	52
French Fries, small, 6.5 oz	360	22	38
Mozzarella Sticks (1), 3.3 oz	300	15	27
Pasta: Entree Size			
Cheese Ravioli	445	20	49
Chicken Parmigiana Platter	1035	34	129
Penne or Spaghetti, plain	650	11	118
Papa Platter: Penne/Spaghetti	995	23	136
Spaghetti & Meatballs	885	19	123
Pizzas: Large (14") Thin Crust ~ Per Slice (1/8)			
Cheese	240	6	36
BBQ Chicken	300	6	44
Buffalo Chicken	260	6	35
Cheeseburger	330	13	37
Chicken Pepper; Garlic Chicken	300	9	37
Hawaiian	295	8	38
Meat Combo	335	14	36
PapaRoni	340	15	36
Pepperoni	285	10	36
Super Veggie	260	7	39
Works; Fenway	320	12	39
Salads: Buffalo Chicken Tender	320	15	31
Caesar Salad	190	8	19
Chicken Bacon Cheddar	480	21	24
Chicken Tender	310	15	29
Garden Salad	140	4	22
Italian Chopped Salad	580	50	10
Caesar Side Salad	70	3	6
Garden Side Salad	65	2	10
Dressings: Blue Cheese, 1 oz	150	15	3
Caesar, 3 oz	400	43	0
Fat Free Ranch, 3 oz	85	0	23
Ranch, 3 oz	385	31	3
Subs (Small): BLT	685	30	75
Italian	775	36	73
Meatball	750	16	81
Seafood Salad	685	34	71
Steak	560	31	45
Tuna	740	38	70
Turkey	600	18	74

Fast–Foods & *Restaurants*

Papa John's®

	C	F	Cb
Original Large Pizza (14") Per Slice (1/8 Whole)			
All the Meats	390	19	37
BBQ Chicken	360	14	43
Cheese; Garden Special, avg.	280	10	38
Chicken Alfredo; Pepperoni	305	12	37
Sausage	325	14	37
Six Cheese	425	21	38
Spinach Alfredo	335	14	35
The Works	345	15	38
Thin Large Pizza (14"): Per Slice (1/8 Whole)			
All the Meats	395	26	22
Cheese; Chicken BBQ	235	13	22
Chicken Alfredo	270	15	21
Garden Special	225	12	24
Pepperoni	265	16	22
Sausage	285	17	22
Six Cheese	375	24	23
Spinach Alfredo	295	17	20
The Works	320	20	24
Sides: Bread Stick (1)	140	2	26
Cheese Sticks (2)	180	8	20
Cheese Sauce, 1 oz	60	5	0
Chickenstrips (1)	85	4	5
Cinnapie, 1 stick	115	6	14
Garlic Sauce, 1 oz	235	26	0
Pizza Sauce, 1 oz	25	2	3

Papa Murphy's®

	C	F	Cb
Pizza: Per Slice			
Deeper Dish: Traditional, 1/8 Pizza	445	24	34
Gourmet: Per Slice (1/12 Family Pizza)			
Chicken Garlic	325	15	30
Classic Italian	365	19	30
Gourmet Veggie	310	14	31
Calzones (1/8 Family): Combo	450	20	45
Italian	485	23	46
Veggie	415	17	46
Papa's (1/12 Family Pizza): All Meat	375	19	31
Cheese	260	10	29
Cowboy	365	19	31
Hawaiian	300	11	34
Murphy's Combo; Papa's Fav.	380	20	32
Pepperoni	315	15	29
Perfect; Veggie Combo	310	13	32
Rancher	330	15	31
Specialty	345	17	31

Papa Murphy's® cont...

	C	F	Cb
Stuffed (1/16 Family): Big Murphy	380	17	39
Chicken & Bacon; Chicago	370	16	38
Salads: Per Container (No Dressing)			
Chicken & Bacon	380	23	9
Italian	265	21	6
Veggie	140	8	7
Cheesy Bread (2)	185	7	23

Penn Station

	C	F	Cb
Litesize Subs: Artichoke	260	7	37
Cheese Bread	255	6	42
Chicken Salad	360	15	41
Chicken Teriyaki	435	13	48
Grilled Vegetarian	255	4	46
Ham Dagwood	265	7	35
Philadelphia Chsesteak, no mayo	400	14	45
Reuben	390	12	37
Tuna Salad	360	16	41
Turkey Dagwood	250	4	35

Perkin's® Family Restaurant

	C	F	Cb
Entrees: Chicken Dinner	620	13	60
Fish Dinner	470	7	60
Fruit Cup	50	0.5	12
'Lite & Healthy'	105	2	15
Omelettes: Country Club	930	79	6
Deli Ham & Cheese	960	79	8
'Everything' Omelette	695	54	9
Granny's Country Omelette	940	82	7
w. 9 oz Hash Browns	1245	90	57
Salads: Chef's, Mini	215	11	7
Muffins: Blueberry	585	26	78
Bran Muffin	560	16	94
Carrot	495	26	55
Chocolate Chips	470	26	81
Pumpkin	625	26	78
Raspberry & Cream	600	26	81
Pancakes: Buttermilk, (3)	440	12	70
Harvest Grain: w. Low-Cal Syrup (5)	475	3.5	93
Short Stack (3)	270	2	56
Pies Per Slice: Apple Pie	520	26	72
Cherry Pie	570	24	84
Coconut Cream Pie	440	21	56
French Silk Pie	550	34	59
Lemon Meringue Pie	395	15	63
Peanut Butter Brownie	455	27	44

228

Restaurants & Fast−Foods

Petro's®

Petros:	C	F	Cb
Pee Wee Petro, avg.	290	16	25
Small Petro: Original	520	30	43
Chicken	470	24	43
Medium Petro: Original	740	43	58
Chicken	670	36	59
Veggie	750	41	70
Large Petro: Original	1080	63	87
Chicken	970	52	88
Veggie	1090	60	105
Lite Petro: Small	380	12	48
Medium	530	16	66
Large	790	24	99
Pasta Petro: Small	410	17	46
Medium	630	27	68
Large	850	37	91
Lite Pasta Petro: Small	335	2.5	52
Medium	495	3.5	80
Large	680	4.5	108
Chili: Per Serving			
Chicken: Medium	275	4	43
Original: Medium	370	14	42
Veggie: Medium	385	11	58
Baked Potatoes			
#1 Lite	365	0.5	74
#2 Butter Sour Cream	480	18	74
#3 Loaded	680	33	78
#4 Loaded w. Chili	780	37	90
#5 Broccoli 3 Cheese	655	30	77
Hot Dogs: Chili	315	17	28
Chili/Cheese; Loaded	350	19	30
Plain	265	14	22
Slaw	350	16	23
Tostitos™ Chips: Queso	500	27	60
Ransalsa	560	35	61
Salsa	415	18	62
Loaded Tostitos™:			
Ultimate Nachos	880	51	79
Petro Salads: Original	570	36	42
Grilled Chicken	740	41	42
Garden Salads: Small	45	0.5	8
Large	85	1	16

Peter Piper® Pizza

	C	F	Cb
Cheese Pizza: Personal Slice	110	3.5	13
Personal Pizza (7")	430	14	51
Small Pizza (10"), 1/6 pizza	160	5	19
Whole Pizza	960	31	114
Medium Pizza (12"), 1/8 pizza	175	5.5	20
Whole Pizza	1385	45	164
Large Pizza (14"), 1/8 pizza	235	8	28
Whole Pizza	1885	61	223
Extra Large Pizza (16"), 1/12 pizza	205	6.5	24
Whole Pizza	2460	79	291
Pepperoni Pizza: Per Slice			
Personal Slice	150	6.5	15
Personal Pizza (7")	600	25	60
Small Pizza (10"), 1/6 pizza	185	8	18
Whole Pizza	425	47	111
Medium Pizza (12"), 1/8 pizza	200	8.5	20
Whole Pizza	1600	68	160
Large Pizza (14"), 1/8 pizza	270	12	27
Whole Pizza	2180	92	218
Extra Large Pizza (16"), 1/12 pizza	235	10	24
Sides: Chicken Wings (4)	210	16	1
Breadsticks (1)	120	4.5	17

For Complete Nutritional Data ~ see CalorieKing.com

P F Chang's®

	C	F	Cb
Beef: Mongolian	360	20	17
Orange Peel	450	25	43
a la Szechwan, 1/3 dish	265	7	33
w. Broccoli	230	12	17
Buddha's Feast: Steamed, 1/3 dish	60	0.5	10
Stir Fried	105	3	13
Chicken & Duck: Crispy Honey	375	19	31
Almond Cashew, 1/3 dish	215	13	10
Cantonese Chicken	255	13	12
Cantonese Duck	255	12	18
Chang's Spicy Chicken	330	14	33
Chef Roy's Favorite	185	9	10
Chow Mein, 1/4 dish	207	7	24
Kung Pao, 1/2 dish	355	18	16
Malaysian, 1/4 dish	180	10	10
Moo Goo Gai Pan	125	5	6
Mu Shu	235	13	19
Orange Peel	340	16	28
Philip's Better Lemon Chkn, 1/4 dish	265	11	24
Spicy Ground Chicken w. Eggplant	220	15	13
Szechwan Chkn Chow Fun, 1/4 dish	290	21	16
w. Black Bean Sauce, 1/3 dish	220	10	12

229

P F Chang's® cont...

	C	F	Cb
Dumplings: Peking (1)	165	9	11
Shrimp (1)	115	4	11
Vegetable (1)	105	1.5	18
Pork: Mu Shu, ¼ dish	245	11	27
Cantonese Pork Medallions (1)	195	4.5	18
Sweet & Sour, ¼ dish	315	21	23
Rice & Noodles: Fried Rice, ⅙ dish	285	13	33
Combo Dble Pan Fried Ndles, ⅙ dish	190	7	22
Dan-Dan Noodles, ⅙ dish	205	7	25
Garlic Noodles, ⅓ dish	250	11	30
Singapore Ndles w. Curry, ⅓ dish	210	9	27
Salad: Ahi Tuna	120	6	5
Cantonese BBQ Chicken, ¼ dish	250	12	17
Cold Cucumber, ½ dish	55	3	3
Oriental Chicken	220	14	14
Peanut-Lime Chicken	220	14	6
Seafood: Crab Wonton (1)	290	16	26
Hot Fish	200	10	15
Lemon Scallops, ⅓ dish	230	8	24
Szechwan from the Sea, ⅓ dish	230	8	19
Paul's Catfish	260	15	6
Salt & Pepper Calamari	320	19	21
Seared Ahi Tuna, ½ dish	125	2.5	1
Shrimp: Crispy Honey, ½ dish	395	24	25
Lemon Pepper, ⅓ dish	190	10	13
Orange Peel, ⅓ dish	265	11	26
Treasures of the Sea:			
w. Shrimp, ⅓ dish	140	7	5
w. Lobster Sauce, ⅓ dish	160	11	5
Vegetables: Coconut Curry	170	11	12
Garlic Snap Peas	260	2	55
Poached Baby Bok Choy	75	1	13
Shanghai Snow Peas, ½ dish	95	2	15
Spinach w. Garlic, serving	120	10	3
Stir-Fried Spicy Eggplant, ⅓ dish	225	16	18
Szechwan Asparagus, ½ dish	165	11	12
Szechwan Long Beans, ⅓ dish	190	8	23
Temple Long Beans, ⅓ dish	155	7	12
Vegetable Chow Fun	180	5	30
Vegetarian: Ma Po Tofu, ¼ dish	180	10	12
Wraps: Per Serving (⅓ Dish)			
Chang's Vege in Lettuce Wraps	175	9	15
Minced Chkn & Cool Lettuce Wraps	180	9	15
Extras: Scallion Pancakes, ⅓ dish	185	9	21
Soup: Hot & Sour	80	6	3
Wonton	70	4	5
Harvest Spring Rolls, ½ roll	170	12	14

For Complete Nutritional Data ~ see CalorieKing.com

Pick-Up-Stix®

	C	F	Cb
California Rolls	200	8	27
Beef Dishes: Beef and Broccoli	510	27	37
House Special	875	27	48
Mongolian	350	20	20
Szechwan	340	20	20
Bowls			
Teriyaki Chicken	1155	22	148
Teriyaki Vegetable	450	1.5	96
Buddah's Feast: Dark	105	0.5	16
Light	80	0.5	16
Chicken Dishes: (Per Cup): Cashew	360	16	33
Garlic	285	12	24
House	755	34	58
Kung Pao	440	22	33
Lemon Twisted	260	3	37
Orange Peel	535	15	76
Sweet n Sour	475	22	60
w. Vegetables	195	3	20
Chow Mein: Per Cup			
Beef	350	10	50
Chicken	355	9	52
House Special	360	9	52
Shrimp	310	5.5	51
Vegetable	270	3.5	49
Fried Rice (Per Cup): Beef	505	16	68
Chicken	475	13	70
Egg	420	8	74
House	480	14	69
Shrimp	430	10	68
Vegetable	390	8	67
Rice: White, 1 cup	205	0.5	45
Salad: Per Serving			
Chicken Salad w/out Dressing	470	20	35
Chinese Chicken Salad			
w. Lime Dressing	675	20	35
Chinese Chicken Salad			
w. Original Dressing	650	22	75
Shrimp: Per Cup			
Black Bean	190	5	23
Garlic	185	5	23
Orange Peel	310	5	54
Szechwan	180	5	21
w/Vegetables	170	5	19
Soup: Per 2 Cup Bowl			
Hot & Sour	290	5	38
Wonton	290	13	27
Vegetables: Szechwan, 1 cup	105	1	21

Restaurants & Fast−Foods

Pizza Hut®

Fit 'N Delicious: Per Slice, (1/8 Medium Pizza)

	C	F	Cb
Diced Chkn, Red On, Green Pep.	170	4.5	23
Diced Chkn, Mushroom, Jalapeno	170	5	22
Ham, Red Onion, Mushroom	160	4.5	22
Ham, Pineapple, Diced Red Tom.	160	4	24
Green Pepper, Red On., Diced Tom.	150	4	24
Tomato, Mushroom, Jalapeno	150	4	22

Pan Pizza: Per Slice (1/8 Medium Pizza)

	C	F	Cb
Cheese	280	13	29
Chicken Supreme	280	12	30
Ham	260	11	29
Sausage Lover's®	330	17	29
Meat Lover's®	340	19	29
Pepperoni	290	15	29
Pepperoni Lover's®	340	19	29
Super Supreme	340	18	30
Supreme	320	16	30
Veggie Lover's®	260	12	30

Personal Pan Pizza: Per Pizza

	C	F	Cb
Cheese	640	28	72
Ham	600	24	72
Pepperoni	680	32	72
Sausage Lover's®	760	40	72
Supreme	760	36	76
Veggie Lover's®	600	24	76

Stuffed Crust: Per Slice (1/12 Large Pizza)

	C	F	Cb
Cheese	360	16	43
Chicken Supreme	380	13	44
Ham	340	11	42
Sausage Lover's®	430	19	43
Meat Lover's	450	21	43
Pepperoni	370	15	42
Pepperoni Lover's®	420	19	43
Super Supreme	440	20	45
Supreme	400	16	44
Veggie Lover's®	360	14	45

Stuffed Crust Gold: Per Slice (1/12 Large Pizza)

	C	F	Cb
Beef Topping	490	24	44
Cheese	440	20	44
Chicken Supreme	440	18	45
Diced Chicken	440	18	44
Ham	410	17	43
Italian Sausage	515	27	44
Meat Lover's®	430	20	43
Pepperoni Lover's®	500	25	44
Pork Topping	495	25	44
Sausage Lover's®	515	27	44
Super Supreme	520	26	46
Supreme	490	24	45
Veggie Lover's®	420	18	46

Thin 'n Crispy: Per Slice (1/8 Medium Pizza)

	C	F	Cb
Cheese	200	8	21
Chicken Supreme	200	7	22
Ham	180	6	21
Sausage Lover's®	240	13	21
Meat Lover's®	270	14	21
Pepperoni	210	10	21
Pepperoni Lover's®	260	14	21
Super Supreme	260	13	23
Supreme	240	11	22
Veggie Lover's®	180	7	23

Hand Tossed: Per Slice, (1/8 Medium Pizza)

	C	F	Cb
Cheese	240	8	30
Chicken Supreme	230	6	30
Ham	220	6	29
Sausage Lover's®	280	12	30
Meat Lover's®	300	13	29
Pepperoni	250	9	29
Pepperoni Lover's®	300	13	30
Super Supreme	300	13	31
Supreme	270	11	30
Veggie Lover's®	220	6	31

P'zone Pizza: Per 1/2 Pizza

	C	F	Cb
Classic	605	21	71
Meat Lover's®	685	28	70
Pepperoni	610	22	69

The Big New Yorker™: Per Serving (1/8 Pizza)

	C	F	Cb
Beef Topping	520	26	47
Cheese	425	18	46
Ham	385	14	46
Italian Sausage	545	29	47
Pepperoni	410	17	46
Pork Topping	510	25	47
Supreme	490	23	48
Veggie Lover's®	500	22	57

The Chicago Dish™: Per Slice

	C	F	Cb
Meat Lover's®	465	27	35
Pepperoni	390	20	34
Pepperoni, Italian Sausage & Mushroom	415	22	35
Supreme	430	23	36
Veggie Lover's®	375	18	36

Pizza Hut® cont...

The Insider: Per Slice (⅛ Medium Pizza)	**C**	**F**	**Cb**
Cheese Pizza	365	17	35
Pepperoni Pizza	360	17	35
Supreme Pizza	415	21	36
Twisted Crust: Cheese	455	16	58
Pepperoni	440	15	58
Supreme	480	18	59
Ultimate Lovers Big New Yorker: Per Slice			
Cheese/Pepperoni Lover's®	470	22	47
Meat Lover's®	580	33	47
Veggie Lover's®	400	16	50
Ultimate Lovers Hand Tossed: Per Slice			
Cheese Lover's®	280	13	28
Meat Lover's®	330	17	28
Pepperoni Lover's®	290	14	28
Veggie Lover's®	230	8	30
Ultimate Lovers Pan: Per Slice			
Meat Lover's®	370	22	29
Cheese Lover's®	330	17	29
Pepperoni Lover's®	300	16	29
Veggie Lover's®	270	12	30
Ultimate Lovers Personal Pan: Per Slice			
Cheese Lover's®	740	35	72
Meat Lover's®	840	45	72
Pepperoni Lover's®	780	39	72
Veggie Lover's®	610	24	75
Ultimate Lovers Stuffed Crust: Per Slice			
Cheese Lover's®	400	19	41
Meat Lover's®	470	26	41
Pepperoni Lover's®	430	22	40
Veggie Lover's®	350	15	42
Ultimate Lovers Thin 'n Crispy: Per Slice			
Veggie Lover's®	200	8	24
Cheese/Pepperoni Lover's®	250	12	28
Meat Lover's®	330	17	28
Sandwiches: Ham & Cheese	550	21	57
Supreme	635	28	62
Dessert Pizza: Apple Dessert	260	3.5	53
Cherry Dessert Pizza	240	3.5	47
Pasta: Cavatini Pasta	475	14	66
Cavatini Supreme Pasta	560	19	73
Spaghetti: w. Marinara	490	6	91
w. Meat Sauce	600	13	98
Meatballs	845	24	120
Sides: Breadsticks, 1.3 oz	150	6	20
Buffalo Wings, Hot (1)	55	3	1
Buffalo Wings, Mild (1)	40	2.5	0
Wing Ranch Dipping Sauce, 1½ oz	210	22	4
Garlic Bread, slice	150	8	16

Pizza Pizza (Canada)

Pizza: Per Slice (⅛ Pizza)	**C**	**F**	**Cb**
Large: BBQ Chicken	240	5	37
Bacon Bonanza/ Dble Chseburger	250	9	32
Canadian	260	9	33
Extreme Cheese	245	7	35
Four Seasons	265	9	37
Four Seasons, no Cheese	170	5	25
Hawaiian	260	7	38
Mediterranean Vegetable	235	7	35
Montreal Smoked Meat	220	5	33
Pepperoni & Mushroom	230	6	33
Sicilian	260	8	34
Super	230	6	33
Vegetarian	215	5	37
Medium Pizza: *Per Slice*			
Deduct 10% fewer calories/fat/carbs from figures for large pizza			
Extra Large Pizza: *Per Slice*			
Add 10% more calories/fat/carbs from figures for large pizza			
Slices: Average all types, 1 slice	800	22	115
vetarian; Big Cheese, 1 slice	700	14	110
Stuffed S'wiches: Avg. all types	360	10	52
Oven Toasted Sandwiches			
BBQ Chicken	470	12	58
no Cheese	280	4.5	58
Deli Classic	560	24	55
Honey Mustard Club	490	15	48
Meatball	550	23	56
Mediterranean Vegetable	440	18	53
Roast Beef Supreme	440	14	53
Chicken Items			
Chicken Wings (6), 200g	420	2.5	28
Dino/Chicken Nuggets (6), 125g	320	29	22
Chicken Strips (4), 170g	350	27	23
X-treme Chicken Sandwich	470	44	18
Fries: Regular, 5 oz	340	47	15
Large, 7 oz	470	66	20
Garlic Stix: Regular (3)	390	13	54
X-treme Cheese (3) w. 1 oz cheese	480	21	54
Garlic Bread: Regular bun	710	38	74
X-treme with Cheese	880	52	74
Drinks			
Crispy Crunch Milkshake, 350mL	350	11	50
Limpton's Brisk, 355mL	135	0	34
Gatorade Orange/Blue Raspb. 500mL	130	0	32
Mountain Dew Code Red, 600mL	320	0	70
Mug Root Beer, 355mL	160	0	39
Orange Crush, 355mL	180	0	45
7-UP, 355mL	140	0	35

Pizzeria Uno® | | C | F | Cb |

	C	F	Cb
Entrees: Veggie Burger Meal	610	15	104
Tomato Basil Chicken	570	8	83
Zesty Pasta Marinara	380	3.5	75
Thin Crust Pizza: 9" Individual			
Vegetarian: w. Cheese	850	22	127
No Cheese	620	5	124
Soup: Light Lunch w. Soup	745	6	150
Tomato Garden Vegetable	125	1	25
Salads: Special House	90	1	17
Light Lunch w. Salad	710	6	141
Pasta Green Salad	410	9	69
Veggie Dip Platter	460	11	77

Pollo Tropical®

	C	F	Cb
Grilled Chicken: 1/4 Chicken White	295	14	1
1/4 White no Skin, 4 oz	170	3	0
1/4 Chicken Dark, 4.5 oz	300	18	0.5
1/4 Dark no Skin, 3.5 oz	170	7	1
Bananas Tropical, 7 oz	500	13	90
Black Beans (combo portion), 5 oz	150	2	24
Black Beans, side, 8.5 oz	270	4	43
Boiled Yucs, 12 oz	330	0	81
Boneless Breast, 5 oz	140	4	1
Chicken Caesar S'wich, 6.5 oz	460	10	36
Chicken Sandwich, 8 oz	440	19	35
Chicken TropiChop	560	10	20
Congri, 7 oz	440	13	69
Corn, 3 oz	140	1.5	34
Grilled Chicken Salad (No Dressing)	210	4	na
Grilled Tropical Shrimp, 1 Skewer	90	1	0
Island Park, 5 oz	210	10	1
White Rice, 7 oz	340	6	65
Yucatan Fries, 5.3 oz	440	24	54

Popeye's®

	C	F	Cb
Chicken: Chkn Breast, Mild/Spicy	530	31	18
Chicken Leg, Mild/Spicy	200	12	7
Chicken Thigh, Mild/Spicy	390	29	12
Chicken Wing, Mild/Spicy	220	15	10
Sides: Biscuit, 2 oz	225	12	25
Cajun Rice	180	7	23
Cinnamon Apple Pie, 3 oz	250	10	37
Coleslaw	235	17	20
Corn on the Cob	255	4	48
French Fries, 4.5 oz	380	18	50
Mashed Potatoes: no Gravy	95	2	17
w. Gravy	120	4	18
Onion Rings, 4 oz	380	20	43
Red Beans & Rice	340	19	33

Port of Subs®

	C	F	Cb
Original Submarines: Per 5" White or Wheat Roll			
No Mayonnaise included in figures below.			
If using mayo, add 1 Tbsp	110	12	0
BLT	400	19	43
Combination of Cheeses	495	25	44
Ham w. American Cheese	475	20	45
Ham & Salami/Turkey w. Provolone	425	15	47
Ham/Salami/Capicolla/Pepp./Prov.	525	26	45
Peppered Pastrami w. Swiss	415	17	44
Roast Beef Turkey w. Provolone	410	14	45
Rstd Chicken Breast w. Provolone	395	13	45
Salami w. Provolone	495	25	45
Salami & Pepperoni w. Provolone	525	27	45
Salami & Turkey w. Provolone	455	20	46
Smkd Ham & Turkey w. Smky Ched.	425	15	47
Smoked Ham w. Swiss	415	16	45
Tuna	420	18	45
Turkey w. Provolone	415	14	45
Vegetarian w. Avoc. & Olives, no chse	350	14	48
Hot Sandwiches: Per 8" White or Wheat Roll			
BBQ Beef	560	6	87
Hot Pastrami	570	17	62
Meatball	645	25	76
Mesquite Chicken	545	11	68
Western Philly Cheese Steak	505	9	78
Breakfast Sandwiches: Per 4" Sub			
Egg & Smoked Ham w. Cheese	250	16	4
Soups, Medium Bowl: Minestrone	50	1	8
Boston Clam Chowder	105	4	13
Broccoli Cheese	125	6	13
Roasted Chicken Noodle	80	2	9
Salads: Includes Vinegar & Oil Unless Indicated			
Antipasto, 12 oz	405	29	14
Chef, 12 oz	395	26	14
Green, 12 oz	125	7	13
Macaroni, no oil, 8 oz	440	30	36
Mesquite Chicken	315	13	16
Potato, no oil, 8 oz	465	26	54
Tuna, 11 oz	280	16	13

Pret A Manager

	C	F	Cb
Bakery: Per Serving			
Almond Croissant	320	22	25
Ham, Cheese & Tomato	400	22	32
Muffin, Seville Orange	470	22	61
Pretzel	370	8	62
Cakes & Slices: Per Serving			
Carrot Cake	380	19	48
Elephant Poo	110	4	17
Pet Brownie	330	17	40
Slice, Orange & Fruit	340	16	45

Fast-Foods & *Restaurants*

Pret A Manager cont...

	C	F	Cb
Sandwiches: Big BLT	540	25	52
Chicken Avocado w. Half Fat Mayo	480	25	38
Smoked Salmon	370	14	50
Super Club	540	25	47
Vegetarian	345	3.5	71
Sushi: Deluxe Sushi	490	8.5	89
Wraps: Avocado	540	37	40
Green Thai Chicken	325	12	34.5
Salads: Noodle & Chicken	295	5	43
Roast Vegetable	60	3.5	6.5
Drinks: Per Serving			
Cappuccino	110	6	8
Cappuccino w. Chocolate	105	6	7.5
Cappuccino, no Chocolate	100	6	7
Hot Chocolate	310	12	39
Latte	195	11	13
Lemon Crush	120	0	30
Lemon Pret Cool	120	0	30
Mango Yogurt	195	6.5	23
Strawberry Lemonade	100	0.5	24
Vanilla Yogurt	230	7	32

Quizno's Subs®

Lowfat Sandwiches: Per Small Sandwich			
Honey Bourbon Chicken	330	6	45
Sierra Smoked Turkey			
w. Raspberry Chipotle Sauce	360	6	53
Turkey Lite	360	6	52
Tuscan Chicken Salad	325	6.5	45
Veggie Lite	300	6	40

Quincy's®

	C	F	Cb
Steak: Chopped, 8 oz	500	42	0
Country Style Steak w. Gravy	530	25	44
Cowboy Steak, 14 oz	580	33	9
Filet w. Bacon	340	17	2
N.Y.Strip Steak, 10 oz	450	26	1
Porterhouse Steak	680	46	0
Ribeye, 10 oz	450	29	0
Sirloin: Large	370	20	2
Regular	285	16	0
Sirloin Junior	195	10	0
Sirloin Tips	205	8	4
Smothered Strip Steak	620	41	12
T-Bone, 13 oz	520	35	0
Soups: Chili with Beans	235	11	21
Clam Chowder	180	9	21
Cream of Broccoli	170	10	18
Vegetable Beef	90	2	14

Quincy's cont...

	C	F	Cb
Entrees: Grilled Chicken	125	2	1
Homestyle Chicken Filet	220	9	21
Grilled Salmon	230	4	1
Sth Breaded Shrimp	545	31	47
Steak & Shrimp	680	39	33
Roasted Herb Chicken	875	65	4
Roasted BBQ Chicken	940	65	21
Grilled Trout	300	12	2
Sandwiches: No Mayo/Extras			
Bacon Cheeseburger	665	41	33
Grilled Chicken Sandwich	325	4	39
Philly Cheese Steak	590	30	38
Smothered Steak	430	15	36
Spicy BBQ Chicken	370	5	45
Breads: Banana Nut	165	7	22
Biscuit	270	15	29
Cornbread	140	5	17
Yeast Roll	160	4	29
Sides: Baked Potatoes	370	0	86
Corn on the Cob	140	1	33
Rice Pilaf	105	2	20
Desserts: Banana Pudding	240	12	30
Brownie Pudding Cake	310	5	66
Chocolate Chip Cookie	60	3	8
Apple Cobbler	255	8	49
Cherry Cobbler; Peach Cobbler	310	8	55
Frozen Yogurt	135	2	25
Sugar Cookie	60	3	8
Fudge Topping; Caramel	105	4	15

Rally's Hamburgers®

Burgers/Sandwiches			
Rallyburger	435	22	35
with Cheese	490	27	35
Big Buford	745	48	35
Chicken Fillet Sandwich	400	15	43
Chili w. Cheese & Onion: 7 oz	360	22	20
13 oz size	670	41	37
Super Barbecue Bacon	595	31	49
Super Double Cheeseburger	760	48	37
French Fries: Regular	210	11	26
Large	320	16	39
X-Large	425	21	52
Shakes: Vanilla, small	320	11	49
Other flavors, small	410	12	73

Restaurants & Fast–Foods

Ranch 1®

	C	F	Cb
Salads: Gourmet Greens, 12½ oz	220	7	31
Chicken on Gourmet Greens, 15 oz	350	11	31
Zesty Caesar Salad, 7 oz	180	3	31
Zesty Chicken Caesar Salad, 9 oz	290	6	31
Sandwiches: American Ranche	390	10	51
Club Sandwich	470	16	53
Grilled Chicken Philly	450	14	53
Ranch Classic	370	5	53
Spicy Grilled Chicken	420	11	58
Side Kicks: Fruit Cup, 8.3 oz	90	0.5	18
Ranch Fries, regular	350	14	51
Specialties: Chicken Tenders	370	15	7
Baked Potato: w. Broccoli	510	0.5	117
w. Cheese	790	25	118
w. Chicken	610	4	114
Grilled Chkn & Vegetable Platter	790	7	129
Grilled Chicken Fajita	330	16	25
Grilled Chicken Hot Pasta	590	10	86

Rax®

	C	F	Cb
Sandwiches: Regular Rax	390	22	31
Deluxe	520	35	34
BBC	715	51	36
Grilled Chicken: Philly Melt	530	33	33
Jr. Deluxe	365	25	25
BBQ Beef	400	20	43
Mushroom Melt	600	37	35
Turk/Bacon Club	680	46	37
Turkey	485	32	32
Cheddar Melt	345	23	26
Potatoes: Plain	205	0	60
w. Butter	305	11	60
w. Sour Topping	255	4	62
Cheese/Broccoli	280	0	71
Soups: Cream of Broccoli	95	4	14
Chicken Noodle	115	1	20
Chili	160	9	11
Salads: Grilled Chicken	160	5	6
Side Salad	40	4	2
Garden	220	9	12
Salad Dressings: Fat Free Italian	10	0	2
Fat Free Catalina; Ranch	30	0	6
1000 Island	130	13	5
Buttermilk Ranch	175	20	1
Blue Cheese; Creamy Caesar	145	16	1
Honey French	140	5	9
Vinaigrette	30	2	4

Rita's®

	C	F	Cb
Cream Ice: Per Serving			
Kids	205	3	45
Regular	330	4.5	72
Large	520	7	115
Quart	880	12	194
Gelati: Regular	320	10	56
Regular w. Cream Ice	345	12	59
Large	545	17	95
Large w. Cream Ice	590	21	101
Italian Ice: Kids	170	0	45
Regular	275	0	73
Large	435	0	115
Quart	735	0	195
Misto: Regular	415	7	90
Regular w. Cream Ice	465	11	88
Large	620	10	135
Large w. Cream Ice	695	17	132
Frozen Custard: Kids	275	14	31
Regular	370	20	42
Large	535	28	60

Rocky Rococo®

	C	F	Cb
Pizza: Per Regular Slice			
Cheese, 5.75 oz	380	9	54
Sausage, 7 oz	495	19	54
Pepperoni, 6.1 oz	430	13	54
Sausage & Mushroom, 7.6 oz	500	19	55
Garden of Eatin', 7.6 oz	390	10	56
Pizza: Per Super Slice			
Average all types	700	27	82
Pasta: Per Serving			
Spaghetti: w. Tomato Sauce, reg.	470	4	87
w. Meat Sce, regular	500	7	87
w. Meatballs, regular	630	16	89
Light Spaghetti: w. Tomato Sauce	235	2	44
w. Meat Sauce, regular	315	8	45
w. Meatballs, regular	250	3	44
Fettuccine: w. Alfredo, regular	460	14	66
Light w. Alfredo Sauce	230	4	33
Can't Decide, 14 oz	465	9	77
Bread: Muffin (1)	200	4	38
Breadsticks (6) w. Marinara Sce	420	7	72
Breadsticks (6) w. Jalapeno Chse	530	18	72

235

Round Table® Pizza

Large Pizza (14"): *Per Slice (1/12 Whole)*	C	F	Cb
Cheese: Thin	210	8	23
Pan	290	10	37
Chicken & Garlic Gourmet™			
Thin	230	9	24
Pan	320	11	38
Chicken Rostadoro™: Thin	250	10	25
Pan	330	12	39
Gourmet Veggie™: Thin	220	9	25
Pan	310	11	39
Guinevere's Garden Delight®:			
Thin	210	7	25
Pan	290	9	38
Hawaiian: Thin	210	7	25
Pan	290	9	38
Hearty Bacon Supreme™: Thin	270	14	22
Pan	360	16	36
Italian Garlic Supreme™: Thin	270	14	23
Pan	360	16	37
King Arthur's Supreme®: Thin	270	14	24
Pan	340	14	38
Maui Zaui™ (Polynesian Sce):			
Thin	240	9	27
Pan	330	11	41
Maui Zaui™ (Red Sce): Thin	240	9	25
Pan	320	11	39
Montague's All Meat Marvel®:			
Thin	290	17	24
Pan	350	16	37
Pepperoni: Thin	240	11	23
Pan	310	12	37
Pepperoni Rostadoro™: Thin	270	12	26
Pan	350	14	40
Roastin' Toastin'™ Chicken Club:			
Thin	260	12	25
Pan	350	14	39
Western BBQ Chicken™: Thin	240	9	23
Pan	320	11	37

16" Pizzas: *Per Slice (1/8 Whole)*			
Aloha Vinnie Pepperoni™	430	14	55
Big Vinnie Pepperoni™	460	19	49
Maui Mama (Polynesian Sce)	570	22	63
Maui Mama (Red Sce)	560	22	61
Mama Zella Pizza	550	23	59

Personal Pizzas: *Per Pizza*	C	F	Cb
Cheese: Thin	580	24	60
Pan	810	36	106
Chicken & Garlic Gourmet™:			
Thin	620	25	64
Pan	850	27	110
Chicken Rostadoro™: Thin	680	29	66
Pan	910	31	112
Hawaiian: Thin	560	19	66
Pan	780	21	109
Gourmet Veggie™: Thin	590	23	67
Pan	820	25	114
Guinevere's Garden Delight®:			
Thin	550	20	66
Pan	760	21	110
Hearty Bacon Supreme™: Thin	700	35	59
Pan	940	37	105
Italian Garlic Supreme™: Thin	760	41	63
Pan	990	43	109
King Arthur's Supreme®: Thin	750	39	64
Pan	900	34	109
Maui Zaui™ (Polynesian Sce): Thin	620	23	71
Pan	850	25	117
Maui Zaui™ (Red Sce): Thin	590	22	66
Pan	820	24	111
Montague's All Meat Marvel®:			
Thin	780	44	61
Pan	1010	46	107
Pepperoni: Thin	640	31	60
Pan	840	29	106
Pepperoni Rostadoro™: Thin	740	35	70
Pan	970	37	116
Roastin' Toastin'™ Chicken Club:			
Thin	710	33	66
Pan	940	35	112
Western BBQ Chicken™: Thin	610	23	61
Pan	840	25	107

Sides/Sandwiches			
Garlic Bread	470	21	59
w. Cheese	630	33	59
Garlic Parmesan Twists, 3 pce	510	14	76
Buffalo Wings, 3 pce	210	14	1
6 pce	420	28	2
Honey BBQ Wings, 3 pce	190	13	4
6 pce	390	25	8
Sandwiches: Chicken Club	820	39	75
Ham Club	810	37	76
RT Pizza	690	34	65
RT Veggie	680	29	79
Turkey Club	800	37	75

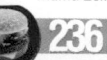

Roy Rogers®

Breakfast Items:	C	F	Cb
Big Country Breakfast: w. Bacon	740	43	61
w. Sausage	920	60	61
w. Ham	710	39	67
Burgers:			
Hamburger	260	9	33
Cheeseburger	300	13	34
1/4 lb Hamburger	430	18	41
1/4 lb Cheeseburger	470	22	42
Sourdough Grilled Chicken	500	21	46
Sandwiches: Roast Beef	260	4	30
Chicken Fillet	500	24	49
Grilled Chicken	340	11	32
Fries: Regular	350	15	49
Large	430	18	59
Desserts: Hot Fudge Sundae	320	10	50

Rubio's Baja Grill®

HealthMex®
All HealthMex® items have less than 20% of calories from fat.

	C	F	Cb
Bean & Cheese	830	37	88
Burrito w. Chicken	530	11	78
Burrito w. Grilled Fish	550	11	77
Salad	180	3	17
Taco with Chicken	170	2.5	23
Taco with Grilled Fish	180	3	24
Veggie	470	8	83
Health Mex® Rice	110	2	21
Tacos			
Carne Asada	250	10	24
Fish Taco	300	16	28
Fish Taco Especial	370	21	30
Grilled Chicken	290	15	24
Grilled Fish	300	15	24
Street Tacos	110	5	14
Quesadillas: Cheese	840	53	55
Grilled Chicken	940	56	56
Carne Asada	990	62	57
Shrimp; Lobster	900	55	56
Burritos			
Baja Carne Asada	690	34	58
Baja Chicken	620	26	56
Especial: Carne Asada	830	40	58
Chicken, Pinto/Black	880	33	111
Carnitas, Pinto/Black	950	38	113

Rubio's® cont...

Burritos (Cont)	C	F	Cb
Fish	830	42	85
Lobster	720	27	89
Mahi	710	34	56
Shrimp	690	27	84
Burritos Chips	210	11	28
Los Otros: Chips	430	22	56
Nachos Grande	1270	78	111
w. Carne Asada	1420	87	113
w. Chicken	1370	81	112
In-Combo Chips & Beans, avg.	480	21	68
Chips	520	27	68
Pinto Beans	220	3	44
Rice	260	3.5	48
Taquitos (3)	330	13	37
Guacamole: Small	190	17	8
Large	370	34	16
Enchiladas:			
Cheese (1)	380	21	27
Chicken (1)	330	15	26
Add Rice, 2 oz	80	1	14
Salads/Bowls: Per Serving			
Grande Asada Black Bowl	770	42	70
Grande Asada Pinto Bowl	750	37	70
Grilled Chicken Chopped Salad	540	33	33
Bowls: Chicken Chipotle Bowl	780	35	76
Chicken Enchilada Bowl	830	32	78
Asada Enchilada Bowl	850	37	78
Grilled Grande chix w. Pinto	700	32	69
Grilled Grande chix w. Bl. Beans	710	31	69
Salsa: Regular, 1.5 oz	15	0	2
Verde, 1.5 oz	5	0	1
Picante, 1.5 oz	30	2	3
Roasted Chipotle, 1.5 oz	10	0	2
Kid Pesky® Meals: Taquitos (2)	240	10	22
Bean & Cheese Burrito	525	21	66
Cheese Quesadilla	360	19	30
Fish Taco	300	16	27
Add Beans	140	3	25
Add Chips	210	11	28
Add Rice	110	2	21
Churro, mini	90	4	12
Desserts: Churro	170	8	23
Zango	510	23	69

Note: Rubio's uses only skinless chicken breast & lean trimmed steak.
Canola oil is used – no lard or MSG.

Fast–Foods & *Restaurants*

Ryan's® Family Steakhouse   C   F   Cb

Mega Bar Buffet: *Per Serving*

	C	F	Cb
Baked Fish, 3.5 oz	75	1.5	1
Black Eyed Peas, 1/2 cup	90	0	17
Breaded Okra, 3/4 cup	90	0	19
Breaded Sweet Potato Nuggets (7)	125	3	22
Chicken Breast, 5.2 oz	230	5	0
Chicken Pot Pie, 3.5 oz	160	6	21
Chicken Salad, 1/3 cup	200	14	4
Chicken Tenders, 3 pieces	225	10	15
Clam Chowder, 8 oz	160	6	18
Corn, 3.5 oz	125	7	14
Crab Salad, 3.5 oz	160	10	10
Glazed Baby Carrots w. Salad, 1/2 cup	105	5	14
Lima Beans, 2/3 cup	120	2	21
Macaroni & Cheese, 8 oz	340	14	38
Marinated 7 Bean Salad, 1/3 cup	165	0	36
Mashed Potatoes, 3.5 oz	110	4.5	14
Meatloaf Patties, 3.5 oz	310	26	8
Mexican Style Beef Casserole, 8 oz	455	25	34
Nacho Cheese Sauce, 1/4 cup	80	5	7
Petite Sirloin, 4.2 oz	230	9.5	0
Pinto Beans, 3.5 oz	85	2	13
Pork Chops, 3.5 oz	235	15	0
Pork Ribs (1 rib)	245	15	5
Salmon, 7 oz	225	7	0
Seafood Pasta Salad, 3.5 oz	145	6	16
Sirloin Tips, Plain, 3.8 oz	190	7.5	0
Sliced Pot Roast w. Gravy, 8 oz	175	8	10
Stewed Tomatoes w. Okra, 3.5 oz	50	0	11
Swt Potato w. M'mallows, 3.5 oz	130	0	32
Taco Meat, 3.5 oz	170	10	8
Turkey Breast, 1.3 oz	60	2	1
Vegetable Beef Soup, 8 oz	100	1.5	17
Vegetable Lasagna, 8 oz	390	20	32
Dressing: Ranch, 3.5 oz	355	36	6
Golden Italian; Blue Cheese 1 oz	125	13	2
Ranch, Fat Free, 2 Tbsp.	45	0	11
Thousand Island, 3.5 oz	140	6	21

Bakery Bar Buffet: *Per Serving*

	C	F	Cb
Pies, average, 1/10 pie	280	8	48
Choc. Pudding, Sugar Free, 1/2 cup	95	5	12
Chocolate Soft Serve, 1/2 cup	125	4.5	19
Cobbler, avg. all varieties	290	12	42
Cookies: Raisin Oatmeal (1)	105	3.5	18
Sugar Free (2)	95	6	10
Avg. other varieties	120	6	16
Frozen Yogurt 1/2 cup	100	0	21

Runza®   C   F   Cb

Sandwiches

	C	F	Cb
Original Runza® Sandwich	545	20	66
Cheese Runza® Sandwich	605	25	68
BBQ Chicken Sandwich	370	11	36
Fish Sandwich	475	23	46
Polish Dog	405	26	25
Smothered Chicken Sandwich	280	9	25
Special Deluxe Chicken Sandwich	295	8.5	29
Kids-Size: Mini Corn Dogs	320	21	25
Chicken Nuggets	310	20	15
Runza® Sandwich	275	10	33
Hamburger	200	10	15

Hamburgers:

	C	F	Cb
Deluxe Hamburger	455	19	50
1/4 lb Hamburger	345	14	28
1/4 lb Cheeseburger	405	18	29
1/2 lb Double Hamburger	510	23	30
1/2 lb Double Cheeseburger	625	32	32
Bacon Cheeseburger Deluxe	515	28	30
Swiss Cheese Mushroom Burger	415	20	30

Onion Rings & Fries

	C	F	Cb
Fries: Regular, 3.3 oz	315	17	35
Large, 3.6 oz	345	19	39
Jumbo, 6.8 oz	640	35	72
Onion Rings: Regular, 4.3 oz	465	29	45
Large, 6.7 oz	715	44	69
Onion Ring Dip, 2 oz	90	6.5	4

Salads & Dressings

	C	F	Cb
Tossed Salad	90	4	4
Tossed Salad w. Chicken	210	8.5	5
Dressing: Ranch, 2.6 oz	290	30	4
Reduced Calorie Ranch, 2.6 oz	175	15	5
French, 2.6 oz	150	0	35
Lite Italian, 2.6 oz	40	1	5
Thousand Island, 2.6 oz	325	30	15

Soups: *Per Serving (9.5 oz)*

	C	F	Cb
Boston Clam Chowder	305	17	30
Broccoli Cheese	280	16	27
Cauliflower Cheese	315	19	30
Chicken Noodle	110	1	16
Homemade Chili	250	8	21
Potato w. Bacon	205	9	27
Vegetable Cheese Medley	250	16	19
Wisconsin Cheese	365	25	27

Desserts & Drinks

	C	F	Cb
Brownie w. Nuts	465	16	74
Vanilla Shake, regular	520	15	84
Oreo® Shake, regular	655	24	97
Pepsi®, medium, 12 fl.oz	160	0	40

7-Eleven®

Hot Dogs	C	F	Cb
1/4 Pound Big Bite Hot Dog	550	34	24
Hot Dog Bun only	120	1.5	22
1/3 Pound Biggest Big Bite	600	47	25
Cheeseburger Big Bite	530	35	25
Spicy Bite (Italian Sausage)	550	40	24
Burritos			
The Bomb (14 oz)	940	42	116
w. Green Chilies	910	42	114
Reynoldos Jumbo Burritos (10 oz):			
Beef & Bean	680	22	93
Beef & Potato	590	20	82
Red Hot Burrito	640	20	88
Green Burrito	710	26	93
Sandwiches (7-Eleven)			
Big Eats Deli Sandwiches:			
Chicken Salad, 7.3 oz	630	35	47
Classic Chicken Caesar, 8.3 oz	540	24	47
Hearty Ham, 8.3 oz	570	30	48
Roast Beef & Bacon, 8.5 oz	650	33	47
Smoked Turkey w. Chse/Mayo	560	27	45
Stacked Turkey & Ham, 7.8 oz	630	34	46
Tuna Salad, 7.5 oz	550	22	56
Hot Pockets: Ham 'n' Cheese, 7 oz	480	19	55
Meatballs w. Mozzarella	490	18	59
The Deli Market (7-Eleven)			
Breakfast Sandwiches:			
Beef, Chse & Bacon Bite w. Bun	390	23	23
Croissant w. Bacon, Egg & Chse	420	26	34
Croissant w. Ham, Egg & Chse	390	22	34
Engl. Muffin w. Saus., Egg, Chse	450	24	37
Sausage, Egg & Chse Biscuit	500	31	34
Bakery Stix™ Treats: Per Stick (3.5 oz)			
BBQ Chicken	230	6	34
Cheese & Steak	290	12	31
Egg, Ham & Cheddar	280	11	35
Egg, Sausage & Cheese	290	12	35
Grilled Chicken & Cheese	270	11	30
Ham & Cheese; Supreme	280	12	32
Pepperoni & Cheese	340	18	30
Sausage & Cheese	300	13	32
Sushi			
California Rolls, 8-Pack	560	8	80

Go-Go Taquitos:	C	F	Cb
Beef Taco & Cheese, 3 oz (1)	250	11	30
Fiesta Chicken, 3 oz (1)	220	12	22
Jalapeno & Cream cheese, 3 oz	240	13	27
Monterey Jack Chkn, 3 oz (1)	280	14	30
Donuts: Blueberry Cake	330	22	31
Chocolate Iced	250	17	23
Glazed	250	16	24
Jelly	420	16	66
Muffins: Apple Spice, 7.5 oz	520	4	114
Banana Nut, 7 oz	660	26	97
Blueberry, 5.6 oz	450	14	73
Fountain Drinks (Figures Assume 1/4 Ice)			
Coca-Cola/Pepsi/Dr.Pepper/7Up:			
Gulp, 20 oz	190	0	48
Big Gulp, 32 oz	300	0	75
Super Gulp, 44 oz	410	0	102
Double Gulp, 64 oz	600	0	150
Diet Coke/Diet Pepsi, 16 oz	1	0	0
Slurpees: Average All Flavors,			
12 oz size	165	0	41
22 oz size	300	0	75
28 oz size	385	0	96
40 oz size	545	0	136
Slurp & Gulp Combo,			
32 oz Big Gulp & 22 oz Slurpee	600	0	150
Café Coolers: Mocha, 12 oz	350	12	63
French Vanilla, 12 oz	380	16	58
Fruit Coolers			
Orange/Strawb. Creme, 12 fl.oz	280	1	68
16 fl.oz size	370	1	90
20 fl.oz size	470	2	113
Arizona Rasp. Green Tea, 12 fl.oz	230	0	56
Cafe Select Coffee: 12 fl.oz	7	0	2
16 fl.oz size	10	0	2
20 fl.oz size	12	0	3
24 fl.oz size	15	0	4
Fresh Fruit Salad, 1 bowl, 10 oz	140	0	32

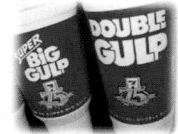

Fast–Foods & *Restaurants*

Sammy's®
Woodfired Pizza

Healthy Dining Meals

	C	F	Cb
Chinese Chicken Salad	480	13	49
Chopped Chicken Salad	385	11	20
Grilled Shrimp Wrap	560	19	57
Grilled Vegetable Penne	620	21	84
Tomato Angel Hair Pasta	670	18	105
Vegetarian Pizza, 1/2 Pizza	860	21	130

Samurai Sam's®

Appetizers: Per Serving

	C	F	Cb
California Rolls	245	1	53
Grilled Egg Rolls	150	5	20

Bowls: Per Regular Bowl

Chicken	605	11	94
Chicken & Steak	610	10	94
Chicken & Steak, all white	565	7	91
Chicken, All White	525	3	89
Steak	615	9	93
Veggie	395	1	88

Salads: Oriental Chicken

	495	8	89

Specialties: Per Serving

Chicken & Prawns	590	9	92
Chicken & Prawns, all white	555	4	92
Steak & Prawns	600	8	92
Teriyaki Prawns	480	2	88
YakiSoba	530	9	96

Sbarro's®

Meals: Per Serving

	C	F	Cb
Baked Ziti, 1 serving	930	42	90
Chicken Parmigiana, 2 pces, 7 oz	365	20	13
Meat Lasagne, 1 serving	825	41	68
Spaghetti w. Sauce, 1 serving	910	23	144

Pizza: Per Slice

Cheeze	485	18	55
Pepperoni	590	27	55
Sausage	640	29	56
Supreme	600	25	59

Stuffed Pizza: Per Slice

Spinach/Broccoli	825	40	85
Sausage Pepperoni	965	47	83

Schlotzsky's®

Bread/Buns

	C	F	Cb
Dark Rye, regular	325	2	68
Sourdough, regular	335	2	68
Wheat, regular	335	3	66
Jalapeno Cheese, regular	355	4	66
Pizza Crust	330	2	68

Original Sandwiches: Per Sandwich

The Original, regular	740	31	79
Large Original, family size	1390	58	152
Deluxe Original, regular	930	42	84
Ham & Cheese Original, regular	750	27	82
Turkey Original, regular	820	32	81

Sandwiches: Per Regular Sandwich

Albacore Tuna	495	10	77
Albacore Tuna Melt	740	29	83
Albuquerque Turkey	920	41	85
All American Angus	900	39	82
BLT	580	24	70
Chicken Breast	500	4	80
Chicken Club	685	23	75
Corned Beef	595	12	78
Corned Beef Reuben	840	33	82
Dijon Chicken	495	6	74
Fiesta Chicken	840	36	79
Pastrami & Swiss	880	36	81
Pastrami Reuben	945	41	83
Pesto Chicken	510	9	73
Roast Beef	625	15	78
Roast Beef & Cheese	855	32	83
Santa Fe Chicken	605	14	81
Smoked Turkey Breast	500	7	75
Texas Schlotzsky's	775	32	76
The Philly	840	29	86
The Vegetarian	480	11	79
Turkey & Bacon Club	835	35	79
Turkey Guacamole	645	19	84
Turkey Reuben	825	34	80
Vegetable Club	540	18	76
Western Vegetarian	610	28	76

Soups: Per Cup (8 oz)

Boston Clam Chowder	235	15	24
Broccoli Cheese w. Florets	250	17	23
Chicken Gumbo	110	5	13
Chicken Tortilla	165	3	24
Chicken w. Wild Rice	380	28	24
Minestrone	90	1	17
Old-Fashioned Chicken Noodle	120	2	18

Schlotzsky's® cont...

Deli Salads: Per 5 oz Container	C	F	Cb
Potato	290	15	35
Mustard Potato	250	13	31
Homestyle Cole Slaw	190	10	24
Elbow Macaroni	275	19	23
California Pasta	60	3	10
Albacore Tuna, small, 4.4 oz	135	9	2
Leaf Salads: w/out Dressing/Croutons/Noodles			
Caesar	30	1	3
Chicken Caesar	110	3	4
Chinese Chicken	130	3	10
Garden Salad	50	1	7
Small	25	1	3
Greek	160	10	11
Ham & Turkey/Smkd Turkey Chef's	200	10	13
8" Pizzas: Bacon, Tom. & Mushr.	610	22	78
Barbeque Chicken	685	15	93
Chicken & Pesto; New Orleans	650	19	78
Double Cheese	580	19	76
Double Cheese & Pepperoni	720	32	77
Fresh Tomato & Pesto	540	16	76
Mediterranean	525	18	72
Smoked Turkey & Jalapeno	625	17	80
Tuscan Herb	540	15	80
Thai Chicken	665	17	89
The Original Combination	625	23	79
Vegetarian Special	550	17	76
Salad Extras: Chow Mein Noodles	75	4	9
Garlic Chinese Croutons, 1/2 oz	45	2	5
Greek Balsamic Vinaigrette, 1.5 oz	170	17	2
Light Italian Dressing, 1.5 oz	90	8	3
Olde World Caesar Dress., 1.5 oz	260	27	1
Ranch Dressing: Traditional, 1.5 oz	270	29	1
Spicy, 1.5 oz	230	25	2
Light Spicy, 1.5 oz	140	11	9
Schlotzsky's Deli Chips, 1.5 oz bag	210	11	26
Sesame Ginger Vinaigrette, 1.5 oz	170	15	8
Thousand Island Dressing, 1.5 oz	220	21	6
Kid's Deals: Cheese Pizza	460	11	72
Cheese Sandwich	400	15	49
Ham & Cheese Sandwich	430	16	50
PBJ Sandwich	470	16	71
Pepperoni Pizza	505	16	72
Desserts/Cookies			
Cookies: Oatmeal Raisin	150	5	24
Cookies w. Real M&M's	140	5	20
Other varieties, average	165	7	23
Cheesecake: Cookies & Crème	330	18	36
Fudge Brownie Cake	410	25	46
New York; Strawberry Swirl	310	18	31

Shakey's® C F Cb

Pizzas (12"): Per Slice (1/10 Pizza)	C	F	Cb
Cheese only:			
Thin Crust	135	5	13
Thick Crust	170	5	22
Homestyle Pan	305	14	31
Onion/Olives/Mushrooms:			
Thin Crust	125	5	14
Thick Crust	160	4	22
Homestyle Pan	320	15	32
Sausage Pepperoni:			
Thin Crust	165	8	13
Thick Crust	205	8	22
Homestyle Pan	375	20	31
Sausage Mushroom			
Thin Crust	140	6	13
Thick Crust	180	6	22
Homestyle Pan	340	17	31
Pepperoni:			
Thin Crust	150	7	13
Thick Crust	185	6	22
Homestyle Pan	345	15	31
Shakey's Special:			
Thin Crust	170	9	13
Thick Crust	210	8	22
Homestyle Pan	385	21	32
Other Items			
3-Piece Chicken & Potato	945	56	51
5-Piece Fried Chicken & Potato	1700	90	130
Hot Ham & Cheese Sandwich	550	21	56
Potato Wedges, 15 pieces	950	36	120
Shakey's Super Hot Hero	810	44	67
Spagh. w. Meat Sce/Garlic Bread	940	33	134

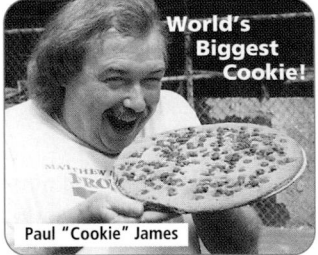

World's Biggest Cookie!

Paul "Cookie" James

Sheetz®

	C	F	Cb
Coffeez™: Per 16 fl.oz			
Hot Chocolate, medium	195	3	39
Cupo'ccino®: Per Medium (16 fl.oz)			
Almond Amaretto; French Vanilla	215	8	34
Fat Free French Vanilla	220	0	47
M.T.O® Cold Subs:			
Per 6" Sub (No Cheese Unless Indicated)			
Cheese Sub w. American Cheese	410	11	75
Chicken, Salad	505	11	85
Club Combo Sub	445	5	76
Cold Cut Sub	520	17	77
Cooked Ham Sub; Roast Beef	410	5	76
Egg Sub	385	6	76
Italian Sub	455	9	77
Tuna Salad	520	12	84
Turkey Sub	405	3	76
Veggie Sub	330	2	75
M.T.O® Hot Subs: Per 6" Sub			
Buffalo/Rstd Chicken, no Cheese	475	6	76
Meatball, no Cheese	535	17	80
Pepperoni Sub	605	28	75
Steak, no Cheese, 10 oz	500	9	77
M.T.O® Bagelz:			
Per Bagel (No Cheese Unless Indicated)			
Cheese Bagel w. American Cheese	385	11	60
Chicken Salad	475	11	71
Club Combo	420	5	62
Cheese Bagel w. American Cheese	385	11	60
Chicken Salad	475	11	71
M.T.O® Bagelz:			
Per Bagel (No Cheese Unless Indicated)			
Club Combo	420	5	62
Cold Cut	495	17	63
Cooked Ham; Roast Beef	380	5	62
Egg	360	6	62
Italian	425	9	63
Tuna Salad	490	12	70
Turkey	375	3	62
Veggie	300	2	61

	C	F	Cb
M.T.O® Burgerz, no Cheese, 8 oz	535	28	41
M.T.O® Hot Dogs (No Cheese)			
Big Deli Dog, 7 oz	675	33	77
Hot Dog, 2 oz	265	15	23
M.T.O® Nachos: Per Serving			
Nachos Bueno/Grande w. Cheese	535	32	42
Nachos Grande, no Cheese	270	12	36
M.T.O® Salads: Per Serving (No Cheese)			
Caesar Salad, 12 oz	20	0	3
Chef Salad, 15 oz	100	3	5
Chicken Caesar; Roasted Chicken	200	4	3
Chicken Salad, 16 oz	195	9	14
Garden Salad, 12 oz	20	0	4
Oriental Chicken, 21 oz	430	12	37
Steak Salad, 16 oz	190	7	6
Taco Salad, 18 oz	215	9	27
Tuna Salad, 16 oz	210	10	13
M.T.O® Breakfast: Per Serving			
Bagels: Bacon Breakfast	490	19	62
Egg	440	15	62
Ham	535	18	64
Italian Meats	480	17	63
Sausage	580	28	62
Steak	610	22	64
Shmiscuits (Includes Cheese):			
Bacon	325	19	26
Egg	275	15	26
Ham	370	18	28
Italian Meats	315	17	27
Sausage	415	28	26
Steak	445	22	28
Shmuffins: (Includes Chse): Egg	285	15	28
Bacon	330	19	28
Ham	380	18	30
Italian Meats	320	17	29
Sausage	425	28	28
Steak	455	22	30
M.T.O® Shpecialties			
Fajita, no cheese	240	5	31
M.T.O® Bavarian Wrapz	530	15	69

For full nutritional data and product updates check the database of the author's website
www.CalorieKing.com

Restaurants & Fast–Foods

Shoney's®

Breakfast	C	F	Cb
All Star Breakfast, no extras	190	14	1
Deluxe Pancake Platter	1610	32	300
Half Stack Pancake Platter	930	14	187
Big Eater Steak Brkfast, no extras	630	41	1
Steak Breakfast	995	66	49
Sunrise Breakfast	970	60	88
Sausage Biscuit (1)	540	34	42
Sausage Biscuits (2)	1055	65	83

Burgers			
All-American: Burger	690	32	44
Bacon Cheeseburger	890	49	44
Mushroom Swiss Burger	970	58	49
Famous Patty Melt	945	60	40
Half O-Pound Burger	1350	53	130

Sandwiches			
Blackened Chicken	885	21	122
Charbroiled Chicken Sandwich	895	22	122
Chicken Parmesan Sandwich	750	30	80
Corned Beef Reuben	790	53	37
Fish Sandwich	830	17	127
Fried Chicken Sandwich	560	15	77
Original Slim Jim Sandwich	1005	34	123
Potatoes & Gravy Sandwich	770	24	95
Raymond's French Dip	500	14	53
Turkey Club/Whole Wheat	950	53	47
Ultimate Grilled Cheese S'wich	895	46	77

Steaks			
BBQ Ribs	1520	78	124
Choice Sirloin, 6 oz	1225	51	127
Half-O-Pound w. Grilled Onions	1335	52	133
Half-O-Pound w. Grilled Mushr.	1315	52	127
Ribeye, 8 oz	1480	75	127
Southwest Half-O-Pound	1305	69	83
T-Bone, 12 oz	1810	100	127
Surf & Turf:			
Ribeye & 5 Fried Shrimp	1640	82	138
Ribeye & 6 Grilled Shrimp	1590	81	128
Sirloin & 5 Fried Shrimp	1380	58	138
Sirloin & 6 Grilled Shrimp	1330	57	128
T-Bone & 5 Fried Shrimp	1965	107	138
T-Bone & 6 Grilled Shrimp	1920	105	128
Rib Combos, w. Fries:			
1/4 Rack & BBQ Chicken	1230	54	103
1/4 Rack & Tenderloins	1370	70	120
1/4 Rack & Fried Shrimp	1145	50	113
1/4 Rack & Grilled Shrimp	1125	52	103

Blue Plate Specials	C	F	Cb
Cajun Whitefish	480	11	56
Baked Whitefish	510	8.5	58
Grandma's Meatloaf w. Glaze	1090	47	93
Grandma's Meatloaf w. Gravy	1090	49	88
Original Country Fried Steak	1150	62	103
Grilled Liver 'n' Onions	710	22	79
Ham Steak Dinner (no veges)	665	26	60
Roast Beef Platter (no veges)	880	30	96
Pasta: Chicken Alfredo	1705	78	170
Italian Feast	1435	45	204
Pasta Ya-Ya	1845	81	176
Shrimp Alfredo	1780	85	171
Spaghetti	495	16	63
Seafood: Fish 'n' Shrimp	1100	39	129
Fried Fish Platter	1050	39	123
Grilled Cod/Salmon Lite	200	4	0
Grilled Salmon	750	19	95
Grilled Shrimp	720	20	96
Grilled Shrimp Lite	315	8	30
Shrimper's Feast	1030	40	128
Shrimp Stir Fry	875	19	131
Sides: Baked Potato, Plain	345	6.5	67
French Fries, 4 oz	215	11	25
Onion Rings, 1 order (7 rings)	500	14	83
Chicken: Chicken Stir Fry	1200	35	172
Charbroiled Blackened Chicken	830	26	100
Charbroiled Chicken Breast	795	23	99
Fried Chicken Tenderloins	1160	61	121
Monterey Chicken	910	40	84
Smothered Chicken	890	34	90
Junior Meals: Fish 'N Chips	310	11	29
All-American Jnr Burger	235	11	20
Junior Chicken	190	10	12
Spaghetti	250	8	32

Desserts, Icecream, Sundaes			
Apple Pie: a la Mode	1205	53	174
w. NutraSweet	455	18	64
Cheesecake, 1 slice, 4 oz	365	26	23
Hot Fudge Sundae	600	30	75
Original Strawberry Pie, 1 slice	330	17	45
Ultimate Hot Fudge Cake	875	37	126
Cherry/Peach Pie w. Nutrasweet	450	21	68
Caramel Sundae	620	27	83
Chocolate/Vanilla Milk Shake	1085	51	141
Strawberry Sundae	610	27	85
Walnut Brownie a la Mode	585	34	61

243

Sizzler®

Hot Entrees

	C	F	Cb
Hamburger	625	33	36
Dakota Ranch Steak: 6 oz	315	20	0
8 oz	420	27	0
9 1/2 oz	500	32	0
Hibachi Chicken Breast			
w. Pineapple	195	3	13
Lemon-Herb Chicken Breast	140	3	0
Malibu Chicken Patty, each	310	19	11
Salmon	250	12	0
Santa Fe Chicken Breast	150	3	0
Shrimp: Broiled	150	6	0
Fried, 4 only	225	2	35
Mini	150	1	24
Shrimp Scampi	145	3	0
Swordfish	315	14	0

Hot Bar

	C	F	Cb
Broccoli Chse Soup, 4 oz	140	9	10
Chicken Noodle Soup, 4 oz	30	1	4
Chicken Wings, 1 oz	75	4	4
Clam Chowder, 4 oz	120	6	11
Focaccia Bread, 2 pces	110	7	9
Meatballs, 4 balls	155	11	5
Minestrone Soup, 4 oz	35	0	7
Pasta: Fettucine, 2 oz	80	1	15
Spaghetti, 2 oz	80	0	16
Potato Skins, 2 oz	160	8	22
Refried Beans, 1/4 cup	60	1	11
Saltine Crackers, 2 crackers	25	1	4
Taco Filling, 2 oz	105	9	3
Taco Shells, each	50	2	7

Dessert Bar: Chocolate Syrup, 1 oz 90 | | 0 | 21 |

	C	F	Cb
Choc/Vanilla Soft Serve, 4 oz	135	4	24
Strawberry Topping, 1 oz	70	0	18
Whipped Topping, 1 Tbsp	10	1	1

Salads & Toppings
Prepared Salads: Per 2 oz

	C	F	Cb
Carrot & Raisin	130	10	10
Chinese Chicken; Teriyaki Beef	55	2	6
Mediterranean Minted Fruit	30	0	7
Mexican Fiesta	55	1	10
Old Fashioned Potato	85	5	10
Red Herb Potato	120	9	9
Seafood	55	3	4
Seafood Louis Pasta	65	2	9
Spicy Jicama	15	0	4
Tuna Pasta	135	10	6

Sides

	C	F	Cb
Cottage Cheese, 2 oz	50	1	2
Eggs, 1 oz	45	3	0
Garbanzo Beans, 1/4 cup	65	1	11
Kidney Beans, 1/4 cup	50	0	10
Olives, 1 oz	60	6	1
Peaches, 1/4 cup	35	0	9
Peas, 1/4 cup	30	0	6
Real Bacon Bits, 1 Tbsp	30	2	1
Turkey Ham, 1 oz	60	5	0

Dressings: Per 1 oz

	C	F	Cb
Blue Cheese	110	12	1
Honey Mustard	160	16	4
Italian, Lite	15	0	2
Japanese Rice Vinegar, Fat Free	10	0	2
Parmesan Italian	100	10	2
Ranch	120	12	2
Ranch, Reduced-Calorie	90	8	4
Thousand Island	145	15	3

Skyline Chili®

Menu Items: Per Serving

	C	F	Cb
Chili (Regular): Plain, 1/2 pint	250	15	4
w. Beans, 1/2 pint	260	12	17
Chili Spaghetti: Regular	400	14	44
Large	540	19	59
Chili Spaghetti w. Onions: Reg.	415	14	47
Large	560	19	63
Chili Spaghetti w. Beans: Reg.	480	14	57
Large	650	19	79
Chili Spaghetti w. Beans/Onions:			
Regular	485	14	60
Large	665	19	82
Burritos: Regular	550	30	42
Deluxe Burrito	610	34	47
Coneys: Regular	270	14	23
Cheese Coney	390	24	23
Chili Sandwich	235	9	25
w. Cheese	340	18	24
Black Beans and Rice	330	12	44
3-Way (Spagh., Chili, Chse): Reg.	715	42	39
Large	1055	61	61
4-Way (3-Way w. Onions): Reg.	725	42	41
Large	1075	61	65
4-Way (3-Way w. Beans): Reg.	785	42	52
Large	1160	61	80

Restaurants & Fast−Foods

Skyline Chili® cont...

	C	F	Cb
5-Way (3-Way + Onions + Beans)			
Regular	795	42	54
Large	1185	61	84
Salads			
Garden Salads: Regular	80	5	4
Large	155	10	7
Greek Salads: Regular	385	36	9
Large	700	68	13
Nacho Salads: Regular	455	25	40
Large	760	42	66

Smoothie King®

	C	F	Cb
Weight Gain Smoothies: Per 20 oz			
Hulk™: Chocolate/Vanilla	870	29	128
Strawberry	980	29	156
Malts	915	41	118
Peanut Power®	535	21	72
Peanut Power Plus™: Grape	730	21	119
Strawberry	665	21	105
Shakes	900	41	117
Lowfat Smoothies: Per 20 oz			
Angel Food™; Mangofest™, avg.	330	0.5	79
Blackberry Dream™	355	0.5	86
Blueberry Heaven™	265	1	58
Celestial Cherry High™	285	0.5	69
Cherry Picker™	420	0.5	98
Cranberry Cooler	535	0	132
Cranberry Supreme™	575	0.5	138
Grape Expectations™; Caribbean®	400	0.5	96
Grape Expectations II™	535	0.5	129
Hearthy Apple™	390	2	81
Immune Builder™; Island Treat®	350	1	80
Instant Vigor™	365	1	87
Lemon Twist® Banana	345	0.5	82
Lemon Twist® Strawberry	405	0.5	97
Light & Fluffy®	405	0.5	98
Muscle Punch®/Plus™	355	1.5	80
Orange Ka-Bam™	425	0	104
Peach Slice™	340	0	80
Peach Slice Plus®	475	0	113
Pep Upper®	340	1	80
Pineapple Pleasure®	315	0.5	76
Pineapple Surf™	455	1	104
Raspberry Sunrise™	360	0.5	85
Slim & Trim™: Chocolate	280	1.5	55
Strawberry	355	1	79
Orange-Vanilla	195	0.5	43
Vanilla	235	1	51

Smoothie King® cont...

	C	F	Cb
Strawberry Kiwi Breeze™	295	0	70
Strawberry X-Treme™	375	0	91
Youth Fountain™	275	0.5	65
Specialty Smoothies: Per 20 oz			
Banana Boat	540	14	93
Coconut Surprise™	480	6	99
Mo'cuccino™	430	12	71
Pina Colada Island™	570	11	102
Yogurt D-Lite®	335	4	58
Workout Smoothies: Per 20 oz			
Activator®: Chocolate	485	1	90
Strawberry	580	1	123
Vanilla	445	1	90
Power Punch™	445	1.5	102
Power Punch Plus®	510	2	113
Super Punch™	390	0.5	95
Super Punch Plus®	485	0.5	118
High Protein Smoothies: Per 20 oz			
Almond Mocha; Chocolate	420	13	45
Banana	440	14	44
Lemon/Pineapple	405	13	41

Snappy Tomato®

	C	F	Cb
Large Pizza: Per Slice (1/12 Pizza)			
Cheese Pizza	160	5	21
Sausage	190	8	22
Pepperoni	200	9	21
Snappy Supreme	425	28	24
Sides: Snappy Wings, 3 pces	160	11	0
Chicken Snappers, 2 pces	150	5	12

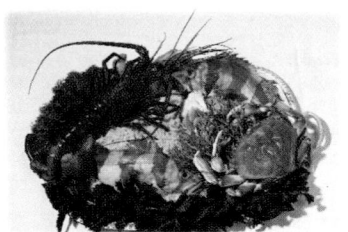

Sonic Drive-In®

Burgers:	C	F	Cb
#1. Burger	550	36	43
#2. Burger	450	25	43
#1. Cheeseburger	625	42	44
#2. Cheeseburger	530	31	44
Bacon Cheeseburger	710	49	44
Super Sonic #1	885	66	45
Super Sonic #2	790	55	46
Jr. Burger	335	21	27
Toaster Sandwiches: BLT	615	41	42
Bacon Cheddar Burger	685	38	60
Chicken Club	715	29	75
Country Fried Steak	730	45	55
Grilled Cheese	310	12	39
Sandwiches: Country Fried Steak	745	47	56
Breaded Chicken	585	23	66
Grilled Chicken	350	13	31
Wraps: Chicken Strip w. Dressing	360	29	55
w/out Ranch Dressing	410	13	53
Grilled Chicken: w. Ranch Dressing	520	27	40
w/out Ranch Dressing	375	12	38
Fritos®Chili Cheese, Wrap	740	42	68
Chicken: Chicken Strip Dinner	760	32	86
Chicken Strip Snack	280	13	22
Coneys: Plain, Regular	265	16	22
Extra Long	475	27	44
Cheese: Regular	365	24	24
Extra-Long	660	42	47
Corn Dog	270	17	23
Breakfast: Breakfast Burrito	620	37	45
Bacon Egg & Cheese Toaster®	535	29	40
Sausage Egg & Cheese Toaster®	595	36	44
Ham Egg & Cheese Toaster®	470	19	41
Sonic Sunrise® Breakfast: Regular	240	0	60
Large	400	0	100
Drinks: Barq's® Root Beer, large	360	0	90
Coca-Cola®, large	325	0	81
Coca-Cola® Float, large	425	17	59

Faves & Craves	C	F	Cb
French Fries: Regular	195	11	22
Large	250	13	30
Super Sonic™	360	18	44
Ched 'R' Peppers®	255	12	29
Cheese Fries: Regular	270	17	23
Large	325	19	31
Chili Cheese Fries: Regular	300	19	24
Large	360	22	32
Fritos® Chili Pie	610	44	36
Mozzarella Sticks	390	19	35
Onion Rings: Regular	340	5	66
Large	520	7	102
Sonic™	720	10	141
Tater Tots: Regular	250	16	27
Large	350	21	40
Supersonic™	465	28	53
Cheese Tater Tots: Regular	325	22	28
Large	435	27	41
Chili Cheese Tater Tots: Regular	360	25	28
Large	530	36	43
Faves & Craves: (Cont)			
Blasts: Regular, all types	520	27	58
Large, all types, average	765	39	89
Slushes: Small, average	230	0	58
Regular, average all flavors	325	0	81
Large, average all flavors	510	0	127
Wacky Pack®, average	200	0	50
Route 44®, average	490	0	123
Slush Floats/CreamSlush™			
Regular, average	340	12	52
Large	485	17	74
Desserts: Banana Split, 12½ oz	425	11	75
Chocolate Sundae, 8½ oz	290	11	41
Dish of Vanilla, 7 oz	195	11	19
Hot Fudge Sundae, 8½ oz	320	15	40
Icecream Cone	215	11	23
Pineapple Sundae, 9 oz	330	11	53
Strawberry Sundae	250	11	32

For Complete Nutritional Data ~ see CalorieKing.com

Souper Salad®

Soups: Per Serving (5 oz)	C	F	Cb
Beef Stroganoff	105	5	10
Chicken Creole	95	2	10
Chicken Tetrazini	110	4	10
Cream of Cauliflower	60	2.5	4
Cream of Spinach	25	1	4
German Potato; Potato Corn	100	5	11
Hungarian Mushroom	115	8	9
Mac and Cheese	100	4	13
New England Clam Chowder	90	3.5	11
Santa Fe Chicken	100	3.5	8
Other varieties, average	80	2	10

Potato Topping: Per 5 oz			
Vegetable Cheese	105	3	3

Bread: Per Serving			
Blueberry, 4 oz	260	5	49
Corn, 4 oz	265	6	49
Focaccia Bread, 3.5 oz	390	7	69
Garlic Bread Stick (2)	120	2	23
Gingerbread, 3.5 oz	290	11	46
Focaccia, all varieties (1)	70	3	10

For Complete Nutritional Data ~ see CalorieKing.com

Souplantation®

Soups: Per Cup			
Low Fat: Chicken Tortilla	100	3	5
Chicken Noodle	160	3	17
Vegetable Medley	90	1	14
Regular Soup: Per Cup			
Chesapeake Corn Chowder	310	13	43
Cream of Mushroom	290	21	15
Irish Potato Leek	260	16	23
Manhattan Clam Chowder	130	4	16
Minestrone w. Italian Sausage	210	11	14
Navy Bean w. Ham	340	10	30
Vegetarian Harvest	190	8	23
Chili: House Chili. 1 cup	230	3	26
Breads: Sourdough	150	0.5	27
Buttermilk Cornbread, 1 pce	140	2	17
Focaccia: Garlic Parmesan	100	3	15
Pizza /Tomatillo	140	6	16
Fresh Tossed Salads: Per Cup			
Antipasto Salad; BBQ, average	140	10	6
Caesar Salad Asiago	190	14	10
Won Ton Chicken Happiness	150	8	12

Souplantation® cont...

Prepared Salads: Per 1/2 Cup	C	F	Cb
Aunt Doris' Red Pepper Slaw	70	0	18
Baja Bean & Cilantro	180	3	29
BBQ Potato	160	8	20
Broccoli Madness	180	14	11
Carrot Raisin	90	3	17
Dijon Potato w. Garlic Dill Vinegar	150	12	9
Greek Couscous w. Feta Cheese	170	9	19
Oriental Ginger Slaw w. Krab	70	3	8
Southern Dill Potato	120	3	20
Thai Noodle w. Peanut Sauce	170	8	17
Dressing & Croutons: Per 2 Tbsp			
Blue Cheese Dressing	140	14	3
Balsamic Vinaigrette	180	19	1
Italian Dressing	120	13	1
Fat Free	20	0	5
Honey Mustard Dressing	150	13	8
Fat Free	45	0	10
Ranch Dressing	130	13	1
Fat Free	10	0	2
Thousand Island Dressing	110	11	3
Croutons, Garlic Parmesan, 5 pcs.	40	3	2
Hot Tossed Pastas: Per Cup			
Bruschetta	260	4	41
Creamy Bruschetta	360	16	43
Garden Vegetable: w. Meatballs	270	7	42
w. Italian Sausage	300	10	42
Italian Vegetable Beef	270	6	43
Vegetarian Marinara w. Basil	260	4	44
Muffins: Chocolate Brownie	170	8	22
Georgia Peach Poppyseed	140	6	20
Lemon	140	4	19
Big Blue Blueberry, small	140	5	22
Fruit Medley Bran	80	0.5	17
Desserts: Per 1/2 Cup			
Apple Cobbler	350	10	64
Apple Medley (fat-free)	70	0	18
Banana Royale (fat-free)	80	0	20
Chocolate Chip Cookie, small	70	3	10
Chocolate Lava Cake	300	8	56
Jello, flavored	85	0	20
Rice Pudding	110	2	20
Vanilla Pudding	150	3	24
Chocolate Syrup, 2 Tbsp	70	0	18
Granola Topping, 2 Tbsp	110	4	16
Soft Serve: Chocolate, 1/2 cup	95	0	21
Vanilla Soft Serve (reduced fat)	140	4	22

For Complete Nutritional Data ~ see CalorieKing.com

Southern Tsunami®

Sushi: Per Serving	C	F	Cb
California Roll, 9 pieces	290	5	54
California Roll & Inari, 7 pieces	325	6	58
California Salad Roll, 6 pieces	570	20	83
Combos: Seaside, 12 pieces	300	3.5	49
Shoreline, 10 pieces	475	5.5	84
Stardust, 11 pieces	305	3	58
Vegetable, 9 pieces	230	4	45
Cream Cheese Roll:			
w. Imitation Crab, 9 pces	530	25	60
w. Salmon, 9 pces	570	29	53
w. Tuna, 9 pces	550	26	53
Crunchy Shrimp Roll, 9 pieces	650	19	83
Dragon Roll, 9 pieces	645	34	63
Eel Roll, 9 pieces	465	18	55
Fullmoon Combo, 6 pieces	305	7	50
Futomaki, 6 pieces	310	1.5	68
Futomaki & Inari, 6 pieces	355	4.5	68
Green River Roll, 9 pieces	490	20	55
Grilled Salmon Roll, 9 pieces	350	6.5	54
Inari, 4 pieces	260	5	46
Mix & Match (M & M) Roll:			
Eel & Carrot, 12 pieces	315	7	51
Imitation Crab & Carrot, 12 pces	245	0.5	53
Tuna & Cucumber, 12 pces	245	1	49
Shrimp & Avocado, 12 pieces	280	4	50
Marina Plate, 6 pieces	425	5	73
Meteor Special, 11 pieces	370	3	67
Nigiri: *Per Piece*			
Eel	85	2	13
Octopus; Salmon; Yellowtail	65	0.5	11
Shrimp	90	1	12
Snapper; Squid; Tuna	60	0	12
Ocean Crab Roll, 9 pieces	345	8	54
Orange Roll, 9 pieces	395	8	65
Rainbow Roll, 9 pieces	480	10	92
Small Roll: *Per 12 Pieces*			
Avocado	295	7	52
Carrot	240	0.5	51
Cucumber	225	0.5	50
Eel	390	13	50
Imitation Crab	250	0.5	53
Salmon	330	6	47
Shrimp	265	1	49
Tuna	260	1.5	47
Yellowtail	290	3	49

Snack Pack: *Per 12 Pieces*	C	F	Cb
Avocado	295	7	52
Carrot-Cucumber	230	0.5	51
Carrot	240	0.5	53
Cucumber	225	0.5	50
Imitation Crab & Cucumber	240	0.5	51
Spicy Roll: *Per 9 Pieces*			
Shrimp	335	5.5	52
Yellowtail	365	8	52
Salmon	360	9	52
Tuna	290	6	45
Sunshine Platter, 15 pieces	815	13	154
Tempura Roll, 9 pieces	605	13	92
Tofu Roll, 9 pieces	250	3	48
Tsunami Roll, 9 pieces	480	15	63
Salads: Per Serving			
Calamari Salad, 4 oz	185	2.5	20
Edamame (soybeans), 4 oz	170	7.5	12
Edamame Salad, 4 oz	60	3	4
Harusame Salad, 2 oz	60	0.5	13
Seabreeze Salad, 2 oz	55	1.5	11
Sauce: AFC Spicy Sauce, 2 oz	50	4.5	2

For Complete Nutritional Data ~ see CalorieKing.com

Spaghetti Warehouse®

Lunch	C	F	Cb
Minestrone Soup	80	1.5	12
Grilled Chicken Marinara	530	8	65
Seafood Marinara	385	5	65
Spaghetti: w. Tomato Sauce	425	5	82
w. Marinara Sauce #12	440	5	84
Spicy Marinara Sce Spaghetti	280	4	52
Vegetable Primavera	340	4	65
Dinner			
Minestrone, 1 bowl	110	2	18
Grilled Chicken Marinara	640	10	85
Grilled Halibut Dinner	880	14	106
Grilled Marinated Chicken Breast	910	17	116
Marinara Sauce #12	520	6	99
Seafood Marinara	520	8	86
Spaghetti w. Tomato Sauce	525	6	101
Spicy Marinara Sce Spaghetti	330	6	60
Vegetable Primavera	610	8	116

Restaurants & **Fast–Foods**

Starbuck's®

Figures Based on Grande (16 fl.oz)
Without Whip Unless Indicated

Classic Favorites: Per 16 fl.oz

	C	F	Cb
Apple Juice	230	0	57
Caramel Apple Cider	300	0	72
Chocolate Milk, Whole Milk	340	15	42
Hot Chocolate, Whole Milk	340	15	42
Steamed Apple Cider	230	10	57
Vanilla Creme	340	14	40
White Hot Chocolate, Whole Milk	480	18	63
Steamed Milk, Whole	270	15	21
w. Nonfat Milk	160	0	23
w. Soy Milk	210	6	28
Cafe Misto/Au Lait, Whole Milk	140	8	11
Caffe Americano	15	0	3
Caffe Latte, Whole Milk	260	14	21
w. Nonfat Milk	160	0	24
w. Soy Milk	210	6	28
Breve	550	47	20
Caffe Mocha, Whole Milk	300	12	41
w. Nonfat Milk	230	2	43
w. Soy Milk	260	6	46
Breve	510	37	40

Espresso (Hot): Per 16 fl.oz

	C	F	Cb
Cappuccino: w. Whole Milk	150	8	13
w Nonfat Milk	100	0	14
w. Soy Milk	120	3	17
Breve	310	27	12
Caramel Macchiato: w. Whole Milk	320	14	37
w. Nonfat Milk	230	2	40
w. Soy Milk	300	8	49
Breve	550	42	36
Caramel Mocca w. Whole Milk	370	11	61
White Choc. Mocha: w. Whole Milk	410	15	56
w. Nonfat Milk	340	5	58
w. Soy Milk	370	14	62
Breve	620	40	55

Espresso (Hot): Per Serving

	C	F	Cb
Espresso: Doppio	10	0	2
Solo	5	0	1
Espresso con Panna: Doppio	40	3	2
Solo	35	3	1
Espresso Macchiato: Doppio	15	0	1
Solo	10	0	1

Espresso (Cold): Per 16 fl.oz

	C	F	Cb
Iced Caffe Americano	20	0	3
Iced Caffe Latte: w. Whole Milk	160	8	13
w. Nonfat Milk	100	0	14
w. Soy Milk	120	3.5	17
Iced Caffe Mocha: w. Whole Milk	220	8	35
w. Nonfat Milk	180	2	36
w. Soy Milk	200	4.5	38
Iced Caramel Macchiato, Whole Milk	270	10	34
Iced White Choc. Mocha, Whole Milk	360	11	56

Frappuccino® Blended Tea: Per 16 fl.oz

	C	F	Cb
Tazo® Chai Creme	370	4.5	69
Tazoberry Creme	330	2	74
Tazoberry	190	0	49

Frappuccino® Blended Coffee: Per 16 fl.oz

	C	F	Cb
Caramel	280	3.5	57
Chocolate Brownie	370	9	69
Coffee	260	3.5	52
Espresso	230	3	46
Mocha	290	4	58
Mocha Coconut	400	10	75
Mocha Malt	430	7	91
White Chocolate Mocha	320	4.5	62

Frappuccino® Blended Creme: Per 16 fl.oz

	C	F	Cb
Chocolate	400	7	73
Chocolate Malt	470	10	87
Vanilla	350	4.5	64

Iced Shaken Drinks: Per 16 fl.oz

	C	F	Cb
Iced Shaken Coffee	80	0	20
Tazo® Iced Tea/Tea	80	0	20
Lemonade	120	0	31

Tazo® Tea: Per 16 fl.oz

	C	F	Cb
Iced Tazo® Chai, Whole Milk	270	7	48
Tazo® Chai, Whole Milk	290	7	50

Drinks Extras: Per Serving

	C	F	Cb
Flav. Sugar Free Syrup, 1 pump	0	0	0
Flavored Syrup, 1 pump	21	0	5
Mocha Syrup, 1 pump	25	0.5	6
Toppings: Chocolate, 4g	5	0	1
Caramel, 15g	15	0.5	2
Sprinkles	0	0	0
Whipped Cream Topping:			
Tall, 25g	90	9	2
Grande/Venti, 35g	130	12	2
Hot Beverage, 27g	100	10	2

Fast-Foods & *Restaurants*

Starbuck's®cont...

C F Cb

Bottled Frappuccino®: Per 9.5 fl.oz Bottle	C	F	Cb
Caramel	200	3	37
Coffee	190	3.5	35
Hazelnut	200	3.5	37
Mocha	200	3.5	37
Bagels: Sesame	440	25	92
Other types, average	440	25	92
Bars: Caramel Apple	310	16	38
Lemon Bar	310	14	44
Peanut Butter Brownie	460	29	45
Raspberry Sammy	310	14	44
Carrot Cake; Enrobed Brownie	430	25	48
Cakes			
Iced Carrot Pound	540	13	101
Apple Walnut Coffee	320	17	41
Banana Pound; Coffee Cake	360	18	48
Choc. Big Baby Bundt	330	15	45
Pumpkin Pullman	370	17	51
Cookies & Biscotti			
Biscotti, 1 oz	110	5	15
Black & White	430	17	68
Crisp Cinnamon Twist	60	2	9
Raisin Cookie Madeline	80	3.5	11
Double Chocolate Chunk	430	21	58
Milk Chocolate Graham	140	8	17
Croissants: Chocolate Filled	350	19	43
Raspberry & Cream Cheese	260	12	34
Other Varieties, average	330	18	39
Muffins: Blueberry	380	19	49
Chocolate Cream Cheese	450	24	53
Cranberry Orange	410	20	53
Morning Sunrise	330	12	54
Scones: Apricot Currant; Blueberry	455	17	67
Butterscotch Pecan	520	27	64
Cinnamon Chip w. Icing	510	23	71
Maple Oat Stone w. Icing	490	22	69
Raspberry	440	18	65
Sweet Rolls:			
Apple Danish	370	19	44
Caramel Pecan	730	40	75
Raspberry Danish	370	19	45

Icecream & Icecream Bars ~ See Page 35
For Complete Nutritional Data ~ see CalorieKing.com

Steak Escape®

C F Cb

Small Sandwiches (7"): No Cheese or Condiments	C	F	Cb
Grand Gobbler	390	2	67
Grand Escape	430	6	64
Grandest Chicken	430	5	64
Great Escape	420	6	63
Hambrosia	395	2	69
Ragin' Cajun	420	5	63
Turkey Club	400	2	65
Vegetarian	305	1	64
Wild West BBQ	460	6	72
Large Sandwiches (12"): No Cheese or Condiments			
Grand Gobbler	680	2	116
Grandest Chicken	775	10	110
Great Escape; Grand Escape	760	12	108
Hambrosia	680	2	119
Ragin' Cajun	760	10	108
Turkey Club	690	4	111
Vegetarian	525	2	109
Wild West BBQ	830	12	126
Fresh Salads & Potatoes: No Cheese or Condiments			
Side Salad	50	0.5	8
Grilled Salad: w. Chicken	190	5	11
w. Ham	125	2	8
w. Steak	190	6	11
w. Turkey	125	2	8
Smashed Potatoes: Plain, 14 oz	255	0	53
w. Chicken	390	4	56
w. Ham	360	2	59
w. Steak	395	5	56
w. Turkey	360	2	59
Loaded: Bacon & Cheddar	650	26	91
Ranch & Bacon	710	34	87
Fresh Cut Fries: Per Serving			
Small, 12 oz	535	26	67
Medium, 16 oz	695	34	87
Large, 25 oz	980	48	123
Loaded: Bacon & Cheddar	820	44	88
Ranch & Bacon	1045	71	84
Condiments			
Mayonnaise, 1 oz	100	11	0
BBQ Sauce, 1 oz	35	0	9
Cheddar Cheese, 1 oz	70	9	1

For Complete Nutritional Data ~ see CalorieKing.com

Restaurants & Fast–Foods

Steak 'N Shake®

Steakburgers & Sandwiches	C	F	Cb
Steakburger	275	7	33
with Cheese	355	13	33
Super	375	12	33
Super with Cheese	450	18	33
Triple	475	17	33
Triple with Cheese	625	30	34
Ham Sandwich	450	22	37
Grilled Cheese Sandwich	250	13	24
Grilled Chicken Sandwich	510	22	53

Other Items			
Baked Beans	175	4	27
Chef Salad	315	18	6
Chili & Oyster Crackers	335	14	37
Chili Mac & 4 Saltines	310	12	34
Chili 3 Ways & 4 Saltines	410	16	45
Cottage Cheese, 1/2 cup	95	4	3
French Fries	210	10	28
Lettuce/Tom/ Salad /1oz 1000 Isl.	170	15	7

Desserts			
Apple Danish	390	24	35
Brownie	260	12	39
Cheesecake	370	11	61
with Strawberries	385	11	65
Pies: Apple	405	18	61
Cherry	335	14	48
Apple, A La Mode	550	25	76
Cherry, A La Mode	475	22	63
Sundaes: Brownie Fudge	645	35	81
Hot Fudge Nut	530	34	51
Strawberry	330	22	29
Vanilla Ice Cream	250	12	23

Shakes & Drinks: Hot Chocolate	685	19	129
Floats: Coca-Cola	515	17	76
Orange	500	17	74
Lemon	555	19	82
Root Beer	530	17	78
Freezes: Lemon	550	25	69
Orange	515	24	63
Shakes: Chocolate/Vanilla	610	38	57
Strawberry	650	40	62

Subway®

7 Under 6™ Salads: Figures include lettuce, tomato, onion, green peppers, olives and pickles.	C	F	Cb
Ham; Turkey Breast & Ham	110	3	11
Roast Beef	115	3	10
Roasted Chicken Breast	140	3	12
Subway Club®	145	3.5	12
Turkey Breast	105	2	11
Veggie Delite®	50	1	9

7 Under 6™ Sandwiches (6"): Figures based on Italian bread and following toppings: Lettuce, tomato, onion, green peppers, olives and pickles.			
Ham; Turkey Breast & Ham	290	5	46
Roast Beef	295	5	45
Roasted Chicken Breast	320	5	47
Subway Club®	325	6	46
Turkey Breast	280	4.5	46
Veggie Delite®	225	3	44

Classic Salads: Figures include lettuce, tomato, onion, green peppers, olives, pickles and cheese.			
Cold Cut Trio	230	15	12
Italian BMT	275	19	12
Meatball	320	20	18
Seafood & Crab	200	11	17
Steak & Cheese	180	8	13
Subway Melt	200	10	12
Tuna	240	16	11

Fresh Salads: Includes Croutons & Bread			
Caesar Salad, no croutons/bread	75	2.5	5
Chicken Caesar Salad	155	5	8
w. Light Caesar Dressing	430	19	40
w. Savory Caesar Dressing	630	38	37
Garden Salad	305	11	41
Mediterranean Salad	215	7	16
w. Mediterranean Vinaigrette	540	28	46
w. Red Wine Vinaigrette	450	12	57
Turkey Bacon Ranch	255	11	16
w. Ranch Dressing, Fat Free	480	16	57
w. Ranch Dressing	710	46	47

Classic Sandwiches (6"): Figures based on Italian bread and following toppings: Lettuce, tomato, onion, green peppers, olives, pickles, cheese, oil, vinegar, salt and pepper.			
Cold Cut Trio	440	21	47
Italian BMT	480	24	47
Meatball	525	26	53
Steak & Cheese	390	14	48
Subway Melt	410	15	47
Subway Seafood & Crab	405	16	52
Tuna	445	16	36

Subway® cont...

	C	F	Cb
Deli Sandwiches (6"): Ham	210	4	35
Roast Beef	225	4.5	35
Tuna	325	16	36
Turkey Breast	215	3.5	36

Select Sandwiches (6"):
Figures based on Italian bread and following toppings: Lettuce, tomato, onion, green peppers, and select sauce.

	C	F	Cb
Chicken Pizziola	405	16	48
Chipotle Southwest Steak & Chse	465	19	49
Chipotle Southwest Turkey Bacon	405	16	49
Dijon Horseradish Melt	470	21	48
Honey Mustard Ham	310	5	52
Red Wine Vinaigrette Club	350	6	53
Sweet Onion Chicken Teriyaki	375	5	59

Select Sauces: *Per 1½ Tablespoon*

	C	F	Cb
Chipotle Southwest	90	9	2
Dijon Horseradish	90	10	1
Fat Free, Honey Mustard	30	0	7
Fat Free, Red Wine Vinaigrette	30	0	6
Fat Free, Sweet Onion	40	0	9

Double Meat Subs (6'): *Per Sub*

	C	F	Cb
Chicken; Subway Club	420	8	50
Cold Cut Trio	610	32	49
Ham; Roast Beef	365	7	47
Italian BMT	675	38	49
Meatball	755	41	61
Steak & Cheese	505	17	51
Subway Melt	535	20	50
Seafood & Crab	520	22	60
Tuna	605	33	48
Turkey Breast	360	6	48
Turkey Breast & Ham	375	7	48

Extreme Subs (6'): *Per Sub*

	C	F	Cb
Dijon Horseradish Melt	550	23	50
Red Wine Vinaigrette Club	455	9	55
Sweet Onion Chicken Teriyaki	470	7	59
Turkey Bacon	475	17	50

Breakfast Deli Sandwiches (6"): *On Italian Bread.*

	C	F	Cb
Bacon & Egg; Cheese & Egg	320	15	34
Ham & Egg	340	13	34
Steak & Egg	330	14	35
Vegetable & Egg; Western Egg	300	12	36

Breakfast Sandwiches (6"): *Based on Italian bread.*

	C	F	Cb
Bacon & Egg; Cheese & Egg	445	19	42
Ham & Egg	435	17	42
Steak & Egg	465	18	43
Vegetable & Egg	420	16	44
Western Egg	435	17	44

	C	F	Cb
Breakfasts: French Toast w. Syrup	355	8	57
Omelets: Bacon & Egg	240	17	2
Cheese & Egg	235	17	2
Ham & Egg	220	14	2
Steak & Egg	245	15	3
Vegetable & Egg	210	14	4
Western Egg	220	14	4

Salad Dressings: *Per Package (2 oz)*

	C	F	Cb
Fat Free, French	70	0	17
Fat Free, Italian	20	0	4
Fat Free, Ranch	60	0	14

Soup: *Per Cup, 8.4 oz*

	C	F	Cb
Black Bean; Clam Chowder	180	4.5	27
Brown & Wild Rice w. Chicken	190	11	17
Cheese w. Ham & Bacon	230	16	13
Chicken & Dumpling	130	4.5	16
Chili Con Carne	240	14	28
Cream of Broccoli	130	6	15
Cream of Potato w. Bacon	210	12	20
Golden Broccoli Cheese	180	12	12
Minestrone	70	1	11
Potato Cheese Chowder	210	10	22
Roasted Chicken Noodle	90	4	7
Tomato Bisque	90	2.5	15
Vegetable Beef	90	1.5	14

Breads:

	C	F	Cb
6" Hearty Italian	210	2.5	41
6" Honey Oat	250	3.5	48
6" Italian Bread, White	200	3	38
6" Italian Herbs & Cheese	255	6	40
6" Monterey Cheddar	240	6	39
6" Parmesan Oregano	210	3.5	40
6" Roasted Garlic	230	3	45
6" Sourdough	210	3	41
6" Wheat Bread	200	2.5	40
Wrap	175	2	39
Deli Style Roll	170	2.5	32

	C	F	Cb
Cookies: Oatmeal Raisin	200	8	30
Peanut Butter	220	12	26
Sugar	230	12	28
Other varieties, average	220	10	29

Fruizle Express: *Small Cup*

	C	F	Cb
Berry Lishus	110	0	28
Peach Pizazz	100	0	26
Pineapple Delight	130	0	33
Sunrise Refresher	120	0	29

For Complete Nutritional Data ~ see CalorieKing.com

Sub Station®

Sandwiches | **C** | **F** | **Cb**

Per 1/2 Sub (Incl. Oil, Vinegar, Salad)

	C	F	Cb
Ham & Cheese	505	30	40
Ham, Turkey & Cheese	510	30	40
Turkey & Cheese	525	31	40
Roast Beef & Cheese	525	31	39
Ham, Salami, Pepperoni, Cappicola, Bologna, Turkey & Cheese	635	42	40

Sweet Tomatoes®

~ Same Menu & Data as Souplantation (See Page 246) ~

Swiss Chalet®

Burgers: Includes Garnishes | **C** | **F** | **Cb**

	C	F	Cb
Bacon Cheese Burger	835	43	52
Big Beef Burger	635	30	48
Veggie Burger	405	11	51
Rotisserie Chicken: Meat Only			
Double Leg	625	34	0
Half Chicken, no Skin	455	18	0
w. Skin	695	39	0
Quarter Chicken: Dark, no Skin	230	10	0
Dark meat w. Skin	315	17	0
White meat, no Skin	225	8	0
White meat w. Skin	380	22	0
Starters: Per Serving			
Baked Garlic Cheese Loaf, 8 oz	695	29	85
Hot Wings, 11.6 oz	955	50	63
Mild Wings, 11.6 oz	915	53	50
Perogies w. Cajun Sauce, 6.5 oz	395	11	62
Ranchero Corn & Chkn Quesadilla	930	42	90
Soup: Chalet Chicken, 1 cup	100	2	11
Creamy Chicken, 1 cup	180	6	17
Entree Garden Salads: Includes Flatbread			
Golden Grilled Chicken Caesar	830	53	41
Santa Fe Grilled Chicken	275	9	17
Warm Chicken Salad Amandine	870	60	42
Side Salads: Garden	35	0	7
Hall Caesar Salad	345	19	12
Fire Grilled: Meat Only Unless Indicated			
Chkn Breast on Rice w. Flatbread	625	9	91
Chicken & Rib Combo	1065	72	5
BBQ Ribs: Feature Cut	500	37	3
Regular	755	55	5
Large	1505	110	10

Swiss Chalet® cont...

Stir Fry/Pot Pie: Per Serving | **C** | **F** | **Cb**

	C	F	Cb
Chicken on Rice w. Flatbread	370	7	40
Veggie on Rice w. Flatbread	220	3	42
Chicken Pot Pie	495	24	53
Sides: Baked Potato	270	0	62
Bread Roll	145	0.5	29
Butter, 1/2 oz	100	11	0
Coleslaw, 2.2 oz	90	6.5	7.5
Corn, 3.5 oz	95	2	16
French Fries, 5.6 oz	470	25	53
Gravy, 3.5 oz	40	1	6
Mashed Potatoes, 6.4 oz	215	8.5	31
Rice Pilaf, 6.2 oz	230	1.5	49
Sour Cream & Chives, 1 oz	50	4	2
Vegetables, 5.5 oz	60	2	7
Sandwiches: Chicken on Kaiser	435	9	37
Chicken on Kaiser and Soup	530	11	48
Club Wrap	620	24	58
Grilled Santa Fe Chicken Breast	525	15	59
Messy Chicken	1010	41	102
Salad Dressings: Per Serving			
Creamy 1000 Isle Dressing, 15 ml	60	6	2
Garlic Peppercorn, 15 ml	65	7	1
Famous Chalet Sauce, 100g	25	0.5	4.5
French Dressing, 15 ml	60	5.5	2
House Dressing, 15 ml	65	6	3.5
Light Italian, 15 ml	30	2	2.5
Mayonnaise, 15 ml	100	11	0
Raspberry Vinaigrette, 15 ml	10	0	3
Dipping Sauce: BBQ, 33 ml	55	0	13
Honey Mustard, 33 ml	75	1	19
Plum, 33 ml	65	0	17
Sweet & Sour, 33 ml	50	0	13
Desserts: Apple Blossom	565	30	67
Apple Pie	425	17	66
Carrot Cake	660	38	73
Chocolate Eruption Cheesecake	785	45	84
Coconut Cream Pie	410	27	41
Colossal Caramel Fudge Chsecake	655	38	68
Cranberry, Raspberry Yogurt	215	4	39
Icecream: Butter Pecan	340	20	38
Chocolate	275	16	26
Vanilla	335	21	32
Sauce: Butterscotch	315	0	78
Chocolate	240	0.5	57
Strawberry	215	0	53
Lemon Meringue	410	16	66
Pecan Pie	410	24	53
Sugar Pie	395	21	52
Tuzedo Truffle Mousse	680	42	66

Taco Bell®

Burritos

	C	F	Cb
7-Layer Burrito	530	22	67
Bean Burrito	370	10	55
Burrito Supreme® Beef	440	18	50
Burrito Supreme® Chicken/Steak	420	16	49
Chili Cheese Burrito	390	18	40
Fiesta Burrito Beef	390	15	50
Fiesta Burrito Chicken; Steak	370	13	48
Grilled Stuft Beef	730	33	79
Grilled Stuft Chicken; Steak	680	27	76
Grilled Stuft Chicken Caesar	700	35	65

Tacos

	C	F	Cb
Taco, regular	170	10	13
Taco Supreme®	220	14	14
Soft Taco Beef	210	10	20
Soft Taco Chicken	190	6	19
Soft Taco Supreme Beef	260	14	22
Soft Taco Supreme Chicken	230	10	21
Soft Taco Steak	280	17	21
Double Decker® Taco	340	14	39
Double Decker® Taco Supreme	380	18	40

Gorditas

	C	F	Cb
Gordita Baja™ Beef	360	19	31
Gordita Baja™ Chicken; Steak	340	16	29
Gordita Supreme® Beef	320	16	30
Gordita Supreme® Chicken; Steak	300	12	28
Gordita Nacho Cheese Beef	310	13	32
Gordita Nacho Cheese Chkn; Steak	290	10	30

Chalupas

	C	F	Cb
Chalupa Baja® Beef	410	27	32
Chalupa Baja® Chicken; Steak	390	25	30
Chalupa Supreme® Beef	370	24	31
Chalupa Supreme® Chicken	350	20	30
Chalupa Supreme® Steak	350	22	29
Chalupa Nacho Cheese Beef	360	22	33
Chalupa Nacho Cheese Chkn; Steak	340	19	31

Breakfast

	C	F	Cb
Breakfast Gordita	400	24	28
Breakfast Burrito	530	25	48
Breakfast Burrito, Steak	530	26	40
Breakfast Quesadilla	420	20	38
Quesadilla, Steak w. Green Sauce	470	23	39

Nachos and Sides:

	C	F	Cb
Nachos, 3.5 oz	330	19	33
Nachos Supreme®	470	26	42
Nachos BellGrande®	760	43	80
Pintos 'n Cheese, 4.5 oz	180	7	20
Mexican Rice, 4.75 oz	190	10	21
Cinnamon Twists, 1.25 oz	150	5	27

Taco Bell® cont...

	C	F	Cb
Specialities: Tostada	250	10	29
Cheese Quesadilla	490	28	39
Chicken Quesadilla	350	14	33
Enchirito® Beef	370	18	35
Enchirito® Chicken; Steak	350	16	33
Meximelt®	290	16	23
Mexican Pizza, 7¹/₂ oz	550	31	46
Taco Salad w. Salsa & Shell	830	42	73
Taco Salad w. Salsa, w/out Shell	410	21	33
Southwest Steak Bowl	660	32	73
Zesty Chicken Border Bowl	720	42	65
w/out Dressing	460	19	60

For Complete Nutritional Data ~ see CalorieKing.com

Taco Cabana®

Grilled Chicken: *Per Serving*	C	F	Cb
¹/₄ Chicken White, 5 oz	300	14	1
No Skin, 4 oz	170	3	0
¹/₄ Chicken Dark, 4.5 oz	300	18	0.5
No Skin, 3.5 oz	170	7	1
Fajitas: Beef, 4 oz	245	12	4
Chicken White, 4 oz	190	6	3
Chicken Dark, 4 oz	235	11	2
Sides: Black Beans, 4 oz	110	0.5	21
Borracho Beans, 4 oz	110	2.5	17
Calabacita, 4 oz	70	5	6
Chips, 2 oz	290	14	36
Elotes (1)	220	11	27
Guacamole, 1 oz; Sour Cream, 1 oz	50	4	2
Queso, 3 oz	170	12	7
Refried Beans, 4 oz	170	6	21
Salsa, all types, 1 oz	10	0	2
Spanish Rice, 4 oz	180	5	30
Tortillas: 6" Flour	130	3.5	22
6" Table Corn	60	1	11
Tortilla Soup: Small, 8.5 oz	250	8.5	26
Large, 19 oz	375	13	32
Tacos: Bean & Cheese	295	12	35
Black Bean	225	5	37
Carne Guisada	210	8	20
Crispy Beef	150	7	13
Soft Chicken	220	9	21
Burritos: Bean & Cheese	695	27	85
Beef	640	24	76
Black Bean	545	11	95
Chicken	650	26	73
Breakfast Tacos: Bacon & Egg	250	12	22
Barbacoa	230	15	2
Chorizo & Egg	245	12	22
Potato & Egg	240	10	21

Taco John's®

	C	F	Cb
Tacos: Taco Bravo®	360	15	40
Taco Burger	270	11	29
Crispy Taco	195	12	13
El Grande Chicken	355	19	21
Sierra Taco™ Beef	500	30	39
Sierra Taco™ Chicken	465	25	37
Softshell Taco	230	10	23
Softshell Chicken	195	6	21
Burritos: Bean Burrito	370	11	53
Beefy Burrito; Super Burrito, avg.	445	20	44
Chicken and Potato	470	19	56
Chicken Fajita	350	11	41
Chicken Festiva	570	29	56
Combination Burrito	410	15	49
El Grande	730	36	69
El Grande Chicken	665	27	66
Meat and Potato Burrito	500	23	58
Ranch Burrito Chicken	405	18	41
Smothered Burrito	515	21	57
Favorites: Bean Tostada	160	7	17
Cheese Crisp	220	16	9
Chilito	445	22	41
Double Enchilada	750	40	59
Mexi Rolls®	460	29	31
Mexican Pizza	560	31	47
Potato Oles w. Nacho Cheese	530	34	50
Sierra Chicken Sandwich	490	27	37
Tostada	200	12	13
Specialities			
Chicken Festiva Salad, no dressing	395	21	27
Chicken Super Nachos	855	55	57
Chicken Taco, no dressing	605	30	55
Potato Oles Bravo	570	35	55
Cheese Quesadilla	480	26	42
Super Nachos	905	60	68
Super Potato Oles®	970	61	82
Taco Salad, no dressing	600	33	50
Platters: Beef and Bean Chimi	730	33	82
Beef Enchilada	795	38	80
Chicken Enchilada	705	33	71
Smothered Burrito	840	34	101
Sides: Mexican Rice	250	5	44
Nachos	440	30	35
Potato Oles: Medium, 7 oz	610	36	67
Refried Beans	360	11	45
Texas Style Chili	310	14	25
Desserts: Apple Grande, 3 oz	260	9	40
Choco Taco, 4 oz	315	17	37
Churros, 1.3 oz	160	11	13
Taco John's Cinn. Mint Swirl (1)	10	0	3

Taco Time®

	C	F	Cb
Burritos			
Beef, Bean & Cheese	630	23	66
Big Juan Beef Burrito	645	25	71
Big Juan Chicken Burrito	630	24	69
Casita Burrito, Beef	650	31	54
Chicken & Black Bean	420	18	45
Chicken BLT	595	39	38
Crisp Burrito: Bean	435	18	53
Meat	560	30	39
Chicken	420	25	32
Soft Bean Burrito	385	10	58
Soft Meat Burrito	505	21	48
Veggie Burrito	510	16	70
Tacos: Crisp Taco	305	17	16
½ lb Chicken Soft Taco	390	16	41
½ lb Soft Taco	525	23	46
Soft Taco	325	15	23
Super Soft Taco	525	23	50
Specialties: Crustos®, 3.5 oz	375	15	47
Cheddar Fries: Small	355	24	27
Large, 9.5 oz	710	48	54
Cheddar Melt	210	11	17
Mexi Fries®: Small, 4 oz	275	17	27
Large, 8 oz	545	34	54
Mexi-Rice, 4 oz	150	2	30
Nachos: Regular, 10.5 oz	690	38	61
Deluxe, 15.25 oz	1060	57	91
Stuffed Fries: Small	500	37	34
Large, 8.5 oz	1075	73	88
Taco Cheeseburger	640	36	48
Refritos, 7 oz	340	10	44
Salads: Per Serving			
Chicken Fiesta, 12 oz	390	19	35
Chicken Taco	375	21	27
Taco Salad, regular	490	28	30
Tostada Salad	635	33	48
Sauces & Dressings: Per 1 oz			
Green Sauce	5	0	1
Original Hot Sauce	10	0	2
Salsa Fresca	65	0	16
1000 Island Dressing	120	12	3
Desserts: Cinnamon Crustos	760	15	47
Fruit Filled Empanadas	250	9	37

For Complete Nutritional Data ~ see CalorieKing.com

Tacone

Gourmet Wrapped Sandwiches:	C	F	Cb
Campfire, 15.1 oz	740	21	92
Pilgrim, 15 oz	770	39	52
Samurai, 19 oz	805	12	124
Thai Cone, 18.5 oz	800	20	106

TCBY®

Icecreams ~ See Page 31

Smoothies	C	F	Cb
Golden Vanilla Yogurt: *Per Serving*			
Banana Berry Blast-off	425	3	95
Latte Cooler	425	7	78
Peanut Butter Fusion	775	36	57
Pina Chill-ada	470	7	97
Raspberry Rush	385	3	85
Strawberry Surge	425	3	95
Tropical Bliss	390	3	87
Smoothies, Juice: *Per Serving*			
Mighty Berry; Passion Power	305	0	75
Pineapple Combustion	355	4.5	77
Raging Raspberry	325	0	79
Smoothies, Non-fat Yogurt: *Per Serving*			
Banana Berry Blast-off	410	0	98
Latte Cooler	405	4.5	79
Peanut Butter Fusion	760	34	61
Pina Chill-ada	455	5	98
Raspberry Rush	360	0	86
Strawberry Surge	405	0	96
Tropical Bliss	370	0	88

T.J. Cinnamons®

Menu Items: *Per Serving*			
Cinnachips, 10 oz	1135	50	157
Cinnamon Twist, 2.5 oz	260	13	33
Mocha Chill: w. Cream, 12.5 oz	290	6	49
w/out Cream, 12 oz	265	3.5	48
Original: w. Icing, 6.5 oz	775	37	103
w/out Cream Cheese Icing	510	17	81
Pecan Sticky, 6.5 oz	695	28	97

The Taco Maker®

	C	F	Cb
Burritos: Bean	295	9	44
Beef	440	17	44
Chicken	370	12	44
Chicken 'n Rice	375	12	51
Crisp Bean	400	27	31
Crisp Beef	425	27	29
Grande: Deluxe Combo	450	19	49
Enchiladas: Beef	375	20	23
Cheese	585	39	26
Chicken	315	13	21
Nachos: Cheese	605	36	49
Chips 'n Beans	295	16	32
Macho Nacho w. Beef	815	50	57
Macho Nacho w. Guacamole	845	55	62
Platters: Combination	870	47	71
Fiesta	1110	53	102
Grande	1235	63	114
Salad: Chicken Fiesta	620	35	39
Taco	680	43	40
Side Orders: Chicken Fajita	225	8	24
Guacamole, 1/2 oz	100	8	6
Sour Cream, 1/2 oz	125	12	2.5
Tostada	160	10	15
Tacos: Crisp	180	9	16
Crisp Super	300	16	25
Soft	180	6.5	21
Soft Super	390	15	43
Tater Gem Fries: *Per Serving*			
Large	975	61	97
Regular	490	31	49
Cheese, Regular	680	44	52

For Complete Nutritional Data ~ see CalorieKing.com

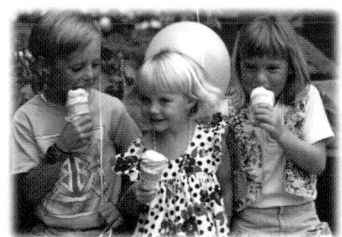

Restaurants & **Fast-Foods**

Tim Horton's®

C F Cb

Sandwiches: *Incl. Dressing Unless Indicated*

	C	F	Cb
Albacore Tuna Salad, no dressing	350	8	49
Black Forest Ham & Swiss	590	27	53
Chunky Chicken Salad, no dressing	380	10	50
Fireside Roast Beef	450	19	48
Garden Vegetable	465	24	50
Harvest Turkey Breast	460	18	53

Soup: *Per Serving (10 oz)*

Chili	325	9	32
Cream of Broccoli	200	7	27
Cream of Mushroom	195	10	21
Hearty Vegetable; Minestrone	130	2	27
Potato Bacon	195	7	29
'Tim's Own' Chicken Noodle	105	3	15
Turkey & Wild Rice	195	2	22
Vegetable Beef Barley	110	2	18

Muffins: Blueberry Bran

Blueberry Bran	305	9	51
Carrot Whole Wheat	425	22	52
Chocolate Chip Plain	405	15	62
Oatbran 'n Apple	360	12	58
Oatbran Carrot 'n Raisin	345	11	57
Oatmeal Raisin	445	11	80
Lowfat Honey	300	2	66
Low Fat Carrot/Cranberry	280	2	60
Raisin Bran	380	10	66
Wild Blueberry	330	11	54

Donuts: Honey Stick

Honey Stick	280	15	34
Sugar Twist	240	10	32
Walnut Crunch	325	18	36
Cake Donut: Chocolate Glazed	350	22	35
Old Fashion Glazed	275	12	39
Old Fashion Plain	220	12	24
Sour Cream Plain	275	18	25
Filled Donut: Angel Cream	275	13	36
Blueberry: Strawberry	220	8	33
Boston Cream; Canadian Maple	230	8	36
Yeast: Apple Fritter	305	14	40
Chocolate Dip; Honey Dip	240	10	33
Dutchie	290	13	39
Maple Dip	250	10	36

Baked Goods

Croissants; Strawberry	220	11	25
Cherry Cheese Danish	370	23	33
Tea Biscuits, average	220	6	36
Southern Country Cran./Rasp., 6 oz	470	19	68

Bagels

	C	F	Cb
Average all types	305	3	59
Cream Cheese: *Per 1 1/2 oz*			
Plain	140	14	1
Plain Light	90	7	3
Garden Vegetable; Strawberry	140	13	3
Timbits: *Each*			
Yeast, average all types	60	2	10
Filled, average all types	50	2	9
Cake: Old Fashion Plain	45	2	7
Chocolate Glazed	70	3	9
Cakes: *Per 1/8 Whole*			
Black Forest	505	21	75
Celebration (white)	500	16	85
Chocolot Fantasy	445	15	72
Shadow, white & chocolate	440	19	63
Pies: *Per 1/4 Whole*			
Apple	545	31	62
Banana Cream	440	26	50
Cherry	575	31	70
Chocolate Cream	495	31	52
Cookies: Chocolate Chip; Oatmeal	155	7	21
Oatcakes	190	10	22
Peanut Butter, all types	170	10	18
Plain Macaroon	130	8	14
Beverages			
Cafe Mocha, 10 fl.oz	240	10	34
Cappuccino Ice, 16 fl.oz	430	23	54
Coffee, w. sugar/cream 10 fl.oz	80	4	10
French Vanilla Cappuccino, 10 fl.oz	140	5	20
Fruit Punch, 300ml	150	0	38
Hot Chocolate, 10 fl.oz	240	6	44

Fast−Foods & *Restaurants*

Togo's Eatery®

	C	F	Cb
Salads: *Per Serving*			
Chicken Caesar, 9 oz	315	13	13
Farmers Market, 9 oz	120	3	18
Oriental Salad, 21.3 oz	390	7	53
Taco, 24.5 oz	1050	66	79
Dressings: *Per Pouch*			
Togo's: Ranch Dressing	100	9	3
Caesar Dressing	125	9	9
Low Fat Balsamic Vin'grett	55	2	9
Oriental Sesame Salad Dressing	140	9	15
Sesame Orange Ginger	330	28	19
Soup: Baked Potato, 8 oz	300	20	23
Black Bean	200	7	27
Broccoli Cheese	200	14	11
Chicken Noodle; Chili, avg.	150	3.5	20
New England Clam Chowder	105	6	6
Sandwiches: *Per Regular*			
Albacore Tuna, 10.8 oz	455	10	69
Avocado & Cucumber, 18 oz	615	26	79
Avocado & Turkey, 16.5 oz	690	27	78
BBQ Beef, 8.5 oz	525	13	64
California Chicken, 11 oz	620	15	68
Cheese, 12 oz	670	30	70
Chunky Chicken Salad, 13.7 oz	1087	63	93
Hot Pastrami, 14 oz	810	42	72
Hummus, 13.3 oz	807	31	104
Meatball, 16.2 oz	690	23	80
Reubin, 12 oz	660	25	69
Roast Beef, 14 oz	670	22	68
The Italian, 13 oz	745	37	68
Turkey & Cheese, 13.7 oz	600	18	71
Turkey, Ham & Cheese, 13.7 oz	600	19	70
Turkey, Roast Beef & Cheese, 14 oz	670	23	70

Topz®

	C	F	Cb
Burger: *Per Burger*			
Ahi Fillet Burger	365	8	42
Cheeseburger	495	23	38
Chicken Breast	315	5	37
Double Cheeseburger	730	36	45
Garden Cheeseburger	485	17	62
Jr. Kids Burger	200	6	21
Spicy Chicken Breast	355	6	43
Topz Burger	425	15	44
Topz Jr Burger	230	9	21
Turkey Burger	390	11	38

Topz® cont...

	C	F	Cb
Chili: Full Order	220	10	8
Half Order	110	5	4
Fries: Aero	380	14	58
Chili Cheese	665	35	68
French Fries	500	22	68
Grilled Cheese on Texas Toast: *Per Serving*			
Cheese	440	20	50
Jr. Kids	220	10	25
w. BBT	740	41	40
w. Bacon	535	29	50
w. Burger	620	32	49
w. Tomato	465	20	54
Hot Dog: Chicken Dog	375	10	49
Double Dog	390	8	60
Jr. Kids Hot Dog	195	4	30
Salad: Grilled Vegetable	230	13	17
Spicy Chinese Ahi Salad	365	17	16
Spicy Chinese Chicken	370	16	23
Topz Chopped Salad	270	16	13
Shakes: Average all flavors	330	1	55

Tubby's

	C	F	Cb
Subs: *Per 6" Sandwich*			
Burger Subs: Big Tub	665	45	41
Cheeseburger	615	41	37
Pizza Burger	630	41	39
Taco Burger	575	31	48
Deli Style Subs: Ham & Cheese	455	24	39
Turkey & Cheese	425	23	37
Turkey Club Sub	480	27	38
Specialty Subs: BLT	530	36	35
Tuna Salad	385	20	35
Veggie Stir Fry	410	20	46
Tubby's Subs: Tubby's Famous	500	29	40
Grilled Chicken Subs: *Per 6" Sub*			
Chicken & Brocolli	460	20	40
Chicken & Cheddar	390	16	38
Chicken Club Sub	445	21	36
Chicken Fajita Sub	350	9	40
Grilled Chicken	240	2	45
Grilled Steak Subs: *Per 6" Sub*			
Mushroom Steak & Cheese	630	42	39
Pepper Steak & Cheese	625	42	38
Pizza Steak & Cheese	620	41	39
Steak & Cheese	610	41	37
Salads: Side, no dressing	50	1	5
Antipasto Salad, no dressing	455	30	18
Chicken Salad	410	23	16
Taco Salad	655	46	25
Tuna Salad	340	26	11

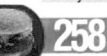

258

Restaurants & Fast-Foods

Una Mas®

	C	F	Cb
Burritos			
Bean & Cheese Burrito	650	25	80
El Cheapo	555	9	98
Fajita Burrito: Chicken	715	21	89
Steak	735	26	89
Fish Burrito Cabo Style	490	14	53
Gallito	590	30	62
Thai Chicken Burrito	500	16	62
Vegetariano Burrito	540	20	69
Una Mas Burrito: Chicken	585	15	76
Steak	605	20	76
Tacos: Crispy Chicken Taco	240	17	12
Fish Taco Cabo Style	265	6	36
Una Mas Taco: Chicken	340	9	48
Steak	345	11	48
Veggie	275	7	45
Favoritos: 5-Layer Dip	345	22	25
Chicken Enchiladas (2)	480	20	37
Nachos	1220	81	91
Quesadilla Grande	635	46	49
Quesadilla Chica	355	18	28
TJ Caesar Salad	355	18	29
w. Chicken	520	26	30
Tortilla Soup: Cup	200	13	4
Bowl	330	20	6
Tostada Salad	475	20	50
w. Chicken	640	29	53
Verde Salad	210	5	19
Side Orders: Beef, 3 oz	190	13	1
Black Beans, 5 oz	150	3	23
Chicken, 3 oz	165	8	1
Corn Tortilla	80	1	17
Fish, 4 oz	195	8	0
Flour Tortilla (12")	150	4	25
Fresh Guacamole, 2 oz	80	7	4
Monterey Jack Cheese, 1 oz	100	7	1
Pinto Beans, 5 oz	170	2	29
Refried Beans, 1/2 Cup	100	2	18
Rice, 5 oz	160	2	31
Sour Cream, 1 oz	60	6	1
The Works	160	14	5
Tortilla Chips, 1 oz	140	7	18
Salsa & Dressing: Chipotle Sce	5	0	1
Salsa Fresca/Ranchero, 1 oz	5	0	1
Mild Sauce; Salsa Verde, 1 oz	10	0	2
Caesar Dressing, 2 oz	140	12	2
Jalapeno Vinaigrette, 2 oz	140	1	16

Wahoo's Fish Taco®

Lower Fat Menu Items	C	F	Cb
Bowls: Carne Asada, Steak	760	22	90
Chicken, Skinless Breast	750	18	90
Fish of the Day	705	16	90
Burrito: Bonzai Chicken	650	18	87
Carne Asada, Steak	690	18	60
Carnitas, Pork	780	27	60
Chicken	510	15	43
Fish of the Day	430	12	44
Veggie	580	13	94
Tacos: Carne Asada, Steak	330	7.5	30
Carnitas, Pork	380	12	30
Chicken, Skinless Breast	260	6	27
Fish of the Day	225	5	27
Veggie	230	4.5	42
Sides: 1/2 Rice, 1/2 Beans	320	6	49
Beans	315	1	46
Rice	335	10.5	52
Salads: Carne Asada, Steak	605	35	12
Chicken, Skinless Breast	575	30	12
Fish of the Day	575	29	12

WAWA

Breakfast & Baked Goods	C	F	Cb
Bagel: Plain	295	1	61
w. Butter	505	23	64
w. Cream Cheese	390	8	66
Avg. other varieties	320	2	66
Bagel Melts: Ham & Cheese	485	13	67
Pepperoni & Cheese	650	26	66
Tomato & Cheese	485	19	68
Turkey Club w. Mayo	675	32	70
Breakfast Bowls: Per Bowl			
Crmd Chipped Beef on a Biscuit	385	19	42
Sausage Gravy on a Biscuit	230	2	41
Croissant: Regular, 2 oz	300	15	35
Hash Brown: (1), 1.7 oz	90	5	10
Muffins: Banana Walnut, 4 oz	435	24	48
Blueberry, 4.2 oz	420	19	55
Chocolate Chip, 4 oz	425	21	52
Corn, 4 oz	395	17	55
Sizzli Bagels: Bacon Egg & Chse	470	19	53
Bacon Egg & Cheese	500	31	37
Sausage Egg & Cheese	515	33	37
Bacon Egg & Cheese	385	21	31
Sausage/Egg & Cheese, average	320	16	31

259

WAWA cont...

Hoagies & Sandwiches: No Cheese Unless Indicated

Specialty Sandwiches

	C	F	Cb
Cold: Ital. w. Pesto & Rstd Peppers	900	64	40
Turkey & Cranberry Mustard	605	18	72
Pepper Turkey w. Rstd Tomato	705	44	41
Roast Beef & Horseradish	460	18	26
Cold Classics: American	670	28	66
BLT	780	42	62
Cheese	780	40	65
Chicken Salad	745	33	69
Egg Salad w. Cheese	970	60	71
Healthy Choice: Chicken	455	6	64
Ham; Roast Beef, average	485	8	65
Honey Smkd Turkey	495	6	69
Ham w. Cheese	615	21	66
Italian	735	32	68
Roast Beef	560	10	62
Seafood Salad	690	31	75
Tuna Salad	720	33	70
Veggie, 7.4 oz	320	3	62
Veggie Supreme, 13.1 oz	515	16	71
Hot Classics: BBQ Pork	880	31	99
Chicken Grilled, no Dressing	665	18	70
Meatball	570	5	81
Roast Beef Homestyle	665	21	67
Sausage & Pepper	905	51	68
Cold Sandwiches: Bologna	565	35	41
Cheese	500	27	38
Chicken Salad	475	22	40
Corned Beef	380	9	36
Egg Salad	520	31	41
Healthy Choice: Chkn on Wheat	295	4	38
Ham on White	255	5	28
Roast Beef on White	255	4	31
Ham	325	7	38
Liverwurst	575	35	38
Seafood Salad	450	21	46
Tuna Salad	465	22	43
Turkey	315	5	43
Veggie	200	2	37
Hot Sandwiches: BBQ Pork Kaiser	560	20	61
Chicken Breaded Club	740	40	53
Cold Shortis: American	425	18	40
BLT; Cheese, average	500	28	37
Chicken Salad	480	22	41
Egg Salad w. Cheese	630	40	43
Healthy Choice: Chicken w. Chse	360	9	39
Ham; Roast Beef	320	6	40
Honey Smoked Turkey	335	5	42
Italian	20	0.5	1.5
Roast Beef	375	7	37

	C	F	Cb
Seafood Salad	450	21	46
Tuna Salad	465	22	43
Veggie	200	2	37
Veggie Supreme	325	11	43
Hot Shortis: BBQ Pork	565	20	62
Chicken Grilled	325	3	42
Meatball	660	37	49
Roast Beef Homestyle	425	14	40
Sausage & Pepper	435	22	38
Wraps: Italian	565	35	39
Turkey w. Cranberry Mustard	345	10	41
Roast Beef & Pepper Jack	430	17	42
Roast Beef Special	380	10	37
Roasted Chicken w. Pesto	340	19	33
Smoked Turkey Supreme	325	7	44
Southwestern Turkey	475	28	33
Turkey Bacon & Colby Jack	455	22	37
Veggie & Colby Jack	550	17	79
Hot Dogs: ¼ lb Beef Frank	210	8	20
All Beef Hot Dog	270	17	20
Big Bacon Cheese Dog	730	50	37
Hot Sausage	300	17	21
Kielbasa	215	17	1
Rice Bowls: Per 12 oz Bowl			
Chicken Teriyaki	550	9	99
Chili; Jambalaya	560	13	88
Pepper Steak	510	9	89
Southwest Chicken Bowl	465	6	85
Sides: Per Medium (11 oz)			
Beef Stew	265	13	24
Chili	275	9	31
Homestyle Chicken & Noodles	325	16	26
Macaroni & Cheese	430	20	45
Mashed Potatoes	520	33	49
Meatballs in a Cup	375	27	14
Shepherd's Pie	400	24	37
Soups: Per Medium (11 oz)			
Boston Clam Chowder	290	15	26
Chicken Corn Chowder	370	24	29
Chicken Gumbo	170	7	18
Chicken Noodle	145	3	23
Cream of Broccoli	265	16	21
Creamy Chicken Rice	260	11	29
Italian Sausage & Vege	160	6	17
Italian Wedding; Maryland Crab	145	5	17
Lumberjack Vegetable	95	1	17
Split Pea w. Ham	235	7	31
Tomato Rice	210	11	26
Tuscan White Bean	175	4	22
Vegetable Beef & Barley	150	5	19

Weinerschnitzel

Breakfast: Per Serving	C	F	Cb
Biscuit: w. Egg	285	18	20
Egg, Sausage & Bacon	410	29	22
Egg, Sausage, Bacon & Cheese	465	34	22
Sausage & Bacon, 3.7 oz	325	23	21
Burrito: Breakfast, 9 oz	575	33	41
Chili Cheese, 9.2 oz	500	24	44
Country Breakfast, 10.1 oz	630	45	31
Croissant, 6.5 oz	580	36	41
French Toast, 5.2 oz	495	30	50
Hash Browns, 2.8 oz	285	25	14
Platter, 9.8 oz	700	48	42
Sandwich, 5.5 oz	370	22	28
Burgers: Chili Cheeseburger	345	13	32
Deluxe Cheeseburger	430	23	33
Deluxe Hamburger	385	19	33
Double Chili Cheeseburger	535	24	35
Dessert: Apple Turnover, 3.2 oz	300	19	31
Fries: Per Serving			
Regular, 4.6 oz	350	25	28
Large, 6.4 oz	480	34	39
Chili Cheese, 8.1 oz	545	38	39
Hot Dogs: BBQ Bacon Dog	370	20	33
Chili Dog	285	13	31
Chili Cheese Dog	335	17	31
Deluxe; Kraut; Mustard; Relish	270	12	30
All Beef: BBQ Bacon Dog	470	28	35
Chili Dog	385	21	33
Chilli Cheese Dog	435	25	33
Deluxe; Kraut; Mustard; Relish	360	20	32
Healthy Choice: BBQ Bacon Dog	320	12	38
Chili Cheese Dog	295	10	36
Chili Dog	235	5	36
Deluxe; Kraut; Mustard; Relish	220	4	35
For Pretzel Bun add extra	140	3	26
Sandwiches: Bacon Ranch Chkn	540	31	41
Bratwurst	335	17	30
Cheddar Sausage Melt	670	38	58
Fish	390	17	48
Italian Sausage	345	17	31
Polish Sausage	495	28	39
Southwest Smoky Sausage	460	27	35
Sides: Jalapeno Poppers	485	32	37
Onion Rings	475	25	56
Ranch Dressing	120	12	2
Tamale: Chili Cheese	445	27	33

Wendy's®

Sandwiches	C	F	Cb
Big Bacon Classic®	580	29	46
Chicken Breast Fillet	435	16	46
Chicken Club	480	19	47
Classic Single with Everything	410	19	37
Grilled Chicken Sandwich	305	7	36
Spicy Chicken Sandwich	430	15	47
Kids' Meal: Jr. Hamburger	275	9	34
Jr. Cheeseburger	310	12	34
Jr. Cheeseburger Deluxe	360	16	37
Jr. Bacon Cheeseburger	380	18	34
French Fries: Medium	395	17	56
Biggie®	445	19	63
Great Biggie®	530	23	75
Kid's Meal	255	11	36
Chicken: Crispy Nuggets, 5 pce	200	14	13
Homestyle Strips (3), no sauce	410	18	33
Sauce: Heartland Ranch, 1 pkt	200	21	0.5
Other varieties, avg., 1 pkt	170	16	5
Garden Sensations Salads			
Caesar Side Salad	70	3	9
w. Croutons/Dressing	290	23	12
Chicken BLT Salad: no Dressing	315	16	10
w. Croutons/Dressing	660	44	30
Mandarin Chicken™: no Dressing	160	1.5	17
w. Dressing/Nuts/Noodles	610	34	50
Side Salad, no Dressing	35	0	7
Spring Mix Salad: no Dressing	530	42	25
w. Dressing/Pecans	290	23	12
Taco Supremo: no Dressing	375	17	29
w. Chips/Sour Cream/Salsa	680	34	61
Hot Stuffed Baked Potatoes™			
Plain	315	0	72
Bacon & Cheese	585	22	79
Broccoli & Cheese	485	14	81
Sour Cream & Chives	375	6	73
Whipped Margarine	65	7	0
Chili: Small, 8 oz	205	6	21
Large, 12 oz	305	9	31
Hot Chili Seasoning	10	0	2
Cheddar Cheese, shredded, 2 Tbsp	75	6	1
Saltine Crackers, 2	25	0.5	4
Frosty™ Dairy Dessert: Per Cup			
Junior, 6 oz	165	4	28
Small, 12 oz	330	8	56
Medium, 16 oz	435	11	73

For Complete Nutritional Data ~ see CalorieKing.com

WesterN SizzliN®

Steaks (Meat Only, Raw Wts)

	C	F	Cb
New York Strip, 14 oz	900	60	0
Ribeye, 10 oz	520	28	0
Sirloin: 8 oz Steak	540	33	0
16 oz Steak	1080	66	0
T-Bone, 20 oz	1230	99	0
Baked Potato, plain, 8 oz	245	0	58

Whataburger®

Burgers/Sandwiches

	C	F	Cb
Whataburger®	605	30	53
Small bun, no oil	425	21	31
Double Meat Whataburger®	850	48	53
Whataburger® w. Bacon/Cheese	790	45	53
Triple Meat Whataburger®	1090	66	53
Justaburger®	315	15	28
Whatacatch®	495	26	45
Whatachick'n®	550	21	63
Whataburger Jr.®	315	15	29
Grilled Chicken S'wich: w. Dressing	495	20	49
Small bun, mustard, no oil	335	8	37
Grilled Chicken Fajita Taco	350	13	35
Boca Burger	530	18	61

Whatameals: Includes Drink & Fries

	C	F	Cb
Whataburger® Meal	1275	50	169
Whataburger® w. Bacon & Chse	1420	62	170
Chicken Strips w. Toast & Gravy	1055	49	127
Chicken Strips Kids Meal	740	38	92
Double Meat Whataburger®	1515	67	169
Grilled Chicken Meal	1115	39	165
Justaburger® Kids Meal	655	26	97
WhataChick'N® S'wich Meal	1240	51	172
Whataburger Jr.® Meal	705	29	110

Sides

	C	F	Cb
French Fries: Small	265	13	33
Medium	400	19	50
Large	535	26	66
Onion Rings: Medium	195	10	23
Large	305	16	35

Chicken & Salads

	C	F	Cb
Chicken Strips (2)	380	24	22
Chicken Strips Salad	425	25	29
w. Cheddar Cheese, no Bacon	610	39	32
Garden Salad	55	0	10
w. Cheddar Cheese	225	15	10
Grilled Chicken Salad	240	7	18
w. Cheddar Cheese	400	21	18

Whataburger® cont...

Dressings: Ranch, 2 oz

	C	F	Cb
Ranch, 2 oz	315	33	3
Low Fat Ranch, 2 oz	80	4	10
Low Fat Vinaigrette, 2 oz	25	1.5	6
Thousand Island, 2 oz	160	13	11

Shakes

	C	F	Cb
Chocolate; Strawberry:			
Small, 20 fl oz	615	16	100
Medium, 32 fl oz	905	25	146
Vanilla: Small, 20 fl oz	535	17	81
Medium, 32 fl oz	800	26	122

Breakfast

	C	F	Cb
Bacon, 2 slices	75	5	1
Biscuit: Buttermilk	300	16	34
w. Bacon	375	22	34
w. Bacon, Egg, Cheese	510	32	35
w. Egg & Cheese	440	27	35
w. Sausage	515	35	34
w. Sausage Gravy	520	33	47
w. Sausage, Egg, Cheese	655	46	35
Breakfast-On-A-Bun®: w. Bacon	400	23	28
w. Sausage	540	36	28
Ranchero: w. Bacon	410	23	29
w. Sausage	545	36	29
Breakfast Platters (Biscuit/Eggs/Hash Brown):			
w. Bacon, 2 slices	685	42	52
w. Sausage, 1 patty	830	56	51
Cinnamon Roll	860	34	126
Egg Sandwich	325	17	28
Hashbrown Sticks (4)	135	8	16
Pancakes: Plain (3)	610	7.5	117
w. Bacon, 2 slices	680	13	118
w. Sausage, 1 patty	835	27	118
Taquito: Bacon & Egg	385	22	25
Potato & Egg	370	20	33
Sausage & Egg	375	23	26
Texas Toast	325	14	42

Desserts: Hot Apple Pie

	C	F	Cb
Hot Apple Pie	240	12	31
Chocolate Chunk Cookie, 2 oz	215	8	33
White Choc Macadamia Cookie	230	11	30

Restaurants **& Fast–Foods**

Winchell's®

Baked Products	C	F	Cb
Bagel	130	1	22
Banana Nut Muffin	560	28	63
Blueberry Muffin	480	25	54
Blueberry Muffin, Low Fat	220	3	42
Bran Muffin	405	20	48
Bran Muffin, Low Fat	230	3	44
Cheese Muffin	485	25	51
Chocolate Chip Muffin	450	22	54
Croissant	285	17	28

Cake Donuts: Per Donut Unless Indicated

	C	F	Cb
Buttermilk Bar Glazed	275	16	29
Cinnamon Crumb Cake	290	18	30
Glazed Old Fashion	290	18	28
Iced Cake	255	15	28
Iced French	230	13	24
Iced Old Fashion	300	19	28
Iced Donut Holes (4)	255	15	28
Plain Donut Holes (4)	235	14	26

Raised Donuts: Apple Fritter

	C	F	Cb
Apple Fritter	615	41	55
Bear Claw	480	30	47
Chocolate Bavarian	330	18	36
Chocolate Rounds/Twist/Bar	275	16	29
Glazed Cinnamon Roll	290	24	18
Glazed Jelly; Sugar Jelly	320	17	36
Glazed Rounds/Twist	250	15	27
Iced Bar	240	16	29
Sugar Rounds/Twist	250	15	27

Drinks: Frozen Orange Chilla — 340 | 8 | 66
Frozen Mocha Cappuccino — 490 | 19 | 74

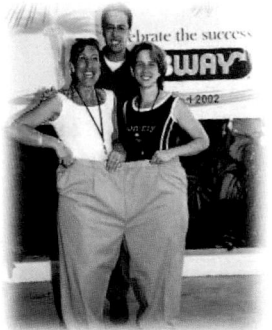

Jared Fogle lost over 200 lbs with Subway® Sandwiches and lots of walking.

White Castle®

Hamburgers	C	F	Cb
Hamburger	140	7	11
Cheeseburger	160	9	11
Bacon Cheeseburger	200	13	12
Double Hamburger	240	14	16
Double Cheeseburger	290	18	16
Sandwiches: Chicken	190	8	21
Fish Sandwich	200	7	27
Breakfast Sandwich	340	25	17
Sides: Cheese Sticks, 3 piece	255	14	22
Chicken Rings, 6 piece	210	14	11
French Fries, small	115	6	15
Onion Rings, 6 piece	260	13	31
Drinks: Coca-Cola, 16 fl.oz	215	0	54
Chocolate/Vanilla Shake, 16 fl.oz	270	8	40
Iced Tea, 16 fl.oz	95	0	24

Yoshinoya®

Bowls

	C	F	Cb
Beef Bowl: Regular, 15 oz	840	30	109
Large, 21 oz	1160	41	153
Kids, 9 oz	340	11	48
Chicken Bowl: Regular, 19 oz	760	15	125
Large, 30 oz	1110	22	180
Kids, 10 oz	370	9	53
Combo Bowl: Regular, 17 oz	750	19	117
Large, 27 oz	1220	36	171
Vegetable Beef Bowl: Reg.,18 oz	770	23	114
Large, 28 oz	1090	32	163
Vegetable Bowl: Regular 19 oz	530	3.5	116
Large, 32 oz	780	5	169
Tempura: Fish Tempura, 22 oz	990	24	168
Fish & Beef Tempura, 30 oz	1450	45	214
Fish & Chicken Tempura, 31 oz	1450	37	225
Shrimp Tempura, 20 oz	890	19	160
Shrimp & Beef Tempura, 28 oz	1350	40	206
Shrimp & Chicken Tempura, 29 oz	1340	32	217
Extras			
Beef, 5¹/2 oz	370	28	6
Chicken & Vegetables, 9¹/2 oz	300	12	21
Rice, 10 oz	460	2.5	104
Vegetable, 9 oz	60	0.5	12

Note: Yoshinoya Beef Bowl Restaurants are based in California.

Zero's Subs®

Oven Baked Subs (6")
(Includes cheese, lettuce, tomato, onions, oil & vinegar)

	C	F	Cb
BLT	410	19	48
BLT, no Mayo	330	12	43
Cosmo Vegetarian	470	23	46
Cosmo Deluxe	500	25	48
Grinder	565	31	48
Grinder, Multigrain	570	32	50
Ham & Cheese	445	19	44
Meatball & Cheese	560	30	50
without Cheese	460	22	50
Pepperoni & Cheese	550	31	42
without Cheese	345	15	41
Roast Beef & Cheese	465	19	45
The Club	505	23	44
Tuna & Cheese	525	26	47
Turkey & Cheese	450	17	44

Subs, 6": Per Sub (No Cheese, Oil or Vinegar)

	C	F	Cb
Cosmo Deluxe	245	3	47
Cosmo Vegetarian	220	2	45
Grilled Veggie	265	3	51
Grinder	400	17	47
Grinder, Multigrain	405	18	49
Ham & Cheese	285	5	43
Roast Beef & Cheese	310	5	45
The Club	360	10	43
Tuna & Cheese	370	12	46
Turkey & Cheese	285	3	43

12" Size Subs: Double the figures for 6" size

Subs From The Grill (6")

	C	F	Cb
Grilled Veggie	410	14	52
Hot Italian Sausage & Cheese	655	37	45
Philly Chicken & Cheese	410	10	48
w. Mushrooms/Green Peppers	415	10	49
without Cheese	325	4	45
Philly Steak & Cheese	495	21	49
w. Mushrooms/Green Peppers	500	21	50
without Cheese	410	15	46

Drinks:

	C	F	Cb
Pepsi (with 25% Ice):			
Small, 12 fl.oz	110	0	29
Medium, 16 fl.oz	150	0	37
Large, 22 fl.oz	210	0	55
Potato Chips, 1 oz pkg.	150	10	15

Zoup!®

Soups: Per Cup (8 fl.oz)

	C	F	Cb
Beef Barley	105	2.5	10
Cajun Chicken & Sausage Gumbo	240	13	18
Chicken Potpie	210	8	25
Chicken & Dumplings	110	1.5	14
Chunky Tomato Chili	110	3.5	16
Collard Green Chicken Barley	140	6	15
Cream of Broccoli	240	14	23
Ginger Chicken	130	6	11
Grilled Chicken Chowder	230	9	27
Mushroom Bisque	180	10	17
New England Clam Chowder	185	7	21
Rock Shrimp and Corn Chowder	220	10	21
Sante Fe' Chicken Chili	140	1.5	21
Shrimp Florentine	180	7	21
Spicy Crab and Rice	155	4.5	20
Spicy Italian Vegetable	110	3	18
Vegetable w. Orzo & Fresh Herbs:	80	0.5	16
Vegetarian Split Pea	160	1	28
White Chicken Chili	150	2	21

12 fl.oz Cup ~ Add 50% to above figures.
16 fl.oz Cup ~ Double the figures for 8 fl.oz cup.

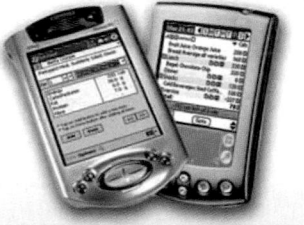

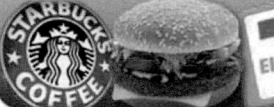

Fats & Cholesterol Guide

Notes on Cholesterol

- **Cholesterol** is a white waxy substance produced mainly by our liver. It is also found in animal food products. Plant foods have no cholesterol.

- **Cholesterol is essential to life.** It is a structural part of every body cell wall and is the building block for vitamin D, sex hormones, and bile acids which help in the digestion of dietary fats.

- **The body makes sufficient cholesterol** for its needs and does not rely on cholesterol in the diet. Dietary fats have a major influence on blood cholesterol levels - more so than dietary cholesterol.

- **A high blood cholesterol increases** the risk of atherosclerosis - the thickening of arteries that can reduce or block blood flow to the heart muscle, brain, eyes, kidneys, sex organs and other body parts.

  This in turn increases the risk of heart attack, stroke, blindness, kidney failure, impotence and other blood circulatory problems.

  Other risk factors which increase the risk of atherosclerosis include high blood pressure, tobacco smoking, obesity and diabetes (uncontrolled).

BLOOD CHOLESTEROL

Check Your Risk!

Cholesterol Level (mg/dL)	Risk of Heart Attack
240 and above	~ High Risk
200 - 239	~ Borderline/High
Below 200	~ Desirable

♥ Know your cholesterol level, particularly if there is a family history of heart disease or stroke. If high, see your doctor.

♥ All adults should have their cholesterol, HDL and triglycerides tested at least every 5 years.

HEART ATTACK WARNING SIGNALS

Many victims die before reaching hospital by ignoring warning signals and delaying medical help.

Symptoms vary and commonly include:

- **Chest pain,** vice-like squeezing or burning sensation in centre of chest or between shoulder blades, or feeling of severe indigestion.

- **Pain** may spread to shoulders, neck, jaw or arms.

- **Sweating,** nausea, dizziness, shortness of breath, irregular pulse.

If you experience any of the above symptoms seek IMMEDIATE medical attention!

Every minute counts.

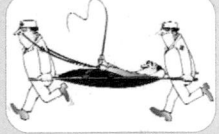

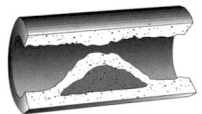

▲ Atherosclerosis can clog arteries and impede blood flow to the heart muscle or other body organs.

▼ A thrombus (blood clot) can form on unstable, festering atherosclerotic plaque and rapidly block blood flow. A heart attack or stroke can result.

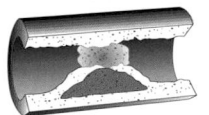

Fats & Cholesterol Guide

The amount and type of dietary fat has the greatest influence on blood cholesterol levels.

Fats in food are a mixture of 3 basic types: saturated, monounsaturated, and polyunsaturated. Animal fats are mainly saturated while plant oils and fish oils are mainly mono- and polyunsaturated.

Saturated fats have subgroups known as long chain, medium chain, and short chain fats. Most of the long chain fats raise blood cholesterol; and increase the risk of blood clots and thrombosis leading to artery blockage.

Long chain saturated fats are found mainly in full cream milk, cheese, butter, cream, fatty meats and sausages, and processed foods.

Monounsaturated fats tend to more selectively lower 'bad' LDL-cholesterol and maintain the protective 'good' HDL-cholesterol in the bloodstream - but only if they replace saturated fats in the diet.

Foods rich in monounsaturates include canola and olive oils, canola margarine, peanuts, and avocados.

Polyunsaturated fats consist of two main classes. **Omega-6** polyunsaturates tend to lower blood cholesterol. Rich sources include safflower, sunflower and corn oils.

Omega-3 polyunsaturated fats can lower blood cholesterol, and also confer extra benefits by lowering blood triglycerides, and reducing the risk of thrombosis, heart arrhythmias, and artery spasm.

Best practical omega-3 sources include canola oil and margarine, soybean oil and fish. (See adjoining chart.)

A balanced intake of the two omega classes is important for optimal health. Increasing slightly omega-3 intake by Americans would help to attain a more ideal balance. Adequate vitamin E intake is also important.

> All fats are high in calories and need to be limited for weight control.

DIETARY FATS COMPARISON

■ Saturated Fat   ■ Monounsaturated Fat
Polyunsaturated Fats:
Linoleic (Omega-6) ■ Alpha-Linolenic (Omega-3)

OILS — PERCENTAGE CONTENT

Oil	Saturated	Monounsaturated	Omega-6	Omega-3
CANOLA OIL	7	63	20	10
LINSEED/FLAX OIL	9	19	17	55
SAFFLOWER OIL	9	14	77	
GRAPESEED OIL	10	22	68	
SUNFLOWER OIL	11	23	66	
CORN OIL	14	32	52	2
OLIVE OIL	14	76		10
SOYBEAN OIL	15	23	54	8
PEANUT OIL	19	45	34	2
COTTONSEED OIL	26	18	58	
PALM OIL	51	39		10

SPREADS & FATS

Saturated Fat includes 'Trans Fats'   ❑ WATER CONTENT

Spread/Fat	Saturated	Monounsaturated	Omega-6	Omega-3	Water
LIGHT MARGARINE	14	14	21		51
CANOLA MARGARINE	18	45	12	6	19
POLYUNSATURATED MARG	24	20	36		20
BUTTER	57	18	2		24
LARD	41	47			12
BEEF FAT	44	37	4		15

GOOD SOURCES OF OMEGA-3 FATS

Plant Sources	Omega-3 Fats (Grams)
Canola Oil, 1 Tbsp, 1/2 fl.oz	1.5g
Flaxseed Oil, 1 Tbsp	8g
Soybean Oil, 1 Tbsp	1.2g
Canola Margarine, 1 Tbsp, 1/2 oz	1g
Soybeans, cooked, 1/2 cup, 4 oz	0.5g
Walnuts, 1/2 oz	0.5g

FISH - Per 4 oz Serving

High Content: Salmon (Chinook), Tuna, Trout (Lake), Sardines, Herring, Mackerel	3g
Medium Content: Salmon (Pink/Red/Coho), 4 oz	2g

Fair Content: Per 4 oz Serving
Bass, Catfish, Cod, Grouper, Hake, Halibut, Kingfish, Perch, Pollock, Shark, Trout (Rainbow), Tuna (Skipjack), Crab, Oysters, Blue Mussel, Shrimp, Squid } 0.5-1g

How Much is Needed?

As little as 1-2 grams daily of omega-3 fats may benefit general health. High doses of fish oil supplements should only be taken as directed by your doctor.

Dietary Cholesterol

Cholesterol in food varies in its effect on blood cholesterol level (BCL) from person to person. Much depends on the amount and type of fat, and fiber eaten at the same meal.

Any elevating effect of dietary cholesterol on BCL is more likely to occur when the diet is high in saturated fat. Little elevation, if any, generally occurs when dietary fats are balanced in favor of mono- and polyunsaturated fats (including omega-3 fats). For example, while fish does contain cholesterol, the omega-3 fats can prevent any increase in BCL. Conversely, a meal containing no cholesterol but rich in saturated fat, may result in a significant increase in BCL.

Consequently, the need to be overly concerned about dietary cholesterol is being de-emphasized in favor of a stricter approach to limiting total fats, as well as saturated fat and trans fats in particular.

The liver usually cuts back its own cholesterol production in response to cholesterol in the diet. Many people can consume normal amounts of high cholesterol foods without concern.

However, it is difficult to identify just who is at risk - the so-called 'hyper-responders' - and because over 50% of Americans have a BCL above ideal levels, the **American Heart Association** advises all Americans to be prudent and limit their cholesterol intake to less than 300mg daily – as well as adopting a heart-healthy diet.

This limitation still allows the inclusion of most foods regularly eaten - even the overly maligned egg.

Note: Eggs contain a modest 5 grams of fat per large egg of which barely 2 grams are saturated, the rest being mono- and polyunsaturated.

By comparison, a cup of whole milk has almost 10g fat of which 6g are saturated.

CHOLESTEROL COUNTER

Cholesterol is found only in foods of animal origin. Plant foods contain no cholesterol. AHA recommends limiting dietary cholesterol to less than 300mg/day.

	Chol mg
Meat - Average all types:	
Lean Meat, cooked, 4 oz	70
Fatty Meat, cooked, 4 oz	105
Fat, thick strip, 2 oz	35
(Note: While lean meat and fat have similar amounts of cholesterol, choose lean meat to limit fat intake.)	
Chicken/Turkey, average, 4 oz	90
Organ Meats: Liver, fried, 4 oz	500
Brains, beef, pan fried, 3 oz	1700
Sausages: Frankfurter, 1.5 oz	25
Salami, 2 slices, 2 oz	40
Bacon: 3 slices, cooked, 1 oz	20
Fish: Fish fillets, average, ckd, 4 oz	70
Tuna/Salmon, canned, 3 oz	30
Scallops, 9 medium, 3 oz	30
Shrimp, 12 large, raw, 3 oz	130
Oysters, raw, 6 medium, 3 oz	45
Lobster, Crab, raw, 3 oz	80
Eggs (Chicken), 1 large	210
1 medium	180
Egg White, *Egg Beaters*	0
Milk/Yogurt: Whole, 1 cup, 8 fl.oz	35
1% Milk, 1 cup	10
Skim/Non-fat, 1 cup	5
Soy Milk, Tofu, Tempeh	0
Cheese: Natural/Hard/Cream 1 oz	30
Cottage, lowfat, 4 oz	5
Ricotta, part skim, 4 oz	25
Fats: Butter, 2 Tbsp, 1 oz	60
Margarine, Oils (vegetable)	0
Mayonnaise, 1 Tbsp	10
Cream: Heavy, whipping, 2 T, 1 oz	40
Half & Half/Sour, 2 Tbsp, 1 oz	10
Icecream: Regular, 1/2 cup, 4 fl.oz	30
Fruit, Vegetables, Avocados	0
Nuts, Seeds, Grains	0
Coffee, Tea, Soda, Beer, Wine	0

For Comprehensive Food Listings ~ see CalorieKing.com

Blood Cholestrol ~ Diet Hints

DIETARY HINTS TO LOWER BLOOD CHOLESTEROL

1. Maintain a healthy weight.
If overweight, lose weight with lowfat eating and daily exercise.

2. Reduce saturated fat intake by:
(a) **eating less dairy fat.** Choose lowfat or fat-reduced varieties of milk, yogurt, cheese, and icecream. Enjoy soy drinks.

(b) **replacing saturated fats** with fats and oils rich in mono- and polyunsaturated fats; and carbohydrate-rich foods. Choose vegetable oils such as canola, olive, sunflower and soybean. Avoid solid frying fats. *Take Control* and *Benecol* (spreads) contain plant stanol esters which can lower total and LDL cholesterol.

(c) **eating less fat from meat** and poultry. Choose lean cuts of meat and skinless chicken. Go easy on luncheon meats, salami and fatty sausages. Enjoy fish.

(d) **eating less saturated and trans fats** from baked and fried fast-foods. Avoid deep-fried foods. Avoid donuts, cakes, pastries and cookies unless made with healthier fats and oils.

3. Increase your 'soluble' fiber intake.
Foods rich in 'soluble' fiber include dried beans, baked beans, lentils, chick peas, hummus, nuts, seeds, psyllium seed husks and psyllium fiber supplements.
Oat bran, rice bran and barley are also useful, as are fruit, veggies and avocados.

4. Eat more soya bean products such as: soy drinks, tofu, tempeh (cultured soya beans), soy flour and soy vegetarian foods.
Soy protein in place of animal protein can significantly decrease high blood cholesterol levels - as well as 'bad' LDL-cholesterol and blood triglycerides. Good' HDL-cholesterol is maintained. For best results, eat at least 25g of soy protein per day (from 3-4 servings)

5. Eat more fruit and vegetables in place of high-fat foods.
Aim for 2 fruits and 5 servings of vegetables per day. They also contain valuable antioxidants.
The fat of avocados (and most nuts and seeds) is mainly unsaturated and lowers blood cholesterol levels.

6. Limit cholesterol to 300mg per day.
(Extra Notes ~ See Previous Page)

7. Avoid brewed unfiltered coffee (espresso; plunger-style). It contains oil compounds (diterpenes) which can raise blood cholesterol. American style filtered coffee is fine.

8. Spread your food intake over the day.
Have 5-6 small meals per day rather than just 2-3 large meals. Nibbling, versus gorging, favors lower blood cholesterol.

ALCOHOL - WINE

Alcohol is a mixed bag. Moderate amounts of 1-2 drinks daily appear to reduce the risk of heart attack and ischaemic stroke in older persons.

However, larger amounts increase the risk of high blood pressure, obesity, heart failure and hemorrhagic stroke; and can aggravate hypertriglyceridemia - in addition to many other health hazards.
(See Alcohol Guide - page 168)

The over-riding harmful effects of excess alcohol do not allow its recommendation for any aspects of health promotion.

Notes On Wine:
Red wine (more so than white) contains antioxidants which may help protect cholesterol in the blood from becoming oxidized.

Many fruits, vegetables and tea also contain protective antioxidants.

How Fats Affect Blood Flow

Fats in the diet not only affect blood cholesterol levels. They can also strongly influence blood clot formation and thrombosis, as well as blood flow and ultimate oxygen delivery to body parts and organs.

While advanced atherosclerosis can impede blood flow to the heart and other organs, it is thrombosis (complete blockage by blood clots) or arterial spasm which commonly result in a heart attack or stroke.

Plant and fish oils rich in omega-3 fats lessen the risk of blood clots, thrombus formation and artery spasm by reducing platelet stickiness and adhesion to artery walls. This reduces the risk of atherosclerotic plaque becoming unstable and reactive.

Omega-3 fats also improve blood flow by reducing blood viscosity; and increasing the flexibility of red blood cells (**RBC**) that need to flex and twist on themselves in order to squeeze through tiny narrow capillaries often half their diameter.

A diet high in saturated fats has the opposite effect by stiffening RBC membranes and increasing blood viscosity thereby hindering blood flow. The stiffening of the RBC membrane also reduces its ability to release vital oxygen to body cells and take up carbon dioxide.

Stiff red blood cells may also form aggregates like coin stacks. In narrow blood vessels, this further impedes blood flow and impairs oxygen release through the much lessened surface area of red blood cell membranes exposed to blood. (Smoking, lack of exercise, and stress can have similar adverse effects on thrombosis, red blood cell flexibility and blood flow.)

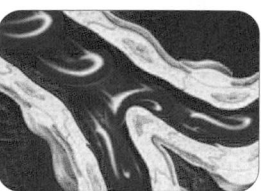

▲ **Picture of Healthy Blood Flow**

Flexible red blood cells twist and slide through tiny capillaries - often half the diameter of red blood cells.

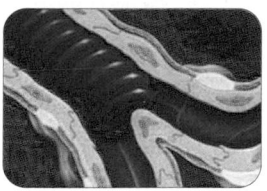

▲ **A Not-So-Healthy Picture!**

Red blood cells have lost their flexibility and ability to twist and slip through capillaries. They are stacked up thereby impeding blood flow.

A diet high in saturated fats can contribute to this picture - as can smoking, lack of exercise and stress.

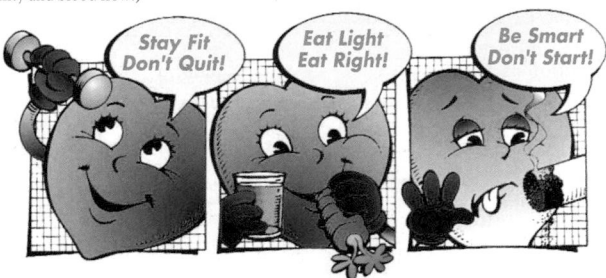

Osteoporosis Guide

Calcium's Role in the Body

Calcium plays a vital role in nerve and muscle function, clotting of blood, enzyme regulation, insulin secretion and overall bone strength. Bones and teeth store 99% of the body's calcium.

The calcium level in blood is kept at a steady level by the continual exchange of calcium between blood and bone. When insufficient calcium is obtained from food the body draws calcium out of the bones.

This bone loss over a period of years may lead to **osteoporosis** - thinning of the bones (*porous bones*).

The bones become weak, brittle and easy to fracture, particularly the bones of the wrist, hips and spine. Loss of height and curvature of the spine may also result, as may periodontal disease - the deterioration of the jaw bones that support the teeth.

Osteoporosis - Common in Women

While osteoporosis also occurs in men, women are particularly vulnerable (1 in 4 by age 60). They have about 30% less bone than men, and a greater bone loss at menopause when estrogen levels drop. Slender framed women are at greater risk. (A woman in her eighties can have lost up to two thirds of her skeleton.)

Insufficient dietary calcium during pregnancy and breastfeeding will see bone reserves drawn upon, increasing the risk of osteoporosis.

Causes of Osteoporosis

The major factors associated with the bone loss of osteoporosis appear to be:

- **Hormone changes of menopause.**
- **Insufficient calcium in the diet.** (Absorption decreases with age.)
- **Insufficient exercise (weight bearing - such as walking, cycling, weight training.)**
- **Family history of osteoporosis.**
- **Other contributing factors may include:** excess amounts of alcohol, protein and phosphorus (from meats and soft drinks); insufficient vitamin D and magnesium; and cigarette smoking.

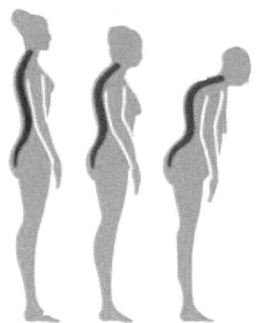

As osteoporosis progresses after menopause, vertebrae may collapse causing the spine to curve and shoulders to hunch.

RECOMMENDED DAILY INTAKE OF CALCIUM

		Calcium
Infants:		
	0-6 mths ~	360mg
	6-12 mths ~	540mg
Children:		
	1-10 yrs ~	800mg
	10-12 yrs ~	1200mg
Teenagers:		
	13-18 yrs ~	1200mg
	16-18 yrs ~	800mg
Adults:	19+ yrs ~	800mg
Women:		
Pre-menopausal	~	1000mg
Menopausal(beginning)	~	1200mg
Post-menopausal	~	1500mg
Pregnancy/breastfeeding:		
	10-18 yrs ~	1600mg
	19+ yrs ~	1200mg

Early Prevention Important

Gradual loss of bone begins in the thirties after maximum bone mass is reached. The stronger the bones at that time, the less trouble is likely to occur later. The earlier that prevention or treatment begins the greater the benefit. **The key to prevention** is to build strong, dense bones early in life. **By age 16**, some 80% of peak bone mass is reached.

Young women may lessen the risk by eating high-calcium foods, not engaging in excessive dieting that results in menstrual period cessation (less estrogen), taking regular exercise and not smoking.

In menopausal women, hormone therapy as well as calcium supplements and exercise, can help retard osteoporosis. Your doctor can advise you.

Dietary Sources of Calcium

Milk, yogurt, calcium-enriched soy drinks and cheese are the richest sources of calcium. (Lowfat and nonfat varieties contain similar amounts of calcium.)

Canned fish with edible bones (salmon/sardines) are high in calcium. Tofu (calcium coagulant), tempeh, broccoli and dried beans are also good sources.

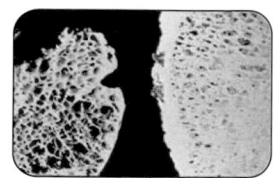

▲ *Osteoporotic Fragile Bone* ▲ *Healthy Dense Bone*

> ### Calculating Calcium ~ Food Labels
> The calcium content of packaged foods and drinks is shown in the Nutrition Facts label as a percentage of the DRI (dietary reference intake) of 1000 mg calcium. To convert this percentage into milligrams of calcium, simply multiply the percent figure by 10 (or add a zero). Examples: 5% = 50 mg calcium; 35% = 350 mg calcium.

Extra Notes on Calcium

Soy drinks (calcium-enriched) may be preferable to cow's milk. Body calcium losses are much greater with animal protein. Soy protein is relatively 'bone-sparing'.

Persons who have difficulty eating sufficient calcium-rich foods should consider a **calcium supplement.** Prescribed high doses of calcium (1500-2000mg/day) may benefit persons with osteoporosis - as well as vitamins D and K, and magnesium.

Calcium in food reduces iron absorption by up to 60% when eaten with iron-containing foods. Ideally, consume calcium-rich foods/supplements at smaller meals and mid-meal snacks. Daily calcium above 2000mg is unlikely to provide any additional benefit.

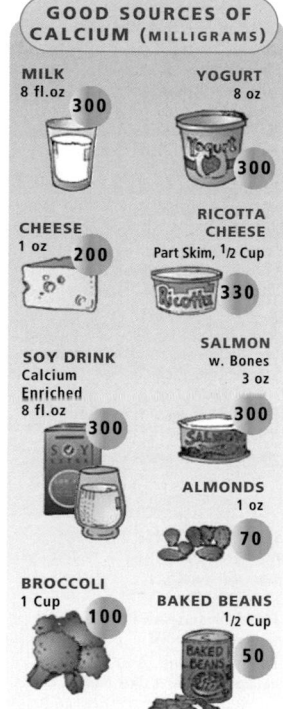

GOOD SOURCES OF CALCIUM (MILLIGRAMS)

MILK 8 fl.oz — 300

YOGURT 8 oz — 300

CHEESE 1 oz — 200

RICOTTA CHEESE Part Skim, 1/2 Cup — 330

SOY DRINK Calcium Enriched 8 fl.oz — 300

SALMON w. Bones 3 oz — 300

ALMONDS 1 oz — 70

BROCCOLI 1 Cup — 100

BAKED BEANS 1/2 Cup — 50

Calcium Counter

Milk & Milk Drinks	Calcium (mg)
Milk Fluid:	
Whole: 1 cup, 8 fl.oz	300
1 small glass, 6 fl.oz	220
1% or 2%: 1 cup, 8 fl.oz	300
Lowfat/Skim: 1 cup, 8 fl.oz	300
Hi-Calcium *(Borden)*, 1 cup	1000
Viva w. extra Calcium, 1 cup	500
Condensed Milk, sweet, 1 fl.oz	110
Evaporated Milk: Skim, 1 fl.oz	90
Whole/Lowfat	80
Dry/Powder: Whole, 1/4 cup	290
Skim/Nonfat, 1/4 cup	380
Other Milks & Milk Drinks	
Buttermilk, average, 1 cup	300
Chocolate Milk, average, 1 cup	300
Nesquik Double Chocolate, 1 cup	400
Goats Milk, 1 cup	320
Malted Milk, 1 cup	350
Milkshakes: Medium, 15 fl.oz	450
Café Latte, 1 cup, 8 fl.oz	220
Cappuccino, 1 cup, 8 fl.oz	150
Milk Drink Powders:	
Malted Milk, dry powder, 1 oz	80
Chocolate, Instant, 3 Tbsp	10
Cocoa Powder: Regular, 1 Tbsp	10
Cocoa Mix: *Hershey*, 1/3 cup	40
Alba High Calcium, 1 envelope	320
Soy & Grain Drinks	
Soy: Regular, non-fortified, 1 cup	60
Enriched/Calcium-fortified, 1 cup	300
Dry Powder, 1 oz	80
Rice/Oat Drinks: Average, 1 cup	10
Yogurt	
Average All Brands, 1 cup, 8 oz	350
Fruit-flavored: 1 cup, 8 oz	250
Small cup, 6 oz	200
4 oz cup	150
Plain: Average, 1 cup, 8 oz	300
Fat Free/Lowfat, 8 oz	350
Custard-style: 6 oz	100
Drinkery (Nouiche)	300
Frozen Yogurt, average, 1/2 cup	150
Fats/Oils	
Butter, Margarine, Spreads, Oils	0
I Can't Believe It's Not Butter	0
w. Sweet Cream and Calcium, 1 Tbsp	100
Country Crock with Calcium, 1 Tbsp	100

Cream	Calcium (mg)
Average: Unwhipped, 1 Tbsp	15
Whipped, 1 heaping Tbsp	15
Half & Half, 1 Tbsp	15
Non-dairy Creamers, 1 tsp	0
Ice Cream & Ices	
Ice Cream: Regular, 1 scoop	65
1/2 cup	90
Premium *(Ben & Jerry's)*, 1/2 cup, 4 oz	150
Soft Serve, 1/2 cup	120
Lowfat, 1/2 cup, 4 oz	150
Ice Milk, average, 1/2 cup	100
Sherbet, average, 1/2 cup	50
Fruit Sorbet	0
Sundae, regular, 6 fl.oz	200
Soy/Tofu Ices, average, 1/2 cup	10
Cheese: Per 1 oz (1 1/2" Cube)	
Natural, Hard: Average, 1 oz	200
Processed Cheese: Average, 1 oz	150
Single-wrapped, 3/4 oz	120
Cheese Substitutes: Average, 1 oz	200
Specific Cheeses:	
Blue, 1 oz	150
Brie, 1 oz	50
Camembert, 1 oz	110
Cheddar, 1 oz	200
Cottage Cheese: 1 round Tbsp, 1 oz	20
1/2 cup, 4 oz	80
Cream Cheese, 1 oz	20
Dorman's Light, average, 1 oz	200
Edam, Gouda, 1 oz	200
Feta, 1 oz	140
Goat, semi-soft, 1 oz	85
Gruyere, 1 oz	290
Kraft Light Naturals, average, 1 oz	250
Light-Line *(Borden)*, singles, 1 oz	200
Monterey Jack, 1 oz	210
Mozzarella, average, 1 oz	170
Parmesan, grated, 1 Tbsp	70
Processed Cheese, average, 1 oz	160
Provolone, 1 oz	210
Ricotta, part skim, 1/2 cup, 4 1/2 oz	330
Swiss, 1 oz	270
Cheese Dishes: Souffle, 4 oz	240
Macaroni & Cheese, 1 cup, 8 oz	150
Ham & Cheese Crepes, 8 oz	350
Quiche, 1 serve, 6 oz	200

Eggs

	Calcium (mg)
1 large Egg	30
Scrambled, with Milk	50
Omelet w. Cheese ($^1/2$ oz)	260

Fish & Seafood

Canned Fish: Tuna, canned, 3 oz	10
Salmon: with bones, 3 oz	190
without bones, 3 oz	10
Sardines, with bones, 3 oz	90
Fresh Fish: cooked, average, 4 oz	35
Seafood: Lobster, cooked, 4 oz	60
Mussels/Oysters (10), 4 oz	95
Crabmeat, cooked, 4 oz	50

Meats & Poultry

Average all types, cooked, 4 oz	20
Vegetarian Soy Burgers:	
Example: *BocaBurger*, 1 pattie, $2^1/2$ oz	100

Soups: *Average all types*

No Milk or Cheese added, 1 serve	30
with Milk, $^1/2$ cup, 1 serve	180
Sauces: Non-Dairy, average, 2 Tbsp	10
Cheese/White Sauce, 2 Tbsp	40
Spices: Average all types, 1 tsp	5

Bread, Bagels

Bread: White, 1 slice, 1 oz	30
Wholewheat, Rye, 1 slice, 1 oz	30
Bagels, average	30
Buns/Rolls: Small	40
Large	90
English Muffins, 2 oz	90
Pita, $6^1/2$ " diameter, 2 oz	50
Tortillas, Corn, 1 oz	40

Breakfast Cereals

Ready To Eat: Average all types, 1 oz	20
with $^3/4$ cup Milk/Soy (enriched)	250
All-Bran, $^1/2$ cup, 1 oz	150
Kashi Heart to Heart, $^3/4$ cup, 1.2 oz	500
Life (Quaker), 1 cup, 1 oz	100
Special K Red Berries, 1 cup	150
Total (General Mills), all types, 1 oz	1000
Wheaties (General Mills), 1 cup, 2 oz	350
Hot Type, cooked: Corn Grits, 1 cup	5
Cream of Wheat, 1 cup	50
Oatmeal/Rolled Oats: Regular, ckd, 1 cup	20
Instant, fortified, 1 pkt	100

Note: Breakfast cereals are a good medium for calcium-rich milk or soy drinks (150mg per $^1/2$ cup).

Flours, Grains

	Calcium (mg)
Wheat Flour: All-purpose, 1 cup	20
Self-rising, 1 cup	330
Whole-wheat, 1 cup	50
Carob Flour, 1 cup, $3^1/2$ oz	360
Corn meal, 1 cup, 4 oz	20
Soybean Flour, 1 cup, 3 oz	170
Grains, Barley, Rice: Cooked, 1 cup	15

Pasta, Spaghetti

Average all types, cooked, 1 cup	15
Lasagne, average, 1 serve	300
Macaroni & Cheese, aver., 1 cup	150
Spaghetti w. Meat Sce, 1 serve	20
with 1 Tbsp Parmesan	90

Sugar & Syrups, Honey

Sugar: White	0
Brown, 1 Tbsp	10
Syrups: Table Syrup, 2 Tbsp	0
Choc., Thin type, 2 Tbsp	5
Fudge type, 2 Tbsp	40
Molasses: Light, 2 Tbsp	70
Blackstrap, average, 1 Tbsp, $^3/4$ oz	270
Honey, Jam, Jelly	0

Cookies & Cakes, Desserts

Cookies: Average all types, 1 cookie	5
Crackers, average, 1 only	5
Cake: Plain, average, 2 oz	40
Carrot Cake with Icing	45
Cheesecake, 1 piece	80
Fruitcake, 1 piece	40
Croissants, average, 2 oz	70
Custard, average, $^1/2$ cup	150
Danish pastry, average, 2 oz	60
Donuts, average, 2 oz	20
Gelatin, plain w. water, $^1/2$ cup	2
Muffins: Regular, average, $1^1/2$ oz	40
English Muffins, 2 oz	90
Pancakes, 4" diameter, average, 1 oz	40
Pies: Apple/Fruit, average, 5 oz	20
Custard Pie, average, 5 oz	140
Pecan Pie, 1 piece, 5 oz	70
Pumpkin Pie, 1 piece, 5 oz	80
w. Icecream, 1 scoop: Add	70
Puddings: Canned, aver., 5 oz	80
Dry Mix, made w. milk, $^1/2$ cup	150
Rice Pudding, $^1/2$ cup	120
Waffles, 7" diameter average	160

Calcium Counter

Candy, Chocolate

	Calcium (mg)
Chocolate: Milk Chocolate, 1 oz	50
Plain/Fruit, 1 oz	65
with Almonds, 1 oz	80
Kit Kat Wafer (1¹/₂ oz); Mars Bar (1.8 oz)	80
Milky Way Bar, 2 oz	60
Carob Bar, average, 2 oz	220
Sugar Candy, Jelly Beans, M'mallow, 1 oz	0

Snacks & Nutrition Bars

Breakfast Bars *(Carnation)*	20
Corn Chips; Tortilla Chips, 1 oz	40
Granola Bars, average	30
Popcorn, 1 cup	5
Potato Chips, 1 oz	10
Nutrition Bars: *Balance Oasis* Bars	350
Dr Soy Bars	350
GeniSoy 'Soy Nutty' Bar	250
Jenny Craig; Power Bars	300
MetRx, After Fx, Pure Protein Bars	500
Slim-Fast 'Meal On The Go'	300
TwinLab Protein Fuel Bars	350
Viactiv Bar	300
Wholefoods Everyday Bars	300

Nuts & Seeds (Shelled)

Almonds, 12-15 nuts, ¹/₂ oz	40
Brazil Nuts, 4 medium, ¹/₂ oz	30
Cashews, 6-8 nuts, ¹/₂ oz	5
Coconut, fresh, ¹/₂ oz	5
Filberts (Hazelnuts), ¹/₂ oz	40
Macadamias, 6 medium, ¹/₂ oz	10
Peanuts, raw, 1 oz	25
Walnuts, 1 oz	20
Seeds: Pumpkin, 1 oz	15
Sesame, 1 Tbsp	10
Sunflower, 1 oz	30
Tahini, 1 Tbsp, ¹/₂ oz	20

Drinks – Alcohol, Soda, Water

Beer, Cider, Wine, 1 glass	5
Spirits, Liqueurs	0
Coffee, Tea, Soda, Fruit Drinks	5
Water: Tap, average, 1 cup	5
Mineral Water *(Perrier)*, 1 glass, 6 oz	20

Fruit & Fruit Juice

	Calcium (mg)
Fresh Fruit: Average all types, 1 serve	20
Apple, 1 medium	10
Avocado, 1 medium	20
Banana, 1 medium	10
Orange, 1 medium	50
Pear, 1 medium	20
Rhubarb, cooked, ¹/₂ cup	170
(calcium largely not available to body)	
Dried Fruit: Average, 1 oz	20
Figs, 3 medium, 1¹/₂ oz	55
Fruit Juice: Average, 1 cup, 8 fl.oz	25
Orange Juice, calcium fortified (8 fl.oz):	
Citrus Hill Plus Calcium, Hi-C	300
Donald Duck	350
Minute Maid (Premium Calcium)	300
Jui2ce, 8 fl.oz	200
Tropicana (Calcium)	350
Welch's Healthy Sensation, 1 cup	350

Vegetables

Average all types, 1 cup	40
Higher Calcium Content:	
Beans, dried: cooked, ¹/₂ cup	50
Baked/Refried Beans, ¹/₂ cup	60
Broccoli, chopped, 1 cup	100
Chickpeas, boiled, ¹/₂ cup	40
Collards, cooked, 1 cup	150
Dandelion Greens, cooked, 1 cup	150
Kale, 1 cup	130
Mustard Greens, 1 cup	100
Soybeans, cooked, ¹/₂ cup, 3 oz	60
Spinach, cooked, ¹/₂ cup	120
Potato: Plain, 1 large	20
Au Gratin, 1 cup	200
Mashed w. Milk, 1 cup	60
Tofu: *Mori Nu:* Silken, 4 oz	90
Azumaya: Silken, 3 oz	20
Firm/Extra Firm, 3 oz	150
Hinoichi: Regular, 1" slice, 3 oz	100
Firm/Extra Firm, 3 oz	150
Soft, 1" slice, 3 oz	60
Nasoya: Firm, Soft, 3 oz	120
Extra Firm, 3 oz	150
Silken, 3 oz	60
Tree of Life: Firm, 3 oz	150
Miso: ¹/₂ cup, 5 oz	100
Tempeh: 4 oz serving	100

Frozen Entrees/Meals

	Calcium (mg)
Authentico:	
Cheese Ravioli w. Alfredo & Broccoli Sce	350
Healthy Choice:	
Cheddar Broccoli Potatoes (Solos)	200
Chicken Broccoli Alfredo (Bowl)	150
Meat Lasagna (Medley)	200
Lean Cuisine:	
Chicken Carbonara (Café Classics)	150
Creamy Chicken/Veges Bowl	250
French Bread Pizza, Cheese, 6 oz	300
Lean Gourmet:	
Cheese Manicotti w. Marinara Sauce	200

Frozen Pizzas ~ Regular Large

Average All Brands: Cheese, 1/4 pizza	350
Meats (Sausage/Pepperoni), 1/4 pizza	250

Nutritional Shakes/Drinks

Atkins Shake, 11 fl.oz can	300
Balanced: Diet, 11 fl.oz can	500
High Protein, 11 fl.oz can	250
Boost, regular, 8 fl.oz can	300
Choice dm (Mead Johnson) 8 fl.oz	330
Ensure High Calcium, 8 fl.oz can	400
Genisoy Shake, 1 scoop, 35g	250
Jevity (w. Fiber) 8 fl.oz	215
Kashi GoLean Shake, 11 oz can	400
Kindercal, 8 fl.oz	240
Met-Rx Protein Shake, 11 fl.oz	950
Myoplex (EAS) Nutrition Shake, 11 oz	400
Optifast 800, Powder or Can (RTD)	200
Slim-Fast Shakes, 325ml can	400
Spiru-Tein, Vanilla, 8 fl.oz can	600
Ultra Slim-Fast: Soy Protein Drink, 11.5 oz	350
Shake, 11 oz can	400
Mix, Meal, 1 scoop, 33g	150
Usana Nutrimeal, 2 scoops, 43g	400
Walgreens, Slim For Less, 11 oz can	400

Calcium Supplements

Caltrate 600, 1 tablet	600
Citracal, 1 tablet	200
Maalox Soft Chews, 1	400
Nature's Life 'Super Cal-Mag', 1	500
Os-cal; 1 tablet	500
Posture Calcium, 1 tablet	600
Tums: Regular, 1 tablet	200
Extra Strength, 1 tablet	300
Viativ Soft Calcium Chews, 1 chew	500

Fast-Foods, Restaurants

	Calcium (mg)
Chicken:	
Grilled/BBQ, 1/4 chicken	20
Battered & Fried, 2 pieces	80
Nuggets, 6 pack	20
Crispy Chicken Deluxe Sandwich	50
Croissant Sandwich: Plain	40
with Cheese, 1 oz	240
Fish Sandwich: no Cheese	60
with Cheese	140
Fish Filet Deluxe	70
Fish, fried, 2 pieces	20
French Fries: Small Serving	10
Hamburgers: Average all outlets,	
Regular, no Cheese	120
Cheeseburger, regular	120
McDonald's: Big Mac	160
Quarter Pounder w. Cheese	120
Egg McMuffin	120
Hot Dog: Plain	60
with Cheese	150
Mexican: Burrito	120
Enchilada	300
Nachos, regular	200
Taco, regular	140
Taco Bell Salad	400
Pizza: Average all types,	
Medium (12"), 2 slices	250
Double Cheese, 2 slices	350
Large (16"), 2 slices	350
Double Cheese, 2 slices	500
Pizza Hut: Cheese, medium, 2 slices	290
Pepperoni, medium, 2 slices	300
Potato: Plain, baked, 8 oz	20
Stuffed w. Cheese Topping	100
with Cheese Filling	300
Sandwiches: no Cheese	60
with 1 oz Cheese (regular)	260
with Cream Cheese	80
Subway: 6" Sandwich, average	100
Cheese & Egg Bkfst Sandwich	150
Steak & Cheese Wrap	150
Cheese (extra fixin'), 3 triangles	150
Pocket Sandwich, no Cheese	150
Salads (Classic), average	100
Salads: Chef, regular	300
Coleslaw, small	20
Shakes, average	330

Fiber Guide

Introduction

Fiber is the general term for those parts of **plant** food that we cannot digest (although bacteria in the large bowel partly digests fiber through fermentation). It is not found in foods of animal origin (meats, dairy products).

Fiber promotes intestinal health, bowel regularity, can benefit diabetes and blood cholesterol levels, and may help prevent colon cancer. High fiber foods also assist weight control.

Most Americans don't eat enough fiber - less than 20 grams/day - instead of a **healthier 25 to 35 grams/day**.

Types of Fiber

Plant foods contain a mixture of different fibers in varying proportions. Insoluble and soluble fiber categories are based on their solubility in water. All types of fiber are beneficial to the body.

◆ **Insoluble fibers** (cellulose, hemi-celluloses, lignin) make up the structural parts of plant cell walls. The **best sources** are wheat bran, corn bran, rice bran, wholegrain cereals and breads, dried beans and peas, nuts, seeds and the skins of fruits and vegetables.

These fibers absorb many times their own weight in water. They create a soft bulk and hasten the passage of waste products through the intestines.

They promote bowel regularity, and aid in the prevention and treatment of uncomplicated forms of **constipation**, **diverticulosis** and **haemorrhoids**.

The risk of colon cancer may also be reduced by fiber's diluting effect of potentially harmful substances.

◆ **Soluble fibers** (pectin, gums, mucilages) are found mainly within plant cells, soy milk (whole bean) and products.

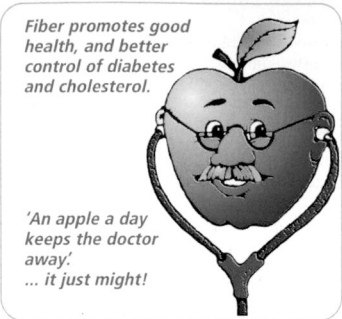

Fiber promotes good health, and better control of diabetes and cholesterol.

'An apple a day keeps the doctor away.'
... it just might!

Types of Fiber (Cont)

Best Sources of Soluble Fiber:
Fruits and vegetables, oat bran, barley, dried beans and peas, psyllium and flax seed.

These fibers form a gel which slows both stomach emptying and the absorption of sugars from the intestines. This helps to control **blood sugar** levels.

Weight control is also aided by the slower emptying of the stomach and the feeling of **fullness provided by soluble fiber**.

Some soluble fibers can lower **blood cholesterol** by binding bile acids and excreting them. More body cholesterol must then be broken down to supply bile acids for emulsification of dietary fats. **Rice bran, while not high in soluble fiber can also lower blood cholesterol.**

◆ **Resistant starch** is that part of starchy foods (approx. 10%) which is tightly bound by fiber and resists normal digestion. Friendly bacteria in the large bowel ferment and change the resistant starch into short-chain fatty acids which are important to bowel health and may protect against colon cancer.

Starchy foods include bread, cereals, rice, pasta, potatoes and legumes.

Fiber & Weight Control

Fiber can assist weight control in several ways. Fiber-rich foods such as fresh fruit and vegetables, potatoes and whole-grain bread contain few calories for their large volume (due to their lowfat, high water content).

Their bulk fills the stomach and satisfies appetite much earlier than fiber-depleted foods. The extra chewing time also contributes to satiety, and gives the stomach time to register a feeling of fullness. Excessive calories are less likely to be consumed.

Fiber-depleted foods and drinks are more concentrated in calories; e.g. fats, sugar, candy, soft drinks, fruit juices, alcohol. They require little or no chewing. Large amounts with excessive calories can be consumed before appetite is satisfied.

Example: Whereas one fresh apple might satisfy our appetite, an apple juice drink with the equivalent sugars and calories of 2-3 apples does little to satisfy appetite. (See illustration below.)

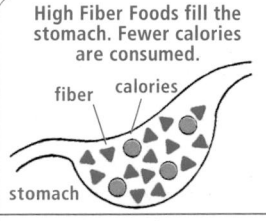

High Fiber Foods fill the stomach. Fewer calories are consumed.

Low Fiber Foods are more concentrated in calories. More food must be eaten to fill the stomach.

EFFECTS OF REMOVING FIBER FROM FOOD

2-3 pieces of fresh fruit produces 1 glass of fruit juice. The removal of fiber concentrates the sugar and calories.

FIBER REMOVED

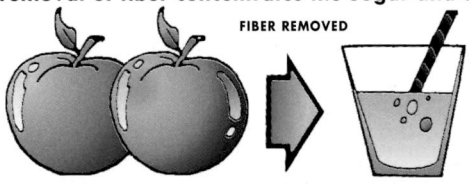

Fresh Fruit		Fruit Juice
High Fiber	←	Negligible Fiber
Low Calorie Density	←	High Calorie Density
Long Eating Time	←	No Eating Time (Drink)
Satisfies Hunger	←	Does Not Satisfy Hunger
Sugar Slowly Absorbed	←	Sugar More Quickly Absorbed
Less Insulin Required	←	More Insulin Required

Fiber Guide - Constipation

Constipation

Constipation can reasonably be defined as a failure to have a bowel movement at least every second day - and just as importantly, without straining or pain.

Typically, stools are too hard, too narrow, and too small ... *sinkers* rather than *floaters*.

The **main cause** is simply a lack of dietary fiber. Other contributing factors include insufficient fluids, too little exercise, emotional stress, gastro-intestinal disease, lack of proper dentition to chew high-fiber foods, and some medications (e.g. some antacids, antidepressants, tranquilizers).

Note: Check with your doctor to rule out any underlying medical problem – especially if you have a change in bowel habits in middle-age or later years.

DESIRABLE FIBER INTAKE

Adults: 25-35gm per day
Children (under 18): Age + 5gm
Example: 6-year old (6 + 5)= 11gm

SAMPLE FOOD QUANTITIES

For 35 Grams of Fiber/Day `Fiber`

Breakfast Cereal (higher-fiber)	5g
plus 4 slices whole-grain Bread	6g
plus 3 servings fresh Fruit	9g
plus 1 medium Potato (w. skin) **or** 1 cup Brown Rice **or** ¹/₂ cup whole-grain Pasta	}4g
plus 3-4 servings Veges/Salad	6g
plus 1 cup Bean Soup **or** ¹/₄ cup Baked/Soy Beans **or** ¹/₂ cup Corn/Peas/Lentils **or** 1¹/₄ oz Almonds (natural) **or** 3 medium Figs	}5g

HINTS TO INCREASE FIBER AND AVOID CONSTIPATION

1. Breakfast is an important contributor to daily fiber intake. Eat high-fiber breakfast cereals (bran-based cereals, oatmeal etc.). Add 1-2 tablespoons of unprocessed bran (wheat/ barley/ rice) and wheat germ if required.

Dried fruits, chopped nuts, soy grits, and seeds are also excellent additions to cereals.

Note: A gradual increase in fiber will prevent bloating, gas or pain. Persons intolerant to bran may benefit from psyllium-based fiber supplements and cereals.

2. Drink 6-8 glasses of water daily. Fiber works by absorbing many times its own weight of water.

3. Eat whole-grain breads, or fiber-enriched breads. One slice of whole-grain bread has over double the fiber of regular white bread.

4. Enjoy fruit as fresh fruit with skins rather than as fruit juice. Enjoy whole-grain pasta, barley, brown rice, nuts and seeds.

5. Eat more vegetables, salads and legumes - especially dried beans, baked beans, lentils, potatoes with skins, avocado, broccoli, brussel sprouts, cabbage, carrots, celery, and peas.

6. Add bran (barley/rice/wheat) or soy grits to soups, casseroles, yogurt, desserts, biscuits, cakes. Also use wholemeal flour or soy flour in place of white flour. Use nuts and seeds.

7. Snack on fresh or dried fruits, carrot or celery sticks, popcorn, nuts or seeds, wholegrain crackers, high-fiber bars (low-fat). Limit amounts if overweight.

8. Exercise regularly to strengthen abdominal muscles and stimulate the gut. Keep up fluids, especially in warm weather.

9. Avoid indiscriminate and regular use of harsh laxatives. They can overstimulate the intestinal muscles and may make normal bowel activity impossible. It may take several weeks to restore normal bowel function.

Fiber Guide

FOODS WITH ZERO FIBER
- **Dairy Products (Milk, Cheese, etc)**
- **Meats, Poultry, Fish, Eggs**
- **Fats/Oils, Sugar/Syrups**

(Only foods of plant origin contain fiber.)

Fiber ~ Fiber (grams)

Breakfast Cereals

General Mills:	Fiber
Basic 4, 1 cup, 2 oz	3
Cheerios (Honey Nut; Multigrain), 1 c., 1 oz	3
Fiber One, 1/2 cup, 1 oz	13
Multi-Bran Chex, 1 cup, 2 oz	8
Oatmeal Crisp Almond, 1 cup, 2 oz	4
Raisin Nut Bran, 3/4 cup, 2 oz	5
Total, average all types, 1 oz	3
Wheat Chex; Wheaties, 1 cup	5
Wheaties Energy Crunch, 1 cup	4

Health Valley:	
10 Bran O's, 3/4 cup, 1.95 oz	4
Amaranth Flakes, 3/4 cup	4
Corn Bran Flakes, 3/4 cup	4
Fiber 7 Flakes, 3/4 cup	4
Golden Flax, 1/4 cup	6
Granola (Fat Free), 2/3 cup	6
Healthy Crunches & Flakes, 3/4 cup	4
Healthy Fiber Flakes, 3/4 cup	4
Oat Bran Flakes, all types, 3/4 cup	4
Real Oat Bran, 1/2 cup	5

Kellogg's: All-Bran, 1/2 cup, 1 oz	10
All-Bran w. Extra Fiber, 1/2 cup, 1 oz	13
Bran Buds, 3/4 cup, 2 oz	12
Corn Flakes, Fruit Loops, Smacks, 3/4 cup	1
Cracklin' Oat Bran, 3/4 cup, 2 oz	6
Cocoa/Rice Krispies Treats, 3/4 cup, 1 oz	0
Complete: Wheatbran Flakes, 3/4 c., 1 oz	5
Oatbran Flakes, 3/4 cup	4
Corn Pops, 1 cup, 1 oz	0
Frosted Mini Wheats, 1 cup, 2 oz	6
Healthy Choice, all types, 1 cup	5
Nutri-Grain Almond, 1 1/4 cup, 2 oz	4
Cereal Bars, 1 bar, 1.3 oz	4
Mueslix (Almond. Raisin Date), 2/3 cup	4
Raisin Bran, 1 cup, 2 oz	8
Smart Start Original, 1 cup	2
Soy Protein, 1 oz	2
Special K; Product 19, 1 cup	1
Special K Red Berries, 1 cup	4
Wheat Chex, 1 cup	3

Breakfast Cereals (Cont)

Kashi: GoLEAN Cereal, 3/4 cup, 1.4 oz	10
GoLEAN Crunch!, 1 cup, 1.8 oz	8
GoLEAN Bars, each	6
Breakfast Pilaf, 1/2 cup, cooked, 5 oz	6
Good Friends, 3/4 cup, 1 oz	8
Cinna-raisin Crunch, 1 cup, 1 3/4 oz	10
Heart to Heart, 3/4 cup, 1.2 oz	5
Puffed Kashi, 1 cup, 0.9 oz	2

Quaker: Cap'n Crunch, 3/4 cup	1
100% Natural Granola, average, 1/2 cup	3
Crunchy Corn Bran, 1 cup, 1 oz	5
Fruity Oh's, 1 cup	2
Honey Nut, 1 cup	3
Life Cereal (3/4 cup), Oat Squares (1/2 c.)	2
Oat Bran, 1/3 cup	6
Oatmeal, average, 1 packet	3
Puffed Rice, 1 cup	1
Puffed Wheat, 1 cup	2
Shredded Wheat, 3 biscuits	3

Post: 100% Bran, 1/2 cup	8
Blueberry Morning, 1 cup, 2 oz	2
Cocoa/Fruity Pebbles, 1 cup	0
Cranberry Almond Crunch, 1 cup, 2 oz	3
Frosted Alpha Bits, 1 cup	1
Fruit & Fibre, 1 cup, 2 oz	5
Grape-Nuts, 1/2 cup	5
Great Grains, 2/3 cup, 1.8 oz	4
Honey Bunches of Oats, 3/4 cup, 1 oz	1
Shredded Wheat 'n Bran, 1/2 cup	3

Brans & Supplements

Oat Bran: 1 Tbsp (level)	0.8
1/3 cup, (5 1/3 Tbsp), 1 oz	4.2
Rice Bran: 1/3 cup, 1 oz	6
Wheat Bran: unprocessed: 1 Tbsp	1.6
2 Tbsp (level), 1/4 oz	3.2
1/4 cup, (4 Tbsp), 1/2 oz	6.4
1/2 cup, 1 oz	13
Corn Germ: 1/4 cup, 1 oz	5
Wheat Germ: 1/4 cup, 1 oz	3
Psyllium Seed Husks, 2 Tbsp	8
Metamucil, 1 dose	3.4

Hot Cereals, Oatmeal

Bulgur (cracked Wheat), ckd, 1 cup	8
Cream of Wheat, ckd, 2/3 cup	1
Hominy Grits, dry, 3 Tbsp, 1 oz	1.2
Oatmeal (uncooked 1/3 cup), ckd, 2/3 cup	2.7

Fiber Guide

Breads & Crackers | Fiber

Bread: White, 1 slice, 1 oz	0.7
Whole-wheat, 1 slice, 1 oz	1.5
Whole-grain, 1 slice, 1 oz	2
Rye, Pumpernickel, 1 oz	1.5
Bagel/Roll/Bun, 1 medium, 2 oz	1.5
Pita, whole wheat, 5" pocket	4.5
Crackers: Graham, average, 2	1.4
Saltine, 4 crackers	0.3
Crispbreads (Rye), average, 2	4
Matzo 1 board, 1 oz	1
Rice Cakes: Average, 1 cake	0.3
Tortilla: Regular, 6"	0.5
Whole-wheat, 6"	1.3

Barley, Pasta, Rice & Flours

Barley, pearled, raw, 1/4 cup, 1.7 oz	5
Rice: White, cooked, 1 cup, 7 oz	1.6
Brown, cooked, 1 cup	3.2
Rice-A-Roni, average, 1 cup	1.5
Spaghetti/Noodles: cooked, 1 cup	2
Whole-grain, cooked, 1 cup	7
Amaranth *(Health Valley),* 1 cup	9
Flour: Wheat, All-purpose, 1 cup, 4 1/2 oz	3.5
Whole-grain, 1 cup, 4 1/2 oz	15
Cornmeal, stone ground, 1 cup, 4 1/2 oz	13
Carob Flour, 1 cup, 3 1/2 oz	13
Rye Flour, 1 cup, 3 1/2 oz	15
Soy Flour: Defatted, 1 cup, 3 1/2 oz	17
Full-fat, raw, 1 cup, 3 oz	8
Soy Meal, defatted, 1 cup, 4 1/2 oz	14

Frozen Entrees & Dinners

Average All Brands: Per Serving	
Beans/Chili base, average	6-10
Potato/Pasta base, average	4-6
Vegetable base, average	3
Meat/Chicken base, average	2-3
Pizzas, 1/4 large, average	3
Vegetarian Soy Burgers, 1 pattie	5

Soups

Chicken Noodle, 1 cup	0
Tomato Soup, average, 1 cup	0.5
Vegetable Soup, average, 1 cup	3
Health Valley: Per 1 Cup Serving	
Black Bean; Minestrone	10
Tomato	4
5-Bean Vegetable; Lentil & Carrots	13
Mushroom & Barley; Split Pea; Vegetable	7
Rotini & Vegetables	4

Fast Foods & Restaurants | Fiber

Hamburgers: Small, average	1.5
Large/Whopper, average	2.5
Hot Dog, Regular	1.5
French Fries: Small serving, 2 1/2 oz	2.5
Regular/Medium, 3 1/2 oz	3.5
Chicken Nuggets, 6 pack	0.5
Chicken Sandwich, average	2
Taco, average	4
Sundaes, Shakes, Soft Drinks	0
Arby's: Baked Potato w. Broc. & Cheddar	7
Roast Beef Sandwich, regular	2
Denny's: Grilled Chicken Caesar Salad	4
Classic Burger w. fries	4
Club Sandwich	3
Grilled Chicken Sandwich	4
Domino's (Classic): Veggie, 2 sl. (12")	3.5
Hawaiian Feast, 2 slices, (12")	3
Pepperoni, 2 slices (12")	3
McDonald's: Big Mac; McChicken	3
Ham/Cheeseburger; Quarter Pounder	2
Egg McMuffin	2
Grilled Chicken Caesar Salad	3
McVeggie Burger	9
Pizza Hut: Per 2 Slices, Medium	
Pan Pizza: Cheese, Pepperoni	2
Supreme	3
Thin 'n Crispy, Supreme	2
Hand-Tossed, average	2.5
Personal Pan Pizza, 1 whole	5
Subway: Sandwich, white roll, avg.	2.5
w. Honey Wheat Roll, avg.	3.2
Footlong w. Wheat Roll, avg.	6.4
Salads, average	3

Cakes, Cookies, Snack Bars

Apple/Fruit Pie, 1 serving	2
Cake: w. plain flour, 1 serving	1
w. whole-wheat flour, 1 serving	3
Carrot Cake, 1 serving	2
Cookies, oatmeal, (3 small/1 large)	3
Donuts	0
Fruit Cake, 1 serving	3
Fig Bars, 2	1.3
Muffins, Oat Bran (2 small, 1 large), 4 oz	5
Granola Bars, average, 1 bar	2
Atkins Advantage Bars, average	9
Cliff Bars, 1.7 oz	5
Fi-Bar Nectar, 1 bar	4
Health Valley: Fruit/Granola Bars	4
Cereal Bars	7
Luna Bars, 1.7 oz	3

Fiber Guide

Chocolate, Chips, Popcorn | Fiber

	Fiber
Cheese Balls/Curls/Twists	0
Chocolate, Hard Candy, Cheese Balls	0
Chocolate with nuts/fruit, 2 oz bar	1
Mars Bar	1
Potato Chips, corn chips, 1 oz	1
Popcorn, 3 cups	2
Pretzels, Twists, 6	1

Nuts, Seeds

	Fiber
Almonds: Natural, 25 kernels, 1 oz	4
Blanched (skins removed), 1 oz	3
Cashews, Filberts, Pecans, 1 oz	1.7
Peanuts, Mixed Nuts, Coconut, 1 oz	2.5
Peanut Butter, 2 Tbsp, 1 oz	1.8
Pistachio Nuts, dried, shelled, 1 oz	3
Walnuts, Black/English, dried, 1 oz	1.5
Seeds: Amaranth, 2 1/2 Tbsp, 1 oz	3.5
Flax Seeds, 3 Tbsp, 1 oz	7
Psyllium Seed Husks, 5 Tbsp, 1 oz	20
Quinoa Seeds, 3 Tbsp, 1 oz	2.7
Sesame Seeds, whole, 1 oz	3
Sesame Butter/Tahini, 2 Tbsp, 1.1 oz	3
Sunflower kernels, 1/4 cup, 1 oz	4.4
Teff Seeds, 1 oz	3.8

Fruit – Fresh

	Fiber
Apples: 1 medium, 6 oz (whole)	
with skin + core	5.5
with skin, no core	4.5
without skin, no core	3.7
Apricots, 2 medium, 4 oz	2
Avocado, average, 1/2 medium	3
Banana, 1 medium, 6 oz (w. skin)	2
Blueberries, raw, 1 1/2 cup, 4 oz	4.4
Cherries, sweet, raw, 10 fruits, 2 1/2 oz	1.5
Grapefruit, average, 1/2 fruit, 8 1/2 oz	1
Grapes, 1 medium bunch, seedless, 7 oz	3
Kiwifruit, 1 medium, 3 oz	3
Mango, 1 medium, 11 oz (whole)	1.6
Melons, cantaloup, 4 oz (edible)	1
Nectarine, 1 medium, 4 oz	1.8
Olives, average all types, 7 jumbo, 2 oz	1.5
Oranges, 1 medium (7-8 oz w. skin)	
5 1/2 oz (peeled)	3.8
Passionfruit, 2 medium, 2 1/2 oz	5
Peaches, 1 large, 6 oz	2
Pears, raw, 1 medium, 6 oz	4.5
Pineapple, 1 slice, 3 oz	1.8
Plums, 2 medium, 6 oz	2.8
Strawberries, 6 medium/3 large, 2 oz	1.5
Watermelon, 4 oz (edible)	0.5

Fruit – Dried, Juice | Fiber

	Fiber
Dried Fruit: Apricots, 8 halves, 1 oz	2.2
Dates (3 med); Raisins (2 Tbsp), 1 oz	1.5
Figs, 3 medium, 1 1/2 oz	5
Prunes, 4 medium, 1 oz	3
Fruit Juice: Orange/Apple etc, 1 glass	<0.5
Prune Juice, 5 oz	1.4
Carrot Juice, 8 oz	1.8

Vegetables

	Fiber
Asparagus, 4 spears	2
Bean Sprouts, 1/2 cup, 2 1/4 oz	1.5
Beans: Snap/Green, 1/2 cup, 2 1/2 oz	2
Baked Beans in Tom Sce, 1/2 c, 4 1/2 oz	10
Dried Beans, ckd, average, 1/2 cup	7
Beets, ckd, slices, 1/2 cup, 3 oz	1.5
Broccoli, cooked, 1/2 cup, 3 oz	2.2
Brussels Sprouts, ckd, 1/2 cup, 3 oz	3.5
Cabbage: White, ckd, 1/2 cup, 2 1/2 oz	1
Red, ckd, 1/2 cup, 2 1/2 oz	1.5
Carrots, 1 medium (7 1/2"), 1/2 cup, 3 oz	2.7
Cauliflower, cooked, 1/2 cup, 3 oz	2.8
Celery, raw, diced, 1/2 cup, 2 1/2 oz	1
Chick Peas (Garbanzos), ckd, 1/2 c., 3 1/2 oz	6
Corn, kernels, ckd, 1/2 cup, 2 1/2 oz	2.5
Cream-style, 1/2 cup, 4 1/2 oz	1.5
Cucumber/Lettuce/Mushrooms, 2 oz	0.5
Eggplant, raw, sliced, 1/2 cup	2.5
Lentils, cooked, 1/2 cup, 3 1/2 oz	4
Onions, 1 medium, 4 oz	2
Spring Onions, chop., 1/4 cup, 1 oz	1.5
Peas: Green, 1/2 cup, 3 oz	3
Cowpeas (Black-eyed), ckd, 1/2 cup	10
Split Peas, ckd, 1/2 cup, 4 1/2 oz	6.5
Peppers, sweet, raw, 1 large, 3 1/2 oz	1.5
Potatoes: 1 medium, with skin, 5 oz	4
without skin	2
1/2 cup mashed, 3 1/2 oz	1.5
French Fries, 3 oz serving	3
Spinach, cooked, 1/2 cup, 3 oz	2
Squash: Summer, cookd, 3 oz	1.2
Winter, cooked, 3 oz	2.4
Tomatoes: 1 medium, 5 oz	2
Tomato Sauce, 1 cup	0.3
Frozen: Mixed Vegetables, ckd, 1/2 cup	3
Soybean Products: Miso, 1/2 c., 5 oz	7.7
Tempeh, 1 piece, 3 oz	2
Tofu, 4 oz	1.4

Salads:
	Fiber
Side Salad, average	1
Bean Salad, 1/2 cup	5
Coleslaw, 1/2 cup	1
Potato Salad, 1/2 cup	2

Protein Guide

General Notes

- **Protein has many important body functions.** It builds and repairs muscle, and is the basis of our body's organs, hormones, enzymes, and antibodies to fight infection.

- **Protein is also an emergency fuel** in the absence of sufficient carbohydrate and fats. For this reason, weight loss should be gradual so as to preserve protein levels in muscle, the heart and other body organs.

- **It is easy to obtain sufficient protein,** even if vegetarian. **Plant proteins are not inferior to animal proteins.** In fact, eating more soy and other plant proteins, and less animal protein, may help to build stronger bones and prevent osteoporosis; and may help to control blood cholesterol levels.

- **When changing to a vegetarian diet,** include soybeans, and other dried beans, soy milk drinks (calcium-enriched), lentils, tofu, tempeh, nuts, and wholegrain breads and cereals. Milk, yogurt, cheese and eggs may enhance nutrient intake.

Protein & Muscle

- Although muscles are built of protein, protein is not a special fuel for working muscle cells - carbohydrates and fats are.

- In fact, a diet high in protein (and fat) and low in carbohydrate, can significantly reduce the performance of endurance sports athletes. **Carbohydrate** is the best fuel for muscles exercised for long periods.

- Any **extra protein** required by athletes and body-builders, can easily be obtained from the extra food eaten to satisfy hunger and energy needs - even allowing an excessive 120g protein daily for a 170 lb athlete (0.7g/lb body wt; twice the RDI).

- Remember, **excess protein** in food will not build bigger muscles. Any excess is converted and stored as fat. Excess protein can also strain the kidneys which excrete the waste products of protein metabolism.

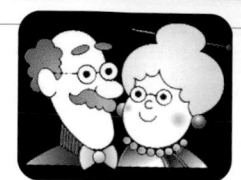

Elderly people (and dieters) must eat sufficient food to ensure adequate protein intake.

Inadequate protein leads to a drop in immune response with greater susceptibility to illness and infections. Muscle strength and muscle mass also drop.

Protein needs are easily met with sensible eating. Athletes who eat enough food for their energy needs, can obtain sufficient protein.

PROTEIN

RECOMMENDED DAILY INTAKE (Grams)

(Figure in brackets - Recommended amount of protein per lb of ideal body weight.)

		Pro	
Infants:	0-6 mths	**9-13g**	(1g/lb)
	6-12 mths	**14g**	(0.7g/lb)
Children:	1-3 yrs	**13g**	(0.6g/lb)
	4-8 yrs	**19g**	(0.5g/lb)
	9-13	**34g**	(0.5g/lb)
Males:	14-18	**52g**	(0.4g/lb)
	19+	**56g**	(0.36g/lb)
Females:	14+	**46g**	(0.36g/lb)
Pregnancy:		**71g**	
Breastfeeding:		**71g**	

Note: Above figures allow for a large safety margin for most persons.

Iron & Anemia Guide

- **Iron deficiency** is one of the most common nutritional deficiencies in women. The risk is increased in dieters who do not eat well-balanced meals. Chronic shortage of iron leads to **anemia**.

- **Women** between 11 and 50 years of age are at greater risk because of the monthly loss of menstrual blood. Pregnancy, growth, and endurance sports also demand extra iron.

- **In red blood cells**, iron combines with protein to form **hemoglobin** - the red pigment which carries oxygen in the blood. A lack of iron limits the production of hemoglobin and hence the amount of vital oxygen delivered to body cells.

Note: A blood test will tell you if your Hb and Iron stores (ferritin) are adequate. (Iron stores can be low even when Hb is normal.)

- **Vitamin C** (in fruits/veges/salads) enhances absorption of 'non-heme' iron in bread, cereals, milk, vegetables, nuts, eggs and iron supplements. Small amounts of meat, fish or poultry also help. (They contain 'heme' iron).

- **Iron absorption is lessened** by up to 60% when high calcium foods are consumed with iron-rich main meals. Tea, coffee, phytates (in bran) and oxalates lessen absorption of non-heme iron.

- **For infants to 1 year**, use iron-fortified milk/soy formula if not breast-feeding. Introduce iron-fortified baby cereals at 4-6 mths.

Note: Iron deficiency in children (even without anemia), can result in lethargy, irritability, repeated infections, and developmental problems.

Iron Supplements

- **Most people** can obtain adequate iron from their diet. **A wide variety** of animal and plant foods contain iron. (See Iron Counter)

- **Iron supplements** are only recommended for women with heavy menstrual blood losses, during pregnancy (if tests show a low-iron status), endurance athletes with low blood ferritin (iron stores) and for persons with diagnosed anemia. Check with your doctor.

- While the 5 mg of iron in multi-vitamin/mineral supplements is safe for most people, large amounts can be toxic, (especially in persons with hemochromatosis iron-overload condition).

ANEMIA SYMPTOMS

Anemia reduces the amount of oxygen carried in the blood. The body tissues become starved of oxygen. Symptoms include:

- **Pale skin; brittle finger nails (may turn up into spoon shape).**
- **Excessive tiredness or fatigue**
- **Breathlessness**
- **Feeling of malaise and irritability.**
- **Always feel cold.**
- **Decrease in attention span.**

Note: Other medical conditions may also cause similar symptoms. Check with your doctor.

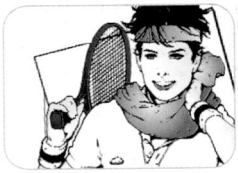

A nutritious diet with adequate iron is important - particularly for women and athletes.

RECOMMENDED DAILY IRON INTAKE (mg)

		Iron
Infants (0-6 mths):		
	Breastfed ~	0.5mg
	Bottlefed ~	3mg
	6-12 mths ~	9mg
Children:	1-11 yrs ~	6-8mg
Males:	12-18 yrs ~	10-13mg
	19+ yrs ~	7mg
Females:	12-50yrs ~	12-16mg
	51+ yrs ~	5-7mg
	Pregnancy ~	22-36mg
	Breastfeeding ~	12-16mg

Protein & Iron Counter

Pro ~ Protein (grams)   **Iron ~ Iron (mg)**

Meat

	Pro	Iron
Steak: Average all cuts, lean (no fat)		
Small (4 oz raw/3 oz ckd)	23	2.3
Medium (6 oz raw/4¼ oz ckd)	34	3.4
Large (10 oz raw/7¼ oz ckd)	57	5.7
Roast Beef: lean, 2 slices, 3 oz	24	2.5
Ground Beef patty, lean, ckd, 3 oz	21	2
Lamb chop, broiled, 3 oz	22	1.5
Liver, cooked, 3 oz	23	5.5
Veal cutlet, 1 medium	23	1
Pork, cooked, lean, 3 oz	24	1
Bacon, 3 medium slices	6	0.3
Ham, roasted, 2 pieces, 3 oz	18	1
Ham, luncheon, 2 slices, 1½ oz	10	0.3
Pastrami *(Oscar Mayer)*, 3 sl., 1¾ oz	10	1.3
Sausages: Bologna, 2 sl., 2 oz	7	1
Braunschweiger, 2 sl., 2 oz	8	5.3
Pork link, thick, 2 oz	6	0.4
Frankfurter, 1⅓ oz	5	0.5
Salami, hard, 3 slices, 1 oz	7	0.5
Vegetarian *(BocaBurger)*, 1 pattie	13	2

Chicken/Turkey

	Pro	Iron
Chicken, ckd; Breast portion, 3 oz	27	1
Leg/Thigh, lean, 3 oz	24	1
½ Whole Chicken	60	2.5
Drumstick, 1 medium, 3 oz	12	0.6
Turkey, cooked: Light meat, 3 oz	24	2
Dark meat, lean, 3 oz	24	2

Fish

	Pro	Iron
Finfish: *Per 4 oz, cooked*		
Cod, Flounder/Sole, Pollock	28	0.5
Catfish, Haddock, Halibut, M/Mahi	28	1.3
Ocean Perch, Swordf., Orange Roughy	28	1.3
Canned Fish: Tuna, Light, 3 oz	25	1.5
White, 3 oz	23	0.5
Salmon, pink, 3 oz	17	1
Salmon, red, 3 oz	17	1
Sardines, 3 whole (3"), 1¼ oz	9	1
Anchovies, 1 can, 1½ oz	13	2
Shellfish: Crabmeat, 3 oz	17.5	0.7
Clams, raw, 4 large/9 sml, 3 oz	11	12
Crayfish, cooked, 3 oz	20	2.7
Lobster, cooked, 3 oz	17	0.5
Oysters, raw, 6 medium, 3 oz	7	5
Scallops, 2 lge/5 small, 1 oz	5	0.1
Shrimp, raw, 6 large, 1½ oz	8.5	1
Fish Products: Fish Sticks, 4 sticks	10	0.5
Fish Portions, in batter, 4 oz	13	0.6
Gefilte Fish, 1 medium ball, 2 oz	8	1

Eggs

	Pro	Iron
1 Large Egg, whole	6	0.7
Egg Yolk	3	0.7
Egg White	3	0
Omelet, 2 eggs	13	1.7
Ham & Cheese	17	3
Egg Substitutes (liquid):		
Eggbeaters, 1 egg equiv.	4.5	1
Scramblers, ¼ cup, 2 oz	6	0.7

Milk, Yogurt, Icecream

	Pro	Iron
Milk: Whole/Lowfat/Skim, 8 fl.oz cup	8	0.1
Protein Enriched, 1 cup	10	0.1
Chocolate Milk, 1 cup	8	0.6
Thick Shake, Chocolate, 10 oz	9	1
Vanilla, 10 oz	11	0.3
Soymilk (fortified), average, 1 cup	7	1
Yogurt: Plain, 6 oz	10	0.1
Fruit flavors: 6 oz	8	0.3
8 oz	11	0.5
Ice-Cream: Rich, ½ cup	2	0
Regular, Vanilla, ½ cup	2.5	0
Sherbet, ½ cup	1	0
Custard, baked, ½ cup	7	0.5

Cheese

	Pro	Iron
Hard Cheeses, average, 1 oz	7	0.2
4 oz piece	28	0.8
Cottage Cheese, ½ cup	13	0.3
Ricotta, part skim, ½ cup	14	1

Bread, Bagels, Biscuits

	Pro	Iron
Bread (w. enriched flour): 1 slice, 1 oz	2	1
4 slices, 4 oz	8	4
4 thick slices, 6 oz	1.2	6
Bagel, plain 2 oz	6	1.5
Biscuits, 1 oz	2	1
Pita Bread, 1 pita, 1½ oz	4	1
Pumpernickel, 1 slice, 1 oz	3	1

Infant/Baby Foods

	Pro	Iron
Infant Formula Milk:		
Enfamil/Gerber/Similac, 5 fl.oz		
Regular/Low Iron	2.2	0.2
With Iron	2.2	1.8
Isomil/Nursoy/ProSobee	3	1.8
Baby Cereals: *Average All Brands*		
Dry, 4 Tbsp, ½ oz	1	7
Jars (w. fruit), 4½ oz	1	7

Breakfast Cereals

	Pro	Iron
Hot Type, cooked:		
Bulgur, cooked, 1 cup, 5 oz	9	2
Oatmeal: Reg., non-fortified, 1 cup	6	1.5
Instant, fortified, average, 1 pkt	4	8
Quaker Extra, all flavors	4	18
Total, all types, 1 pkt	4	18
Corn/Hominy Grits: Reg., 1 cup	3	1.5
Quaker: Reg., 3 Tbsp, 1 oz	2	0.8
Instant White, 1 packet	2	8
Cream of Wheat, 1 cup	4	10
Ready-To-Eat: *Per 1 oz Serving Unless Shown*		
Arrowhead: Average, all varieties	3	1
General Mills, Basic 4, 1 cup, 2 oz	4	3.8
Cheerios, regular, 1 cup, 1 oz	3	6.8
Cocoa Puffs, 1 cup, 1 oz	1	4.5
Fiber One, 1/2 cup	2	3.8
Kix, 1 1/3 cups; 1 oz	2	6.8
Multi-Bran Chex, 1 cup, 2 oz	4	16
Total Corn Flakes, 1 1/3 cups, 1 oz	2	6.8
Total Raisin Bran, 1 cup, 2 oz	4	18
Wheaties Energy Crunch, 1 cup, 1.95 oz	6	18
Health Valley: 10 Bran O's, 3/4 cup	3	0.9
Amaranth Flakes, 3/4 cup	3	0.6
Bran Cereal w. Raisins, 3/4 cup	5	1.5
98% Fat Free Granola, 2/3 cup	5	1.2
Real Oat Bran, 1/2 cup	6	0.6
Golden Flax, 1/4 cup	6	1.2
Kashi GoLean: 3/4 cup, 1.5 oz	8	1.5
Crunch!, 1 cup, 1.9 oz	9	1.8
Kellogg's: All Bran, 1/2 cup	4	4.5
Complete Oatbran Flakes, 3/4 cup	3	8.5
Cocoa Krispies, 3/4 cup	2	1.8
Corn Flakes, 1 cup	2	8.4
Just Right, 1 cup	4	16
Nutrigrain Almond Raisin, 1 1/4 cup	4	1.4
Product 19, 1 cup, 1 oz	2	18
Raisin Bran, 1 cup, 2 oz	6	4.5
Rice Krispies, 1 1/4 cup	2	1.8
Special K, 1 cup	6	8
Post: Raisin Bran, 1/2 cup, 1 oz	3	4.5
Grape Nuts, 1/2 cup, 1 oz	3	1
Quaker: Crunchy Corn Bran, 1 cup, 1 oz	2	8
Oatmeal Squares, 1 cup, 1 oz	4	6
100% Natural Granola, 1/2 cup	3	1
Life, 1/4 cup, 1 oz	3	4.5
Puffed Rice/Wheat, 1 cup, 1/2 oz	1	0.5
Shreaded Wheat, 3 biscuits	4	1

Brans & Wheatgerm

	Pro	Iron
Oat Bran, raw, 1 Tbsp	2	0.5
Rice Bran, raw, 2 Tbsp	1	1
Wheat Bran, unprocessed, 2 Tbsp	1	1
Wheat Germ, 2 Tbsp, 1/2 oz	4	1.3

Grains & Flours

	Pro	Iron
Amaranth, 1 cup, 1/2 oz	10	3
Barley, 1/2 cup, 3 1/2 oz	8	2
Buckwheat Flour, dark, 1 cup	11.5	2.7
light, 1 cup	6	1
Carob Flour, 1 cup	5	3
Corn Flour, 1 cup, 4 oz	9	2
Corn Meal, enriched, 1 cup	11	3.5
Flour: White, enriched, 1 cup, 4 1/2 oz	13	6
Wholegrain, 1 cup, 4 1/4 oz	16	5
Millet, wholegrain, 1 cup, 3 1/2 oz	10	7
Rye Flour, dark, 1 cup, 4 1/2 oz	21	6
light, 1 cup, 3 1/2 oz	10	1
Soy Flour, full fat, 1 cup, 3 oz	32	5.5
Yeast: Brewer's, dry, 1 Tbsp	3	1.5

Rice, Spaghetti

	Pro	Iron
Rice: Brown/White, average		
1 cup cooked, 6 1/2 oz	5	1
Spaghetti/Macaroni/Noodles (enriched):		
Cooked, 1 cup, 4 1/2 oz	7	2
Canned: in Tomato Sauce, 1/2 cup	2	0.5
w. Meatballs, 1 cup, 8 oz	9	2

Soups

	Pro	Iron
With Noodles/Vegetables, 1 cup	3	0.5
With Meat/Beans/Peas, 1 cup	8	1.5

Fruit

	Pro	Iron
Fresh/Canned: Average, all types, 1 serving		
1 medium/2 small fruit	1	0.5
Avocado, 1/2 medium	2	1
Dried Fruit: Apricots, 8 halves, 1 oz	1	1.3
Dates, 6 dates, 2 oz	1.5	0.7
Figs, 4 medium figs, 2 oz	2	1.7
Prunes, 5 medium, 1 1/2 oz	1	1
Raisins, 1 oz	1	0.7
Fruit Juice: Average, 1 cup	0.5	0.5
Prune Juice, 6 fl.oz	1	2.5
Tomato Juice, 6 fl.oz	0.5	1

King Kong was a vegetarian!

Protein & Iron Counter

Vegetables

	Pro	Iron
Beans: Snap/green, 1/2 cup	1	0.8
Dried: Average all types, cooked, 1/2 cup	7	2.5
Baked Beans, 1/2 cup 4 1/2 oz	5	2
Bean Sprouts, mung, 1 cup	3	1
Broccoli, 3/4 cup pieces, 4 oz	4	1.4
Cabbage; Cauliflower, 1 cup	1	0.6
Corn, 1/2 cup kernels, 3 oz	2.5	0.3
1 ear trimmed to 3 1/2"	2	0.4
Lentils, cooked, 1/2 cup, 3 1/2 oz	9	3.3
Mushrooms, raw, 1/2 cup, sliced	0.5	0.5
Peas: green, 1/2 cup, 3 oz	4	1.2
Split Peas, cooked, 1 cup	16	2.5
Potatoes, cooked:		
1 medium, with skin, 5 oz	3.3	2
without skin, 4 oz	2.3	1
French Fries, 3 oz	3	1
Potato Salad, 1/2 cup	3.5	2.5
Pumpkin, 1/2 cup mashed	1	2.5
Seaweed, kelp, 1 oz	<1	2.5
Spinach, cooked, 1/2 cup, 3 oz	2.7	2.5
Squash, ckd, all types, 1/2 cup	1	0.3
Tomatoes, 1 medium, 4 1/2 oz	1	0.6
Vegetables, mixed, ckd, 1 cup	2.5	0.7
Soybeans, cooked, 1/2 cup, 3 oz	14	4.4

Tofu, Tempeh, Miso

	Pro	Iron
Tofu, raw, firm, 1/2 cup, 4 1/2 oz	10	1.5
Tempeh, 1/2 cup, 3 oz	16	2
Miso, 1/2 cup, 5 oz	16	4
Miso Soup, 1 cup	3	0.4
Soybean Protein (TVP), 1 oz	18	3

Cakes, Pastries, Pies

(Made with enriched flour)

	Pro	Iron
Carrot w. cream cheese frosting, 4 oz	4	1.3
Cheesecake, 1 piece, 3 1/2 oz	5	0.5
Chocolate, 1 piece, 2 oz	2	2
Fruitcake, 1 piece, 1 1/2 oz	2	1.2
Plain, 1 piece, 3 oz	4	1.2
Croissant, plain, 2 oz	5	2
Danish Pastry, 1 pastry, 2 1/4 oz	4	1.3
Donuts, average, 2 oz	4	1.2
Muffins, average, 1 medium, 1 1/2 oz	3	1
Pancakes, 4" diam., two, 2 oz	4	1
Pies: Fruit, 1 piece, 5 1/2 oz	4	1.5
Pecan, 1 piece, 5 oz	7	4.5
Puddings, average, 1/2 cup, 4 1/2 oz	4	0.3
Waffles, 1 large, 2 1/2 oz	7	1.5

Sugar, Honey, Jam

	Pro	Iron
Sugar: White	0	0
Brown, 1 Tbsp	0	0.3
Molasses: Light/Medium, 1 Tbsp	0	1
Blackstrap, 1 Tbsp, 3/4 oz	0	3
Corn Syrup, 1 Tbsp, 3/4 oz	0	1
Honey, Jams, Jelly	0	0.2

Candy, Chocolate, Carob

	Pro	Iron
Candy, sugar-based	0	0
Chocolate: Plain, 2 oz bar	4	0.8
with nuts, 2 oz bar	6	0.8
Carob, plain, 2 oz	6	0.7

Cookies, Crackers, Chips

	Pro	Iron
Cookies, average, 4 cookies	2	1
Crackers: Graham, 2 1/2" sq., 2	1	0
Rice Cakes, average, one	1	0
Corn/Potato Chips, 1 oz	2	0.3

Nuts:

	Pro	Iron
Almonds, shelled, 20-25 nuts	6	1
Brazil Nuts, 7-8 medium nuts, 1 oz	4	1
Cashews, 12-16 nuts, 1 oz	5	1.5
Macadamias, 1 oz	2	0.5
Peanuts, dry roasted, 40 nuts, 1 oz	6	0.5
Pecans, 24 halves, 1 oz	2	0.5
Walnuts, 15 halves, 1 oz	4	0.7
Peanut Butter, 1 Tbsp	4	0.5

Seeds:

	Pro	Iron
Sesame Seeds, dry, 1 Tbsp	2	0.6
Pumpkin Kernels, dry, hulled, 1 oz	7	4.2
Sunflower Seeds, dried, hulled, 1 oz	6	2
Tahini, 1 Tbsp, 1/2 oz	2.5	1.4

Granola & Food/Protein Bars

	Pro	Iron
Granola Bars, average, 1 bar, 2 oz	2	0.5
Balance Oasis Bars, 1.76 oz	9	6.3
Bariatrix: Nutra Bars, 1	11	3.6
Choice dm Bar, 1.23 oz	6	3.6
Dr Soy Protein Bars, 1.76 oz	11	18
Ensure Nutrition Energy Bar	9	3.6
Gatorade Bars, Chocolate, 2.3 oz	7	3.5
Genisoy Nature Grains, 2.3 oz	14	4.5
IDN: proGram-16, 65g	16	3.6
Jenny Craig Bars, 1.97 oz	10	3.6
Met-Rx Bar, 100g	27	7.2
Planters Peanut Bar, 1.6 oz	7	0.7
Power Bar, 1 bar, 2.3 oz	10	6.3
Slim-Fast Bar, 34g	6	4.5
Source One Bar, 2.2 oz	15	4.5
Sweet Success Snack Bar, 33g	2	2.7
Twin Lab Protein Fuel, 3 oz	35	4.5
High Energy Bars, 2 oz	15	1.5

Nutritional & High Protein Drinks

	Pro	Iron
Atkins Shakes, 11 fl.oz can	20	2.7
Bariatrix Shakes, dry, 1 oz	15	3.6
Proti-Max Meal Replacement, 67g	35	6.3
Boost Ready To Drink, 8 oz can	10	3.6
Carnation Instant Breakfast, 10 oz	12	4.5
Ensure High Protein, 8 oz can	12	2.3
GeniSoy Shake, 1 scoop, 35g	14	3.6
Kashi GoLean Shake (RTD), 11 oz can	15	2.7
Kindercal, 8 fl.oz	7	2.5
Met-Rx Protein Shake, 11 oz	25	4.5
Myoplex (EAS), Nutrition Shake, 11 oz	20	5.4
Nature's Best, Protein Shake, 11 oz	20	3.6
Optifast 800, made-up, 8 oz	14	3.6
Resource (Novartis) Standard, 8 fl.oz	9	4.5
Revival Soy, Plain, 58g pkt	20	3.6
Slim Fast Shakes 325 ml can	10	3.6
Sweet Success (Nestle), 10 fl.oz can	10	4.5
Ultra Slim Fast, powder, 1 scoop, 33g	5	6.3
Usana Nutrimeal Mix, 2 scoops, 1^1/$_2$ oz	12	6
Walgreens Slim For Less, 11 oz can	10	2.7
Weider: Muscle Builder, 2 scoops	18	9

Coffee, Tea, Soda

	Pro	Iron
Coffee, Coffee Substitutes, 1 cup	0	0.1
Tea (all types); Soft Drinks/Soda	0	0
Hot Chocolate, 6 fl.oz	2	2.2

Beer, Wine, Spirits

	Pro	Iron
Beer, 12 fl.oz	1	0
Wines, red/white, 1 glass	0	0.4
Spirits/Liquor	0	0

Fast-Foods/Burgers

For extra listings ~ see CalorieKing.com

	Pro	Iron
Arby's: Roast Beef Sandwich, reg.	21	4
Giant Roast Beef S/wich	32	6
Italian Sub	29	2
Roast Chicken Club	29	3
Burger King: Whopper S/wich	29	2.5
Hamburger	19	1.5
Bacon Double Cheeseburger	41	2.5
Chicken Sandwich; Big Fish Sandwich	25	2
Carl's Jr: Famous Star Hamburger	24	4
Carl's Jr (Cont): Ranch Crispy Chicken	24	2
Super Star Hamburger	41	3
Charbroiled Chicken Club Sandwich	35	2

Fast Foods/Burgers (Cont)

	Pro	Iron
Domino's Pizza: Deep Dish (12"), 2 sl.		
Cheese, 2 slices	42	4
Pepperoni, Sausage, Ham	41	4
X-tra Cheese & Pepperoni	50	4.5
KFC: Original, Wing & Breast	35	0.4
3-Pce. Dinner, Original	51	4
Crispy Strips, 3	26	0.4
Original Recipe Sandwich	29	1.5
McDonald's: Big Mac	24	4.5
Cheeseburger	15	3
Chicken McNuggets (6)	15	1
Crispy Chicken Burger	22	3
Filet-O-Fish	15	2
Grilled Chicken Caesar Salad	26	2
Hamburger	12	3
Quarter Pounder w. Cheese	28	4.5
French Fries: Small, 2.4 oz	3	0.4
Large, 6 oz	8	1
Breakfast: Egg McMuffin	18	3
Bacon, Egg & Cheese McGriddles	19	3
Ham, Egg & Cheese Bagel	26	4.5
Sausage McMuffin w. Egg	19	3
Pancakes: Average all outlets, 3	8	2
Pizza Hut: Per Medium, 2 slices		
Pan Pizzas, average	26	4
Thin 'n Crispy: Supreme	24	2
Hand Tossed: Pepperoni	26	3
Personal Pan Pizza: Beef	26	4
Shakes, Chocolate	12	0.4
Subway: 6" Subs, average	20	2
Meatball	-	-
Roast Chicken Breast	25	3.5
Steak & Cheese, 6"	23	6
Subway Club	22	3.5
Sundaes: Average all outlets	7	0.3
Taco Bell: Bean Burrito	13	3.5
Beef Burrito Supreme	17	3.5
Tostado	10	1.5
Enchirito; Chicken; Steak	22	3
Taco Supreme	10	2
Gordita Baja Beef	13	2.5
Chicken Quesadilla	25	3
Wendy's: Single w. Everything	25	3
Big Bacon Classic	34	3
Jr Hamburger Kid's Meal	14	2
Grilled Chicken Sandwich	24	1.5

High Blood Pressure

High Blood Pressure

Many American adults have hypertension (high blood pressure), and are unaware of it. It is generally symptomless, so **have your blood pressure checked annually** - particularly if it runs in the family.

Untreated hypertension overworks the heart, damages arteries and promotes atherosclerosis. This in turn greatly increases the risk of heart disease, stroke, blindness, kidney disease and impotence. The earlier hypertension is detected, the sooner it can be brought under control.

BLOOD PRESSURE CLASSIFICATIONS

National High Blood Pressure Educ. Prog. (2003)

	DIASTOLIC		**SYSTOLIC**
Normal ►	Below 80	and	Below 120
Prehypertension			
►	80-89	or	120-139
Stage 1 ►	90-99	or	140-159
Stage 2 ►	100 or more	or	160 or more

Treating Hypertension

Prehypertension (in the chart above) means you don't have high blood pressure now but are likely to develop it in the future.

You can take steps to prevent it with healthy lifestyle habits: reducing sodium intake, eating adequate fruit and vegetables, losing weight if overweight, limiting alcohol to 2 drinks or less daily, quitting smoking, exercising regularly, and managing stress.

Stage 1 hypertension can often be treated with the above lifestyle changes.

Stage 2 hypertension usually requires drug therapy. However, salt restriction, abstaining from alcohol and the above lifestyle changes will improve the success of drug therapy, and enable smaller drug doses to be prescribed.

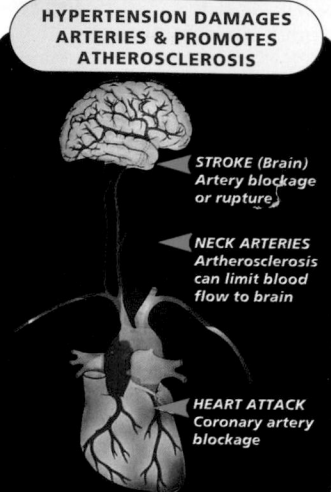

HYPERTENSION DAMAGES ARTERIES & PROMOTES ATHEROSCLEROSIS

STROKE (Brain) Artery blockage or rupture

NECK ARTERIES Artherosclerosis can limit blood flow to brain

HEART ATTACK Coronary artery blockage

STROKE
KNOW THE WARNING SIGNS!

If you notice one or more of these signs, **call your doctor immediately**. They may be signalling a possible stroke or transient ischemic attack:

- **Sudden weakness** or numbness in your face, arm or leg on one side of your body.
- **Sudden dimness**, blurring or loss of vision, particularly in one eye.
- **Loss of speech**, or trouble talking or understanding speech.
- **Sudden severe headache** - 'a bolt out of the blue' - with no apparent cause.
- **Unexplained dizziness**, unsteadiness or a sudden fall, especially if accompanied by any of the other symptoms.

Salt & Sodium

- **Sodium is a mineral element** most commonly found in salt (sodium chloride). It also occurs naturally in much smaller amounts in animal and plant foods, and water - normally sufficient for our needs without having to add salt.

- **Sodium is required** for nerve and muscle function as well as to balance the amount of fluid in our tissues and blood.

  Sodium acts like a sponge to attract and hold fluids in body tissues.

- **Excess sodium** can cause water retention, and increase the risk of developing hypertension. Very high salt intake may also increase the risk of stomach cancer.

- **Too little sodium** may cause low blood pressure (hypotension), and decrease blood flow to the heart, brain and kidneys - especially during exercise. (A certain blood volume is required to sustain the blood pressure needed for adequate blood flow in the capillaries.)

Salt-Sensitive Persons

- **Normally, our kidneys** excrete excess dietary sodium. The thirst we feel after a salty meal is the body calling for water to dilute the sodium, and enable the kidneys to flush out excess sodium.

- **However, 'salt sensitive' persons** (perhaps 1 in 2-3 adults) tend to retain excess sodium (above approximately 3000mg daily) instead of excreting it. Such persons are more likely to develop hypertension and would most benefit from sodium restriction. Assume you are susceptible if there is a family history of hypertension.

- **Although not everyone will benefit,** all Americans are being asked to **moderate their salt and sodium intake** as a public health measure - particularly that so many do not know whether or not they have hyper- tension; and also because we do not know just who is salt-sensitive.

SAFE SODIUM LEVELS

The American Heart Association recommends a **maximum sodium intake of 2400mg per day** for adults with normal blood pressure. However, people who consume less than 1500mg sodium have the lowest blood pressure levels.

Persons with hypertension and kidney ailments are usually restricted to as little as **1000mg sodium per day**. Your doctor will discuss the correct sodium level for you.

Persons engaged in prolonged strenuous work or exercise may lose sodium through heavy sweating - especially in hot, humid weather. Adequate salt (and fluids) is necessary to avoid dehydration. A little extra salt at mealtimes is usually sufficient to satisfy any extra need. Do not take salt tablets.

FINDING HIDDEN SODIUM

On average, **only one third of our sodium intake comes from the salt shaker**. The rest is hidden in processed foods that have salt added during manufacture.

Sodium compounds added to food or medicinals can also contribute significant sodium.

Sodium bicarbonate in particular is widely used in antacid tablets and powders, and saline drink powders (such as *Alka Seltzer*). Sodium bicarbonate contains 27% sodium by weight. Each gram contributes 270mg sodium. Large amounts of sodium can be unwittingly consumed – up to 600mg per tablet (See Antacids ~ Page 293).

Other sodium compounds include monosodium glutamate (MSG), sodium ascorbate, sodium nitrite, and sodium citrate.

ALCOHOL DANGER

Excess alcohol causes up to 20% of hypertension in America.

Susceptible persons should abstain to normalize their blood pressure.

Salt & Sodium Guide

Sodium accounts for only 40% of the weight of salt (sodium chloride). Examples:
1 gram (1000mg) Salt has 400mg Sodium
1 teaspoon (5g) Salt has 2000mg Sodium

Hints to Reduce Sodium

● **Watch the salt shaker.** Start with an easy 50% cut in sodium by using Lite Salt (*Morton*) or *Cardia* Salt. Then gradually cut back until you can leave the salt shaker off the table.

● **Taste your food before salting.** Use the pepper shaker (small holes) for more controlled sprinkling of salt.

● **Choose low sodium**, sodium free, and reduced sodium products in place of regular salted products.

● **Check labels for sodium levels.** The following sodium descriptors may appear on labels:

  Reduced Sodium: At least 75% less sodium than the original product.
  Low Sodium: 140 mg or less/serving.
  Very Low Sodium: 35mg or less/serving.
  Sodium Free: Less than 5mg per serving.

● **Use reduced-sodium breads**, butter and margarine. Regular varieties contain up to 2% salt. This is considered high in view of their significant contribution to our diet.

● **Go easy on condiments and sauces** such as tomato ketchup, mustard, soy sauce and spaghetti sauces, plus salad dressings. Use low sodium varieties.

● **Limit pizzas and salty fast-foods.** Check *CalorieKing.com* food database.

● **Avoid salty snack foods** such as potato chips, corn chips, salted nuts, pretzels and cheesy-flavored snacks. **Choose unsalted** popcorn, nuts or seeds. Eat more fruit.

● **Don't salt children's food** to your taste.

● **Limit or avoid antacids and saline powders** with sodium bicarbonate (such as *Alka-Seltzer*). They are high in sodium.

FOODS HIGH IN SODIUM

- Cheese, Butter, Margarine
- Pickles, Sauerkraut, Olives
- Condiments, Sauces
- Salad Dressings
- Canned vegetables/salads/beans
- Deli Salads (with dressing)
- Frozen/Packaged Meals/Entrees
- Soups: Canned/dry; bouillon cubes
- Meats: Ham, bacon, sausage, luncheon meats, smoked meats
- Canned Fish (in brine/salt)
- Sea Salt, Garlic/Celery Salt
- Snack Foods (potato chips, pretzels)
- Tomato Juice (Canned), V8 Vegetable Juice
- Fast Foods: Pizza, Burgers, Chicken
- *Alka-Seltzer* Antacid

MODERATE SODIUM

- Bread (Reduced Salt)
- Meat, Fish, Poultry - Unprocessed
- Milk, Yogurt, Soy Drinks, Eggs
- Peanut Butter
- Breakfast Cereals (<200mg/serving)
- Chocolate Candy, Fruit/Nut Bars
- *Reduced & Low-Sodium* Products

FOODS LOW IN SODIUM

- Products labelled *Very Low Sodium*, or *Sodium Free*
- Fresh fruits and vegetables
- Canned and Dried Fruits
- Potatoes, Rice, Pasta
- Dried Beans & Lentils, Tofu
- Nuts & Seeds (unsalted)
- Corn & Popcorn (unsalted)
- Pepper, Spices, Herbs
- Jam, Honey, Syrup
- Candy, Gum
- Hard & Jelly Candy
- Coffee, Tea, Alcohol
- Fresh Fruit Juices, Water

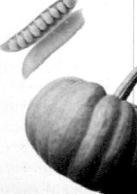

The American Heart Association recommends a sodium intake of **less than 2400mg/day**

Sodium ~ Sodium (mg)

Milk & Dairy Products

	Sodium
Milk: Whole/lowfat/skim, average	
1 cup, 8 fl.oz	120
Whole, low sodium, 1 cup	5
Choc Milk (*Hershey's*), 1 cup	130
Soy Milk, 8 fl.oz	30
Buttermilk, cultured, 8 fl.oz	250
Dry/Powder, skim, 1/4 cup, 1 oz	110
Yogurt: with fruit aver., 8 oz	130
Cheese: Blue, 1 oz	330
Parmesan, 1 oz	450
Kraft: Cheddar, 1 oz	180
Philadelphia Brand Cream Cheese	85
Process Cheese., average,1 oz	430
Swiss, 1 oz	40
Cottage Cheese, 1/2 cup, 4 oz	450
Ricotta Cheese, 1/2 cup, 4 oz	150

Icecream, Frozen Yogurt

Icecream, average,1/2 cup	50
Frozen Yogurt, 1/2 cup	50

Fats/Oils

Butter/Margarine:	
Regular, 2 Tbsp, 1 oz	230
Unsalted, reg., 2 Tbsp, 1 oz	5
Mayonnaise, aver., 2 Tbsp, 1 oz	160
Oils/Lard/Dripping	0
Cream, average, 1 Tbsp	6
Coffee-Mate: Powdered, 1 tsp	2
Liquid, 1 Tbsp	5

Eggs

Whole, 1 large	70
Omelet, 2 egg, plain	220
w. cheese	400
Egg Beaters (*Fleischmann's*), 1/4 cup	80

Meats

Meat, average all types, cooked	
(Beef/Lamb/Veal/Pork), 4 oz	80
Corned Beef, cooked, 3 oz	800
Bacon, cooked, 2 slices, 1/2 oz	270
Ham, 3 oz	1100

Chicken & Turkey

Chicken/Turkey, cooked, unsalted, 4 oz	80
Stuffing Mixes, average., 1/2 cup	500

Sausages & Meats

	Sodium
Bologna, 1 oz	280
Frankfurter, 2 oz	640
Ham, chopped, 3/4 oz slice	290
Liverwurst (Braunschweiger), 1 oz	320
Pepperoni, 5 slices, 1 oz	570
Salami, cooked, 1 oz	350
dry/hard, 1 oz	600
Sausage, 1 oz link	220
Pork, 2 oz patty	260
Turkey Roll, 1 oz	160

Fish:

Fresh Fish, average, plain	
Cooked, 4 oz (no bone)	60
Broiled w. butter, 4 oz	150
Breaded & fried, 4 oz	320
Fish fillets, bat.-dipped 3 oz	350
Fish sticks, 1 oz stick	160
Gefilte Fish (w. broth), 1 pce, 1 1/2 oz	220
Herring, pickled, 2 pces, 1 oz	260
Lobster, meat only, 4 oz	180
Oysters, fresh, 6 med., 3 oz	95
Salmon, canned, 3 oz	460
No Salt Added, 3 oz	65
Smoked fish, average, 3 oz	650
Tuna, canned, 3 oz	330
No Added Salt, 3 oz	40

Entrees & Meals

Frozen Meals, average	600-900
Lean Cuisine, average	700
Stouffer's, average	580
Dinners, average	900-1200
Side Dishes, average	400-600
Pizza, frozen, 1/4 large, 6 oz	800-1200
Microwave Cup Meals	900-1400
Cup O'Noodles, average	1500

Fast-Foods & Restaurants

Cheeseburger	750
Chicken Dinner (3 piece)	2200
Chicken Nuggets w. Sauce	800
Fish/Chicken Sandwich	1000
French Fries, small, 2 1/2 oz	150
Hamburger: Regular	500
Large with cheese	1100
Hot Dog (Frankfurter)	800
Pizza, 2 medium slices	1200
Shake, chocolate	250
Taco	400

Extra Listings ~ see CalorieKing.com

Sodium Counter

Sodium ~ **Sodium (mg)**

		Sodium
Soups: Condensed, 1 c., 8 oz		800-1000
Low Sodium		70
Chicken Noodle, 1 cup		900
Bouillon Cube, average		950
Cup-A-Soup, average		850
Lite, average		450
Soup Mixes, average, 1 cup		900

Condiments, Sauces, Dressings

A-1 Sauce, 1 Tbsp	270
Barbecue Sauce, 1 Tbsp	130
Bragg Liquid Aminos, 1 tsp	220
Chili Sauce, 1 Tbsp	230
Ketchup: tomato, 1 Tbsp	180
Low Sodium, 1 Tbsp	20
Mayonnaise, 1 Tbsp	80
Mustard, 1 tsp	70
Pizza Sauce, 1/2 cup	700
Salad Dressings, 2 Tbsp, 1 oz	160-400
Spaghetti Sauce, 1/2 cup	500
Soy Sauce, 1 Tbsp	900
Lite *(Kikkoman)*, 1 Tbsp	600
Sweet & Sour, 1/2 cup	250
Tabasco, 1 tsp	25
Vinegar, Lemon Juice	0
Worcestershire, 1 Tbsp	200
Tomato: Sauce, 1 cup	1200
Paste/Puree (salted), 1/2 cup	1000
No Salt Added, 1/2 cup	25

Salt & Salt Substitutes

Table Salt: 1 teaspoon, 6g	2400
Single Serve package, 1 g	400
Cardia Salt, 1 teaspoon	1080
Lite Salt *(Morton)*, 1 teaspoon, 6g	1200
Morton Salt Substitute	5
No Salt Salt Substitute, 1 teaspoon	5
Garlic/Seasoned Salt 1 teaspoon, 4g	1300
Sea Salt, 1 teaspoon, 5g	2250

Seasonings, Herbs & Spices

Baking Powder, 1 tsp, 3g	340
Baking Soda (Sodium bicarb), 1 tsp, 3g	810
Accent (Flavor Enhancer), 1 tsp	600
Chili Powder, 1 tsp, 3g	25
Herbs/Spices: Curry Powder	0
Lemon Pepper *(Lawry's)*, 1 tsp	340
Meat Tenderizer, 1 tsp, 5g	1750
MSG (Monosodium glutamate), 5g	500
Mrs Dash (Herb/Spice Blend), 1 tsp	0
Pepper, Mustard (dry), 1 tsp	1
Yeast, Nutritional, 1 Tbsp	10

Breakfast Cereals

		Sodium
Kellogg's: All-Bran, 1/3 cup, 1 oz		260
Oatbran Flakes, 3/4 cup, 1 oz		220
Corn Flakes, 1 cup, 1 oz		290
Just Right, 1/2 cup, 1 oz		200
Mini Wheats Frosted, 3/4 cup,		-
Health Valley Cereals, 1 serving		5
Quaker: Cap'n Crunch, 3/4 cup, 1 oz		-
Crunchy Corn Bran, 1 cup, 1 oz		320
100% Natural Granola, 1/2 cup, 1 oz		15
Puffed Rice/Wheat, 2 cups, 1 oz		1
Total, 1 cup, 1 oz		140
Oatmeal: Regular, 3/4 cup		1
Instant *(Quaker)*, 2/3 cup (1 pkt)		270

Breads, Bagels, Crackers

Bread: Average all types, 1 oz	140
Low Sodium, 1 oz	10
Bagels, plain, 2 oz	200
Sara Lee, 3 oz	500
Biscuits, average, 1 oz	180
Bun/Roll, 1 medium, 1 1/2 oz	200
Crackers: Saltine, 2 crackers	70
Low Salt (Premium), 2	45
Graham, 2 regular	50
Croissant, average, 2 oz	280
Rice Cakes, average	25
RyKrisp Crispbread, Sesame, 2	100

Cookies, Cakes, Desserts

Cookies, average, 2-3 cookies, 1 oz	100
Mrs Fields', average, 2 1/2 oz	180
Baked Custard, 1/2 cup	100
Brownie, 1/4 oz piece	75
Cake, average, 3 oz piece	250
Cinnamon Sweet Roll, 2 oz	250
Danish, Apple	250
Donut, average	150
Muffins, 1 medium, 2 oz	150
Sara Lee, average, 2 1/2 oz	300
Pancakes, 3 x 4"	360
Pie, average, 1/6 of 9" pie	300
Pudding, average, 1/2 cup	160
Jell-O (Mix), Instant, 1/2 cup	400
Waffles: Home-made, 7", 2 1/2 oz	350
Frozen, average, 1 1/4 oz	260
Aunt Jemima, avg, 2 1/2 oz	630

Sodium Counter

Fruit & Juices	Sodium
Fresh Fruit, average all types, 1 serving	1
Dried/Canned Fruit, 1/2 cup	1
Fruit Juice: Fresh, sqz'd, 6 fl.oz	1
Commercial, aver., 6 fl.oz	20
Carrot Juice (*Ferraro's*), 8 fl.oz	230
Tomato Juice (*Campbell's*), 6 fl.oz	570
Low Sodium (No Salt Added)	20
V8 Vegetable (*Campbell's*), 6 fl.oz	600
(No Salt Added) 6 fl.oz	45

Vegetables

Fresh/Frozen (No Salt Added), 1/2 cup	
Asparagus, Bean Sprouts, Corn	3
Beets, Carrots, Celery, 1/2 cup	40
Broccoli, Cabbage, Cauliflower	10
Cucumber, Green Beans, Mushroom, Okra	3
Onions, Peas, Potato, Pumpkin, Squash	3
Peppers, Hot Chili, raw, each	3
Spinach, Turnips, 1/2 cup, ckd	40
Tomato, 1 medium, 5 oz	10
Canned: Asparagus, 4 spears	300
Beans, baked in tomato sauce	450
Beets, 1/2 cup, 3 oz	240
Corn Kernels, 1/2 cup, 3 oz	190
Creamed, 1/2 cup, 4 1/2 oz	330
Mushrooms w. butter sce, 2oz	550
Peas, 1/2 cup, 3 oz	250
Sauerkraut, 1/2 cup, 4 oz	750

Pickles, Olives

Olives, pickled: Green, 1 large	90
Ripe/black, 1 large	40
Pickles: Bread & Butter, 4 sl., 1 oz	200
Dill, 1 pickle, 2 1/2 oz	900
Sweet, 1 gherkin, 1/2 oz	130

Soybean Products

Miso (Soy Paste), 1/4 c., 2 1/2 oz	2500
Soybean Protein Isolate, 1 oz	280
Tempeh, 1/2 cup, 3 oz	5
Tofu, average, 1/2 cup, 4 oz	5

Jam, Honey, Syrups

Jam/Jelly, 1 Tbsp	2
Honey/Maple Syrup, 1 Tbsp	1
Log Cabin Syrup, 1 fl.oz	35
Lite, 1 fl.oz	90

Peanut Butter

Peanut Butter, regular, 1 Tbsp	70
Unsalted, 1 Tbsp	1

Snacks, Nuts	Sodium
Cheese Balls/Curls, 1 oz	280
Corn/Tortilla Chips, aver., 1 oz	220
Granola bars, aver., 1 bar	80
Nuts: Plain, unsalted, 1 oz	1
Lightly salted, 1 oz	80
Salted or Honey Roasted, 1 oz	160
Popcorn: Plain (unsalted), 1 cup	1
Flavored, average, 1 cup	60
Salt added, 1 cup	180
Potato Chips, plain, 1 oz	160
Flavored, average, 1 oz	250
Pretzels, regular, 3, 1 oz	450

Candy, Chocolate

Chocolate, milk, 1 oz	30
Carob Milk Bar, 1 oz	55
Fudge, chocolate, 1 oz	55
Candy Bars, average, 1 1/2 oz	60
Hard Candy, Jelly Beans, 1 oz	10
Licorice, 1 oz	30

Beverages, Alcohol

Coffee (& Substitutes), Tea, 1 cup	1
Cocoa, dry, plain, 1 Tbsp	0
Mix, average, 1 envelope	120
Quik (*Nestle*), 2 tsp	35
Soft Drinks, average, 8 fl.oz	20
Mineral Water, Perrier, 8 fl.oz	5
Gatorade Thirst Quencher, 8 fl.oz	110
Water, average, 1 cup, 8 fl.oz	5
Drier regions, 1 cup	20+
Alcohol: Beer, average, 12 fl.oz	15
Wines, average, 4 fl.oz	10
Spirits (distilled), 1 1/2 fl.oz	1

Antacids – Alka-Seltzer

Alka-Seltzer (Per Tablet):	Sodium
Alka-Seltzer P.M., 1 tablet	500
Original (Light Blue Box)	570
Extra Strength (Dark Blue Box)	590
Flavored Lemon/Lime & Cherry	500
Antacid (yellow Box)	310
Gelatine Capsule, 1	0
Alka-Mints, chewable	0
Bromo Seltzer, 3/4 capful	760
Rolaids: All types	0
Tums: Regular/Extra Strength	0
Sodium Bicarbonate (27% sodium), 1g	270

Index A - B

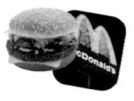

FAST-FOOD RESTAURANTS INDEX
~ SEE PAGE 183 ~

Index C - F

Index I - M

FAST-FOOD INDEX
~ PAGE 183 ~

Index P - S

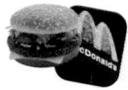

FAST-FOOD RESTAURANTS INDEX
~ SEE PAGE 183 ~

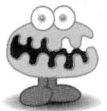

Index V - Z

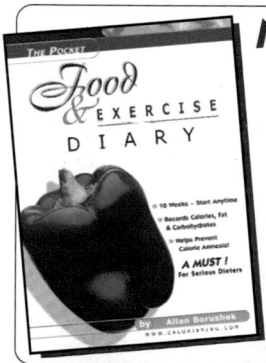